TEACHING PATIENTS WITH

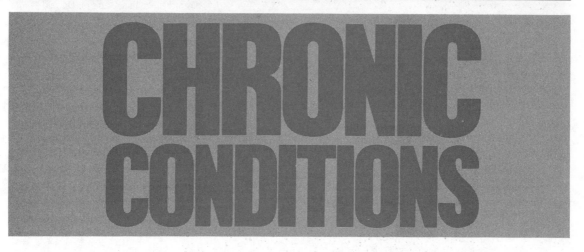

CHRONIC CONDITIONS

Springhouse Corporation
Springhouse, Pennsylvania

STAFF

Executive Director, Editorial
Stanley Loeb

Editorial Director
Matthew Cahill

Clinical Director
Barbara F. McVan, RN

Art Director
John Hubbard

Senior Editor
June Norris

Clinical Editor
Joan E. Mason, RN, EdM

Drug Information Editor
George J. Blake, RPh, MS

Editor
Edith McMahon

Copy Editors
Jane V. Cray (supervisor), Christina
Price

Designers
Stephanie Peters (associate art
director), Kristina Gabage, Donald
Knauss, Doug Miller (photographer)

Typography
David Kosten (director), Diane Paluba
(manager), Elizabeth Bergman, Joyce
Rossi Biletz, Phyllis Marron, Robin
Rantz, Valerie L. Rosenberger

Manufacturing
Deborah Meiris (manager), T.A. Landis

Production Coordination
Colleen M. Hayman

Editorial Assistants
Maree DeRosa, Beverly Lane, Mary
Madden

The clinical procedures described and recommended in this publication are based on research and consultation with nursing, medical, and legal authorities. To the best of our knowledge, these procedures reflect currently accepted practice; nevertheless, they can't be considered absolute and universal recommendations. For individual application, all recommendations must be considered in light of the patient's clinical condition and, before administration of new or infrequently used drugs, in light of the latest package-insert information. The authors and the publisher disclaim responsibility for any adverse effects resulting directly or indirectly from the suggested procedures, from any undetected errors, or from the reader's misunderstanding of the text.

TPCC-020693

Library of Congress Cataloging-in-Publication Data

Teaching patients with chronic conditions.
    p. cm.
    Includes bibliographical references and index.
    1. Patient education—Study and teaching.
2. Chronic diseases. 3. Nurse and patient.
I. Springhouse Corporation.
    [DNLM: 1. Chronic Disease—nursing.
    2. Patient Education—methods—nurses' instruction. WY 152 T2533]
RT90.T422 1992
615.5'07—dc20
DNLM/DLC
                                                    92-2171
ISBN 0-87434-497-2   CIP

Contents

INTRODUCTION

Today, nurses find themselves caring for more gravely ill patients than ever before. Although many of these patients are hospitalized for acute conditions, others are admitted for flare-ups or complications of chronic conditions. Oftentimes, these flare-ups or complications result when a condition follows its inevitable course. At other times, they result from preventable causes, such as a patient's failure to comply with treatment or inadequate patient teaching. Frequently, nurses don't have the time or the resources to help address these problems. Fortunately, they can turn to *Teaching Patients with Chronic Conditions* for help.

In this valuable book, you'll find virtually everything you need—from background information for you to reproducible instructional materials for your patients. The book's 10 chapters use the same easy-to-follow format. Organized primarily by body system, each chapter begins with a definition of the condition and identifies any difficulties to expect in teaching.

Following this introductory section, you'll find a discussion of the condition's causes and pathophysiology. Then, you'll read about the complications that may occur if the patient doesn't comply with the prescribed treatment regimen. Next, you'll find a discussion of the diagnostic workup that the patient may undergo, including what you must teach him about specific tests. In the section about treatments, you'll review activity, diet, drug, procedural or surgical therapies.

At the end of each chapter, after a list of pertinent sources of information and support, you'll find reproducible patient-teaching aids. Printed in large, easy-to-read type and often illustrated, these teaching aids can be photocopied and distributed to your patients. No longer will you have to write out patient instructions from scratch or use incomplete forms. At your fingertips you'll have a wealth of resources for teaching patients to cut down on cholesterol, exercise safely, perform chest physiotherapy, prepare for diagnostic tests, and much more.

Besides patient-teaching aids, you'll find other features to help you teach quickly and effectively. These features include:
• sample teaching plans
• convenient and brief drug charts identifying adverse reactions and highlighting teaching points
• timesaving teaching tips
• answers to questions patients commonly ask.

With the help of all these features, you'll meet your goal of effectively teaching patients—even when you have little time available.

CHAPTER

1

Cardiovascular Conditions

Contents

Coronary artery disease

Year after year, coronary artery disease (CAD) claims more lives in the United States than any other disorder. It most commonly results from a hardening of the arteries on the heart's surface that begins in childhood and progresses throughout life. Most patients remain asymptomatic until middle age or later, when the heart's blood supply can no longer meet the heart's needs.

Many patients with CAD first seek medical help after experiencing angina. They may confuse this classic symptom of CAD with the chest pain of myocardial infarction (MI) and turn to you for advice. How can your teaching help them? First of all, you'll need to prepare each patient for diagnostic tests, which sometimes are complex and frightening. Then you'll need to identify angina-provoking activities and teach patients how to take prescribed antianginal drugs. Your teaching must also focus on other treatment measures to relieve angina or, if necessary, to reopen or bypass occluded coronary arteries.

Most important, however, your teaching can help the patient identify risk factors and develop a strategy for modifying them. Many CAD risk factors, such as smoking, high serum cholesterol level, hypertension, obesity, sedentary life-style, and stress, are within the patient's control. Modifying them can halt or even reverse CAD's course. (See *Tailoring your teaching for the CAD patient,* pages 4 and 5.)

Discuss the disorder
Begin this discussion by describing how the heart and blood vessels work (see *Explaining cardiac physiology,* page 6). Inform the patient that CAD is characterized by narrowing or blockage of one or more of the coronary arteries, resulting in diminished blood flow to the heart. This deprives the heart of vital oxygen and nutrients, causing tissue damage.

Explain that atherosclerosis—the buildup of fatty, fibrous plaques on inner arterial walls—usually causes CAD. These plaques constrict the vessels and reduce the volume of blood that can be pumped through them (see *Atherosclerosis stages,* page 7).

To facilitate discussion of risk factors linked to atherosclerosis, have the patient complete the *CAD risk factor survey* (see page 8). This survey shows where you'll need to focus your teaching and will help you to develop a plan for each CAD patient.

Next, discuss how lack of oxygen triggers the classic symptom

Richard K. Gibson, RN, MN, JD, CCRN, CS, wrote this chapter. He's a clinical nurse specialist in the surgical intensive care unit at Veterans Administration Hospital, San Diego.

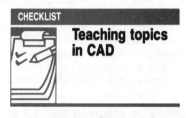

CHECKLIST

Teaching topics in CAD

☐ An explanation of disease mechanisms: atherosclerosis and coronary artery spasm
☐ Cardiac physiology, with emphasis on coronary arteries
☐ Risk factor analysis
☐ How angina develops and how to treat and prevent it
☐ Importance of treating coronary artery disease to prevent complications, such as myocardial infarction
☐ Preparation for diagnostic tests, such as cardiac catheterization, electrocardiography, angiography, and serum lipid studies
☐ Recommended exercise program
☐ Dietary restrictions to lower serum low-density lipoprotein level and control hypertension
☐ Use of prescribed drugs
☐ Preparation for percutaneous transluminal coronary angioplasty or coronary artery bypass grafting, if ordered
☐ Modifying risk factors: reducing stress, controlling weight, and quitting smoking

Tailoring your teaching for the CAD patient

When teaching your coronary artery disease (CAD) patient, you'll probably find a standard teaching plan to be a useful starting point. But you'll also need to modify this plan to help meet your patient's distinctive needs. Let's look at how to modify a standard CAD teaching plan.

Suppose you're caring for Martin Feldman, a 52-year-old computer analyst who lives with his wife and two teenage children. Mr. Feldman was admitted complaining of chest pain. A myocardial infarction has been ruled out.

The doctor plans to prescribe nifedipine and nitroglycerin for Mr. Feldman, as needed. Before discharge, Mr. Feldman is scheduled for an exercise ECG with a thallium scan. If his chest pain recurs, he'll have to undergo cardiac catheterization.

Mr. Feldman is relieved that his heart muscle isn't damaged. He acknowledges that he should start making life-style changes now. His wife seems concerned and eager to help her husband. However, Mr. Feldman and his wife know little about the disorder.

What are Mr. Feldman's learning needs? What will you teach him and his wife first? Because the Feldmans know little about CAD, you decide to teach them about cardiac anatomy and atherosclerosis. Then you'll proceed to the risk factor assessment and preparation for the upcoming thallium scan. Using the *CAD risk factor survey* (see page 8), you help identify three major risk factors: smoking, hypercholesterolemia, and a sedentary life-style.

You prepare a set of learning outcomes with Mr. Feldman (see next page), and organize the teaching points in order of importance. Once again, Mr. Feldman expresses his willingness to change his life-style, if it will improve his condition. You welcome his enthusiasm, but carefully explain that he mustn't set his expectations too high. Otherwise, he'll feel like a failure if he can't make all the changes right away. You point out to him that lifelong habits don't disappear overnight. His focus right now should be on making a strong beginning.

Standard teaching plan for coronary artery disease

CONTENT	TOOLS AND ACTIVITIES	EVALUATION METHODS
Understanding the heart muscle • Anatomy • Blood flow • Oxygen demand and supply	Heart diagrams, discussion	• Questions and answers
Coronary artery disease • Atherosclerosis • Ischemia • Angina • Complications	Discussion, printed material on CAD	• Questions and answers
Risk factors • Modifiable • Nonmodifiable	Risk factor survey	• Risk factor survey score • Discussion
Diagnostic tests • Blood tests • Cardiac angiography • Cardiac blood pool imaging • Cardiac catheterization • Echocardiography • ECG • Exercise ECG • Thallium scan	Discussion, printed material and patient-teaching aid on cardiac tests	• Questions and answers • Discussion
Treatments • Diet • Exercise • Risk factor modification • Medications • Percutaneous transluminal coronary angioplasty • Coronary artery bypass grafting	Discussion, coronary artery bypass grafting, attendance in stop-smoking support group, diet planning with spouse, guidelines for taking cardiac drugs	• Questions and answers • Menu selection • Patient demonstration of pulse-taking techniques • Patient demonstration of nitroglycerin administration

Tailoring your teaching for the CAD patient—*continued*

Learning outcomes
Mr Feldman will be able to:
- identify modifiable risk factors
- describe how atherosclerosis upsets the balance of oxygen demand and supply in his heart
- list five foods from his usual diet that are high in cholesterol and saturated fats
- demonstrate how to use nitroglycerin spray
- complete the registration form for the next series of stop-smoking classes
- plan three nonsedentary activities he and his wife can pursue together in the evening, instead of watching television
- describe what steps to take if chest pain interrupts sexual activity
- explain the purpose of a thallium scan and the test procedure.

of angina by stimulating the pain fibers that surround the heart. Angina is typically described as a burning, squeezing, or crushing sensation in the chest. This pain may also radiate to the arm, shoulder blades, neck, or jaw. Inform the patient that angina doesn't always herald an MI, although it's a significant warning symptom. Tell him that certain activities tend to precipitate angina: physical exertion, exposure to extreme heat or cold, emotional stress, and even eating a large, heavy meal. (One type of angina occurs during rest and isn't related to stress. This variant, known as Prinzmetal's angina or the nocturnal variant, is associated with coronary artery spasm rather than with atherosclerosis.)

Complications
Emphasize that strict adherence to the treatment plan can reduce the risk of serious complications, including MI, dysrhythmias, congestive heart failure, and death.

Describe the diagnostic workup
Explain any ordered diagnostic tests to the patient. These may include blood tests, cardiac angiography, cardiac blood pool imaging, cardiac catheterization, echocardiography, electrocardiography (ECG), and exercise ECG and thallium scan.

Blood tests
Tell the patient that blood tests can detect and classify hyperlipemia, including total cholesterol level, serum triglyceride level, lipoprotein phenotyping, and lipoprotein-cholesterol fractionation. Instruct him not to eat for 12 to 14 hours and not to drink alcohol for 24 hours before the test. Inform him that periodic blood tests help evaluate the effectiveness of drug and dietary therapy in reducing serum lipid levels.

6 Coronary artery disease

Explaining cardiac physiology

To better understand coronary artery disease, your patient may require an explanation of cardiac physiology. Begin by telling him that the heart is a muscle that pumps oxygen-filled blood through the *aorta,* the largest artery in the body. Explain that all major arteries branch from the aorta, carrying blood to all parts of the body. Blood vessels called *veins* return blood to the heart. Mention that after picking up oxygen from the lungs, the blood is pumped throughout the body again.

Tell the patient that like other muscles, the heart requires oxygen to work. It relies on the *coronary arteries* to supply it with oxygenated blood.

Describe the three major coronary arteries—the *circumflex artery, the right coronary artery, and the left anterior descending artery*—which branch from the aorta close to the heart's surface and then split off into smaller arteries that distribute blood throughout the heart muscle.

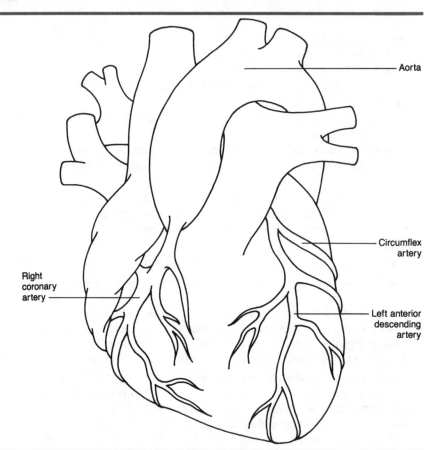

Aorta

Circumflex artery

Right coronary artery

Left anterior descending artery

Cardiac angiography

Tell the patient that angiography examines arteries for atherosclerotic obstruction. Explain that the test can take 30 minutes to 4 hours, depending on which blood vessels are examined.

Inform the patient that an area of his groin or armpit or another location will be shaved and cleansed in preparation for the test. After a local anesthetic is injected, the doctor will insert a catheter into a vessel, advancing it as necessary. A contrast dye will be injected into the blood vessels; then a series of X-rays films will be taken to enable the doctor to follow the dye's passage. The patient may be asked to turn on his side or to elevate an arm or leg for the X-rays.

Instruct the patient to remain perfectly still to avoid distorting the X-ray image. Reassure him that if he feels flushed or nauseated or develops an unusual taste, these feelings will pass quickly.

Inform the patient that after the catheter is removed, pressure is applied over the insertion site for 15 to 30 minutes; then a bulky dressing is applied and a sandbag may be rested against it. He must keep his arm or leg extended and immobile for 4 to 24 hours. Mention that he'll have his pulse and circulation in the affected limb checked often.

Cardiac blood pool imaging

Explain to the patient that this 30- to 45-minute test evaluates the function of his heart's left ventricle. Tell him that before the test begins, electrodes will be attached to various sites on his body.

Atherosclerosis stages

When explaining atherosclerosis to the patient, be sure to point out that the disorder doesn't just happen; it occurs in stages. As shown in the illustrations below, atherosclerosis starts with an injury to the intimal layer of the arterial wall. This makes the wall permeable to circulating lipoproteins.

Next, lipoproteins invade smooth muscle cells in the intimal layer, forming a fatty streak—a nonobstructive lesion. Eventually, a fibrous plaque develops, impeding blood flow through the artery. Plaques contain lipoprotein-filled smooth muscle cells, collagen, and muscle fibers.

In the final stage of atherosclerosis, a complicated lesion develops, marked by calcification or rupture of the fibrous plaque. Thrombosis can occur, with near-total occlusion of the arterial lumen.

INJURY TO INTIMAL LAYER

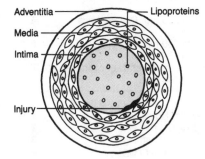

FORMATION OF LESION

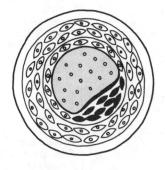

PLAQUE DEVELOPMENT

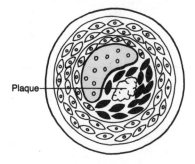

NEAR-TOTAL OCCLUSION OF ARTERIAL LUMEN

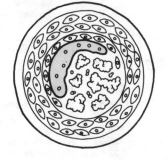

CAD risk factor survey

Researchers recognize certain factors that can increase the risk of developing coronary artery disease and its complications. To assess your patient's risk, help him complete this survey. In each category, circle the number that applies to him; then add the circled numbers to get his score. Compare his score to the ranges at the bottom of the chart to get an idea of his overall risk. Explain that some factors can be controlled if he's willing to make changes in his life-style.

FACTOR	SCORE
Age	
10 to 20	1
21 to 30	2
31 to 40	3
41 to 50	4
51 to 60	6
61 and over	8
Heredity	
Include parents, grandparents, and siblings	
No known history of cardiovascular disease	1
One relative with cardiovascular disease after age 60	2
Two relatives with cardiovascular disease after age 60	3
One relative with cardiovascular disease before age 60	4
Two relatives with cardiovascular disease before age 60	6
Three relatives with cardiovascular disease before age 60	7
Weight	
More than 5 lb (2.2 kg) below standard weight	0
−5 to +5 lb of standard weight	1
6 to 20 lb (2.7 to 9 kg) overweight	2
21 to 35 lb (9.5 to 15.8 kg) overweight	3
36 to 50 lb (16.3 to 22.6 kg) overweight	5
More than 50 lb overweight	7
Smoking	
Add 1 point if you inhale deeply and smoke cigarettes to the end. (Don't subtract any points if you do not inhale or if you smoke only part of a cigarette.) Subtract 1 point if you smoke but exercise regularly.	
Nonsmoker	0
Smoke cigar or pipe	1
Smoke 10 cigarettes or less a day	2
Smoke 20 cigarettes a day	4
Smoke 30 cigarettes a day	6
Smoke 40 or more cigarettes a day	10

FACTOR	SCORE
Exercise	
Intensive occupational and recreational exertion	1
Moderate occupational and recreational exertion	2
Sedentary work and intense recreational exertion	3
Sedentary work and moderate recreational exertion	5
Sedentary work and light recreational exertion	6
Complete lack of exercise	8
Serum cholesterol level and percentage of fat in diet	
Use your cholesterol level if you know it. Otherwise, estimate your intake of dietary fats—primarily animal fats. The U.S. average, 40%, is too high for good health.	
Cholesterol level of 180 mg or less. Diet contains no animal or solid fats.	1
Cholesterol level of 181 to 205 mg. Diet contains 10% animal or solid fats.	2
Cholesterol level of 206 to 230 mg. Diet contains 20% animal or solid fats.	3
Cholesterol level of 231 to 255 mg. Diet contains 30% animal or solid fats.	4
Cholesterol level of 256 to 280 mg. Diet contains 40% animal or solid fats.	5
Cholesterol level of 281 mg or higher. Diet contains 50% or more animal or solid fats.	7
Blood pressure	
Systolic pressure of 100 mm Hg or less	1
Systolic pressure of 101 to 120 mm Hg	2
Systolic pressure of 121 to 140 mm Hg	3
Systolic pressure of 141 to 160 mm Hg	4
Systolic pressure of 161 to 180 mm Hg	6
Systolic pressure over 180 mm Hg	8
Sex or physique	
Female under age 40	1
Female aged 40 to 50	2
Female over age 50	3
Male	5
Stocky male	6
Bald, stocky male	7

SCORE	RISK
6-11	Well below average
12-17	Below average
18-24	Average
25-31	Above average
32-40	Well above average
41-62	Exceptionally high—see a doctor now

During the test he'll lie supine while a slightly radioactive contrast dye is injected into a vein, and a scintillation camera records the dye's passage through the heart. Instruct the patient to remain still during scanning. Explain that by synchronizing the camera with an ECG, the doctor can correlate subsequent images with ECG waveforms.

Cardiac catheterization
Tell the patient that this test evaluates the function of his heart and its vessels. It reveals coronary artery stenosis or evaluates left ventricular function before coronary artery bypass surgery. The test usually takes 2 to 3 hours.

Inform the patient that the doctor will inject a local anesthetic into the patient's groin area and thread a catheter either through an artery to the left side of the heart or through a vein to the right side of the heart and to the lungs. Next, the doctor will inject a contrast dye through the catheter. Instruct the patient to follow directions to cough or breathe deeply, and inform him that he may receive nitroglycerin during the test to dilate coronary vessels and aid visualization. For more information on what to teach patients undergoing this procedure, see the patient-teaching aid *Preparing for cardiac catheterization,* pages 20 to 22.

Echocardiography
Inform the patient that echocardiography is a safe and painless method of evaluating the size, shape, and motion of various cardiac structures. Mention that the procedure usually takes 15 to 30 minutes and that he may undergo other tests, such as an ECG or phonocardiography, simultaneously. Explain that before the test conductive jelly will be applied to his chest. Emphasize that he must remain still during the test because movement may distort results.

Explain that during the test, a technician will angle a transducer over the patient's chest to observe different parts of the heart, and may reposition him on his left side. While changes in heart function are recorded, the patient may be asked to slowly breathe in and out, to hold his breath, or to inhale a gas with a slightly sweet odor (amyl nitrite). Amyl nitrite may cause dizziness, flushing, and tachycardia. Reassure the patient that these effects quickly subside.

Electrocardiography
Explain to the patient that this 15-minute test evaluates the heart's function by graphically recording its electrical activity. It usually doesn't cause discomfort. Before the test, the technician will cleanse, dry, and possibly shave different sites on the patient's body, such as his chest and arms, and will apply a conductive jelly over them. Then he'll attach electrodes at these sites.

Point out that talking or limb movement will distort the ECG recordings and require additional testing time. The patient must lie still, relax, breathe normally, and remain quiet.

Exercise ECG
Tell the patient that exercise ECG (also known as a stress test or a treadmill or graded exercise test) evaluates the heart's electrical activity while he walks a treadmill or pedals a bicycle. It usually takes about 30 minutes. Inform him that he mustn't eat or smoke for 2 hours before the test. Mention that the test will make him perspire and that he should wear loose, lightweight clothing and snug-fitting shoes. Men usually don't wear a shirt during the test, and women usually wear a bra and a lightweight short-sleeved blouse or a patient gown with front closure.

Encourage the patient to express any fears regarding the procedure. Reassure him that a doctor and a nurse will be present at all times. Emphasize that he can stop if he feels chest pain, leg discomfort, breathlessness, or severe fatigue. Tell the patient that before he begins, a technician will cleanse, shave (if necessary), and abrade sites on his chest and, possibly, his back. Then he'll attach electrodes at these sites.

If the patient is scheduled for a multistage treadmill test, tell him that the treadmill speed and incline increase at predetermined intervals and that he'll be told of each adjustment. If he's scheduled for a bicycle ergometer test, tell him that resistance to pedaling gradually increases as he tries to maintain a specific speed. Typically, he'll feel tired, out of breath, and sweaty during the test. Still, encourage the patient to report any of these reactions. He can expect to have his blood pressure and heart rate checked periodically.

Inform the patient that he may receive an injection of thallium during the test so the doctor can evaluate coronary blood flow on a scanner. Reassure him that the injection involves negligible radiation exposure.

Inform the patient that after the test, his blood pressure and ECG will be monitored for 10 to 15 minutes. Explain that he should wait at least 1 hour after the test before showering, and then he should use warm water.

Teach about treatments
Treatment will probably include increased exercise, dietary changes, and other risk factor–reduction measures along with drug therapy. If these measures don't improve or eliminate angina, the patient may need to undergo percutaneous transluminal coronary angioplasty (PTCA) or coronary artery bypass grafting (CABG).

Activity
Explain how a sedentary life-style contributes to CAD. Tell the patient that it encourages overeating, leads to obesity and hypertension, and unfavorably alters the ratio of high-density lipoprotein (HDL) to low-density lipoprotein (LDL).

Next, discuss the benefits of regular exercise. Tell him that it increases serum HDL level, promotes weight loss, lowers blood pressure, and tones the entire cardiovascular system. Encourage aerobic exercises, such as walking, jogging, bicycling, or swimming (see the patient-teaching aids *Tips for exercising safely* on page 23 and *Personalizing your exercise program* on pages 24 and 25). Teach the patient how to monitor his pulse during exercise (see the patient-teaching aid *How to take your pulse,* page 26). Advise against isometric exercises, such as weight lifting, which elevate blood pressure and tax the heart and coronary arteries. Warn that occasional strenuous exercise may be more dangerous than no exercise.

Tell the patient to take his prescribed medication before engaging in any activity that normally provokes angina, including exercise and sex. If angina occurs, he should stop the activity immediately, sit or lie down with his head elevated, breathe deeply and slowly to relax, and take his prescribed medication. Tell him to have someone take him to the hospital emergency room if his angina persists for longer than 10 minutes after he takes three spaced doses of his medication.

Diet

Explain to the patient how dietary adjustments can help modify three of the important CAD risk factors you have helped him identify: high serum cholesterol level, obesity, and hypertension. First, point out the need to limit fat intake to no more than 30% of total calories, with saturated fats making up less than 10% of total calories. (See *Teaching tips for healthful eating.*) Emphasize the importance of limiting cholesterol intake (see the patient-teaching aid *Cutting down on cholesterol,* page 27). Explain the difference between desirable HDL and undesirable LDL and the benefits of a favorable HDL:LDL ratio.

Specifically, advise the patient to limit red meat, processed meat, lard, whole milk products, and saturated tropical oils (coconut, palm, and palm kernel), found mostly in processed foods. Tell him to trim visible fat from red meat, to remove the skin from poultry before cooking, and to substitute fish and margarine for meat and butter. Remind him that broiling, microwaving, grilling, or roasting meat on a rack is preferable to deep-frying. If he eats at fast-food restaurants, suggest that he ask whether the food is fried in animal fat or unsaturated vegetable oils. Recommend that he eat no more than three egg yolks a week, including yolks in prepared foods.

Discuss with the patient the possible value of including fiber, fish oils, and olive oil in his diet. Explain that soluble fiber, such as oat bran (but not wheat bran), may reduce the absorption of saturated fats in the intestines. Intake of fish oils, also known as omega-3 fatty acids or marine oils (found in salmon, mackerel, herring, and tuna), may improve his HDL:LDL ratio. But advise him that the effectiveness of fish oil capsules hasn't yet been proven, only the eating of fish, especially as a substitute for red meat. Suggest that he substitute the monounsaturated olive oil for other dietary oils, keeping in mind the overall reduction in dietary fat. Advise the patient who already drinks alcohol that up to two drinks a day can also improve his HDL:LDL ratio, but that more than this amount can adversely affect his heart.

The second risk factor that you can help the patient modify by

---

Teaching tips for healthful eating

Food habits play an important part in determining a person's risk of heart disease. Offer your patient the following tips for healthier eating. Advise him to:
• drink a glass of water before each meal.
• start with a smaller portion than usual. If he wants more, he should wait 4 or 5 minutes; he'll feel less hungry.
• avoid placing serving dishes on the table, which makes having seconds too easy.
• avoid rushing the meal. Suggest that he put his fork down between bites and wait until he finishes chewing before picking it up again.
• hold a conversation as he eats; doing so will slow down his eating pace.
• try cutting down on salt. He should take the salt shaker off the dining table and avoid cooking with salt. Or, if this seems too difficult, suggest using low-sodium salt.
• avoid fried food and food prepared with rich sauces when eating in restaurants. Such foods may contain saturated fat and too many calories. Recommend that he consider ordering broth or vegetable soup rather than a cream soup, an oil and vinegar dressing for his salad rather than a creamy one, broiled fish or fowl (skip the sauce), and fresh fruit.
• stop eating as soon as he's no longer hungry—not continuing until he feels stuffed, even if he must leave food on his plate.

Relieving occlusions with PTCA

Percutaneous transluminal coronary angioplasty (PTCA) offers a nonsurgical alternative to coronary artery bypass surgery. It can open an occluded coronary artery without opening the chest. If your patient will be undergoing PTCA, use the information below to help you explain the procedure to him.

After coronary angiography has confirmed the occlusion's location, the doctor threads a guide catheter through the patient's femoral artery into the coronary artery.

When the guide catheter is positioned at the occlusion, the doctor inserts a smaller, double-lumen balloon catheter through the guide catheter and directs it through the occlusion. A marked pressure gradient occurs.

The doctor alternatively inflates and deflates the balloon until angiography verifies successful arterial dilation and the pressure gradient has decreased.

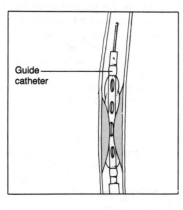

Guide catheter

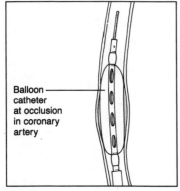

Balloon catheter at occlusion in coronary artery

diet is hypertension. Instruct him that eliminating caffeine and lowering sodium intake usually lowers blood pressure.

The third risk factor, obesity, is closely linked to several other factors. Explain how losing excess weight by itself affects CAD, and also helps to lower hypertension. Tell him that the two best ways to lose weight are to limit caloric—especially fat—intake and to exercise, an activity that also corrects a sedentary lifestyle. Advise against fad diets or pills, but refer him to a weight control group for additional information and support.

Finally, be sure the patient knows how to read food labels for information on types of fat and amount of sodium.

Medications

Explain the purpose of all prescribed medications, including antilipemics and antiplatelet drugs, beta blockers, calcium channel blockers, and nitrates. (See *Teaching patients about drugs for CAD*.) Explain, for instance, that antilipemics reduce the levels of certain protein and fat combinations in the patient's blood. Antiplatelets, such as aspirin and dipyridamole, hinder blood clotting. Beta-adrenergic blockers lower blood pressure, reduce the frequency of anginal attacks, and control rapid heart rate. Calcium channel blockers reduce the frequency and severity of chest pain and lower blood pressure, and nitrates prevent or alleviate anginal pain. If appropriate, provide the patient with a copy of the patient-teaching aid *How to use nitroglycerin,* pages 28 and 29. Teach the patient to examine labels of nonprescription medications for sodium, caffeine, and aspirin content.

Procedures

If drug therapy fails to relieve angina, the doctor may order PTCA. Explain that *percutaneous* means that the procedure involves going through the skin, *transluminal* indicates that the procedure is done inside the artery, *coronary* defines the treated artery as one that involves the heart, and *angioplasty* means the technique of repairing the narrowed or blocked artery.

Inform the patient that the doctor may introduce the catheter into either the arm (brachial approach) or the groin (femoral approach). Tell him that the doctor will numb the site with a local anesthetic and then insert a thin, balloon-tipped catheter into a peripheral artery. Guided by fluoroscopy, he'll thread the catheter through the constricted coronary artery to the site of obstruction. After verifying the catheter's placement by instilling contrast dye, the doctor will inflate the balloon tip (see *Relieving occlusions with PTCA*). This compresses the obstruction against the arterial walls, expanding the vessel to increase blood flow. Tell the patient that the doctor will then deflate the balloon but may leave the catheter in place temporarily to repeat the procedure or to administer drugs.

Inform the patient that he'll be given a sedative before the procedure to help him relax and that he'll be asked to cough several times during the procedure to help clear contrast dye from his heart. Warn him that he may feel flushed and experience angina

continued on page 16

Teaching patients about drugs for CAD

DRUG	ADVERSE REACTIONS	TEACHING POINTS
Antilipemics		
cholestyramine (Cholybar, Questran)	Be alert for severe constipation, rash, black or tarry stools, severe stomach pain, and unusual weight loss. Other: bloating, mild constipation, diarrhea, flatulence, nausea, and vomiting.	• Explain to the patient that this drug should reduce the levels of certain protein and fat combinations in his blood. • Emphasize that he is still responsible for limiting his intake of cholesterol and saturated fat. Encourage him to increase fluid and fiber intake and to use a bulk laxative, as needed. • Tell the patient to mix powder with liquids, applesauce, or crushed pineapple to prevent GI erosion. • Instruct him to take the drug 1 hour before or 3 hours after a meal. • If the patient takes fat-soluble vitamins (A, D, E, K, or folic acid), he should stagger administration times, since cholestyramine interferes with vitamin absorption. • If the patient is taking prescription drugs, advise him to check with the doctor or pharmacist for administration guidelines. Cholestyramine may interfere with absorption of several prescription drugs. • Tell the patient to take a missed dose as soon as possible, but warn him not to double-dose.
clofibrate (Atromid-S)	Be alert for bloody or painful urination, chest pain, chills, dyspnea, fever, irregular heart rate, leg and ankle edema, and sore throat. Other: abdominal fullness, decreased libido, diarrhea, flatulence, flulike aches and pains, nausea, and weight gain.	• Explain to the patient that this drug should reduce the levels of certain protein and fat combinations in his blood. • Emphasize that he is still responsible for limiting his intake of cholesterol and saturated fats. Encourage him to increase fluid and fiber intake and to use a bulk laxative, as needed. • Reassure the patient that any GI distress is transient. • Tell him to take a missed dose as soon as possible, but warn him not to double-dose.
gemfibrozil (Lopid)	Be alert for abdominal and epigastric pain, blurred vision, diarrhea, dizziness, dry mouth, dyspepsia, flatulence, headache, nausea, and vomiting. Other: dermatitis, extremity pain, pruritus, and rash.	• Explain to the patient that this drug should reduce the levels of certain protein and fat combinations in his blood. • Emphasize that he is still responsible for limiting his intake of cholesterol and saturated fats. Encourage him to increase fluid and fiber intake and to use a bulk laxative, as needed. • Stress the importance of close monitoring by the doctor, reporting any adverse reactions, and complying with prescribed regimen and diet. • Tell patient to take gemfibrozil with food to minimize GI discomfort. • Warn him not to exceed the prescribed dose.
lovastatin (Mevacor)	Be alert for abdominal pain or cramps, blurred vision, constipation, diarrhea, dysgeusia, dyspepsia, flatus, heartburn, muscle cramps, myalgia, and nausea. Other: dizziness, headache, myositis, peripheral neuropathy, pruritus, and rash.	• Explain to the patient that this drug should reduce the levels of certain protein and fat combinations in his blood. • Emphasize that he is still responsible for limiting his intake of cholesterol and saturated fats. Encourage him to increase fluid and fiber intake and to use a bulk laxative, as needed. • Instruct the patient to take lovastatin with his evening meal and to notify the doctor of any adverse reactions, particularly muscle aches and pains. • Advise him to restrict alcohol intake because taking this drug with alcohol may cause liver toxicity.

continued

14 Coronary artery disease

Teaching patients about drugs for CAD—*continued*

DRUG	ADVERSE REACTIONS	TEACHING POINTS
Antilipemics—*continued*		
niacin	Be alert for activation of peptic ulcer, bloating, blurred vision, burning, diarrhea, dizziness, excessive peripheral vasodilation, flatulence, flushing, hypotension, nausea, stomach pain, tingling, transient headache, vomiting, and warmth. Effects may depend on the dosage. Other: dry skin, rash, syncope, and tachycardia.	• Explain to the patient that this drug should reduce the levels of certain protein and fat combinations in his blood. • Emphasize that he is still responsible for limiting his intake of cholesterol and saturated fats. Encourage him to increase fluid and fiber intake and to use a bulk laxative, as needed. • To help ensure compliance, explain the rationale for therapy. Stress that niacin, though a vitamin, is used to treat hyperlipidemia or dilate peripheral vessels. • Cutaneous flushing and warmth commonly occur during the first 2 hours after taking niacin. Tell the patient these reactions will cease with continued therapy. For severe reactions, the doctor may prescribe taking aspirin 30 minutes before taking niacin. • Instruct the patient to avoid drinking hot liquids when initially taking the drug (to minimize flushing), to avoid making sudden changes in position (to minimize effects of postural hypotension), and to consider taking the drug with meals (to reduce GI irritation).
probucol (Lorelco)	Be alert for abdominal pain, angioneurotic edema, decreased hemoglobin and hematocrit, diarrhea, dizziness, fetid sweat, flatulence, headache, indigestion, insomnia, itching, nausea, petechiae, rash, thrombocytopenia, tinnitus, and vomiting. Other: conjunctivitis, ecchymoses, eosinophilia, GI bleeding, hyperhidrosis, impotence, paresthesias, and peripheral neuritis.	• Explain to the patient that this drug should reduce the levels of certain protein and fat combinations in his blood. • Emphasize that he is still responsible for limiting his intake of cholesterol and saturated fats. Encourage him to increase fluid and fiber intake and to use a bulk laxative, as needed. • Advise the patient to take the drug with meals to enhance absorption. Explain to him that probucol is not curative. • Inform him that GI effects usually disappear with continued use.
Antiplatelets		
aspirin	Be alert for bleeding gums, easy bruising, hearing loss, hematemesis, tarry stools, and tinnitus. Other: GI upset and headache.	• Explain to the patient that aspirin hinders blood clotting. • To relieve mild GI distress, advise the patient to take aspirin with food or milk or to use a buffered or enteric-coated form of the drug. • When taking aspirin, he should avoid antacids, which can reduce the drug's effectiveness. He should also avoid drinking alcohol during therapy because GI bleeding may occur. • Also warn against substituting acetaminophen, which doesn't share aspirin's antithrombotic effects. • Tell him to take a missed dose within 12 hours, but warn him not to double-dose.
dipyridamole (Persantine)	Be alert for chest pain or tightness, vomiting, and weakness. Other: GI upset and heartburn.	• Explain to the patient that this drug hinders blood clotting and dilates his coronary arteries. • Instruct him to take drug 1 hour before or 3 hours after a meal. • Tell him to take the drug with a light snack or a glass of milk to help reduce GI distress. • To minimize dizziness, advise the patient to rise slowly from a sitting or lying position. • Tell him to take a missed dose as soon as possible, but warn him not to double-dose. • Warn against drinking alcohol during therapy. Dizziness may result.

continued

Teaching patients about drugs for CAD—*continued*

DRUG	ADVERSE REACTIONS	TEACHING POINTS
Beta-adrenergic blockers		
acebutolol (Sectral) **atenolol** (Tenormin) **labetalol** (Trandate) **metoprolol** (Lopressor) **nadolol** (Corgard) **pindolol** (Visken) **propranolol** (Inderal) **timolol** (Blocadren)	Be alert for depression, dizziness, dyspnea, rash, very slow heart rate, and wheezing. Other: decreased libido, diarrhea, fatigue, headache, insomnia, nasal stuffiness, nausea, vivid dreams and nightmares, and vomiting.	• Explain that this drug can lower blood pressure and reduce the frequency of angina attacks. • If the patient takes one dose daily, instruct him to take a missed dose within 8 hours. If he takes two or more doses each day, instruct him to take a missed dose as soon as possible. However, warn him never to double-dose. • Teach him to take his pulse before taking the drug and to notify his doctor if it falls below 60 beats/minute. • Instruct him to take labetalol, metoprolol, and propranolol with foods to increase drug absorption. • Warn him against suddenly discontinuing the drug. He must taper the dosage, as directed, to avoid complications. • If the patient complains of insomnia, suggest that he take the drug no later than 2 hours before bedtime.
Calcium channel blockers		
diltiazem (Cardizem) **nifedipine** (Procardia) **verapamil** (Calan, Isoptin)	Be alert for ankle edema, chest pain, dyspnea, fainting, and very slow or fast heart rate. Other: constipation, dizziness, flushing, headache, and nausea.	• Explain to the patient that this drug can reduce the frequency and severity of his chest pain and lower his blood pressure. It won't relieve acute chest pain; he must continue to use nitroglycerin, if prescribed. • Reassure him that he can continue to eat and drink calcium-containing foods in reasonable amounts. • Teach him to prevent constipation by increasing fluid and fiber intake and by using a bulk laxative, as necessary. • Advise him to limit alcohol intake to prevent dizziness. • Tell him to take a missed dose within 4 hours, but warn him not to double-dose. • To minimize dizziness, tell him to rise slowly from a sitting or lying position. • Advise checking with his doctor or pharmacist before taking over-the-counter cold or allergy preparations. Many contain drugs that will increase blood pressure and decrease the effectiveness of calcium channel blockers.
Nitrates		
erythrityl tetranitrate (Cardilate) **isosorbide dinitrate** (multiple forms and brands) **nitroglycerin** (multiple forms and brands) **pentaerythritol tetranitrate** (Duotrate, Peritrate)	Be alert for blurred vision, extreme dizziness, dry mouth, rapid heart rate, and skin irritation or rash. Other: headache, flushing, mild dizziness, nausea, and vomiting.	• If nitroglycerin tablets are prescribed for acute angina attacks, instruct the patient to take one tablet every 5 minutes up to a maximum of three tablets. Tell him to hold each tablet under his tongue until it dissolves. Meanwhile, he should sit down and try to relax. If the tablets bring no relief, tell him to call his doctor immediately or have someone take him to an emergency department at once. • If he uses nitrates to prevent angina, teach him to maintain a self-administration schedule. He should also take the drug before any activity that induces angina, such as exposure to cold, exertion, or sex. • Advise him to avoid overly hot showers. Vasodilation might make him dizzy and faint. To prevent dizziness, tell him to rise slowly from a sitting or lying position. • Reassure him that headaches should diminish with continued use of nitrates. If they don't, tell him to notify his doctor. • Tell him to take a missed dose as soon as possible, but warn him not to double-dose. • Because nitroglycerin tablets must be fresh to be effective, tell the patient to cap the bottle quickly and tightly after each use and to replace an opened bottle after 3 months, even if some tablets remain. • Instruct him to shield tablets from light.

16 Coronary artery disease

Speeding recovery after PTCA

Before your patient leaves the hospital after percutaneous transluminal coronary angioplasty (PTCA), the doctor will give him instructions for activities, diet, and medications. In addition, you'll need to provide directions to speed the patient's recovery. Tell him to:
• avoid heavy lifting and other strenuous activities for at least a week.
• resume his usual daily activities and return to work according to the doctor's orders.
• carefully follow the doctor's instructions about taking medication. He should contact the doctor if any medication causes adverse reactions, but he shouldn't stop taking the medication unless instructed to do so.
• keep all scheduled follow-up medical appointments.
• feel free to discuss his concerns about his illness with the doctor, nurse, or both.

---

when the contrast dye is instilled; reassure him that these effects are transient.

Explain that after PTCA, the patient will be on bed rest for 1 or 2 days and will require periodic blood tests to evaluate blood coagulation, cardiac enzymes, and electrolytes. He'll receive I.V. nitroglycerin (to prevent coronary artery spasm) or anticoagulants (to prevent clot formation), or both. Inform the patient that his blood pressure and pulses will be checked frequently and that he may be connected to a cardiac monitor. Instruct him to increase his fluid intake to help the kidneys excrete the test dye more readily.

Warn the patient that mild chest pain is common immediately after PTCA, but should subside in 1 to 2 hours. However, if his chest pain worsens or returns, advise him to call you immediately. If the femoral approach was used, tell the patient that some short tubes or sheaths may be left in his groin until the next day. Instruct him to keep the affected leg straight to prevent the tube from kinking. Reassure him that he'll be able to bend his leg and then stand for a few hours after the tubes are removed.

Tell the patient to have someone take him home rather than drive himself. (For more advice to give the patient, see *Speeding recovery after PTCA*.) Make sure he understands that the procedure doesn't cure CAD. The expanded artery can eventually reocclude if he fails to modify his risk factors.

Surgery
If the doctor schedules CABG to relieve angina and, possibly, prevent MI, explain the surgery to the patient, and teach him about pertinent preoperative and postoperative care measures. Provide encouragement by mentioning that CABG eliminates anginal pain, improves heart function, and may increase life expectancy.

Explain the procedure. Tell the patient that CABG will restore normal blood flow to his heart. As necessary, clarify and reinforce what the doctor has told him. Explain that the doctor will remove a portion of a healthy vessel from another part of the body (usually a portion of a saphenous vein or a mammary artery) and then graft it above and below the blocked coronary artery (see *Learning about CABG*). Tell him that his circulation will then be diverted through the graft. Reassure him that circulation won't be disrupted in the area from which the graft was excised.

Next, tell the patient where he'll be taken to recover after the procedure. If possible, arrange a tour for the patient and his family before surgery. Explain the complex, and often frightening, equipment that will support the patient's vital functions after surgery. For example, prepare the patient for intubation and mechanical ventilation. Mention that he won't be able to speak while intubated, but he will be able to communicate by gesturing or writing.

Explain to the patient that an intra-aortic balloon pump may be inserted to provide circulatory support for several hours postoperatively. He'll also have a nasogastric tube, a mediastinal chest

Learning about CABG

If your patient is scheduled for coronary artery bypass grafting (CABG), show him a heart model or a drawing of the heart and coronary arteries to demonstrate the procedure.

In this example of bypass grafting, the surgeon has used saphenous vein segments to bypass occlusions in three sections of coronary artery.

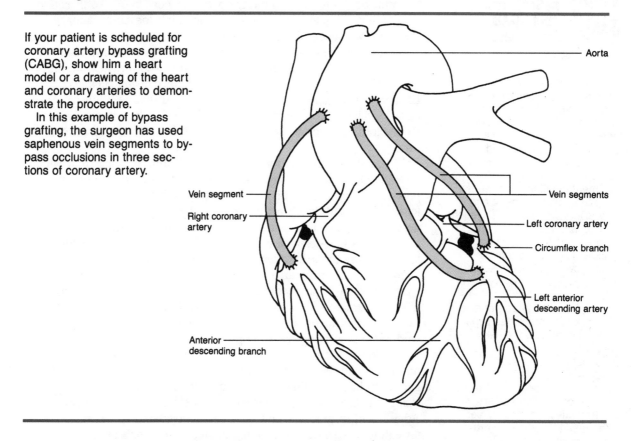

Aorta

Vein segment

Right coronary artery

Vein segments

Left coronary artery

Circumflex branch

Left anterior descending artery

Anterior descending branch

tube, and an indwelling catheter in place for the first day or two. In addition, he'll be connected to a cardiac monitor.

Describe preoperative care. The afternoon before surgery, teach the patient about preoperative care measures. Explain that he'll be asked to shower with a special antiseptic soap and may be shaved from his neck to his toes. Tell him that he won't be allowed to eat or drink anything after midnight, although he can request a sleeping pill. Inform him that he may receive a sedative the morning of surgery to help him relax.

If indicated, prepare the patient for preoperative pulmonary artery catheterization. Explain that the catheter will remain in place after surgery, but reassure him that the catheter, arterial lines, and epicardial pacing wires will cause minimal or no discomfort.

Teach about postoperative care. After surgery, teach the patient about short-term postoperative care measures and his role in implementing them. Start with the expected course of his hospital stay—how many days he'll spend in the critical care area, stepdown unit, and regular room before discharge.

Emphasize that his priority is to relax and rest; stress and anxiety will only hinder his recovery. Encourage him to request pain medication to promote relaxation. When the endotracheal and nasogastric tubes are removed, he'll be able to sit up and swallow liquids. Tell him that solid foods will then gradually be reintroduced to his diet.

Questions patients ask about CAD treatments

Why is coronary artery bypass surgery done on some patients but not on others?
Candidates for coronary artery bypass usually fall into one of three groups: patients with severe angina that doesn't respond to medication or other treatments; patients who've developed complications of coronary artery disease (CAD), such as myocardial infarction; and patients who are scheduled for artificial heart valve replacement. However, bypass surgery isn't appropriate for everyone in these groups. In some patients, the number and degree of arterial blockages precludes bypass surgery; in others, the risk of the surgery outweighs its possible benefits. The doctor will consider all the available information on your condition before deciding on bypass surgery. As an alternative, he may try percutaneous transluminal coronary angioplasty (PTCA).

Will bypass surgery cure me?
No, surgery can't cure CAD. The vein grafts can develop atherosclerosis just like your arteries did. You should feel relief from angina, though, and have more energy. But you'll need to carefully follow postoperative and long-term care instructions to reduce the risk of developing new blockages.

What happens to fatty arterial deposits after a PTCA?
Although we don't know for sure, we do know that they don't float "downstream" to lodge somewhere else. Inflation of the balloon inside the artery breaks up the hard protective coating of the fatty plaque deposits and flattens the deposits against the arterial wall. Then, over the course of several months, "scavenger" cells in the bloodstream presumably remove most of the debris.

To help prevent pulmonary complications, encourage the patient to perform coughing and deep-breathing exercises. Teach him how to splint his incision to minimize pain and how to use an incentive spirometer. Reassure him that coughing won't loosen or damage the graft or reopen his chest incision.

Next, discuss other self-care measures. About 6 days after surgery, the patient will probably be allowed to shower. Instruct him to use warm, not hot, water and to wash all incision sites gently. Explain that complete healing takes time and that he'll always have a scar (although it will fade). Suggest that he wear soft, loose clothing, such as cotton T-shirts, at first for maximum comfort.

To enhance circulation and reduce swelling in a leg from which a saphenous vein graft was taken, he may also need to wear support stockings, elevate his leg frequently, and avoid crossing his legs. Tell him to watch for and report any new tenderness, redness, swelling, or drainage from his chest and leg incisions.

Discuss long-term care. As the patient gains strength, begin teaching him about long-term care measures. Review his prescribed exercise program. Emphasize the need to increase his activity gradually, and encourage him to set realistic goals. Teach him to alternate light and heavy tasks and to rest between tasks. Reinforce the doctor's restrictions on such activities as lifting, working, and driving, as appropriate.

Address the patient's concerns about sex after surgery. Reassure him that once the doctor has given his okay, sex is no more dangerous to his heart than walking up a couple flights of stairs. Point out that a satisfying sex life can help speed his recovery. Advise him to reduce strain on his heart by avoiding sex right after eating a big meal or drinking alcohol, when he's fatigued or emotionally upset, or when he's in an unfamiliar and stressful situation—in a strange environment or with a new partner, for example. Tell him to choose a position that doesn't restrict his breathing; he should also avoid any position in which he has to support himself or his partner with his arms. Explain that impotence is fairly common but that it's almost always temporary and is no cause for concern.

Because medications form an important part of postoperative care, make sure the patient understands their administration schedules and possible adverse effects. Also discuss dietary restrictions with the patient, emphasizing that he can reduce the risk of arterial reocclusion by adhering to a diet that's low in cholesterol and saturated fats. With his doctor's permission, he can have up to two alcoholic drinks a day beginning 2 to 3 weeks after surgery.

Before discharge, teach the patient to watch for and report warning signs of reocclusion or other serious complications: angina, persistent fever, swelling or drainage at the incision site, dizziness, shortness of breath at rest, rapid or irregular pulse, and prolonged recovery time from exercise or sex. Also prepare him for postoperative depression, which may not set in until he's home. Reassure him that depression is usually temporary.

Other care measures

Tell the patient that smoking and stress are also CAD risk factors. Explain that smoking reduces his serum HDL level, constricts his arteries (thereby elevating blood pressure), and reduces the blood's oxygen-carrying capacity. Encourage him to quit by noting that most of these effects will cease shortly after he quits. Refer him to a support group, such as a local chapter of the American Lung Association or the American Cancer Society, if necessary.

Also discuss how stress aggravates hypertension and overstimulates the heart. Help the patient identify stressors and develop strategies to cope with them. No one can eliminate stress altogether, but the patient can learn to reduce it by avoiding noise and crowds; by modifying aggressive, hard-driving behavior; by changing a stressful job; by learning to relax through such measures as yoga, walking, or deep-breathing exercises; by getting adequate exercise and rest; and by taking up an enjoyable hobby. If appropriate, consider referring the patient to an assertiveness training workshop to help him reduce aggression and frustration. Also refer the patient to a local chapter of the American Heart Association.

Sources of information and support

American Cancer Society (ACS)
90 Park Avenue, New York, N.Y. 10016
(212) 599-8200

American Heart Association
7320 Greenville Avenue, Dallas, Tex. 75231
(214) 750-5300

American Lung Association
1740 Broadway, New York, N.Y. 10019
(212) 315-8700

Further readings

Braunwald, E., et al., eds. *Harrison's Principles of Internal Medicine.* St. Louis: C.V. Mosby Co., 1987.
Cowley, M., et al. "The Angioplasty Option for CAD," *Patient Care* 21(17):34, October 30, 1987.
Kern, L. "Advances in the Surgical Treatment of Coronary Artery Disease," *Journal of Cardiovascular Nursing* 192-98, November 1986.
Marshall, J., et al. "Structured Postoperative Teaching and Knowledge and Compliance of Patients Who Had Coronary Artery Bypass Surgery," *Heart & Lung* 15(1):76-82, January 1986.
National Heart, Lung, and Blood Institute. *Report of the Expert Panel on Detection, Evaluation, and Treatment of High Cholesterol in Adults.* NIH Publication 88-2925. Bethesda, Md.: National Institutes of Health, 1988.
Streff, M. "Exercise in the Prevention of Coronary Artery Disease," *Journal of Cardiovascular Nursing* 1(4):42-53, August 1987.

Preparing for cardiac catheterization

Dear Patient:

Your doctor has scheduled you for cardiac catheterization, a procedure that allows him to look at the inside of your heart. He does this by first making a small incision in a blood vessel near your elbow or groin and then inserting a long, thin, flexible tube called a catheter into the vessel.

After inserting the catheter, the doctor will slowly thread it through your bloodstream into your heart. When the catheter is in place, the doctor will perform certain tests that may include injection of a special dye. What the doctor sees will help him to decide what additional treatment might improve your heart's functioning.

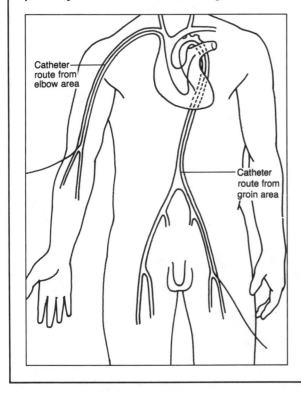

Catheter route from elbow area

Catheter route from groin area

Before the procedure

If your catheterization is scheduled for early morning, you probably won't be allowed to eat or drink anything after midnight of the evening before the procedure.

To protect against infection, the nurse may shave the area where your incision will be made. Before you go to the catheterization laboratory for the procedure, she'll also ask you to urinate. Then she'll help you into a hospital gown. Depending on the doctor's orders, she may start an I.V. line in your arm.

When you reach the catheterization lab, you'll be placed on a padded table and probably strapped to it. During catheterization, the doctor will tilt the table to view your heart from different angles. The straps will keep you from slipping out of position. Special foam pads, called leads, may be connected to a monitor and put on your chest so that your heartbeat can be monitored.

Cardiac catheterization usually takes 1 to 2 hours. You'll be awake throughout the procedure, although the doctor may order medication to help you relax. You may feel flushed or nauseated during catheterization or you may feel pain in your chest. These sensations should pass quickly. (Some patients even doze off.)

continued

PATIENT-TEACHING AID

Preparing for cardiac catheterization—*continued*

During the procedure

When the doctor is ready to begin, he'll inject a local anesthetic at the catheter insertion site. The injection may hurt a little, but it will numb the area before he puts in the catheter. When the catheter is going in, you should feel a little pressure but no pain. You may receive nitroglycerin during the test, to enlarge your heart's blood vessels and help the doctor get a better view.

If the catheter's passage is blocked—where atherosclerosis has narrowed a blood vessel, for example—the doctor will pull back the catheter and start from another insertion area.

When the catheter enters your heart, you may feel a fluttering or flip-flop sensation. Tell the doctor if you do, but don't worry; this is a normal reaction.

You're also likely to feel a warm sensation, some nausea, or the urge to urinate if dye is injected, but these feelings will quickly pass. Throughout the catheterization, remember to let the doctor or the nurse know if you have chest pain.

During the catheterization, your doctor may ask you to cough or to pant like a dog. Coughing and panting help to move the dye through your heart. The doctor may also ask you to breathe deeply, which will give him a better view of your heart.

When the test is finished, the doctor will slowly remove the catheter and put a special bandage on your arm or groin. Chances are the anesthetic will still be working, so you shouldn't feel anything.

continued

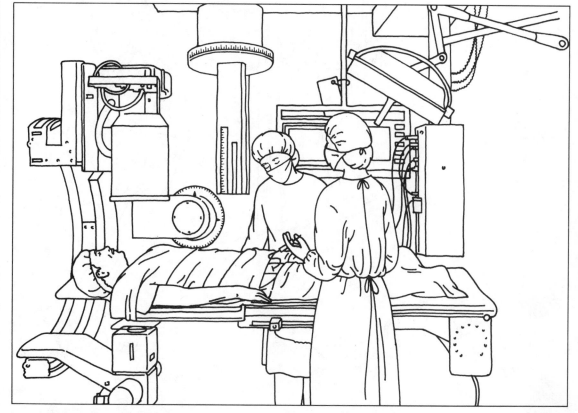

Preparing for cardiac catheterization—*continued*

After the procedure

When you're back in your room, the nurse will probably do an electrocardiogram if you're not already on a cardiac monitor. She'll check your bandage and your temperature, pulse, breathing, and blood pressure frequently. This frequent checking is done for everyone who has had cardiac catheterization, so don't be concerned.

At this point, we'll need your special cooperation. Your bandaged arm or leg must stay completely still for up to 24 hours. To help you keep from moving, the nurse may splint your arm or leg or weigh it down with a sandbag. She'll check the site frequently for swelling as well as check the blood flow in your arm or leg. She'll probably ask you to wiggle your toes or fingers once an hour or more.

As your anesthetic wears off, you'll probably feel some pain at the insertion site. Let the nurse know so she can give you pain medication.

As soon as the test results are available, the doctor will talk to you and your family about them. Don't hesitate to ask him or the nurse any questions.

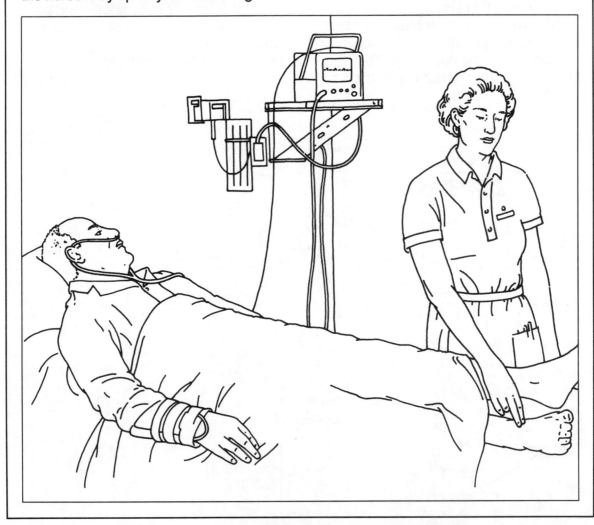

PATIENT-TEACHING AID

Tips for exercising safely

Dear Patient:

The following tips will help you exercise safely. Remember that your goal is to pace yourself, not to overdo it.

What you should do
• If you've been inactive for a long time, return to exercise gradually.
• Take part in fitness activities, such as walking and swimming, rather than competitive sports, such as tennis.
• Wait 2 to 3 hours after a heavy meal before exercising. A light snack warrants a 1- to 2-hour wait. Also avoid hot or cold showers immediately before or after exertion.
• Wear comfortable, lightweight clothes and shoes with adequate support. Dress in layers and remove articles of clothing as you warm up.

What you shouldn't do
• Exercise in extreme heat or cold, windy weather, high humidity, or heavy pollution, or at a high altitude.
• Exercise if you have a fever or don't feel well.

When to slow down
You may be exercising too hard if you have symptoms of angina, muscle cramps, side "stitch," and excessive shortness of breath or fatigue. Slow down.

When to stop exercising
Stop exercising and check with your doctor immediately if you experience chest pain, a cold sweat, dizziness, nausea or vomiting, heart palpitations, fluttering, or an abnormal heart rhythm.

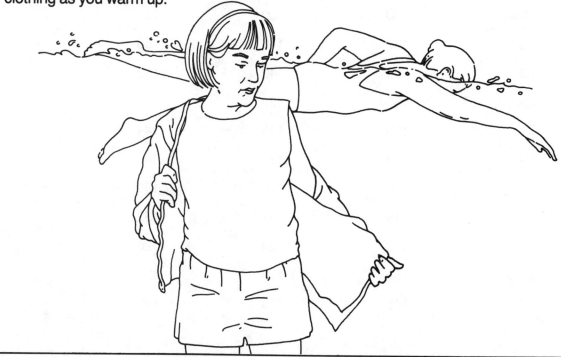

Personalizing your exercise program

Dear Patient:

You can make your exercise program suit your individual needs by determining your aerobic training level, adjusting your pace accordingly, and allowing adequate time for warm up and cool down.

Finding your pace

How do you determine the aerobic training level that's best for you?

Your target heart rate provides a guideline for achieving the greatest benefits during exercise while reducing risk.

First, find your maximum heart rate. To do this, subtract your age from 220. To determine your target heart rate, calculate 75% of your maximum rate (multiply your maximum rate times .75). For example, if your maximum rate is 180, your target rate is 135 beats per minute.

To determine your heart rate range, calculate the range between 70% and 80% of your maximum heart rate. By monitoring your pulse and staying in this range, you will achieve the greatest benefits from aerobic exercise. The chart below provides heart rate ranges according to age.

continued

HEART RATE RANGE

AGE	MINIMUM	TARGET	MAXIMUM
20	140	150	160
25	137	146	156
30	133	143	152
35	130	139	148
40	126	135	144
45	123	131	140
50	119	128	136
55	116	124	132
60	112	120	128
65	109	116	124
70	105	113	120

PATIENT-TEACHING AID

Personalizing your exercise program—*continued*

Keep in mind, however, that these numbers provide a measure of what a healthy heart can do. Gradually slow down if you begin to experience any pain.

Warming up
Before starting any kind of demanding physical activity, you'll want to perform warm-up exercise to stretch muscles and loosen joints. This will lessen the risk of muscle strain or ligament damage. A good warm-up offers psychological benefits as well. Use this time to focus on the activities ahead and to get rid of tension. First, take your pulse and then do 5 to 10 minutes of stretching exercises and light calisthenics.

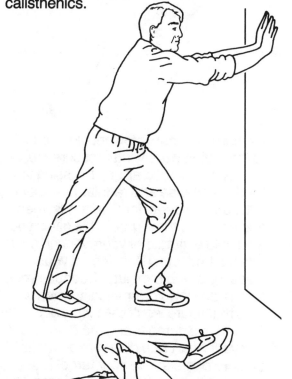

Adjusting the pace
Gradually work toward your optimal aerobic training level. During your exercise period, take your pulse two or three times as your doctor directs. Adjust your pace according to your pulse rate and how you feel. If you exceed your target rate, or if you have chest discomfort, breathlessness, or palpitations, slow down *gradually*. Don't stop suddenly.

Cooling down
Never stop exercise abruptly. Otherwise, the amount of blood circulating back to the heart, which is still beating rapidly, won't be adequate to meet your body's needs. You need a cool-down period much as a horse needs to be walked after a race.

Gradually decrease the pace of your exercise for 5 to 10 minutes. Then do 5 minutes of light calisthenics and simple stretching exercises. At this point your pulse should be no more than 15 beats above your resting pulse. If you feel dizzy or faint after exercise, you may need a longer cool-down period.

Keeping records
Keep an exercise diary. List the date and time, the activity and its duration, your heart rate, and any symptoms you experience. Tracking your progress will help you keep up your motivation, and the record you develop will help you and your doctor.

How to take your pulse

Dear Patient:

The doctor wants you to take your pulse—the number of times your heart beats per minute. Take your pulse at rest and during exercise. By comparing these two pulse rates, the doctor can evaluate how well your heart is pumping.

Taking your pulse at rest
Don't check your resting pulse right after exercising or eating a big meal. When you're ready to take your *resting* pulse rate, be sure you have a watch or a clock with a second hand. Sit quietly and relax for 2 minutes. Then place your index and middle fingers on your wrist, as shown here.

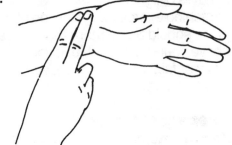

Count the pulse beats for 30 seconds and multiply by 2. (Or count for 60 seconds, but do not multiply, if your doctor has so instructed because of your irregular heart rhythm.) Record this number and the date.

Taking your pulse during exercise
By taking your pulse during exercise, you can help ensure the most benefit from your exercise program.

As soon as you stop exercising, find your neck (carotid) pulse. To do this, place two or three fingers on your wind pipe and move them 2 to 3 inches (5 to 8 cm) to the left or right. Feel for the pulse point low on your neck and don't press

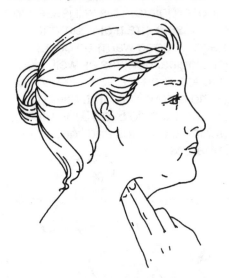

too hard. You can interrupt blood supply to the brain by applying pressure too high on the carotid artery. Pressing too hard may cause an irregular heartbeat.

Count the beats for 6 seconds; then add a zero to that figure. This gives you a reliable estimate of your *working* heart rate for 1 minute. (Don't count your pulse for a whole minute. Because your heart rate slows dramatically when you rest, that figure won't be accurate.) Record this number and the date.

If your heart rate during exercise is 10 or more beats above your target rate, don't exercise so hard the next time. But if your working heart rate is lower than your target rate, exercise a little harder next time.

Cutting down on cholesterol

Dear Patient:

By changing your diet, you can help reduce your cholesterol level and ensure better health in the years to come. You'll also need to reduce the amount of saturated fats you eat. This means cutting down drastically on eggs, dairy products, and fatty meats. Rely instead on poultry, fish, fruits, vegetables, and high-fiber breads.

Use this list as a starting point for your new diet. If you do a lot of home baking, adapt your recipes by using modest amounts of unsaturated oils. Remember to substitute two egg whites when a recipe calls for one whole egg.

FOOD	ELIMINATE	SUBSTITUTE
Bread and cereals	Breads with whole eggs listed as a major ingredient	Oatmeal, multigrain, and bran cereals; whole-grain breads; rye bread
	Egg noodles	Pasta, rice
	Pies, cakes, doughnuts, biscuits, high-fat crackers and cookies	Angel food cake; low-fat cookies, crackers, and home-baked goods
Eggs and dairy products	Whole milk, 2% milk, imitation milk	Skim milk, 1% milk, buttermilk
	Cream, half-and-half, most non-dairy creamers, whipped toppings	None
	Whole milk yogurt and cottage cheese	Nonfat or low-fat yogurt, low-fat (1% or 2%) cottage cheese
	Cheese, cream cheese, sour cream, light cream cheese, light sour cream	None
	Egg yolks	Egg whites
	Ice cream	Sherbet, frozen tofu
Fats and oils	Coconut, palm, and palm kernel oils	Unsaturated vegetable oils (corn, olive, canola, safflower, sesame, soybean, and sunflower)
	Butter, lard, bacon fat	Unsaturated margarine and shortening, diet margarine
	Dressings made with egg yolks	Mayonnaise, unsaturated or low-fat salad dressings
	Chocolate	Baking cocoa
Meat, fish, and poultry	Fatty cuts of beef, lamb, or pork	Lean cuts of beef, lamb, or pork
	Organ meats, spare ribs, cold cuts, sausage, hot dogs, bacon	Poultry
	Sardines, roe	Sole, salmon, mackerel

How to use nitroglycerin

Dear Patient:

Your doctor has prescribed nitroglycerin to control angina. By temporarily widening your veins and arteries, nitroglycerin brings more blood and oxygen to your heart when it needs it most. This drug is available in ointment, disk, tablet, and spray forms. To ensure its effectiveness, follow these directions for the form of medication you're taking.

Ointment

1 Measure the prescribed amount of nitroglycerin ointment onto the special paper.

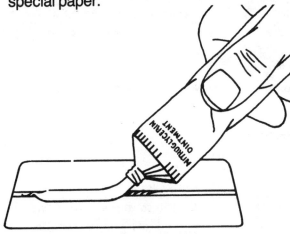

Spread it lightly over the area specified by the doctor—usually the upper arm or chest. Don't rub it into your skin. For best results, spread the ointment to cover an area about the size of the application paper (roughly 3½ by 2¼ inches [9 by 6 cm]).

2 Cover the ointment with paper and tape it in place. You may want to cover the paper (including the side edges) with plastic wrap to protect your clothes from stains. If you get a persistent headache or feel dizzy while using the ointment, call your doctor.

Disk

1 Apply the disk to any convenient skin area—preferably on the upper arm or chest, but never below the elbow—touching only the back of the disk. If necessary, shave the site first.

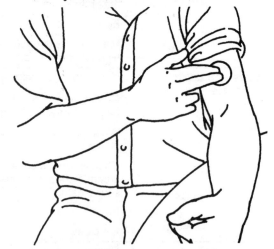

Avoid applying the disk to skin folds, scars, calluses, and any damaged or irritated skin. Use a different site every day.

2 After application, wash your hands. Avoid wetting the disk. If the disk should leak or fall off, throw it away and apply a new disk at a different site.
   To ensure 24-hour coverage, set a routine for applying a new disk each

continued

How to use nitroglycerin—*continued*

day. Also, apply the new disk 30 minutes before removing the old one. If you get a persistent headache or feel dizzy while using the disk, tell your doctor.

Sublingual tablets

1 Place one tablet under your tongue and let it dissolve. Avoid swallowing while the tablet's dissolving.

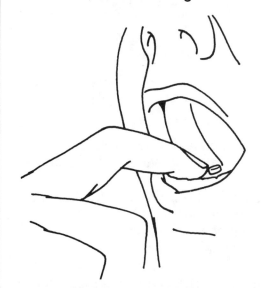

2 If your angina lasts longer than 5 minutes after taking the first tablet, take another tablet. Then take a third one after 5 more minutes, if necessary.

3 If three tablets don't provide relief, call your doctor and have someone take you to the nearest hospital. *Never* take more than three tablets.

Get new tablets after 3 months, even if you have some left in the container.

Spray

1 Hold the spray canister upright as close as possible to your open mouth.

2 Press the button on the canister's top to release the spray onto or under your tongue.

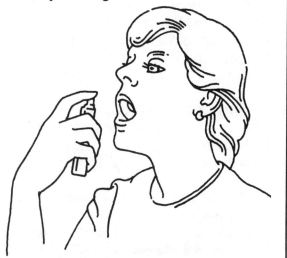

Release the button and close your mouth. Avoid spraying into your eyes. And don't swallow immediately after spraying.

3 If your angina lasts longer than 5 minutes, spray again. Then spray a third time after 5 more minutes, if necessary.

Don't take more than three sprays within any 15-minute period. If your angina continues, call your doctor and have someone take you to the nearest hospital.

Learning about propranolol

Dear Patient:

The medication you're taking is called propranolol. (The label may also read Inderal or Inderal LA.)

Your doctor has prescribed this medication to help relieve your angina. The medication will do this by taking some of the strain off your heart.

Taking your medication

Take propranolol exactly as the label directs. And take it at the same time each day, so you'll be less likely to forget it.

Once a day, preferably before the first dose, take your pulse. If your pulse is less than 60 beats a minute, don't take the next dose. Instead, contact the doctor as soon as possible. Don't skip more than one dose.

Some restrictions

Before taking any over-the-counter cold medications, check with your doctor or pharmacist.

Be sure to call your doctor if you feel depressed or dizzy or can't sleep at night. Also call him if you have trouble breathing, start wheezing, develop a rash, or have a very slow heart rate.

Special instructions

• To increase absorption, take the drug with meals.

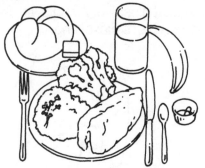

• Don't stop taking this drug suddenly— doing so may increase angina or cause a heart attack.
• To minimize dizziness, rise slowly from a sitting or lying position and avoid sudden position changes.
• Don't permit others to take your medication, and don't try any of theirs. The doctor's prescription is meant for your specific needs.
• Store your medication in a cool, dry area. Avoid keeping it in the bathroom medicine chest.
• Throw away any unused portion of your medication that is several years old.
• To prevent insomnia, take the drug no later than 2 hours before bedtime.

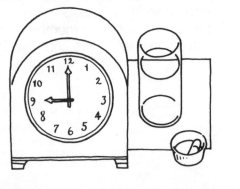

Hypertension

An insidious disorder, hypertension affects roughly one of every four black Americans and one of every six white Americans—in all, about 60 million Americans. But because the patient is typically asymptomatic, hypertension may go undetected until it's revealed during a routine checkup.

Consequently, your first teaching session may find you persuading a patient who feels fine that he has a serious disorder, and, most important, that he must take steps to control it. You'll start by defining blood pressure and describing how elevated blood pressure taxes the heart and other vital organs.

Because your teaching plan aims to promote compliance with long-term treatment, you'll emphasize adhering to a prescribed medication, diet, exercise, and behavior modification regimen. And because research links stress with hypertension, you'll teach the patient techniques to help him reduce and relieve daily stress. You'll also show the patient (or a family member) how to monitor blood pressure. (For more information, see *Teaching the recalcitrant hypertensive patient,* page 32.)

Discuss the disorder

Explain that blood exerts pressure against arterial walls as the heart pumps it through the body. Hypertension—or high blood pressure—simply means that this pressure is greater than it should be. Explain further that a complex system involving the kidneys, brain, and nerves regulates blood pressure. Sensing when the pressure is too high or too low, this system makes adjustments by releasing certain hormones into the bloodstream. Other elements governing blood pressure include the heart's strength and pumping ability, circulating blood volume, and arterial condition.

Tell the patient that blood pressure is measured in millimeters of mercury (mm Hg) and that two values constitute a blood pressure reading. The first, or systolic, value measures maximum pressure, or that exerted when the heart contracts or beats (the heart at work). The second, or diastolic, value measures minimum pressure, or that exerted when the heart relaxes between beats (the heart at rest). For more information, see *Classifying hypertension: Where does your patient fit in?* page 33.

Explain that blood pressure normally fluctuates with age, activity, and emotional stress and that it rises and falls many times daily. For example, it rises during exercise and returns to normal with rest.

Richard K. Gibson, RN, MN, JD, CCRN, CS, and **Barbara A. Todd, RN,C, MSN,** wrote this chapter. Mr. Gibson is a clinical nurse specialist in the surgical intensive care unit at Veterans Administration Hospital, San Diego. Ms. Todd is director of cardiothoracic surgery services at Temple University Hospital, Philadelphia.

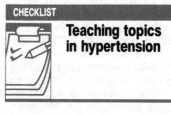

CHECKLIST

Teaching topics in hypertension

☐ An explanation of hypertension, including normal and high blood pressure and factors that affect blood pressure
☐ An explanation of the patient's type of hypertension: primary or secondary
☐ Importance of adhering to treatment to prevent complications, such as myocardial infarction, renal failure, and stroke
☐ Diagnostic tests to rule out secondary hypertension
☐ Exercise program and precautions
☐ Dietary restrictions, including reduced salt intake, increased potassium intake, if necessary, and weight loss
☐ Use of antihypertensives, diuretics, and other prescribed medications
☐ Home blood pressure monitoring
☐ Other measures to reduce long-term complications, such as smoking cessation and stress reduction
☐ Sources of information and support

TEACHING PLAN

Teaching the recalcitrant hypertensive patient

Typically, patients with hypertension don't feel ill, even though they have a serious disorder. So teaching about the disorder and necessary life-style changes can be a challenge. You can start with a standard teaching plan and adapt it to fit your patient's specific needs. Suppose you're caring for Daryl Jordan, a 40-year-old construction foreman.

Assess first
Two days ago, Mr. Jordan was admitted to your medical unit. He was brought in by a co-worker after he complained of a severe headache and then fainted. His initial blood pressure was 200/100 mm Hg. After ruling out secondary causes, the doctor diagnosed primary hypertension and prescribed medication. After 2 days on medication, Mr. Jordan's blood pressure has dropped to 150/90 mm Hg.

Your assessment reveals that Mr. Jordan weighs 200 lb and stands 5'7". He describes himself as a "meat-and-potatoes man" and admits that he's smoked two packs of cigarettes a day for 22 years. He says that he gets enough exercise on the job.

When you meet Mrs. Jordan, you observe that she's overweight, too. You learn that she takes pride in her cooking. "I hope Daryl doesn't have to go on a diet," she says. "It'll kill him to do without my good cooking." Mr. Jordan agrees and adds, "I don't think anything's wrong with me now. I feel fine. And I don't think I need this blood pressure medicine, either. I've heard it can make me lose my 'nature.'"

Define the patient's learning needs
Clearly, Mr. Jordan and his wife need instruction. What should you teach them? To find out, compare their knowledge of hypertension with the content of a standard teaching plan, which includes:
• definitions of normal and high blood pressure
• factors that contribute to primary hypertension and causes of secondary hypertension
• complications of vascular damage to vital organs
• signs and symptoms of hypertension and its complications
• treatments, such as diet, exercise, and medications
• importance of life-long follow-up care.

You decide that the Jordans know little about hypertension. Your initial goal? Getting Mr. Jordan to admit that he has hypertension, accept his disorder, and tell you how it affects his life.

Your next goal involves persuading the Jordans to comply with treatment. Inform Mr. Jordan that the doctor may switch his medication if he experiences adverse reactions, such as impotence.

Using the standard teaching plan as an outline,

work with the Jordans to set learning outcomes. Together, you agree that Mr. and Mrs. Jordan will be able to:

```
-discuss their feelings about hypertension
-describe how smoking, obesity, and high sodium
intake contribute to hypertension
-list the names of Mr. Jordan's medications and
possible adverse effects
-describe how to take the medications
-identify foods high in sodium
-develop a meal plan incorporating prescribed
diet restrictions
-voice their willingness to perform home blood
pressure monitoring
-demonstrate that they can take blood pressure
accurately
-explain the risks of uncontrolled hypertension
-verbalize the need for regular follow-up care.
```

Choose teaching tools and techniques
To teach about hypertension, you'll use *explanation and discussion* of the disorder's course and treatments, focusing first on diet. You'll include *demonstrations* of blood pressure monitoring and of stress-reducing relaxation, meditation, or biofeedback techniques; *printed materials,* such as booklets on hypertension, menus, and recipe pamphlets about low-sodium diets; *videotaped materials,* presenting healthful diet and exercise programs; and ideally, *consultations* with a dietitian.

Does Mr. Jordan acknowledge that he has hypertension? Is his wife willing to change her cooking habits? The answers to these questions and others will influence your teaching strategies.

Don't overwhelm them with information—offer only what they can absorb readily. Allow them time to think about adjusting their life-style and hypertension's impact on their lives if they don't comply with treatment. Encourage Mr. Jordan to express his feelings about a changing self-image and altered life-style.

Evaluate your teaching
Does Mr. Jordan accept his illness? Are the Jordans complying with treatment? For answers, look to your ongoing evaluation and assessment.

Simple observation will reveal whether Mr. Jordan is complying with dietary restrictions. Using a variation of the *question-answer* technique, ask Mrs. Jordan to share her husband's favorite new recipe with you. Also use *return demonstration*. Have both Jordans show you how to take a blood pressure reading. Your findings will help you estimate their progress and refocus your teaching, if necessary.

Classifying hypertension: Where does your patient fit in?

Inform your patient that hypertension classifications range from high normal to severe. Explain that the higher the blood pressure reading—especially the diastolic value—the greater and more imminent the health danger. Use this information to persuade your patient to schedule regular blood pressure evaluations.

Explain that normal systolic pressure ranges from 100 to 135 mm Hg; normal diastolic pressure, from 60 to 80 mm Hg. A blood pressure reading of 120/80 mm Hg is commonly accepted as normal pressure for adults; a reading of 140/90 or above is high and requires monitoring. Unless a single reading is extremely high, at least three separate elevated blood pressure readings on different days are necessary to confirm a diagnosis of hypertension.

BLOOD PRESSURE RANGE (mm Hg)	CLASSIFICATION	RECOMMENDED ACTION
Diastolic		
85 to 89	High normal	Recheck blood pressure within 1 year
90 to 104	Mild hypertension	Confirm blood pressure value within 2 months
105 to 114	Moderate hypertension	Refer to doctor for evaluation within 2 weeks
$\geq$ 115	Severe hypertension	Refer to doctor for immediate evaluation
Systolic (when diastolic value is < 90)		
140 to 159	Borderline isolated systolic hypertension	Confirm blood pressure value within 2 months
$\geq$ 160	Isolated systolic hypertension	Confirm blood pressure value within 2 months
$\geq$ 200	Severe hypertension	Refer to doctor for evaluation within 2 weeks

Discuss which type of hypertension the patient has. More than 95% of cases have no known cause, though certain factors (notably diet, stress, and heredity) contribute to its development. Although incurable, this type—known as *primary hypertension*—can be controlled with proper treatment. Less common is hypertension that results from an identifiable (and usually curable) cause. Causes of *secondary hypertension* include renal arterial or parenchymal disease, various endocrine disorders, coarctation of the aorta, and pheochromocytoma.

Complications
Emphasize the importance of strict compliance with treatment by explaining the dangers of untreated or improperly treated hypertension. Sustained hypertension eventually damages blood vessels and reduces blood flow to tissues. (See *How hypertension damages blood vessels,* page 34.) This can lead to widespread organ damage, especially to the heart, brain, kidneys, and eyes. Cardiovascular damage increases the risk of potentially fatal congestive heart failure, myocardial infarction, or cerebrovascular accident.

How hypertension damages blood vessels

Point out to your patient how sustained, untreated hypertension causes insidious damage to his arteries and other blood vessels. Explain that vascular injury begins with alternating dilation and constriction in the arterioles—the smallest branches of the arteries. This increased intra-arterial pressure and strain weakens and damages the endothelium.

Independently, angiotensin, a vasopressive enzyme, induces endothelial wall contractions, which allow plasma to permeate the interendothelial spaces. These plasma constituents (platelets, fibrinogen, and proteins) deposited in the vessel wall cause necrosis and, eventually, occlusion, aneurysm, or ruptured vessels.

NORMAL VASCULAR STRUCTURE

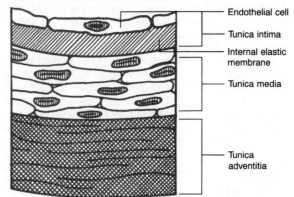

- Endothelial cell
- Tunica intima
- Internal elastic membrane
- Tunica media
- Tunica adventitia

VASCULAR DAMAGE

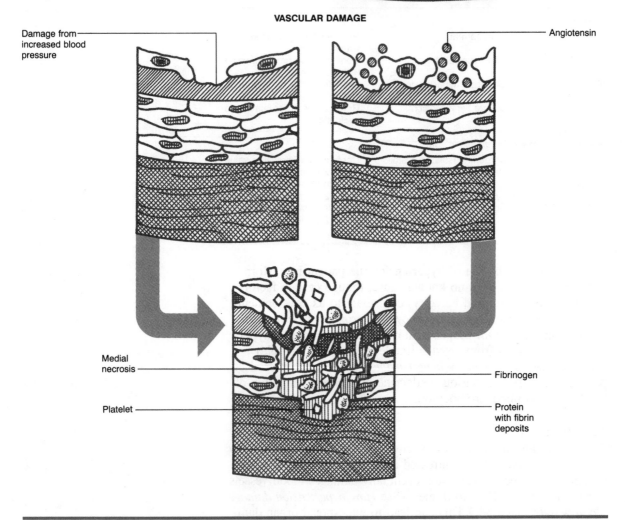

Damage from increased blood pressure

Angiotensin

Medial necrosis

Platelet

Fibrinogen

Protein with fibrin deposits

(For more information, see *Warning signs and symptoms of hypertension*.) Explain further that in hypertensive crisis, a rare but life-threatening complication, blood pressure rises sharply to more than 200/120 mm Hg. Untreated hypertensive crisis can cause brain damage and death.

Describe the diagnostic workup

Inform the patient that consistently elevated blood pressure readings confirm hypertension. Then, if appropriate, the doctor may order various diagnostic studies to rule out secondary causes of high blood pressure.

If ordered, prepare the patient for venipuncture and urine collection. Blood tests that detect abnormal plasma renin and cortisol activity and abnormal serum aldosterone, calcium, and parathyroid hormone levels may point to certain disorders that cause hypertension. And so can urine tests that detect vanillylmandelic acid (VMA), aldosterone, catecholamines, and 17-hydroxycorticosteroids.

Explain the procedure for collecting a 24-hour urine specimen to measure VMA levels. Instruct the patient to restrict foods and beverages containing phenolic acid (such as bananas, citrus fruits, chocolate, vanilla, coffee, and tea) for 3 days before urine collection. Also tell him to avoid physical and emotional stress during the collection period.

Prepare the patient for other tests to confirm secondary causes or to detect complications of hypertension. For example, a chest X-ray can evaluate whether the heart's size and shape show changes consistent with hypertension. Angiography can reveal renal artery stenosis or coarctation of the aorta, and electrocardiography, echocardiography, and cardiac catheterization can detect cardiac complications, such as ventricular hypertrophy. If appropriate, give the patient the teaching aids *Preparing for cardiac catheterization*, pages 20 to 22, and *Preparing for echocardiography*, page 85.

Teach about treatments

Inform the patient with newly diagnosed mild hypertension that the doctor will try managing the disease with a low-sodium diet. He'll advise weight loss, too, if appropriate, and a regular exercise program. If these measures fail, the doctor will prescribe medications to lower blood pressure. And rarely, if the patient has a pheochromocytoma, surgery may correct this disorder, which causes hypertension.

Activity

Encourage the patient to exercise regularly to help lower his blood pressure. Tell him that the doctor will recommend an exercise program based on the patient's medical history, age, and medication regimen. The program will emphasize aerobic exercise, such as walking, jogging, or swimming, which helps to tone the cardiovascular system and lower blood pressure. However, the program won't include isometric exercise, such as weight lifting, which raises blood pressure by elevating serum catecholamine levels.

Warning signs and symptoms of hypertension

Tell your patient that hypertension is called "the silent killer" because most people have no symptoms. However, explain that some patients do experience signs and symptoms, including the following:

• *Headache.* Most severe in the morning, headache occurs occipitally.

• *Dizziness, faintness, numbness, weakness, and vision changes.* These cerebrovascular symptoms may result from hypertension alone or from concurrent atherosclerosis.

• *Chest pain, palpitations, dyspnea, paroxysmal nocturnal dyspnea, orthopnea, and peripheral edema.* Such cardiovascular symptoms may accompany hypertension associated with coronary artery disease, which may lead to congestive heart failure. *Intermittent claudication* may also occur, resulting from peripheral vascular disease linked to atherosclerosis.

• *Nocturia, polyuria, hematuria, urinary tract infection, excessive urinary sediment, fatigue, weakness, muscle cramps, and peripheral edema.* These signs and symptoms may signal kidney damage caused by hypertension.

• *Nosebleeds.* When associated with hypertension, epistaxis may be a safety mechanism that relieves severe hypertension and prevents cerebral hemorrhage.

Questions patients ask about hypertension

My father had high blood pressure, and now I have it. Could I have done anything to prevent getting it?
Probably not. It is known that the tendency to develop hypertension is inherited. However, people in high-risk families may be able to prevent it by decreasing salt in their diet and avoiding obesity from an early age, but this remains unproved.

If my blood pressure's normal, why can't I stop taking my medication?
Because even though your blood pressure falls within acceptable limits, it's not really normal—it's just controlled. If you discontinue your medication, your pressure may rise again. You may always need to take some medication. Of course, other measures may also help keep your pressure in check—for ex-

ample, regular exercise, stress reduction, and a low-salt diet.

Can my blood pressure get too low?
It might, if your treatment regimen is changed—for example, if the doctor increases your drug dosage or gives you a different drug. So check your blood pressure regularly, and report any of these symptoms of low blood pressure to the doctor: dizziness, light-headedness, fatigue, and weakness.

I've heard that garlic helps lower high blood pressure. Can I use this instead of medication?
No. Although garlic is sold in various forms as a "treatment" for heart problems and high blood pressure, no documented evidence has proved that it works to lower blood pressure.

Advise the patient that exercise should be frequent (at least three times a week), vigorous (sufficient to raise the heart rate to between 70% and 80% of maximum capacity), and sustained (gradually building up to about 30 minutes a session). But warn him not to overdo it. Caution him to stop before he reaches exhaustion. Also, urge him to stop exercising immediately and call the doctor if he becomes dizzy. Give him copies of the teaching aids *Tips for exercising safely,* page 23, and *Personalizing your exercise program,* pages 24 and 25.

Diet
Because excessive sodium intake contributes to hypertension, instruct the patient to avoid or limit salty foods, including most processed foods, luncheon meats, canned soups and vegetables, and most snack foods and condiments. Tell him to read package labels for sodium content. Suggest that he use alternatives to table salt, such as herbs, spices, or sodium-free salt substitutes. And give him a copy of the patient-teaching aid *Cutting down on salt,* page 43.

Remember to advise him to limit his caffeine and alcohol intake. Most alcoholic beverages are high in calories, and beer contains considerable sodium. So he may need to avoid alcohol entirely, depending on his prescribed medications.

If the patient's medications include potassium-depleting diuretics, advise him to ask his doctor about following a potassium-rich diet. Mention that many foods naturally high in potassium contain little sodium. To direct the patient further, offer him the teaching aid *Learning about potassium-rich foods,* page 44.

If the patient's overweight, discuss how obesity raises blood pressure by increasing blood volume, thus adding to the heart's work load. Tell him that overweight people are three times more likely to have hypertension than are people who maintain normal weight. Add that research shows that weight loss lowers blood pressure.

Under the doctor's supervision, encourage the patient to begin a weight-reduction program that emphasizes a balanced diet, regular exercise, and gradual weight loss. Explain that he'll have to modify his eating habits but that eating can still be pleasurable. Tell him to set realistic goals for weight loss, and impress on him that fad and crash diets and diet pills seldom work.

When teaching about diet, include the patient's family, especially if the patient doesn't usually shop for groceries or cook for the household.

Medication
If dietary restrictions and exercise fail to lower blood pressure sufficiently, inform the patient that drug therapy may be necessary. Initial therapy usually consists of a diuretic, a beta-adrenergic blocker, an angiotensin-converting-enzyme inhibitor, or a calcium channel blocker. Later, a combination of these drugs or other antihypertensive agents may be prescribed if his blood pressure still isn't under control. Explain, too, that the doctor may step down drug therapy, depending on the patient's response (see *Teaching about antihypertensive drugs,* pages 38 to 41, and *Understanding stepped care*).

Stress the importance of strict compliance with the prescribed drug regimen to treat primary hypertension. Make sure the patient understands that drugs can only control, not cure, his hypertension and that he'll probably have to take an antihypertensive drug for the rest of his life. Advise him to continue taking his drugs even when he feels well. Explain that reducing or discontinuing them without his doctor's guidance may lead to severe rebound high blood pressure, possibly precipitating hypertensive crisis.

Instruct him not to take any over-the-counter medications without first checking with his doctor. Many medications, especially cold and allergy remedies, contain ingredients that can counteract the effectiveness of antihypertensives. Remind him, too, that many over-the-counter drugs are high in sodium—particularly antacids, laxatives, diet pills, and cold and allergy medications.

Procedures
If appropriate, teach the patient how to measure his own blood pressure. And show family members how to measure blood pressure as well. Provide copies of the teaching aids *How to take your blood pressure,* page 45, and *How to take another person's blood pressure,* page 46, to reinforce your instructions.

Surgery
If the patient has secondary hypertension, you may need to prepare him for thyroidectomy, excision of a pheochromocytoma, or angioplasty.

continued on page 42

Understanding stepped care

Explain to the patient the "stepped care" approach to treatment for hypertension. The doctor goes "up the steps" until a patient's hypertension is controlled. Then after mild hypertension has been controlled for 1 year, the doctor may try going back *down* the steps, reducing the dosage or the number of antihypertensives the patient takes.

Step 1
Restrict sodium and alcohol intake and control weight and cardiovascular risk factors.

Step 2
Start drug therapy with an angiotensin-converting-enzyme inhibitor, beta blocker, calcium channel blocker, or a diuretic.

Step 3
Increase the dosage of the initial drug, substitute a different drug, or add another drug from another class.

Step 4
Substitute for the second drug or add a third drug from a different class.

Step 5
Add a third or fourth drug or refer patient for further evaluation.

Teaching about antihypertensive drugs

DRUG	ADVERSE REACTIONS	TEACHING POINTS
Angiotensin-converting-enzyme inhibitors		
captopril (Capoten) **enalapril** (Vasotec) **lisinopril** (Prinivil, Zestril)	• Watch for chest pain, diaphoresis, dyspnea, fever, mouth sores, orthostatic hypotension, persistent cough, rapid heart rate, rash, severe diarrhea and vomiting, and sore throat. • Other reactions include altered taste, dizziness, fatigue, headache, and palpitations.	• Instruct the patient to take a missed dose as soon as he remembers but not to double-dose. • To minimize hypotension, advise him to rise slowly from a sitting or lying position. • Instruct him to limit his intake of high-potassium foods. • Tell him to notify the doctor if fever, sore throat, or other signs of infection develop.
Beta-adrenergic blockers		
acebutolol (Sectral) **atenolol** (Tenormin) **carteolol** (Cartrol) **labetalol** (Trandate) **metoprolol** (Lopressor) **nadolol** (Corgard) **penbutolol** (Levatol) **pindolol** (Visken) **propranolol** (Inderal) **timolol** (Blocadren)	• Watch for depression, dizziness, dyspnea, rash, very slow heart rate, and wheezing. • Other reactions include decreased libido, diarrhea, fatigue, headache, insomnia, nasal stuffiness, nausea, nightmares, vivid dreams, and vomiting.	• If the patient takes one dose daily, instruct him to take a missed dose within 8 hours. If he takes two or more doses daily, tell him to take a missed dose as soon as possible. He should never double-dose. • Warn him against suddenly discontinuing the drug. To avoid serious complications, the doctor will taper the dosage. • Teach him to check his pulse before taking the drug and to notify the doctor if his pulse rate falls below 60 beats/minute. • To help prevent insomnia, advise him to take the drug no later than 2 hours before bedtime. • Suggest he take the drug with food to increase its absorption.
Calcium channel blockers		
diltiazem (Cardizem) **nicardipine** (Cardene) **nifedipine** (Procardia) **verapamil** (Calan, Isoptin)	• Watch for ankle edema, chest pain, dyspnea, fainting, and very slow or fast heart rate. • Other reactions include constipation, dizziness, flushing, headache, and nausea.	• Instruct the patient to take a missed dose as soon as he remembers but not to double-dose. • To minimize dizziness, tell him to rise slowly from a sitting or lying position. • Reassure him that he can continue to eat and drink reasonable amounts of calcium-containing foods. • To prevent constipation, suggest he increase his fluid and fiber intake and use a bulk laxative. • Advise him to limit alcohol intake.
Centrally acting antihypertensives		
clonidine (Catapres)	• Watch for ankle edema, skin pallor, vivid dreams, and nightmares. • Other reactions include constipation, drowsiness, insomnia, mouth dryness, and slow heart rate.	• Advise the patient to take one dose just before bedtime to take advantage of the drug's tendency to cause drowsiness. • To avoid constipation, tell him to increase his fluid and fiber intake and use bulk laxatives. • To relieve mouth dryness, suggest he use sugarless gum, hard candy, or mouth rinses. • Instruct him to limit his alcohol intake. • Warn against stopping the drug even if he feels better. • If he's using a transdermal patch, instruct him to wear it 24 hours a day, 7 days a week. He should reapply it once a week to a hairless area on his upper arm or torso, changing the site weekly.

continued

Teaching about antihypertensive drugs—*continued*

DRUG	ADVERSE REACTIONS	TEACHING POINTS
Centrally acting antihypertensives—*continued*		
guanabenz acetate (Wytensin)	• Watch for difficulty breathing, dizziness, mouth dryness, orthostatic hypotension, slow heart rate, and weakness. • Other reactions include breast enlargement in men, chest pain, decreased libido, depression, diarrhea, hair loss, nasal congestion, nausea, numbness, vomiting, and weight gain.	• Tell the patient to avoid activities that require mental alertness, such as driving a car or operating heavy machinery, until his reaction to the drug is known. • Instruct him to take a missed dose as soon as he remembers but not to double-dose. • Tell him to limit his alcohol intake because alcohol may exacerbate drowsiness.
guanethidine monosulfate (Ismelin)	• Watch for difficulty breathing, dizziness, mouth dryness, orthostatic hypotension, slow heart rate, and weakness. • Other reactions include chest pain, decreased libido, depression, diarrhea, hair loss, nasal congestion, nausea, numbness, vomiting, and weight gain.	• Tell the patient to avoid activities that require mental alertness, such as driving a car or operating heavy machinery, until his reaction to the drug is known. • Instruct him to take a missed dose as soon as he remembers but not to double-dose. • Tell him to limit his alcohol intake because alcohol may exacerbate drowsiness.
guanfacine (Tenex)	• Watch for chest pain, irregular heartbeat, mouth dryness, runny nose, sedation, shortness of breath, and slow pulse. • Other reactions include confusion, constipation, depression, dry or itchy eyes, and sexual dysfunction.	• Advise the patient to take the drug at bedtime unless the doctor directs otherwise. • Tell him to limit his alcohol intake. • Tell him to avoid activities that require mental alertness until his reaction to the drug is known. • Instruct him to take a missed dose as soon as he remembers but not to double-dose.
methyldopa (Aldomet)	• Watch for chest pain, depression, edema, fever, impotence, syncope, very slow heart rate, weakness, and weight gain. • Other reactions include decreased libido, diarrhea, dizziness, drowsiness, mouth dryness, nasal stuffiness, nausea, orthostatic hypotension, slightly slow heart rate, and vomiting.	• Instruct the patient to take a missed dose as soon as he remembers but not to double-dose. • Advise him to take one dose at bedtime to take advantage of the drug's tendency to cause drowsiness. • Reassure him that drowsiness is usually temporary. • To minimize orthostatic hypotension, advise him to rise slowly from a sitting or lying position. • To relieve mouth dryness, suggest he use sugarless gum or hard candy or mouth rinses. • Tell him to limit his alcohol intake.
pargylene (Eutonyl Filmtab)	• Watch for edema, fainting, headache, nausea, nightmares, rash, sleeplessness, sweating, tremors, vomiting, and weakness. • Other reactions include constipation, diarrhea, dizziness, and increased appetite.	• Tell the patient to avoid activities that require mental alertness until his reaction to the drug is known. • Instruct him to take a missed dose as soon as he remembers but not to double-dose. • Tell him to limit his alcohol intake. • Caution him to avoid foods high in tyramine—they can cause increased blood pressure even weeks after discontinuing the drug. Such foods include cheese, sour cream, yogurt, liver, pickled or dried fish, certain fermented sausages (including bologna, pepperoni, salami, and summer sausage), avocados, yeast extracts, beer and ale (especially imported and dark beers), and red wines (especially Chianti).
prazosin (Minipress) **terazosin** (Hytrin)	• Watch for chest pain, dyspnea, edema, rapid heart rate, and syncope. • Other reactions include drowsiness, gastric upset, headache, and slight dizziness.	• Instruct the patient to take a missed dose as soon as he remembers but not to double-dose. • Advise him to take his first dose at bedtime because dizziness is most severe after this dose. • Tell him to limit his alcohol intake to prevent dizziness. • Caution him not to drive a car or operate heavy machinery during the first week of therapy in case he should feel faint.

continued

40 Hypertension

Teaching about antihypertensive drugs — *continued*

DRUG	ADVERSE REACTIONS	TEACHING POINTS
Centrally acting antihypertensives — *continued*		
reserpine (Serpasil, Serpalan)	• Watch for chest pain, depression, diarrhea, difficulty breathing, dizziness, headache, heartburn, loss of appetite, nervousness, nightmares, rash, and shortness of breath. • Other reactions include breast swelling, constipation, difficult or painful urination, edema, flushing or skin redness, hearing difficulty, impotence, loss of libido, mouth dryness, nasal stuffiness, nausea, vomiting, and weight gain.	• Tell the patient to avoid activities that require mental alertness, such as driving a car or operating heavy machinery, until his reaction to the drug is known. • Instruct him to take a missed dose as soon as he remembers but not to double-dose. • Tell him to limit his alcohol intake because alcohol may exacerbate drowsiness. • To minimize GI upset, advise him to take the drug with food or milk.
Diuretics		
Loop diuretics **bumetanide** (Bumex) **ethacrynic acid** (Edecrin) **furosemide** (Lasix)	• Watch for fatigue, fever, hearing loss, increased thirst, jaundice, muscle cramps, nausea, tinnitus, urgent or burning urination, vomiting, and weakness. • Other reactions include anorexia, blurred vision, diarrhea, dizziness, muscle aches and cramps, orthostatic hypotension, and weight loss.	• Explain to the patient that the drug should lower his blood pressure by helping his kidneys filter out excess body fluid. • Instruct him to take a missed dose as soon as he remembers, but remind him never to take a double dose of the drug. • If he takes the drug twice a day, tell him to take the second dose in late afternoon rather than at night. This schedule will prevent possible sleep interruption from nocturia. • To prevent GI distress, advise him to take the drug with meals. • Encourage him to eat potassium-rich foods (for example, citrus fruits, tomatoes, bananas, dates, apricots, halibut, salmon, canned sardines, carrots, and potatoes) and to take potassium supplements, as ordered. • Advise him to limit his alcohol intake to prevent dizziness. • To minimize orthostatic hypotension, instruct him to rise slowly from a sitting or lying position. • Instruct the patient to record his weight daily to help monitor fluid loss.
Potassium-sparing diuretics **amiloride** (Midamor) **spironolactone** (Aldactone) **triamterene** (Dyrenium)	• Watch for confusion, irregular heart rate, muscle flaccidity, numbness, tingling in hands and feet, and weight changes. • Other reactions include decreased libido, diarrhea, headache, nausea, stomach cramps, vomiting, and weakness.	• Explain that this drug is a potassium-sparing diuretic; therefore it should lower his blood pressure without depleting the body of potassium. • Tell the patient to take a missed dose within 8 hours; otherwise he should skip it. Warn him not to double-dose. • To relieve GI distress, advise him to take the drug with food. • Instruct him to limit his potassium intake by avoiding foods with extremely high potassium levels, such as salt substitutes and low-salt milk. • Tell him to weigh himself at least every other day and to report any unusual weight changes.

continued

Teaching about antihypertensive drugs — *continued*

DRUG	ADVERSE REACTIONS	TEACHING POINTS
Diuretics — *continued*		
Thiazide and thiazide-like diuretics		
bendroflumethiazide (Naturetin) **benzthiazide** (Aquatag, Exna, Hydrex, Marazide) **chlorothiazide** (Diuril) **chlorthalidone** (Hygroton, Thalitone) **cyclothiazide** (Anhydron) **hydrochlorothiazide** **hydroflumethiazide** (Saluron) **indapamide** (Lozol) **methyclothiazide** (Aquatensen, Enduron) **metolazone** (Diulo, Zaroxolyn) **polythiazide** (Renese) **quinethazone** (Hydromox) **trichlormethiazide** (Diurese)	• Watch for excessive thirst, fever, irregular heart rate, lethargy, mouth dryness, muscle cramps, skin rash, urgent or burning urination, weakness, and weak pulse. • Other reactions include anorexia, diarrhea, dizziness, GI distress, and restlessness.	• Tell the patient to take a missed daily dose within 8 hours; otherwise, he should skip it. Warn him not to double-dose. • To prevent nocturia, instruct him not to take an evening dose just before bedtime. • Advise him to eat potassium-rich foods, such as bananas and citrus fruits. • Caution him that this drug may elevate blood glucose levels. • Instruct the patient to record his weight daily to monitor fluid loss. • Tell him to avoid large doses of calcium supplements.
Vasodilators		
hydralazine (Apresoline)	• Watch for chest pain, numbness, palpitations, rapid heart rate, systemic lupus erythematosus–like syndrome (fever, joint pain, malaise, skin rash), and tingling. • Other reactions include anorexia, diarrhea, headache, nasal stuffiness, and nausea.	• If he's taking four doses a day and he misses a dose, tell the patient to take the missed dose no later than 2 hours before his next scheduled dose. Warn him not to double-dose. • Advise him to take the drug on an empty stomach — either 1 hour before or 3 hours after a meal.
minoxidil (Loniten)	• Watch for distended neck veins, dyspnea, edema, rapid heart rate, and weight gain. • Other reactions include lengthening and darkening of fine body hair.	• Tell the patient to take a missed dose within 8 hours of the scheduled time. Warn him not to double-dose. • Suggest that he remove unwanted hair by shaving or using a depilatory. • If the doctor has prescribed beta blockers to control reflex tachycardia, or diuretics to control sodium and water retention, remind the patient to take all the drugs on schedule to ensure their safety and effectiveness. • Instruct him to weigh himself at least every other day and to report any sudden weight gain.

Other care measures

Because stress and hypertension go hand in hand, teach the patient stress-reducing techniques, such as relaxation breathing or meditation. Then advise him to practice these techniques twice a day for 10 to 20 minutes. If appropriate, suggest using biofeedback techniques to reduce stress. Explain that with this technique he'll use a biofeedback device to help measure how well he can control his blood pressure.

If your patient smokes, give him information to encourage him to quit. Explain how nicotine constricts arterioles, which further increases blood pressure. As appropriate, refer him to community programs, agencies, or support groups that can help him stop smoking and provide follow-up services after he stops. Also direct him to the local chapter of the American Heart Association for more information about hypertension.

Last, schedule the patient for a follow-up appointment. Emphasize the importance of keeping these appointments, and remind him to take his blood pressure often and to keep a record to bring with him each time. Encourage him to ask you and the doctor questions about his condition and treatment during these office visits.

Sources of information and support

American Heart Association
7320 Greenville Avenue, Dallas, Tex. 75231
(214) 750-5300

Citizens for the Treatment of High Blood Pressure
1990 M Street, NW, Suite 360, Washington, D.C. 20036
(202) 296-7747

High Blood Pressure Information Center
National Institutes of Health
4733 Bethesda Avenue, Bethesda, Md. 20814
(301) 952-3260

Further readings

Abbott, S.D. "Assessing the Quality of Life in Hypertensive Patients," *Canadian Journal of Cardiovascular Nursing* 1(1):28-31, April 1989.

Beare, P.G., et al. "Hypertension: Weight, Sodium, and Alcohol Do Make a Difference in Management," *Consultant* 29(6):95-99, June 1989.

Lesko, W.A., and Summerfield, L.M. "The Effectiveness of Biofeedback and Home Relaxation Training on Reduction of Borderline Hypertension," *Health Education* 19(5):19-23, October-November 1988.

Linas, S.L. "Potassium: Weighing the Evidence for Supplementation," *Hospital Practice* 23(12):73-79, 83-84, 86, December 15, 1988.

Mann, K.V. "Promoting Adherence in Hypertension: A Framework for Patient Education," *Canadian Journal of Cardiovascular Nursing* 1(1):8-14, April 1989.

Pickering, T.G. "Blood Pressure Monitoring Outside the Office for the Evaluation of Patients with Resistant Hypertension," *Hypertension* 11(3):96-100, March 1988.

Tanji, J.L. "Exercise for Hypertensives," *Consultant* 28(9):123-25, 128, 130, September 1988.

Tolman, J. "Dietary Control of Hypertension: What Should We Be Teaching?" *Health Education* 19(5):61-63, October-November 1988.

PATIENT-TEACHING AID

Cutting down on salt

Dear Patient:

You need to cut down on salt because too much salt causes your body to retain water. This can lead to hypertension or can worsen it. Even a moderate reduction in salt can lower blood pressure by 10 to 15 mm Hg.

Reducing your salt intake isn't hard to do. The following information and suggestions will help you get started.

Facts about salt
- Table salt is about 40% sodium.
- Americans consume about 20 times more salt than their bodies need.
- About three-fourths of the salt you consume is already in the foods you eat and drink.
- One teaspoon of salt contains 2 grams (2,000 milligrams) of sodium — the recommended daily amount for people with high blood pressure.
- You can reduce your intake to this level simply by not salting your food during cooking or before eating.
- Some people are so sensitive to salt that even a moderate amount causes their blood pressure to rise.
- The more salt you eat, the more medication you'll need to control your blood pressure if you are a salt-sensitive hypertensive.

Tips for reducing salt intake
Reducing your salt intake to a teaspoon or less a day is easy if you:
- read labels on medicines and foods.
- put away your salt shaker, or if you must use salt, use "light salt" that contains half the sodium of ordinary table salt.
- buy fresh meats, fruits, and vegetables instead of canned, processed, and convenience foods.
- substitute spices and lemon juice for salt.
- watch out for sources of hidden sodium — for example, carbonated beverages, nondairy creamers, cookies, and cakes.
- avoid salty foods, such as bacon, sausage, pretzels, potato chips, mustard, pickles, and some cheeses.

Know your sodium sources
Canned, prepared, and "fast" foods are loaded with sodium; so are condiments, such as ketchup. Some foods that don't taste salty contain high amounts of sodium. Consider the values below:

Food	mg sodium
1 can tomato soup	872
1 hot dog	639
1 cheeseburger	709
1 tablespoon ketchup	156
1 dill pickle	928
1 cup corn flakes	256

Other high-sodium sources include baking powder, baking soda, barbecue sauce, bouillon cubes, celery salt, chili sauce, cooking wine, garlic salt, onion salt, softened water, and soy sauce.

Surprisingly, many medicines and other nonfood items contain sodium, such as alkalizers for indigestion, laxatives, aspirin, cough medicine, mouthwash, and toothpaste.

Learning about potassium-rich foods

Dear Patient:

Your doctor has prescribed a diuretic (water pill) to help control your blood pressure. Because this diuretic can lower your potassium level, you may need to add potassium to your diet.

How much potassium do you need?

Doctors recommend 300 to 400 mg of potassium daily. Not enough potassium can cause leg cramps, weakness, paralysis, and spasms. Too much can cause heart problems and fatigue.

The chart below lists potassium-rich foods along with their potassium content (the number of milligrams in a 3½-oz serving). Because some of these foods are also high in calories, check with your doctor or dietitian if you're on a weight-reduction diet.

Potassium content of common foods

Meats	mg
Beef	370
Chicken	411
Lamb	290
Liver	380
Pork	326
Turkey	411
Veal	500

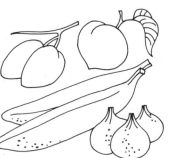

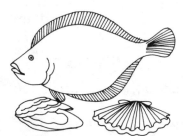

Fish	mg
Bass	256
Flounder	342
Haddock	348
Halibut	525
Oysters	203
Perch	284
Salmon	421
Sardines, canned	590
Scallops	476
Tuna	301

Fruits	mg
Apricots	281
Bananas	370
Dates	648
Figs	152
Nectarines	294
Oranges	200
Peaches	202
Plums	299
Prunes	262
Raisins	355

Vegetables	mg
Asparagus	238
Brussels sprouts	295
Cabbage	233
Carrots	341
Endive	294
Lima beans	394
Peppers	213
Potatoes	407
Radishes	322
Spinach	324
Sweet potatoes	300

Juices	mg
Orange, fresh	200
reconstituted	186
Tomato	227

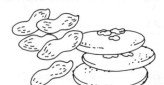

Other foods	mg
Gingersnap cookies	462
Graham crackers	384
Oatmeal cookies with raisins	370
Ice milk	195
Milk, dry (nonfat solids)	1,745
Molasses (light)	917
Peanuts	674
Peanut butter	670

How to take your blood pressure

Dear Patient:

To take your own blood pressure, you can use a digital blood pressure monitor. (You can also use a standard blood pressure cuff and stethoscope, but you'll probably need help from someone else to do so.)

Before you begin, review the instruction booklet that comes with the blood pressure monitor. Operating steps vary with different monitors, so be sure to follow the directions carefully.

Start by taking your blood pressure in both arms. It is common for blood pressure readings to differ by as much as 10 points from arm to arm. If the readings stay consistently similar, the doctor will probably suggest that you use the arm with the higher reading. Here are some guidelines:

1 Sit in a comfortable position and relax for about 2 minutes. Rest your arm on a table so it's level with your heart. (Use the same arm in the same position each time you take your blood pressure.)

2 Wrap the cuff securely around your upper arm just above the elbow. Make sure that you can slide only two fingers between the cuff and your arm. Next, turn on the monitor.

3 Inflate the cuff, as the instruction booklet directs. When the digital scale reads 160, stop inflating. The numbers on the scale will start changing rapidly. When they stop changing, your blood pressure reading will appear on the scale.

4 Record this blood pressure reading, with the date and time. Then deflate and remove the cuff, and turn off the machine.

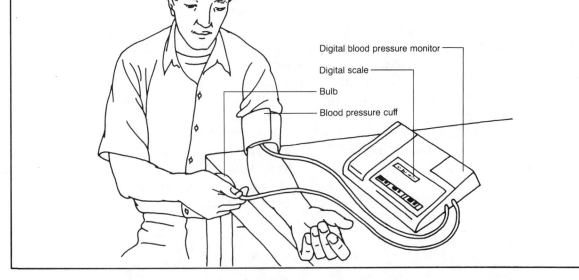

Digital blood pressure monitor

Digital scale

Bulb

Blood pressure cuff

How to take another person's blood pressure

Dear Caregiver:

You can use a standard blood pressure cuff and stethoscope to take the blood pressure of the person in your care. If you're using an aneroid model, you may need to have it calibrated every 6 months. Just follow these steps:

1 Ask the person to sit comfortably and relax for about 2 minutes. Tell him to rest his arm on a table so it's level with his heart. (Use the same arm in the same position each time you take his blood pressure.) While the person relaxes, hang the stethoscope around your neck.

2 Push up the person's sleeve, and wrap the cuff around his upper arm (just above the elbow) so you can slide only two fingers between cuff and arm.

3 Then, using your middle and index fingers, feel for a pulse in the wrist near the person's thumb.
   When you find this pulse, turn the bulb's screw counterclockwise to close it; then squeeze the bulb rapidly to inflate the cuff. Note the reading on the gauge when you can no longer feel his pulse. (This reading, called the *palpatory pressure,* is your guideline for inflating the cuff.) Now, deflate the cuff by turning the screw clockwise.

4 Place the stethoscope's earpieces in your ears. Then place the stethoscope's diaphragm (the disc portion) over the brachial pulse, in the crook of the person's arm.

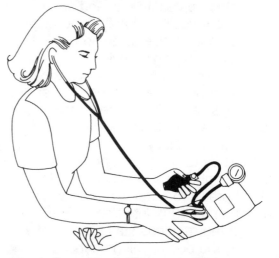

5 Inflate the cuff 30 points higher than the palpatory pressure (the reading you obtained in step 3). Then loosen the bulb's screw to allow air to escape from the cuff. Listen for the first beating sound. When you hear it, note and record the number on the gauge: this is the *systolic* pressure (the top number of a blood pressure reading).
   Slowly continue to deflate the cuff. When you hear the beating stop, note and record the number on the gauge: this is the *diastolic* pressure (the bottom number of a blood pressure reading). Now, deflate and remove the cuff. Record the blood pressure reading, date, and time.

Congestive heart failure

As with many cardiovascular disorders, the prognosis for the patient with congestive heart failure (CHF) depends not only on the disorder's underlying cause and severity but also on how strictly he adheres to prescribed treatment. Although you can't guarantee compliance, you can encourage it by helping the patient understand the pathophysiology of CHF and by clarifying the reasons for activity limitations, sodium and fluid restrictions, drug therapy, and other measures to relieve symptoms and prevent complications. You also must emphasize the relation between CHF and other cardiovascular disorders and teach the patient how to minimize common risk factors and improve cardiovascular fitness.

When teaching about CHF, you'll encounter two groups of patients: those with acute CHF, commonly triggered by myocardial infarction, and those with chronic CHF, associated with renal retention of sodium and fluids. Of course, you'll have to tailor your teaching plan to fit each patient's needs and condition.

Discuss the disorder

Tell the patient that his heart's ability to pump blood has become impaired. Most commonly, patients will experience failure in the heart's left side—the side most vulnerable to coronary artery disease, hypertension, and valvular problems. Explain that when the left ventricle fails to pump enough blood, it triggers compensatory mechanisms: strengthened cardiac contractions, increased blood pressure and venous return, and increased blood volume. However, as CHF progresses, these compensatory mechanisms fail, causing decompensation (see *Understanding CHF,* page 48).

In left-sided heart failure, increased work load and end-diastolic volume enlarge the left ventricle. This impairs left ventricular function, allowing blood to pool in the ventricle and atrium. Eventually, blood backs up into pulmonary veins and capillaries, leading to elevated capillary pressure. In response, sodium and water enter the interstitial space, resulting in pulmonary edema.

As vascular pressure rises and left ventricular function deteriorates, the right ventricle shows signs of stress, such as hypertrophy, increased conduction time, and dysrhythmias. When the patient lies down, pulmonary edema worsens because excess fluid from the legs pools in the pulmonary circulation. Blood also pools in the right ventricle and atrium, causing pressure and congestion in the vena cava and elevating general circulation. Blood backup also distends visceral veins, and the liver and spleen become en-

Richard K. Gibson, RN, MN, JD, CCRN, CS, wrote this chapter. He is a clinical nurse specialist in the surgical intensive care unit at Veterans Administration Hospital, San Diego.

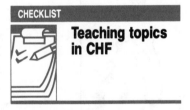

CHECKLIST

Teaching topics in CHF

☐ Explanation of the disorder, including compensation and decompensation, left heart failure, and right heart failure
☐ Preparation for chest X-ray, electrocardiography, cardiac blood pool imaging, and other diagnostic tests
☐ Activity restrictions and energy conservation methods
☐ Sodium and fluid restrictions
☐ Medications and their use
☐ Preparation for pulmonary artery catheterization, rotating tourniquets, or other necessary procedures
☐ Measures to relieve symptoms and minimize complications
☐ Source of information and support

Understanding CHF

Tell the patient that CHF typically begins in the left ventricle when the heart fails to pump sufficient blood to meet the body's needs. This lowers cardiac output, elevates venous pressure, and reduces arterial pressure, triggering a series of *compensatory* mechanisms (shown here) to ensure perfusion of vital organs. However, these mechanisms can't sustain themselves indefinitely. When they begin to fail (a phenomenon known as *decompensation*), CHF progresses, resulting in pulmonary edema if blood backs up and sodium and water enter the interstitial space.

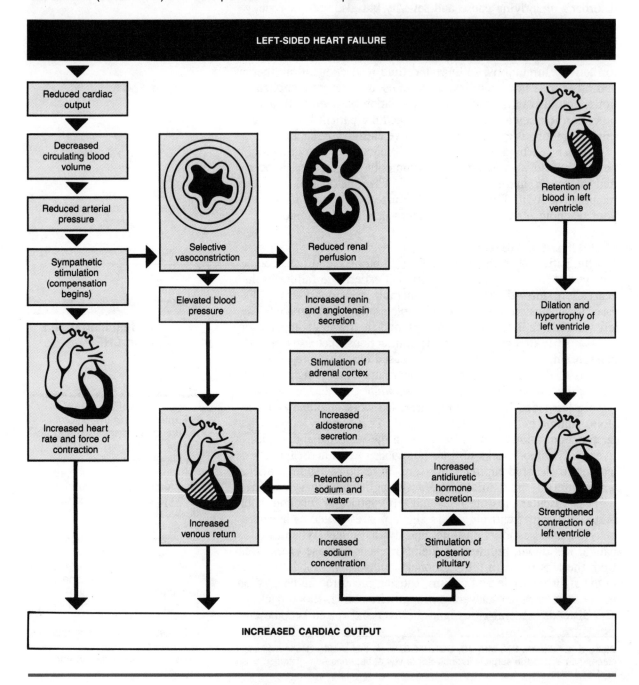

gorged. In response to rising capillary pressure, capillary fluid flows into the interstitial space. This causes tissue edema, especially in the lower legs and abdomen.

Sometimes left- and right-sided heart failure develop simultaneously (see *Comparing signs of left- and right-sided heart failure*).

Complications

Explain that noncompliance with treatment can cause severe complications, including pulmonary edema, susceptibility to pneumonia and other respiratory infections, thromboembolism, and exacerbation of CHF. It can also result in damage to other organs, notably the liver, kidneys, and brain.

Describe the diagnostic workup

No single test confirms CHF. As a result, the patient may undergo various tests to confirm CHF and gauge its severity, type, and cause. Such tests may include arterial blood gas analysis to evaluate oxygenation and a chest X-ray to detect fluid in the lungs or cardiac enlargement. You may also need to prepare the patient for cardiac blood pool imaging or echocardiography to evaluate valvular and ventricular function, electrocardiography (ECG) to reveal conduction abnormalities, and cardiac catheterization to assess coronary artery blood flow and valvular and ventricular function.

Cardiac blood pool imaging

Tell the patient that this 30- to 45-minute test evaluates how well the left ventricle pumps. Describe how a technician will attach electrodes to various sites on the patient's body before the test begins. During the test, the patient will be placed in a supine position, and a mildly radioactive contrast dye will be injected into a vein. A scintillation camera will record the dye's passage through the heart and then will be synchronized with the ECG to correlate subsequent images with ECG waveforms. Stress the need to remain still during scanning.

Echocardiography

Explain that this safe and painless 15- to 30-minute test evaluates the size, shape, and motion of various cardiac structures. Mention that other tests, such as an ECG and phonocardiography, may be performed simultaneously.

Tell the patient that conductive jelly will be applied to his chest. Then during the test, a technician will angle a transducer over his upper body to observe different parts of the heart, and he may ask the patient to lie on his left side and to breathe in and out slowly, to hold his breath, or to inhale a gas with a slightly sweet odor (amyl nitrite) while changes in heart function are recorded. Amyl nitrite may cause dizziness, flushing, and tachycardia, but these effects quickly subside.

Instruct the patient to remain still during the test because movement may distort the results.

Comparing signs of left- and right-sided heart failure

In left-sided heart failure, the patient will experience mainly *pulmonary* signs. In right-sided heart failure, he'll develop *systemic* signs.

Left-sided heart failure
- Paroxysmal nocturnal dyspnea, dyspnea on exertion, orthopnea
- Bronchial wheezing
- Hypoxia, respiratory acidosis
- Crackles
- Cough with frothy pink sputum
- Cyanosis or pallor
- Elevated blood pressure
- S_3, S_4 sounds
- Palpitations, dysrhythmias
- Elevated pulmonary artery diastolic and pulmonary capillary wedge pressures
- Pulsus alternans

Right-sided heart failure
- Dizziness, fatigue, syncope, weakness
- Hepatomegaly, with or without pain
- Ascites
- Pitting peripheral edema
- Jugular vein distention
- Hepatojugular reflux
- Oliguria
- Dysrhythmias
- Elevated central venous and right atrial pressures
- Abdominal distention, anorexia, nausea, vomiting
- Weight gain

Electrocardiography (ECG)

Inform the patient that an ECG evaluates the heart's function by recording its electrical activity. It takes about 15 minutes and usually causes no discomfort.

Describe test preparation: A technician will cleanse, dry, and possibly shave different sites on the patient's body, such as his chest and arms, and will apply a conductive jelly over them. Then the technician will attach electrodes at these sites.

During the test, the patient will need to lie still, to relax and breathe normally, and to remain quiet. Talking or limb movement will distort the ECG recordings and require additional testing time.

Cardiac catheterization

Inform the patient that this 2- to 3-hour test evaluates the function of his heart and its vessels. Instruct him not to eat or drink anything for 6 hours beforehand.

Tell the patient that he'll be placed on a padded table, and his groin area will be shaved and cleansed. The technician will insert a peripheral I.V. line and attach electrodes at various sites. Tell the patient that he'll receive a mild I.V. sedative to help him relax.

After a local anesthetic is injected into the patient's groin, the doctor will insert a catheter and thread it up through an artery to the left side of the heart or through a vein to the right side of the heart and to the lungs. Next, the doctor will inject a contrast dye through the catheter. When he does so, the patient may feel flushed or nauseated or may experience chest pain; reassure him that these sensations should pass quickly. Tell the patient that he may be asked to cough or breathe deeply and may receive nitroglycerin to dilate coronary vessels, thus aiding visualization.

When the catheter is removed, a nurse will apply pressure and a bulky dressing to the site to control bleeding. The nurse will check the site frequently for swelling. The patient must keep his leg straight for several hours. Once he's allowed to resume his diet, he should drink plenty of fluids. To monitor the patient's response to therapy, the doctor may leave the pulmonary catheter in place for a few days.

Teach about treatments

Treatment will vary with CHF's severity and cause. However, its goals are always the same: to identify or prevent precipitating or aggravating factors, to reduce cardiac work load, to improve pump performance, and to control sodium intake and fluid retention.

Be sure to highlight the significance of life-style changes. Emphasize the need to strictly adhere to the prescribed treatment plan and keep medical appointments.

Activity

Explain that excessive physical activity can further weaken the patient's heart, possibly exacerbating CHF. Stress the need to obtain adequate rest and avoid overexertion.

If the patient has acute CHF, you may have to help him sit up in bed. Inform him that sitting up allows his lungs to function better. Describe how dangling his legs over the edge of bed will help drain fluid from his chest.

If the patient's on bed rest, instruct him to alternately flex and extend his toes several times an hour and to perform range-of-motion leg exercises as scheduled. These exercises can help prevent deep vein thrombosis caused by vascular congestion.

To help the recovering patient function as normally as possible and maintain independence, teach him to gradually increase walking and other physical activities. He must pace himself. To help avoid excessive fatigue, instruct him to alternate light and heavy tasks and to rest frequently. If possible, suggest that he shorten his workday and set aside a daily rest period.

Instruct the patient to maintain his activity level provided it doesn't cause shortness of breath, palpitations, or severe fatigue. If these symptoms appear or worsen, instruct him to notify his doctor.

Diet

Reinforce the importance of adhering to the prescribed diet. Inform the patient that he must restrict sodium intake. This will help diminish fluid retention, thereby decreasing the heart's work load. Collaborate with the patient on developing a low-sodium diet (see *Planning low-sodium meals*).

If the doctor orders fluid restrictions, arrange a mutually acceptable schedule for allowable fluids. Tell the patient he can relieve a dry mouth with rinses or sugarless gum or hard candy. Humidifying room air can also help.

Depending on the patient's prescribed medications, the doctor may order a high- or low-potassium diet. Guide the patient in identifying foods that are high in potassium, including certain salt substitutes and colas.

Medication

In acute CHF, drug therapy may include rapid-acting I.V. diuretics, such as furosemide. Explain to the patient how diuretics rid the body of excess fluid.

In chronic CHF, long-term therapy is likely to include cardiac glycosides, diuretics, and angiotensin-converting enzyme (ACE) inhibitors.

Cardiac glycosides. Tell the patient that the cardiac glycoside digoxin strengthens cardiac contractions and, by slowing down his pulse, regulates his heart rate. Instruct him to check his pulse daily before taking digoxin, and to call the doctor immediately if the rate is less than 60 beats per minute or the rhythm is irregular. Encourage him to promptly report abdominal pain, dizziness, drowsiness, fatigue, or headache. He should also report loss of appetite, malaise, nausea, visual disturbances, or vomiting. (See *Digoxin toxicity: Common patient problem*, page 52.)

Planning low-sodium meals

Help the patient with CHF adjust to a low-sodium diet. Typically, the doctor will tell him how many milligrams of sodium he's allowed each day. To help the patient comply, instruct him to:
• read food labels for sodium content (200 mg of salt equals 80 mg of sodium chloride).
• avoid using salt in cooking and at the table.
• stay away from salty foods, such as potato chips, pretzels, and snack crackers; canned soups and vegetables; prepared foods (for example, TV dinners and frozen entrees); luncheon meats, cheeses, or pickles; and foods preserved in brine.
• include unsalted meat, broth, soups, and butter in his diet. Inform him about low-salt milk, canned vegetables, soups, and baking powder.
• use herbs and spices to enhance the flavor of food. Warn the patient that not all flavor enhancers are salt-free. Some, such as monosodium glutamate and horseradish, are notoriously high in sodium.
• be aware that many over-the-counter medications contain sodium. Examples include Alka-Seltzer, Di-Gel, and Rolaids. Have him consult his doctor or pharmacist about the sodium content of over-the-counter medication before taking it.
• seek his doctor's approval before using a salt substitute. Many products contain a salt other than sodium chloride. They may contain potassium or ammonium salt that could be harmful if the patient has kidney or liver disease.
• order baked, broiled, or roasted foods at restaurants and skip gravies, juices, soups, and cheesy dressings.
• be aware that bottled soft drinks may be high in sodium. In low-calorie beverages, substituting sodium saccharin for sugar increases the sodium content even more.

52   Congestive heart failure

Explain that some foods can change the way digoxin works. For instance, high-fiber foods, such as bran, raw and leafy vegetables, and most fruits, can reduce its absorption. Advise the patient to avoid antacids; antidiarrhea medications, such as Kaopectate; and laxatives because these nonprescription medications decrease digoxin absorption. Warn him not to substitute one brand of digoxin for another without first consulting his doctor.

Potassium-sparing diuretics. If the patient's taking amiloride (Midamor), spironolactone (Aldactone), or triamterene (Dyrenium), explain that the drug should relieve edema and lung congestion. Tell him to be alert for confusion, irregular heart rate, muscle flaccidity, numbness and tingling in the hands and feet, and weight changes. Other reactions include decreased libido, diarrhea, headache, nausea, abdominal cramps, vomiting, and weakness.

Instruct the patient to limit his intake of high-potassium foods (citrus fruits, tomatoes, bananas, dates, and apricots) as well

---

Digoxin toxicity: Common patient problem

Inform the patient that digoxin is the most commonly used drug for treating congestive heart failure. Significantly, nearly one-third of the patients taking it will experience digoxin toxicity. That's because of the narrow range between therapeutic and toxic blood levels.

What causes toxicity?
Toxicity may result from overdosage or from accumulation of digoxin in the myocardium after changes in the patient's condition or treatment. For example, GI disorders may cause potassium loss and so increase the heart's sensitivity to digoxin. Hypothyroidism and acid-base and electrolyte disturbances can also increase sensitivity to digoxin. Hepatic and renal disorders may reduce digoxin excretion.

Treatment, such as cardioversion, can influence the patient's response to digoxin. For elective cardioversion, digoxin is typically withheld for 1 to 2 days before the procedure and the dosage is adjusted after it. Concurrent treatment with amphotericin B, I.V. calcium or glucose, potassium-wasting diuretics, propantheline, or quinidine predisposes the patient to digoxin toxicity.

Detecting toxicity
Instruct the patient to report these extracardiac symptoms of toxicity: abdominal pain, anorexia, diarrhea, fatigue, headache, nausea, vomiting, and weakness. He should also report visual disturbances, such as blurring, yellow-green halos around lights, and double vision.

If the patient complains of these symptoms, be alert for heart failure. Check his pulse for bradycardia or tachycardia. Monitor the ECG for premature ventricular contractions, atrial fibrillation, accelerated junctional nodal rhythm, atrioventricular dissociation, or heart block.

Confirming toxicity
To confirm digoxin toxicity, the doctor will order serum samples for measuring drug levels at least 6 hours after an oral dose, the duration necessary for serum and tissue levels to reach equilibrium. Digoxin's therapeutic level ranges from 0.5 to 2.0 ng/ml; a level greater than 2.5 ng/ml causes toxicity.

Digibind: Treating digoxin toxicity
If appropriate, explain that Digibind is an antidote to digoxin toxicity. It comes in powder form and after being reconstituted is usually administered I.V. The dosage depends on how much digoxin needs to be neutralized. Note that its use is reserved for severe overdoses. Mention that digoxin therapy won't be resumed until Digibind has been eliminated from the body—several days for most patients.

as some salt substitutes. Advise him to take the drug with food to relieve GI distress and to weigh himself at least every other day and to report any unusual changes. Tell him to check with the doctor or pharmacist before taking nonprescription cold or allergy preparations. Many contain drugs that will elevate blood pressure and counteract the diuretic's effectiveness.

Loop diuretics. If the patient's taking bumetanide (Bumex), ethacrynic acid (Edecrin), or furosemide (Lasix), explain that the drug should help his kidneys filter excess fluid, thereby clearing fluid from his lungs. Tell him to be alert for fever, increased thirst, jaundice, muscle cramps, nausea, unusual fatigue or weakness, urgent or burning urination, and vomiting. He should also be alert for hearing loss or tinnitus. Other reactions include anorexia, blurred vision, diarrhea, dizziness, muscle aches and cramps, and weight loss.

Advise the patient to limit his alcohol intake to prevent dizziness. If he takes the drug twice daily, tell him to take the second dose late in the afternoon rather than at night to prevent interrupting sleep from nocturia. Instruct him to take the drug with meals to prevent GI distress. Encourage intake of high-potassium foods and remind him to take potassium supplements, if ordered. Instruct the patient to record his weight daily to monitor fluid loss. To minimize postural hypotension, tell him to rise slowly from a lying or sitting position.

Thiazide diuretics. Tell the patient taking chlorothiazide (Diuril), chlorthalidone (Hygroton), hydrochlorothiazide (Esidrix, HydroDIURIL), or metolazone (Diulo) that the drug should relieve lung congestion and edema. Instruct him to be alert for dry mouth, excessive thirst, fever, irregular heart rate, lethargy, muscle cramps, rash, urgent or burning urination, weakness, and weak pulse. Other reactions include anorexia, diarrhea, dizziness, GI distress, and restlessness.

Instruct the patient to take an evening dose early in the evening to prevent sleep interruption from nocturia. He should record his weight daily to monitor fluid loss. Tell him to avoid large doses of calcium supplements but to increase his intake of high-potassium foods, such as bananas and citrus fruits. Advise him to consult his doctor before taking any nonprescription drugs, such as cold or allergy remedies. Many contain drugs that may elevate his blood pressure and decrease the diuretic's effectiveness.

ACE inhibitors. If the patient's taking captopril (Capoten), enalapril (Vasotec), or lisinopril (Prinivil), explain that this drug should relieve symptoms of heart failure. Tell him to be alert for chest pain, diaphoresis, severe diarrhea, dyspnea, fever, mouth sores, rapid heart rate, rash, sore throat, and severe vomiting. Other reactions include altered taste, dizziness, fatigue, headache, and palpitations.

Teach him to minimize postural hypotension by rising slowly from a sitting or lying position. Tell him to drink 2 to 3 quarts of fluid daily, unless otherwise directed, to prevent hypotension. Advise him to limit high-potassium foods and low-salt milk and salt substitutes. Instruct him to consult his doctor before taking any over-the-counter drugs, such as cold or allergy remedies. Many contain drugs that may elevate his blood pressure and decrease the ACE inhibitor's effectiveness.

Procedures
If the patient requires *supplemental oxygen,* explain that this will help to ease breathing difficulty caused by lung congestion. If the patient with severe pulmonary involvement requires *endotracheal intubation and mechanical ventilation,* reassure him that these measures won't be needed once his respiratory status stabilizes. To help him communicate while intubated, provide pencil and paper; explain that he'll be able to speak once the tube is removed.

Explain that *pulmonary artery catheterization,* if ordered, will help to evaluate heart function and allow the doctor to tailor treatment accordingly. Tell the patient that a sheath will be inserted into the subclavian, jugular, or femoral vein under local anesthesia and then sutured in place. Next, a thin balloon-tipped catheter will be introduced through the sheath and carried by the circulation through the right atrium and right ventricle into the pulmonary artery. There, hemodynamic pressures and cardiac output will be measured until the patient's condition stabilizes.

If *rotating tourniquets* are necessary, inform the patient that this procedure reduces venous return and relieves pulmonary congestion, thus helping him to breathe more easily. Warn him that the skin on his extremities may become slightly discolored during this procedure.

Surgery
Although not generally indicated for CHF, open-heart surgery may benefit a patient with associated coronary artery disease or structural abnormalities.

Other care measures
Review steps for preventing complications and enhancing comfort.

Preventing complications. Anxiety may raise blood pressure and heart rate and reduce urine output. So coach the patient in relaxation techniques to help him reduce his anxiety level. Instruct him to watch for and report early signs of pulmonary edema: cough, difficulty breathing, fatigue, restlessness, anxiety, and increased pulse rate.

Unexplained weight gain often constitutes an important early sign of recurrent CHF. Encourage the patient to weigh himself daily. He should do this at the same time each day, on the same scale, and while wearing the same amount of clothing. Tell him to keep an accurate record of daily weights and to notify the doctor if he notices a gain. Other reportable signs include anorexia, dyspnea on exertion, persistent cough, frequent urination at night, and swelling of the ankles, feet, or abdomen.

The patient's condition makes him more susceptible to pneumonia and other respiratory infections. Warn him to limit his exposure to crowds and to people with infections. Suggest asking the doctor about pneumonia and influenza vaccinations.

Enhancing comfort. By elevating his legs, the patient can minimize leg and ankle edema. Note if the patient complains of awakening with shortness of breath shortly after going to bed. This results from fluid in his legs returning to his circulation. Encourage him to elevate his feet for an hour before lying down. This will protect his lungs while allowing his kidneys to clear the extra fluid.

To avoid dizziness, teach the patient to change positions slowly. Because extreme heat can make breathing difficult, recommend that he stay in a cool environment whenever possible. Performing activities in the cooler part of the day will also help.

Because extreme cold interferes with circulation, advise the patient to dress warmly in cold weather, reminding him to avoid restrictive clothing. Suggest that he wrap a scarf over his nose and mouth to warm the air and make breathing easier.

Finally, refer the patient to a local chapter of the American Heart Association.

Source of information and support
American Heart Association
7320 Greenville Avenue, Dallas, Tex. 75231
(214) 750-5300

Further readings
Bernard, R. "Heart Failure: Can Earlier Diagnosis and Vasodilators Boost Survival?" *Emergency Medicine* 20(5):299-302, 340, March 15, 1988.
"Beta-blockers in Congestive Heart Failure," *Nurses Drug Alert* 12(4):29-30, April 1988.
Poindexter, S., et al. "Nutrition in Congestive Heart Failure," *Nutrition in Clinical Practice* 1(2):83-88, April 1986.
Valle, G., et al. "Effective Technique of Controlling Volume in Refractory Congestive Heart Failure," *Heart & Lung* 16(16):712-717, November 1987.
Watson, J. "Fluid and Electrolyte Disorders in Cardiovascular Patients," *Nursing Clinics of North America* 22(4):797-803, December 1987.

Living with congestive heart failure

Dear Patient:

Recognizing the common early symptoms of your condition is one way for you to monitor yourself and help prevent any complications. Keep your doctor posted on the symptoms you experience. Then follow his directions. Of course, continue to follow your diet, activity, and medication regimens as directed.

Common early symptoms of heart failure appear below. You'll also find tips for living with them.

Breathing difficulties

You may have difficulty breathing when blood and fluids don't move fast enough through your lungs. Shortness of breath may occur with exertion, such as climbing the stairs or lifting a grandchild. If you feel short of breath, stop what you're doing and steady yourself. Then rest until you feel better.

If you feel short of breath when you're resting or lying down, try raising your head with several pillows. Or, if you're short of breath when you get up after a nap or a night's sleep, try sitting up, dangling your legs over the bedside, and wiggling your feet and ankles. You can also stand up and walk around a bit to promote circulation.

Swelling

You may have swelling if your body doesn't get rid of extra salt and fluid. You probably have some swelling if you press your finger to your skin and the impression remains briefly.

You may also notice puffiness in your hands, ankles, or feet. Or you may see marks on your skin from the elastic in your socks or rings on your fingers. Try elevating your feet, ankles, or hands above the level of your heart. This may help the swelling go down.

Be sure you weigh yourself every day at about the same time. Use the same scale and wear about the same amount of clothing. If you notice a sudden, unexplainable gain (perhaps 2 pounds or more in a day), let your doctor know. He may prescribe medication or suggest other relief measures.

Other symptoms

Other symptoms to report to your doctor include:
• a dry cough
• frequently getting up during the night to urinate
• increased weakness and fatigue
• upper abdominal pain or a bloated feeling.

A word of caution

If at any time you feel as if you can't breathe at all and your heart is pounding, call your doctor right away. Also call him right away if you cough up pink, frothy sputum.

Chronic arterial occlusive disease

Most commonly affecting elderly patients, especially men, chronic arterial occlusive disease often goes undetected until symptoms of arterial insufficiency force the patient to seek treatment. Typical symptoms include painful intermittent claudication from leg artery occlusion or transient ischemic attacks from carotid artery occlusion.

Unfortunately, by the time symptoms appear, arterial damage is often extensive, limiting the effectiveness of treatment. Nevertheless, your teaching can help the patient cope with the demands of his chronic disorder. For example, you'll need to teach him about relieving symptoms through proper exercise, nutrition, and positioning. If necessary, you'll also teach him about arterial bypass grafting or other surgical procedures. To reduce the risk of long-term complications, you'll emphasize scrupulous skin care, correct use of anticoagulant drugs, and appropriate life-style changes.

Discuss the disorder

Explain to the patient that arterial occlusive disease involves the obstruction or narrowing of the aorta and its major branches. (For details, see *Sites of arterial occlusion,* page 58.) As a result, interrupted blood flow, usually to the legs and feet, prevents oxygen and nutrients from reaching the tissues. Occlusion can cause severe ischemia, skin ulceration, and gangrene (see *Signs and symptoms of arterial occlusive disease,* page 59).

Point out the vascular changes—primarily arteriosclerotic and atherosclerotic—that produce chronic arterial occlusive disease. (Although arterial occlusion is commonly chronic, it can be acute. For more information, refer to *What causes acute arterial occlusion?* page 60.) Tell the patient that one or both of these vascular changes may cause his condition. In arteriosclerosis, calcification and occlusion of the arteries stem from a progressive loss of vessel elasticity associated with such factors as aging, hypertension, and diabetes. Atherosclerosis, the gradual buildup of fatty, fibrous plaques on the inner arterial walls, results from lipoprotein abnormalities, arterial wall injury, and platelet dysfunction. Both disorders produce varying degrees of arterial occlusion.

Next, explain how intermittent claudication results from these arterial changes. Insufficient blood flow through occluded arteries leads to oxygen deficiency in the leg muscles—usually in the

Richard Gibson, RN, MN, JD, CCRN, CS, and **Rosanne Hopson, RN, BSN,** wrote this chapter. Mr. Gibson is a critical care clinical nurse specialist at the Veterans Administration Hospital in San Diego. Ms. Hopson is a clinical research study coordinator in electrophysiology at the University of Iowa Hospitals and Clinics in Iowa City.

CHECKLIST

Teaching topics in arterial occlusive disease

☐ Major causes of reduced arterial blood flow—atherosclerosis and arteriosclerosis
☐ How intermittent claudication and arterial ulcers develop
☐ Preparation for arteriography, Doppler ultrasonography, blood clotting studies, and possibly serum lipid and lipoprotein measurements
☐ Relief of intermittent claudication with rest or by placing leg in a dependent position
☐ Activity and dietary recommendations
☐ Anticoagulants and other drugs—proper use and precautions
☐ Preventing infection and ulcers
☐ Caring for ulcers, including dressing changes
☐ Preparation for procedures, such as percutaneous transluminal angioplasty or laser-assisted angioplasty
☐ Preparation for possible surgery: arterial bypass grafting, sympathectomy, or endarterectomy

Sites of arterial occlusion

Show the patient this anatomic diagram to help him understand the arterial system. Point out the location of the aorta, its major branching arteries, and the body areas affected by the blood flow from these arteries. Remember to pinpoint the site of the patient's occlusion on the diagram.

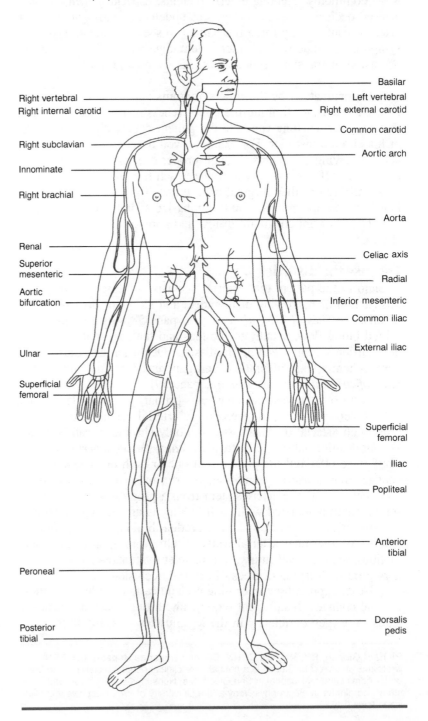

Right vertebral

Right internal carotid

Right subclavian

Innominate

Right brachial

Renal

Superior mesenteric

Aortic bifurcation

Ulnar

Superficial femoral

Peroneal

Posterior tibial

Basilar

Left vertebral

Right external carotid

Common carotid

Aortic arch

Aorta

Celiac axis

Radial

Inferior mesenteric

Common iliac

External iliac

Superficial femoral

Iliac

Popliteal

Anterior tibial

Dorsalis pedis

Signs and symptoms of arterial occlusive disease

SITE OF OCCLUSION	SIGNS AND SYMPTOMS
Carotid arterial system • Internal carotids • External carotids	A blockage in this area reduces cerebral blood flow and can cause transient ischemic attacks (TIAs), which may produce unilateral sensory or motor dysfunction. These effects may involve transient blindness in one eye or weakness on one side of the body. Other characteristic symptoms include possible loss of the ability to produce or comprehend speech (aphasia) or difficulty speaking (dysarthria), confusion, decreased mentation, and headache. Such recurrent symptoms usually last 5 to 10 minutes but may persist up to 24 hours. Instruct the patient to notify the doctor because these symptoms may herald a stroke. Other clinical features include an absent or decreased pulsation with an auscultatory bruit over the affected vessels.
Vertebrobasilar system • Vertebral arteries • Basilar arteries	Less common than carotid TIA, brain stem and cerebellum TIAs produce the following characteristic signs and symptoms: binocular visual disturbances, vertigo, difficulty speaking, and "drop attacks" (falling down without loss of consciousness).
Innominate • Brachiocephalic artery	Signs and symptoms of occlusion in this area are the same as those for a vertebrobasilar occlusion: binocular visual disturbances, vertigo, difficulty speaking, and drop attacks. The patient also may experience claudication in his right arm.
Subclavian artery	Subclavian steal syndrome is characterized by blood backflow from the brain. Blood travels through the vertebral artery on the same side as the occlusion into the subclavian artery distal to the occlusion. Other features of this syndrome include binocular visual disturbances, vertigo, difficulty speaking, and drop attacks. The patient also may experience exercise-induced arm claudication and may develop gangrene in his fingers.
Mesenteric artery • Superior (most commonly affected) • Celiac axis • Inferior	Occlusion in this area causes ischemia, necrosis, and gangrene in the bowel. Signs and symptoms include sudden, acute abdominal pain, nausea and vomiting, diarrhea, and shock, resulting from massive intraluminal fluid and plasma loss.
Aortic bifurcation (saddle block occlusion, a medical emergency associated with cardiac embolization)	Muscle weakness, numbness, paresthesia, and paralysis characterize occlusion in the aortic bifurcation. The patient also may experience symptoms of ischemia: sudden leg pain and cold, pale legs (with decreased or absent peripheral pulses).
Iliac artery (Leriche's syndrome)	With this area of occlusion, intermittent claudication may develop in the thighs. It's relieved by rest. Pain also may occur in the lower back and buttocks. Male patients also may be impotent.
Femoral and popliteal arteries (associated with aneurysm formation)	Signs and symptoms of occlusion in these arteries include intermittent claudication of the calves on exertion, painful feet, leg pallor and coolness, and gangrene. The patient also may notice pain associated with necrosis and ulceration and blanching on elevating the feet. Palpable pulses are absent in ankles and feet.

What causes acute arterial occlusion?

Inform the patient that the most common cause of acute arterial occlusion is obstruction of a major artery by a clot. Such obstruction usually stems from an embolus originating in the heart.

Emboli typically lodge in the arms and legs, where blood vessels narrow or branch. In the arms, emboli usually lodge in the brachial artery but may occlude the subclavian or axillary arteries. Common leg sites include the iliac, femoral, and popliteal arteries. Emboli originating in the heart can cause serious neurologic damage if they enter the cerebral circulation.

Atheromatous debris (plaques) from proximal arterial lesions also may intermittently obstruct small vessels (usually in the hands or feet). These plaques also may develop in the brachiocephalic vessels and embolize to the cerebral circulation, where they lead to transient cerebral ischemia or infarction.

If *thrombosis* occurs in a patient with preexisting atherosclerosis and marked arterial narrowing, acute intrinsic arterial occlusion may occur. This complication typically arises in areas with severely stenotic vessels, especially in a patient who also has congestive heart failure, hypovolemia, polycythemia, or traumatic injury. Thrombosis has become the most common cause of acute arterial occlusion.

Acute arterial occlusion also may stem from *insertion of a medical device,* such as a catheter, or from *intra-arterial drug abuse* or *peripheral arterial injection of foreign material.*

Extrinsic arterial occlusion can result from *direct blunt or penetrating arterial traumatic injury.*

calves, the most distal leg muscles—causing a painful cramp. The patient usually feels no symptoms while resting; pain and weakness develop in the calf muscle after he walks a certain distance without resting. When he does rest, his symptoms disappear as the supply of blood to the calf muscle is restored.

Complications

Stress the importance of strict compliance with treatment in helping prevent complications of arterial occlusive disease, such as painful and slow-healing arterial ulcers. (However, because vascular changes from underlying arteriosclerosis and atherosclerosis may be irreversible, the patient is still susceptible to complications even with compliance and successful surgery.) Arterial ulcers can form wherever a blocked or constricted artery produces ischemia in distal tissues. As ischemia worsens, capillary perfusion drops, metabolic exchange decreases, and the skin becomes increasingly fragile and susceptible to disruption and eventual infection from direct injury, pressure, and irritation (for more information, see *Using hyperbaric oxygen for chronic leg ulcers*).

Extremely dangerous, though rare, complications of arterial occlusive disease include embolism and aneurysm.

Describe the diagnostic workup

Prepare the patient for diagnostic tests to evaluate the extent of arterial occlusion and collateral circulation. These include arteriography, Doppler ultrasonography, and blood chemistry studies.

Arteriography
Explain to the patient that arteriography evaluates arteries for abnormalities. Tell him that the test may take 30 minutes to 4 hours, depending on the number of blood vessels examined.

Inform the patient that an area on his groin, armpit, or another location will be shaved and cleaned. After a local anesthetic is injected, a catheter will be inserted into a vessel and advanced as necessary. Then a contrast dye will be injected into the blood vessels, and several X-rays will be taken to follow the dye's passage. Warn the patient that he may feel flushed or nauseated, or that he may have an unusual taste in his mouth. Assure him that these feelings will pass quickly. Tell him that he may be asked to turn on one side or to elevate an arm or leg for the X-rays. Instruct him to remain perfectly still when asked, to avoid distorting the X-ray image.

Explain that after the test the catheter will be removed and pressure will be applied over the insertion site for 15 to 30 minutes. Tell the patient that a bulky dressing will then be applied and that a sandbag will be placed against the insertion site for additional pressure. Instruct him to keep his arm or leg extended and immobile for 4 to 24 hours (as ordered) after the test and to expect frequent evaluations of the pulse rate and circulation in his limb.

Doppler ultrasonography
Explain to the patient that Doppler ultrasonography will help to evaluate the blood flow in his arms, legs, or neck. Tell him that the test takes about 20 minutes, is painless, and doesn't involve risk. Mention that he'll be asked to uncover his arm, leg, or neck and to loosen or remove any constrictive clothing. He'll also be required to move his arms to different positions and to perform breathing exercises to vary blood flow while measurements are taken.

Point out that a transducer resembling a microphone will be placed at various sites along specific arteries and that his blood pressure will be checked at several sites, including his arms, calves, and thighs. Tell the patient that the transducer (which will be covered with a conductive jelly) will be moved along the artery being examined. Explain that the transducer directs sound waves through the skin to detect arterial obstruction.

Blood chemistry studies
Prepare the patient for blood coagulation studies, such as partial thromboplastin time and prothrombin time, to investigate possible clotting abnormalities or to evaluate the effectiveness of anticoagulant therapy. If ordered, prepare the patient for serum cholesterol, triglyceride, and lipoprotein studies to assess for atherosclerosis. Instruct him to abstain from alcohol for 24 hours

Using hyperbaric oxygen for chronic leg ulcers

When chronic leg ulcers complicate your patient's condition, hyperbaric oxygenation may be recommended. Explain that this new therapy, which uses 100% oxygen administered in a pressurized chamber, promotes healing by improving circulation and stimulating capillary return.

Tell the patient that he may undergo one treatment a day for 20 to 30 days. Usually after about 10 treatments, his progress will be evaluated.

Special instructions
Orient the patient to the treatment chamber's confined space. Then discuss special precautions. For example, tell him that he may feel pressure in his ears similar to that felt during an airplane landing. Advise him to yawn or swallow to relieve this discomfort.

Additionally, warn him that he may experience visual changes, such as nearsightedness or double vision. Reassure him, though, that normal vision will return soon after each therapy session.

and from exercise for 12 hours before the tests. If ordered, tell the patient to discontinue all thyroid, antilipemic, and oral contraceptive drugs.

Teach about treatments

Explain that treatment may be medical or surgical or a combination, depending on the cause, location, and size of the obstruction. Medical management may include risk-factor reduction (such as cessation of smoking), exercise, foot and leg care, medication, and angioplasty procedures. Surgery may involve techniques such as bypass grafting, sympathectomy, or endarterectomy.

Activity

Tell the patient that regular exercise is essential to prevent further arterial occlusion and to promote development of collateral circulation, which helps reduce intermittent claudication and formation of arterial ulcers. Depending on the patient's age and capabilities, encourage him to walk, swim, or bicycle daily. Instruct him to exercise until claudication forces him to stop. Advise him to rest and then to resume exercising when the pain subsides. Daily progressive exercise of this type may gradually reduce the severity of claudication and increase the distance the patient can walk without pain.

If the patient with severe intermittent claudication is ambulatory, instruct him to walk for about 10 minutes each hour and to rest the remainder of the time. Reinforce the need to balance exercise and rest. Explain that overly vigorous exercise generates excessive heat in the leg muscles and places inordinate demands on already compromised leg circulation, increasing the risk of infection and exacerbating leg pain. For the same reasons, instruct him to avoid crossing his legs and elevating or applying heat to the affected leg.

Teach the patient to relieve persistent leg pain by periodically placing his legs in a dependent position, such as dangling them over the side of a bed. This position improves blood flow to the legs and relieves symptoms. Advise him to report any excessive leg or ankle swelling resulting from this practice.

Diet

Depending on the underlying cause of arterial occlusive disease, review dietary restrictions on cholesterol, saturated fats, and sodium. Give the patient a copy of the teaching aid *Cutting down on cholesterol*, page 27.

To help maintain skin integrity and reduce the chance of infection and ulceration, stress the importance of adequate intake of protein, vitamin B_{12}, and vitamin C. Point out good sources of these nutrients. Nutritional yeast is high in vitamin B_{12} and protein, and it comes in a powder form that can easily be added to foods. Sources of vitamin C include citrus fruits, strawberries, cantaloupe, tomatoes, bean sprouts, broccoli, cabbage, peppers, and brussels sprouts. Because traditional protein sources—meats, dairy products, and eggs—also contain high levels of cholesterol or saturated fats (or both), teach the patient about alternative sources of protein: legumes, nuts, seeds, and grains.

Medication
Discuss prescribed anticoagulant therapy. Explain that an anticoagulant reduces the blood's ability to clot. Emphasize the need for precautions while taking anticoagulants, and warn the patient about any possible adverse reactions. (See *Do's and don'ts of anticoagulant therapy,* page 70.) Review the purpose, possible adverse effects, and special considerations for other prescribed drugs. Inform the patient that antiplatelet agents, such as aspirin or dipyridamole, reduce the formation of clots by interfering with platelet function, and vasodilators, such as isoxsuprine, decrease symptoms by dilating the arteries. If the doctor orders pentoxifylline (Trental), tell the patient that this hemorrheologic agent decreases the viscosity of blood, which improves blood flow through his blood vessels. Reinforce your teaching with the patient-teaching aid *Learning about pentoxifylline,* page 71. For more specific teaching points, see *Teaching about drugs for arterial occlusive disease,* pages 64 and 65.

Also tell the patient what pain medications are available to him, and if necessary, teach him how to apply topical antibiotics to areas of skin breakdown and ulceration.

Procedures
Stress meticulous skin care to prevent infection, and describe percutaneous transluminal angioplasty (PCTA) or laser-assisted angioplasty to open occluded arteries.

Self-care. Advise the patient to avoid any activity that could cause skin injury or irritation or that could apply pressure or heat to his skin. Emphasize the importance of daily foot and leg care to prevent infection and ulceration. For further information, see *Foot care guidelines,* page 66.

If appropriate, teach the patient proper care of arterial ulcers. Explain that wet-to-dry dressings will mechanically debride ulcers and help them heal. Instruct him to take his prescribed pain medication about ½ hour before changing dressings. List the supplies he'll need to care for his ulcers at home, and tell him where he can get them. Mention that an Unna's boot may be prescribed to treat his leg ulcer. (See *Applying a medicated boot,* page 72.)

Percutaneous transluminal angioplasty. Inform the patient that PCTA allows the doctor to open a blocked or narrowed artery. This procedure involves introducing a catheter into either the patient's arm or groin. Tell him that first the doctor will numb the site with a local anesthetic and then will insert a thin, balloon-tipped catheter into a peripheral artery. Guided by fluoroscopy, he'll thread the catheter through the constricted artery to the site of obstruction. After instilling contrast dye to verify the catheter's placement, he'll inflate the balloon tip. This compresses the obstruction against the arterial walls, expanding the vessel to increase blood flow. Multiple balloon inflations (each taking 30 to 60 seconds) achieve dilatation. The doctor will then deflate the

Teaching about drugs for arterial occlusive disease

DRUG	ADVERSE REACTIONS	TEACHING POINTS
Anticoagulants		
warfarin (Coumadin, Panwarfin)	• Watch for bleeding nose or gums, chills, dark blue toes, discolored urine, excessive menstrual flow, fatigue, fever, prolonged bleeding from cuts or bruises, prolonged diarrhea, red or black stool, sore throat, and vomiting (sometimes bloody). • Other reactions include bruising, diarrhea, nausea, and slight hair loss.	• Instruct the patient to avoid over-the-counter drugs containing aspirin and high doses of vitamins A and E; he may take an occasional dose of ibuprofen with the doctor's permission. • Tell him to limit alcohol consumption to one or two drinks per day. • Instruct the patient to maintain a consistent diet because both vitamin K and fat absorption affect how the drug is absorbed. Emphasize that the drug dosage is adjusted to meet his specific needs (and is based on a consistent diet), so he shouldn't alter his diet radically without first consulting the doctor. • Tell him to take a missed dose within 8 hours, but warn him not to double-dose. • Inform him that he'll need frequent blood tests to monitor the drug's effects. • Teach measures to reduce the risk of bleeding, such as always wearing shoes, placing a nonskid mat in the bathtub, shaving with an electric razor, using a soft toothbrush, and wearing gloves for yard work. • Help him obtain a Medic Alert tag or card, identifying him as a warfarin user. • If the patient's a female of childbearing age, emphasize the need for practicing birth control. That's because warfarin can adversely affect fetal development and cause placental bleeding.
Antiplatelet agents		
aspirin (multiple forms and brands)	• Watch for bleeding gums, dyspnea, easy bruising, hearing loss, tarry stools, tinnitus, and vomiting blood. • Other reactions include GI distress and heartburn.	• To avoid excessive GI bleeding, warn the patient not to take aspirin with alcohol. • To relieve mild GI distress, advise him to take aspirin with food or milk or to use a buffered or enteric-coated form of the drug. • Tell him to take a missed dose within 12 hours, but warn him not to double-dose. • Teach him that acetaminophen doesn't have the same antithrombotic effect as aspirin and cannot be substituted.
dipyridamole (Persantine)	• Watch for chest pain and rash. • Other reactions include dizziness, GI distress, and headache.	• Tell the patient to take a missed dose as soon as possible, but warn him not to double-dose. • To minimize dizziness, tell him to rise slowly from a sitting or lying position. • To avoid dizziness, instruct him not to combine the drug and alcohol. • Advise him to take dipyridamole with a light snack or a glass of milk to reduce GI distress.
Hemorrheologic agent		
pentoxifylline (Trental)	• Watch for chest pain, flushing, nausea, palpitations, persistent GI distress, rapid heartbeat, shortness of breath, swollen feet and ankles, and vomiting. • Other reactions include agitation, dizziness, drowsiness, headache, insomnia, nervousness, and tremor.	• If the patient is also taking warfarin, stress the need for more frequent monitoring of prothrombin time. Trental may prolong prothrombin time. • Tell him to take Trental with meals to minimize GI distress. • Teach him to take a missed dose as soon as possible, but not to double-dose. • Instruct him to swallow the pills whole. Tell him not to crush or break the extended-release tablets.

continued

Teaching about drugs for arterial occlusive disease — *continued*

DRUG	ADVERSE REACTIONS	TEACHING POINTS
Vasodilators		
cyclandelate (Cyclospasmol)	• Watch for dizziness, headache, rapid heartbeat, sweating, tingling, and weakness. • Other reactions include flushing, heartburn, and stomach upset.	• Advise the patient that flushing, headache, and rapid heartbeat may occur within the first week of therapy and may require a dose reduction. • Tell him to take the drug with meals or with an antacid, if prescribed, if stomach upset occurs. • Advise him that improvement is gradual and that prolonged therapy may be necessary.
isoxsuprine hydrochloride (Vasodilan)	• Watch for dizziness, fainting, light-headedness, muscular weakness, nervousness, palpitations, postural hypotension, and severe rash. • Other reactions include GI distress, nausea, and vomiting.	• Advise the patient to report any adverse reactions; they can usually be controlled by a dose reduction. • Point out the importance of proper care for his toenails and the skin on his legs and feet. Emphasize the importance of weight control and stopping smoking as adjuncts to drug therapy.

balloon, remove the catheter, and apply manual pressure to the puncture site to stop any bleeding.

Laser-assisted angioplasty. Explain that this alternative to standard angioplasty can be used to open vessels that are totally occluded or obstructed with dense, calcified plaque. Before the procedure, instruct the patient to fast for 8 to 12 hours. Tell him that he may have an I.V. inserted and that he will receive a sedative. Mention that an arterial site on either his arm or leg will be cleaned and shaved.

Then the patient will be positioned on an examination table in the operating room or a special procedures room and will be covered with sterile drapes; the room will be darkened. The doctor will numb the arterial site and make a small incision to expose the artery or will insert a needle through the skin and into the artery. Next, he'll insert a small catheter into the artery, advancing it to the blockage site. The patient will then receive several contrast medium injections to outline the occluded area. Warn him that he may experience mild burning with each injection.

Explain that once the occluded area is identified, the doctor will open the blood vessel with a laser catheter alone, or if some occlusion remains, he may also use a balloon-tipped catheter. Describe the laser as a special type of light that focuses energy, or heat, to remove a blockage. Warn the patient that he may feel an uncomfortably warm sensation in the affected limb from the laser. Assure him that this sensation will last only seconds to minutes, although repeated laser applications may be required. The procedure usually lasts from 1 to 3 hours.

Inform the patient that afterward the doctor will remove the catheters and apply either direct pressure or use stitches to close the puncture site. The patient may receive I.V. fluids to help his kidneys remove the contrast medium. Tell him that he'll remain in bed for several hours or even overnight, keeping his affected limb as still as possible.

Foot care guidelines

Does your patient overlook proper foot care? Review these guidelines with him to help him safeguard his feet from injury and subsequent infection. Emphasize daily foot care, precautions against injury, and when to contact the doctor.

Daily care
• Instruct your patient to wash his feet daily with mild soap and warm water. (To prevent burns, he should never use hot water.) Remind him to dry his feet carefully, especially between the toes.
• If his skin is dry, tell him to apply lanolin ointment. If his feet tend to sweat, recommend a mild foot powder, making sure it doesn't cake.
• Stress inspecting the feet daily—around the nails, between the toes, and on the soles too. Tell the patient to look for corns, calluses, redness, swelling, bruises, or breaks in the skin.
• To treat corns or calluses, tell your patient to soak his feet, gently pat them dry with a towel, and apply lanolin ointment. Advise him to repeat these steps once or twice a day until he sees improvement. If corns or calluses don't improve, he should visit a podiatrist.
   Warn him never to use nonprescription corn remedies and never to cut corns or calluses with a razor or knife.

Special precautions
• Instruct the patient to cut his toenails straight across and file them carefully to eliminate rough edges. He should do this under good light after washing his feet. Are his toenails too thick to cut? Or do they tend to crack when they're cut? Tell him to have a podiatrist cut them.
• Advise the patient to make sure new shoes fit comfortably and support, protect, and cover his feet completely. Recommend breaking them in gradually.
• Caution the patient never to go barefoot.
• Warn the patient not to use hot-water bottles, heating pads, or ice on his legs or feet. Explain that decreased blood flow to the legs and feet reduces sensation in the feet; he could burn or chill them without feeling it.
• If a foot injury causes a break in the skin, teach the patient to wash the affected area with soap and water immediately and cover it with a dry sterile gauze bandage. Instruct him to change the bandage daily and inspect the area for redness, swelling, and drainage.

When to notify the doctor
Tell your patient to call the doctor if any foot injury doesn't improve in 72 hours. He should also call him if he notices any of these signs of impaired circulation when examining his feet:
• new sores or ulcers that take unusually long to heal
• unusual, persistent warmth or coolness
• numbness or muscle weakness
• swelling that doesn't resolve after raising the leg.

Surgery
Point out that surgery usually is performed for chronic arterial occlusive disease when claudication interferes with ambulation, when carotid artery occlusion produces neurologic deficits, or when the procedure will improve blood supply to an ulcerated area. (See *Teaching about vascular repair*, page 68.)

Bypass grafting. Explain that this procedure uses a graft to divert blood flow around the occlusion. Inform the patient that bypass graft surgery is the most effective surgical treatment. Depending on the occlusion site, surgery may involve an aortofemoral bypass, an axillofemoral bypass, or a femoropopliteal bypass graft.

If the patient's scheduled for an *aortofemoral bypass,* explain that he'll receive a general anesthetic, and he may have two or three incisions: one midline abdominal and one groin site for each femoral graft done.

If the patient's scheduled for an *axillofemoral bypass,* he'll have a general anesthetic, and he may have up to three incisions at one axillary and one or two groin sites. Postoperatively, tell the patient not to lie on the side of the graft; this could result in graft occlusion. Also advise him to avoid heavy lifting, carrying, any sudden or forceful use of the arm on the affected side, and reaching high overhead—these maneuvers could dislodge the graft from the donor site.

Help the patient gradually to regain use of the affected leg by teaching a family member how to perform passive range-of-motion exercises: alternately flexing and extending the patient's legs, wiggling his toes, and rotating and flexing his feet. Then, as the patient's condition allows, have him begin active exercises. He'll also need to avoid sitting or standing for prolonged periods to prevent graft occlusion.

Instruct the patient not to wear any tight or constrictive garments (belts, girdles, or suspenders) over the graft. Demonstrate how to check the graft pulse, placing the patient's index and middle fingers on the graft where it passes over the rib cage into the femoral area. Instruct the patient to notify the doctor promptly if he can't detect a graft pulse or if he experiences intermittent claudication.

Tell the patient undergoing revascularization with a *femoropopliteal bypass* that this procedure can be done under general or spinal anesthesia.

Sympathectomy. Inform the patient that a sympathectomy may be done in conjunction with other revascularization procedures. Explain that he'll receive a general anesthetic and that selected sympathetic nerve fibers will be surgically excised. If successful, this surgery will allow arterial dilatation and increased blood flow to the limbs.

Endarterectomy. Inform the patient that an endarterectomy will improve cerebral circulation by removing the atherosclerotic plaque that has built up in the artery and occluded blood flow. Explain that he'll remain in the critical care unit for at least 24 hours and that he'll have a bulky dressing and, possibly, a drain on his neck for the next 24 to 48 hours.

Tell the patient that frequent neurologic checks will be done to assess nerve function near the surgical site. Before he's dis-

68 Chronic arterial occlusive disease

Teaching about vascular repair

If your patient is a candidate for vascular repair to restore circulation to the occluded area, tell him what to expect. As necessary, discuss removal techniques or bypass grafts.

REMOVAL TECHNIQUES

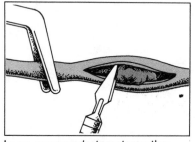

In an *open endarterectomy*, the surgeon cuts the diseased artery lengthwise over the involved segment, then removes the occlusion.

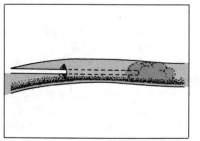

In a *closed endarterectomy*, the surgeon inserts an intra-arterial stripper to remove the atherosclerotic lining of the vessel.

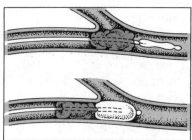

To remove an occlusive embolus, the surgeon may perform a *balloon catheter embolectomy* by threading a deflated catheter through the embolus, inflating the device, then withdrawing it and the embolus.

BYPASS GRAFTS

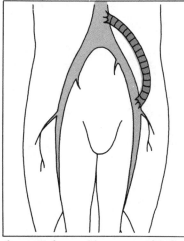

An *aortofemoral bypass graft* helps treat a patient with disabling claudication. Surgery involves major abdominal dissection and aortic manipulation. The surgeon sutures the graft to the aorta and then to the femoral artery, creating a bypass around a femoral artery occlusion.

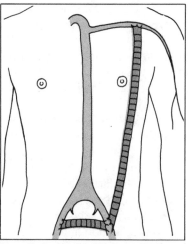

In *axillofemoral bypass graft* surgery, the surgeon sutures a graft to the patient's axillary artery and threads it down along his side in a tunnel created just under his skin to the femoral artery.

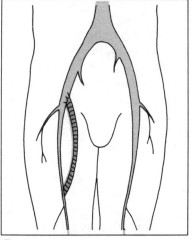

Femoropopliteal bypass graft surgery is used for a patient with disabling intermittent claudication, resulting from occlusion between the femoral and popliteal arteries (associated with atherosclerosis). This procedure can prevent leg loss. The surgeon makes several incisions from ankle to groin, depending on the specific procedure.

charged from the hospital, instruct him to call the doctor immediately if he experiences any changes in speech or level of consciousness, difficulty swallowing, hoarseness, paralysis or weakness in the extremities, or facial drooping—these symptoms could signal developing neurologic damage.

After any of these types of surgery, teach the patient proper incision care. Also advise him to report promptly any early signs of infection, such as fever and pain, redness, swelling, warmth, or drainage at the incision site. Explain that he'll probably be walking within 1 to 5 days after surgery, depending on the extent of the procedure. Ambulation will begin gradually, and he may need to use a cane or walker at first.

Point out that surgery may relieve symptoms, but it won't cure chronic arterial occlusive disease. The patient will still need to follow prescribed treatment measures to prevent further disease progression.

Other care measures

Counsel the patient about long-term management of arterial occlusive disease. If his job involves standing for prolonged periods or working outdoors in cold weather, he may consider changing to an indoor, sedentary occupation or, if possible, retiring early. If the patient agrees, refer him to available social service agencies for counseling.

Also advise the patient of other steps to reduce risk factors for this and other cardiovascular diseases: controlling his weight, minimizing his dietary intake of salt and cholesterol, quitting smoking, learning to reduce stress, and if applicable, receiving proper treatment for hypertension and diabetes.

Finally, teach the patient to recognize and report early warning signs of embolism and aneurysm: sudden onset of excruciating pain, mottling or pallor, difficulty breathing, loss of pulse, and paralysis in the affected extremity.

Further readings

"Femoral Popliteal Disease," *British Journal of Theatre Nursing* 26(11):19, November 1989.

"Fish Oil After PTCA Not Beneficial. . .Percutaneous Transluminal Coronary Angioplasty," *Nurses' Drug Alert* 13(10):78, October 1989.

Grasch, A.L., and Roberts, H.E. "Carotid Bruits: Clinical Significance, Implications, Diagnosis, and Management," *Journal of American Academy of Physician Assistants* 2(6):447-60, 49A, November-December 1989.

Leavitt, V., and Hilton, C.S. "An Uncommon Condition That Nurses Can Spot First," *RN* 52(8):20-22, August 1989.

Sliwa, J.A., et al. "Concurrent Musculoskeletal Pain in a Patient with Symptomatic Lower Extremity Arterial Insufficiency," *Archives of Physical Medicine and Rehabilitation* 70(12):848-50, November 1989.

Stern, P.H. "Occlusive Vascular Disease of Lower Limbs: Diagnosis, Amputation, Surgery, and Rehabilitation: A Review of the Burke Experience," *American Journal of Physical Medicine and Rehabilitation* 67(4):145-54, August 1988.

Young, H.L. "Peripheral Vascular Disease: Arterial Disease of the Lower Limb," Part 1, *British Journal of Occupational Therapy* 52(4):127-29, April 1989.

Do's and don'ts of anticoagulant therapy

Dear Patient:

To hinder your blood's ability to clot, your doctor has prescribed an anticoagulant drug. Follow this list of do's and don'ts when taking this drug.

Do's
• Carry Medic Alert identification stating that you're taking an anticoagulant.
• Use an electric razor to shave or a depilatory to remove unwanted hair.
• Place a rubber mat and safety rails in your bathtub to prevent falls.
• Wear gloves while gardening.

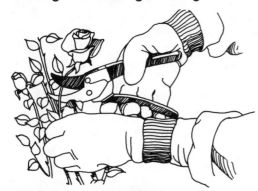

• Use a soft-bristled toothbrush.
• Ensure adequate intake of foods high in vitamin K: green leafy vegetables, tomatoes, bananas, and fish.
• Avoid sharp objects and rough sports. Report abdominal or joint pain or swelling to your doctor.
• Draw a line around the margins of new bruises. If the bruises extend outside of the line, notify your doctor.
• Maintain pressure on all cuts for 10 minutes. If you cut your arm or leg, also elevate it above heart level. If the bleeding doesn't stop, call for help. Then call your doctor immediately.
• Check your urine and stool for any signs of blood.
• Notify your doctor of bleeding gums, nosebleeds, bleeding hemorrhoids, reddish or purplish skin spots, or excessive menstrual flow. Also report vomiting, diarrhea, or fever that lasts longer than 24 hours.
• Keep all appointments for blood tests.
• Refill your prescription at least 1 week before your supply runs out.
• Take your medication at the same time each day, as prescribed. Change your dosage only as directed by your doctor.
• Store your medication away from extreme heat or cold.

Don'ts
• Avoid taking aspirin, drugs containing aspirin, or any other drug (including nonprescription cough and cold remedies and vitamins) without checking with your doctor or pharmacist.
• Don't take an extra dose of your anticoagulant. If you forget to take a dose, just take your next dose at the scheduled time. If you miss two doses, call your doctor.
• Never put toothpicks or sharp objects into your mouth.
• Avoid walking barefoot.
• Don't trim calluses and corns yourself; instead, consult a podiatrist.
• Never use power tools.
• Avoid heavy alcohol consumption.

Learning about pentoxifylline

Dear Patient:

Poor circulation caused by arterial occlusive disease commonly causes leg pain. To help relieve this pain, your doctor has prescribed the drug pentoxifylline (also called Trental). This drug will allow you to walk farther before having to rest because of leg cramps.

Follow instructions
• Take this drug exactly as the label directs.
• Take it with meals to lessen the risk of upsetting your stomach.
• Swallow the tablets whole. Don't crush or break them. Why? Because they are extended-release tablets. This means the drug is designed for slow, steady release into your bloodstream.

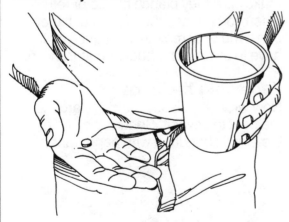

• Don't stop taking the drug if you think it isn't working. Up to 2 weeks may pass before you see any improvement. So it's important to continue taking the drug unless your doctor tells you otherwise.

Report side effects
Let your doctor know if you experience:
• dizziness or headaches
• tremor, agitation, or nervousness
• drowsiness
• insomnia.
   Also call him if you have:
• chest pain
• rapid or irregular heartbeat
• flushing
• swelling in your feet and ankles
• shortness of breath
• persistent upset stomach
• nausea or vomiting.
   If you are elderly, be especially alert for any of the side effects mentioned here. Aging hinders the way your body uses and excretes this drug. As a result, you have a higher risk for side effects.

Use other drugs cautiously
Check with your doctor or pharmacist before taking any other drugs. If you go to more than one doctor or pharmacist, make sure that each one knows about *all* of the drugs you are taking—even those prescribed by another doctor.

Important reminders
• If you're also taking warfarin (Coumadin), you'll need to have more frequent laboratory tests to measure your blood's ability to clot. Remember to keep your blood test appointments.
• Store the drug in a cool, dry place. Also, never let someone else take the drug that your doctor has prescribed for you.

Applying a medicated boot

Dear Patient:

A medicated boot (called an Unna's boot) can protect and medicate your leg ulcers while it prevents swelling. The boot is a bandage containing calamine, glycerin, zinc oxide, and gelatin. Here's how to apply it.

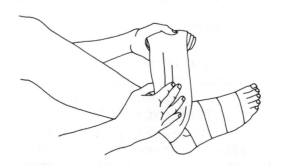

Getting ready
Gather the equipment that you'll need. This includes a scrub sponge with hexachlorophene, normal saline solution, a gauze bandage saturated with medicated paste (Unna's boot), an elastic bandage, paper tape, and moisturizer.

Now, wash your hands thoroughly.

Cleaning the area
Gently clean the lower half of your leg with the scrub sponge. Rinse with normal saline solution. If the skin of your upper calf is dry, apply moisturizer.

Wrapping the boot
Place your foot at a right angle to your leg. Begin wrapping the bandage by making a circular turn around your foot. Then slant the bandage over your heel. Cut the bandage and smooth the edges.

Repeat this procedure, making sure to overlap the bandage in spiral fashion as you wrap.

Next, circle the medicated bandage up and around your leg, moving toward your knee. Use less pressure now than you did when wrapping your foot and ankle. Stop wrapping at 1 or 2 inches below your knee. To cover the area

completely as you wrap, make sure you overlap the previous turn by half the bandage's width.

Repeat this procedure twice more so that your bandage has three layers.

Mold the boot as you apply the bandage to make it smooth and even.

Is the boot too tight?
Wait 30 minutes as the boot dries and hardens. Periodically pinch your toes to make sure they blanch but color returns when you release the pressure. If they don't, the boot may be too tight (you'll have to unwrap the boot and start over).

Fastening the boot
Now wrap the elastic bandage around the boot to cover it. Secure the end of the elastic bandage with paper tape.

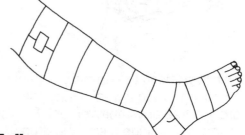

Follow-up
Make sure to remove the boot and repeat this procedure every 5 to 7 days.

Valvular heart disease

When teaching a patient about valvular heart disease, perhaps your greatest challenge will be to convince him that regular follow-up assessment and treatment are critical to preserve his health. That's because the patient may have few symptoms and health problems—at least in the early disease stages. As a result, he may not believe his condition warrants such serious concern.

To help convince him, you'll need to describe how the disease causes extra stress on his heart, leading to possible heart failure, dysrhythmias, and other life-threatening complications. If valvular heart disease causes symptoms, you'll also cover activity and dietary guidelines and any prescribed medications. If indicated, you'll discuss valvular repair or replacement. And you'll stress the importance of recognizing symptoms of worsening disease and, if the patient smokes, of giving up the habit.

Discuss the disorder

Teach the patient how heart valves work to provide efficient blood flow. Explain that the heart has four chambers separated by valves that propel blood by opening and closing in synchrony with the heart's contractions. (For more information, see *How heart valves control blood flow,* page 74.)

Classify the patient's form of valvular heart disease—valvular insufficiency (valvular regurgitation or valvular incompetence), valvular stenosis, or mitral valve prolapse. Mention that valvular insufficiency or stenosis can affect any heart valve.

Inform the patient with valvular *insufficiency* that his valve leaflets fail to close securely, permitting backward blood flow. If the patient has valvular *stenosis,* his valve opening is too narrow, restricting forward blood flow. With either insufficiency or stenosis, the heart's work load increases and blood pools in the heart's chambers. If the patient has both insufficiency and stenosis, explain both functional impairments and possible complications.

Reassure the patient with *mitral valve prolapse* that this form of valvular heart disease is usually benign, although in a few patients the condition may lead to mitral insufficiency.

Describe the patient's particular disorder, including its signs and symptoms and complications. Refer to *Understanding valvular heart disease,* pages 75 and 76, for more information.

Complications

Warn the patient with valvular heart disease that even if he's symptom-free, he'll need continuing assessment and care to prevent or slow heart valve deterioration. Explain that complications may occur despite treatment. Emphasize, though, that treatment

Rosanne Hopson, RN, BSN, a nurse clinician in the cardiology department, University of Iowa Hospitals and Clinics, Iowa City, wrote this chapter.

CHECKLIST

Teaching topics in valvular heart disease

☐ Explanation of normal heart valve function
☐ Causes, signs and symptoms, and complications of the patient's specific valve disease
☐ Importance of complying with treatment to control the disease and prevent complications
☐ Diagnostic tests, including echocardiography, electrocardiography, and cardiac catheterization
☐ Activity restrictions and dietary guidelines
☐ Drugs to control valvular heart disease, such as digoxin, diuretics, beta blockers, nitrates, anticoagulants, and others
☐ How to obtain an accurate pulse rate
☐ Valve repair and replacement surgery, including preoperative and postoperative care
☐ Importance of smoking cessation
☐ Source of information and support

How heart valves control blood flow

Using a model heart or a simple diagram, show your patient the heart's valves and chambers. Point out how the valves regulate blood flow through the heart.

Mention that heart valves are made of endothelium and are covered by fibrous tissue. This makes them sturdy and flexible enough to open and close in response to pressure changes in the heart chambers.

Outline how the blood travels from the body to the right atrium and passes through the tricuspid valve into the right ventricle. As the right ventricle contracts, blood flows through the pulmonic valve into the lungs where it picks up a new supply of oxygen. This newly oxygenated blood then flows from the lungs into the left atrium and passes into the left ventricle through the mitral valve. Finally, when the left ventricle contracts, blood pumps through the aortic valve and into the body.

Explain that when atrial pressure exceeds ventricular pressure, the atrioventricular (AV) valves open (like a swinging door), allowing blood to flow into the ventricles. During systole (when the heart contracts and the valves open to eject the blood), rising ventricular pressure forces the valves closed. The chordae tendineae help keep the valves closed during diastole — also called the filling stage or the rest between heart muscle contractions.

Inform the patient that the semilunar valves (with their three half-moon-shaped cusps) control blood outflow from the ventricles. When right ventricular pressure exceeds pulmonary arterial pressure, the pulmonic valve opens. Similarly, when left ventricular pressure exceeds aortic pressure, the aortic valve opens, allowing blood to flow into the systemic circulation.

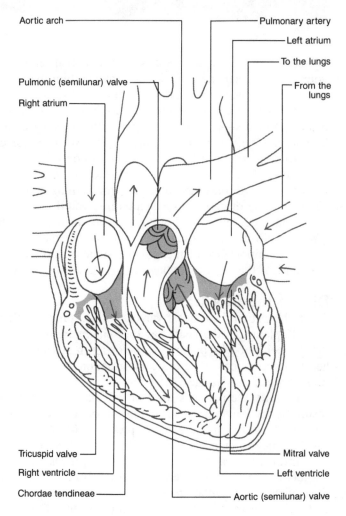

Aortic arch — Pulmonary artery — Left atrium — To the lungs — From the lungs — Pulmonic (semilunar) valve — Right atrium — Tricuspid valve — Right ventricle — Chordae tendineae — Mitral valve — Left ventricle — Aortic (semilunar) valve

can help to relieve symptoms and prevent some complications.

Discuss why the patient is especially at risk for bacterial endocarditis. Explain that slowed, disrupted blood flow may lead to the pooling of blood—a fertile breeding ground for bacteria. As a result, bacteria may colonize on damaged valves, causing inflammation of the cardiac endothelium (the heart muscle's innermost layer), which further damages the heart.

Point out that another complication, an enlarged heart, results from the additional work load. Valvular insufficiency forces the heart to pump harder to propel back-flowing blood forward. Valvular stenosis forces the heart to increase pressure to overcome the resistance to blood flow. As a result of this increased work load, the chambers dilate or the heart muscle enlarges. These effects can cause congestive heart failure, dysrhythmias, and pulmonary edema.

Understanding valvular heart disease

Use this chart as a guide when describing the patient's particular dysfunction, the signs and symptoms he should watch for, and possible complications. Be sure to use terms that he can readily understand.

DISEASE AND CAUSES	PATHOPHYSIOLOGY	SIGNS, SYMPTOMS, AND COMPLICATIONS
Left-sided valve disease		
Mitral stenosis Results from rheumatic fever (most common cause) and congenital disorders, such as tetralogy of Fallot	Thickening and contracture of valve leaflets progressively impede blood flow from the left atrium to the left ventricle. To adequately fill the ventricle and maintain cardiac output, the left atrium must pump more forcefully to push blood through the narrowed opening.	The patient may be asymptomatic or may exhibit dyspnea on exertion, fatigue, rapid, irregular pulse, palpitations, increased left atrial pressure, and pulmonary hypertension. Complications include congestive heart failure, atrial fibrillation, and an enlarged heart.
Mitral insufficiency Results from congenital defects, rheumatic fever, trauma, myxomatous degeneration, valve calcification and stretching of the mitral valve secondary to ventricular dilation, rupture of papillary muscle or chordae tendineae, endocarditis, or rarely, mitral valve prolapse	Valve leaflets fail to close tightly, permitting blood to flow back into the left atrium during left ventricular contraction. This forces the heart to pump harder so that the extra blood from the left atrium will flow into the left ventricle, which eventually dilates to accommodate the additional blood volume.	The patient may be asymptomatic or may develop dyspnea and fatigue (late in chronic insufficiency), symptoms of pulmonary edema, palpitations, and chest pain. Complications include congestive heart failure and an enlarged heart.
Mitral valve prolapse Also called floppy mitral valve syndrome, Barlow's syndrome, and billowing mitral valve syndrome — usually idiopathic and commonly inherited	Enlarged valve leaflets bulge backward into the left atrium during ventricular systole.	Usually no symptoms, but patient may experience sharp chest pain unrelated to exercise, fatigue, palpitations, lightheadedness, syncope, dyspnea, anxiety, and panic attacks. Complications include supraventricular and ventricular dysrhythmias, chordae tendineae rupture, and mitral insufficiency (occasionally).
Aortic stenosis Results from rheumatic fever (most common cause between ages 30 to 70), degenerative calcification of aortic valve (after age 70), and congenital malformation of aortic valve (symptoms after age 60)	Fibrosis or calcification of the aortic valve obstructs blood flow from the left ventricle into the aorta during ventricular contraction. With increasing resistance to ventricular emptying, the pressure work of the left ventricle rises. To compensate, the left ventricle hypertrophies to generate more pressure and maintain peripheral perfusion.	The patient may experience angina pectoris and syncope upon exertion and may develop left ventricular failure with signs of pulmonary congestion, dyspnea, orthopnea, and paroxysmal nocturnal dyspnea.
Aortic insufficiency Usually results from valve damage from rheumatic fever, syphilis or endocarditis, but sometimes associated with Marfan's syndrome, rheumatoid arthritis, ankylosing spondylitis, severe hypertension, or congenital defects, such as tetralogy of Fallot	Aortic valve fails to close properly, causing blood backflow into the left ventricle during diastole.	The patient may experience an unusually forceful heartbeat with visible carotid pulse, dyspnea on exertion, progressing to paroxysmal nocturnal dyspnea and orthopnea (pulmonary congestion), angina (beginning about 2 years after onset of dyspnea), and dysrhythmias. Complications include left ventricular failure and pulmonary edema.

continued

Understanding valvular heart disease – *continued*

DISEASE AND CAUSES	PATHOPHYSIOLOGY	SIGNS, SYMPTOMS, AND COMPLICATIONS
Right-sided valve disease		
Tricuspid stenosis Results from rheumatic fever (most common cause), mitral stenosis, congenital disorders, endocarditis (uncommon cause)	Stiffened tricuspid valve leaflets open improperly, impairing blood flow from the right atrium to the right ventricle during diastole.	The patient may experience fatigue, fluttering sensation in neck, cyanosis, and signs of right heart failure: peripheral edema, liver enlargement, ascites, nausea, vomiting, and anorexia.
Tricuspid insufficiency Occurs secondary to right ventricular failure or infarction or pulmonary hypertension. Also related to tricuspid stenosis from rheumatic fever, endocarditis, papillary muscle dysfunction, and myxomatous degeneration	Diseased valve closes improperly, causing blood backflow from the right ventricle into the right atrium during systole.	Patient may develop signs of right heart failure: peripheral edema, liver enlargement, ascites, nausea, vomiting, and anorexia.
Pulmonary stenosis (rare) Results from congenital defects, rheumatic fever, endocarditis, and trauma	Stiffened pulmonic valve leaflets impair blood flow from the right ventricle into the lungs.	The patient may be asymptomatic or have dyspnea, fatigue, syncope, chest pain, and right heart failure symptoms: peripheral edema, liver enlargement, ascites, nausea, vomiting, and anorexia.
Pulmonary insufficiency Results from pulmonary artery hypertension related to left-sided valvular heart disease, pulmonary artery dilation, endocarditis, and congenital disorders	Diseased pulmonic valve closes improperly, causing blood backflow into the right ventricle during diastole.	Patient is asymptomatic unless right-sided heart failure develops with peripheral edema, liver enlargement, ascites, nausea, vomiting, and anorexia.

Describe the diagnostic workup

Explain that the doctor searches the patient's health history for evidence of rheumatic heart disease or endocarditis, both of which damage the valves. He'll also perform a thorough cardiac examination, listening carefully for heart sounds associated with valvular heart disease.

Teach about noninvasive tests, such as chest X-ray, electrocardiography (ECG), and echocardiography to diagnose valvular heart disease. Also prepare the patient for cardiac catheterization, an invasive test that confirms the diagnosis.

Chest X-ray

Explain that a chest X-ray shows the heart's size and the blood vessels within the lungs. Mention that this test takes only minutes but that the technician may need additional time to check the quality of the X-ray film. Before the test, instruct the patient to remove his clothing above the waist and to put on a gown without snaps. Tell him to remove all jewelry and metal objects from his neck and chest.

For an X-ray study performed in the radiology department, inform the patient that he'll stand or sit in front of a machine. If the X-ray study's done at bedside, someone will help him to a sitting position and place a cold, hard film plate behind his back.

In either place, he'll be instructed to take a deep breath, hold it, and remain still for a few seconds while the film is taken. Reassure him that radiation exposure is minimal.

Electrocardiography
Explain that electrocardiography (ECG) evaluates cardiac function. Tell the patient that by recording the heart's electrical activity, an ECG may show conduction and rhythm abnormalities associated with valvular heart disease and signs of cardiac enlargement, too.

Inform the patient that an ECG takes about 15 minutes. Just before the test, the doctor (or a technician) will cleanse, dry, and possibly shave different sites on the patient's body, such as the chest and arms. Then he'll apply a conductive jelly to the patient's skin where he'll attach electrodes.

During the test the patient will lie still, relax, breathe normally, and remain quiet. Explain that talking or moving will distort the ECG recordings and require extra testing time.

Echocardiography
Inform the patient that echocardiography can confirm and evaluate valvular abnormalities and show heart chamber size, wall motion, and valve movements. Explain that the test takes 15 to 30 minutes, and is safe and painless. Mention that other tests, such as an ECG, may be performed simultaneously. Give the patient the teaching aid *Preparing for echocardiography*, page 85.

Cardiac catheterization
Inform the patient that this invasive test can evaluate blood flow through the heart, pressures within its chambers, valve structure, and pumping ability.

Tell the patient that the test is done in the cardiac catheterization laboratory and may take up to 3 hours. Instruct him not to eat or drink anything for 6 hours before the test. Explain that he'll lie on a padded operating room table, and his groin area will be cleansed and shaved to allow the doctor to insert a peripheral I.V. line and to attach electrodes to various body sites. Mention that he'll receive a mild I.V. sedative to help him relax.

After the doctor injects a local anesthetic to numb the patient's groin, he'll thread a catheter through an artery to the left side of the patient's heart or through a vein to the right side of the heart and to the lungs. Next, he'll inject a contrast medium through the catheter. Then the patient may feel flushed or nauseated or experience chest pain. Explain that the contrast medium outlines specific structures on the X-ray film. Assure him that the sensations from its infusion should pass quickly.

Tell him that he may be directed to cough or breathe deeply and that he may receive nitroglycerin during the test. This drug will dilate his coronary vessels to aid visualization.

Advise the patient that the doctor will remove the catheter when the test ends and apply pressure and a bulky dressing to control bleeding. The nurse will monitor the site for swelling. Instruct the patient to keep his leg straight for several hours and, once he's allowed to resume his diet, to drink plenty of fluids.

Teach about treatments

If the patient has symptoms of valvular heart disease, outline activity and diet restrictions and teach about medication. (Refer to *Teaching about drugs for valvular heart disease* for further information.) If indicated, discuss valvular repair—valvuloplasty, annuloplasty, or commissurotomy—or replacement with a prosthetic valve. Cover other important care measures.

Activity

Advise the patient that while he's symptom-free, he won't have to limit his activities. But once symptoms occur, the doctor may restrict strenuous activities, such as heavy lifting. Warn the patient that disregarding prescribed activity guidelines could worsen his disease or lead to complications, such as dysrhythmias.

Diet

Point out ways to restrict salt if the patient suffers from fluid retention. Advise him to avoid or limit most processed foods, luncheon meats, canned soups and vegetables, snack foods, and condiments. Suggest that he use alternative table-salt flavorings, such as herbs, lemon juice, or a sodium-free salt substitute.

Medication

If the doctor prescribes digoxin for an aortic or mitral valve disorder, tell the patient that this drug should strengthen his heart's pumping ability.

If the doctor prescribes the beta-blocker propranolol, inform the patient that this drug helps stabilize the irregular heart beat associated with atrial fibrillation, occurring in mitral stenosis. Give him a copy of the patient-teaching aid *Learning about propranolol,* page 30. With either digoxin or a beta blocker, explain how to obtain an accurate pulse rate. Reinforce your instruction with the patient-teaching aid *How to take your pulse,* page 26.

Tell the patient with atrial fibrillation that his doctor may also prescribe anticoagulants, such as warfarin, or antiplatelets, such as aspirin and dipyridamole, to reduce the blood's clotting ability. Explain that atrial fibrillation can cause blood to pool in the heart, making it more vulnerable to clot formation. Inform the patient with a valve replacement that he is also vulnerable to clots and will be taking anticoagulants for life. Provide a copy of the patient-teaching aid *Learning about warfarin,* page 86.

If the patient experiences shortness of breath and fatigue (especially if these symptoms limit his daily activities), the doctor may prescribe a diuretic, such as furosemide. Explain that diuretics help reduce cardiac work load by decreasing blood volume. Warn the patient that he will probably urinate frequently because the drug removes excess fluids from the body.

For the patient with an aortic valve dysfunction, such as stenosis, the doctor may prescribe an oral nitrate, such as nitroglycerin, to relieve chest pain. Explain that nitrates enhance vasodilation, causing more blood to remain in the veins and reducing the volume of blood that returns to the heart. This lightens

Teaching about drugs for valvular heart disease

DRUG	ADVERSE REACTIONS	TEACHING POINTS
Anticoagulant		
warfarin (Coumadin, Panwarfin)	• Watch for back pain, bleeding nose or gums, chills, constipation, dark blue toes, discolored urine, dizziness, excessive menstrual flow, fatigue, fever, pain or swelling in joints or stomach, prolonged bleeding from cuts or bruises, prolonged diarrhea, red or black stool, sore throat, severe or continuing headache, and vomiting (sometimes bloody). • Other reactions include bruising, diarrhea, nausea, and slight hair loss.	• Explain to the patient that this drug should prevent blood clots in his legs, lungs, and heart. • Inform him that he'll need frequent blood tests to monitor the drug's effects. • Help him obtain a Medic Alert tag or card, identifying him as a warfarin user. • Teach measures to reduce the risk of bleeding, such as always wearing shoes, placing a nonslip mat in the bathtub, shaving with an electric razor, using a soft toothbrush, and wearing gloves for yard work. • If the patient's female of childbearing age, emphasize the need for practicing birth control. That's because warfarin can adversely affect fetal development and cause placental bleeding. • Instruct the patient to avoid over-the-counter drugs containing aspirin or acetaminophen and high doses of vitamins A and E. • Tell the patient to limit alcoholic beverage consumption to one or two drinks daily. • Because vitamin K counteracts warfarin, stress the need to maintain a consistent intake of vitamin K and of fats, which enhance vitamin K absorption. Explain that this is necessary to adjust his warfarin dosage precisely. • Tell him to take a missed dose as soon as possible, but warn him not to double-dose. If he misses a day, instruct him not to take the missed dose at all.
Antiplatelets		
aspirin	• Watch for bleeding gums, easy bruising, hearing loss, hematemesis, tarry stools, and tinnitus. • Other reactions include GI upset and headache.	• Explain to the patient that aspirin hinders platelet function, which prevents clot formation. • To relieve mild GI distress, advise the patient to take aspirin with food or milk or to use a buffered or enteric-coated form of the drug. • When taking aspirin, he should avoid antacids, which can reduce the drug's effectiveness. He should also avoid drinking alcoholic beverages during therapy because GI bleeding may occur. • Also warn against substituting acetaminophen, which doesn't share aspirin's antithrombotic effects. • Tell him to take a missed dose within 12 hours, but warn him not to double-dose.
dipyridamole (Persantine)	• Watch for chest pain or tightness, vomiting, and weakness. • Other reactions include dizziness, GI upset, and heartburn.	• Explain to the patient that this drug hinders platelet function, which prevents clot formation. • Instruct him to take the drug 1 hour before or 3 hours after a meal. • Tell him to take the drug with a light snack or a glass of milk to help reduce GI distress. • To minimize dizziness, advise the patient to rise slowly from a sitting or lying position. • Tell him to take a missed dose as soon as possible, but warn him not to double-dose. • Warn against drinking alcohol during therapy. Dizziness may result.

continued

Teaching about drugs for valvular heart disease — *continued*

DRUG	ADVERSE REACTIONS	TEACHING POINTS
Beta-adrenergic blockers		
acebutolol (Sectral) **atenolol** (Tenormin) **labetalol** (Trandate) **metoprolol** (Lopressor) **nadolol** (Corgard) **pindolol** (Visken) **propranolol** (Inderal) **timolol** (Blocadren)	• Watch for depression, dizziness, dyspnea, rash, very slow heart rate, and wheezing. • Other reactions include decreased libido, diarrhea, fatigue, headache, insomnia, nasal stuffiness, nausea, vivid dreams and nightmares, and vomiting.	• Explain that this drug can reduce the frequency of angina attacks. • If the patient takes one dose daily, instruct him to take a missed dose within 8 hours. If he takes two or more doses each day, instruct him to take a missed dose as soon as possible. However, warn him never to double-dose. • Teach him to take his pulse before taking the drug and to notify his doctor if it falls below 60 beats/minute. • Instruct him to take labetalol, metoprolol, and propranolol with foods to increase drug absorption. • Warn him against suddenly discontinuing the drug. He must taper the dosage, as directed, to avoid complications. • If the patient complains of insomnia, suggest that he take the drug no later than 2 hours before bedtime.
Cardiac glycoside		
digoxin (Lanoxicaps, Lanoxin)	• Watch for abdominal pain, anorexia, visual disturbances, dizziness, drowsiness, fatigue, headache, irregular heart rate, loss of appetite, malaise, nausea, and vomiting. • Other reactions include breast enlargement.	• Explain that this drug controls the rate and rhythm of the patient's heartbeat. • Teach the patient to take his pulse before taking digoxin and to report an unusually low pulse rate to his doctor. • Tell him to avoid antacids, kaolin and pectin mixtures, antidiarrheals, and laxatives, which decrease digoxin absorption. Also instruct him to limit his fiber intake, as dietary fiber can decrease digoxin absorption. • If he is also taking cholestyramine (Questran or Cholybar), advise him to wait at least 2 hours after taking digoxin before taking this medicine. • Tell him to establish a regular routine for taking digoxin each day. • Warn him not to take another person's tablets because different generic digoxin tablets are absorbed at different rates. • Instruct him to take a missed dose within 12 hours, but warn him not to double-dose.
Loop diuretics		
bumetanide (Bumex) **ethacrynic acid** (Edecrin) **furosemide** (Lasix)	• Watch for fever, hearing loss, increased thirst, jaundice, muscle cramps, nausea, tinnitus, unusual fatigue or weakness, urgent or burning urination, and vomiting. • Other reactions include anorexia, blurred vision, diarrhea, dizziness, muscle aches and cramps, and weight loss.	• Explain to the patient that this drug should reduce his cardiac work load. • If the patient takes the drug twice daily, tell him to take the second dose in late afternoon rather than at night to prevent sleep interruption from nocturia. • Advise him to take the drug with meals to prevent GI distress. • Encourage intake of high-potassium foods (citrus foods, tomatoes, bananas, dates, and apricots). Remind him to take potassium supplements if ordered. • Instruct him to record his weight daily to monitor fluid loss. • To minimize postural hypotension, tell him to rise slowly from a lying or sitting position. • Advise him to limit alcohol intake to prevent dizziness. • Instruct him to take a missed dose as soon as possible. Warn him not to double-dose.

continued

Teaching about drugs for valvular heart disease — *continued*

DRUG	ADVERSE REACTIONS	TEACHING POINTS
Nitrates		
erythrityl tetranitrate (Cardilate) **isosorbide dinitrate** (multiple forms and brands) **nitroglycerin** (multiple forms and brands) **pentaerythritol tetranitrate** (Duotrate, Peritrate)	• Watch for blurred vision, extreme dizziness, dry mouth, rapid heart rate, and skin irritation or rash. • Other reactions include headache, flushing, mild dizziness, nausea, and vomiting.	• If nitroglycerin tablets are prescribed for acute angina attacks, instruct the patient to take one tablet every 5 minutes up to a maximum of three tablets. Tell him to hold each tablet under his tongue until it dissolves. Meanwhile, he should sit down and try to relax. If the tablets bring no relief, tell him to call his doctor immediately or have someone take him to an emergency department at once. • If he uses nitrates to prevent angina, teach him to maintain a self-administration schedule. He should also take the drug before any activity that induces angina, such as exposure to cold, exertion, or sex. • Advise him to avoid overly hot showers. Vasodilation might make him dizzy and faint. To prevent dizziness, tell him to rise slowly from a sitting or lying position. • Reassure him that headaches should diminish with continued use of nitrates. If they don't, tell him to notify his doctor. • Because nitroglycerin tablets must be fresh to be effective, tell the patient to cap the bottle quickly and tightly after each use and to replace an opened bottle after 3 months, even if some tablets remain. • Instruct him to shield tablets from light. • Tell him to take a missed dose as soon as possible, but warn him not to double-dose.
Thiazide and thiazide-like diuretics		
chlorothiazide (Diuril) **chlorthalidone** (Hygroton, Thalitone) **hydrochloro-thiazide** (multiple brands) **metolazone** (Diulo, Zaroxolyn)	• Watch for dry mouth, excessive thirst, fever, irregular heart rate, lethargy, dry mouth, muscle cramps, rash, urgent or burning urination, weakness, and weak pulse. • Other reactions include anorexia, diarrhea, dizziness, GI distress, and restlessness.	• Explain that this drug reduces cardiac work load. • Instruct the patient not to take an evening dose just before bedtime, to prevent sleep interruption from nocturia. • Caution the diabetic patient that this drug may elevate his blood glucose level. • Instruct him to record his weight daily to monitor fluid loss. • Advise him to avoid large doses of calcium supplements. • Tell him to check with his doctor or pharmacist before taking over-the-counter cold or allergy preparations. Many contain drugs that may increase his blood pressure and decrease the effectiveness of this medication. • Tell him to increase intake of potassium-rich foods, such as bananas and citrus fruits. • Tell him to take a missed daily dose within 8 hours. Otherwise, he should skip the missed dose. Warn him not to double-dose.

the heart's work load, permitting more effective pumping action. If appropriate, give him the patient-teaching aid *How to use nitroglycerin,* pages 28 and 29.

Reinforce the need for antibiotics to prevent endocarditis before and after any dental procedure or surgery. After exposure to the streptoccoccus bacteria, advise the patient to contact the doctor for treatment with pencillin or sulfonamides to prevent a recurrence of acute rheumatic fever, which can further damage his heart valves.

Surgery
Tell the patient that surgery to repair or replace a valve is usually done only if medication fails to relieve symptoms. If appropriate,

Explaining types of prosthetic heart valves

Before the doctor chooses the patient's new heart valve, he'll evaluate its design, durability, and hemodynamic qualities. He'll also consider the patient's ability to comply with lifelong anticoagulant therapy.

Here's why. Mechanical valves encourage thrombus formation, so the patient must take anticoagulants for the rest of his life and undergo regular prothrombin time testing. For a patient who's unlikely to comply, the doctor may select a bioprosthetic valve instead because it doesn't require long-term anticoagulant therapy.

Mechanical valve features
The *ball cage* mechanical valve, such as the Starr caged-ball valve (by Baxter-Edwards), can withstand

considerable stress. However, its large size makes it sometimes difficult to implant, and blood flow is turbulent through the valve.

Bioprosthetic valve features
The biological prosthetic heart valve, such as the Carpentier valve (by Baxter-Edwards), doesn't obstruct blood flow as much as a mechanical valve and is less likely to cause thrombus formation. In addition, a biological prosthetic valve doesn't require prolonged anticoagulant therapy. However, the valve is difficult to insert and less durable (prone to degeneration or calcification, especially in patients with renal disease) than its mechanical counterpart.

STARR VALVE   **CARPENTIER VALVE**

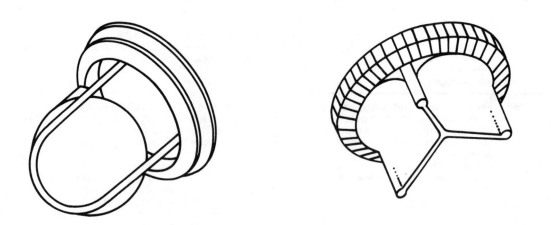

explain that *valvuloplasty* repairs the valve and sutures the torn leaflets, *annuloplasty* tightens and sutures the annulus ring of the malfunctioning valve, and *commissurotomy (or valvotomy)* dilates the valve's commissures to enlarge the valve opening.

If the patient will undergo valve replacement, inform him that the surgeon will remove his diseased valve and replace it with a prosthetic device. Explain the two kinds: mechanical devices and bioprostheses. Add that he could receive a homograft—the aortic valve of a human cadaver—if one is available (see *Explaining types of prosthetic heart valves*).

Inform the patient that valve repair or replacement will take place during open heart surgery. Explain that the surgeon will open the mediastinum and expose the heart and great vessels. Then he'll place the patient on a cardiopulmonary bypass machine, which removes blood from the body just before it reaches the heart. The machine oxygenates the blood and then returns it to the body through the ascending aorta—just as the heart does normally. To prepare the patient, discuss preoperative, postoperative, and long-term care.

Preoperative care. Inform the patient that he'll be asked to shower with a special antiseptic soap and may be shaved from his neck to his toes. Tell him that he won't be allowed to eat or drink anything after midnight, although he can request a sleeping pill. He may receive a sedative the morning of surgery to help him relax.

Postoperative care. Tell the patient where he'll be taken to recover after the procedure. If possible, arrange a tour for the patient and his family before surgery.

Explain the complex and often frightening equipment that will support the patient's vital functions after surgery. For example, prepare the patient for intubation and mechanical ventilation. Mention that he won't be able to speak while intubated but that he will be able to communicate by gesturing or writing.

Explain to the patient that an intra-aortic balloon pump may be inserted to provide circulatory support for several hours postoperatively. He'll also have a nasogastric tube, a mediastinal chest tube, and an indwelling catheter in place for the first day or two. In addition, he'll be connected to a cardiac monitor.

Teach the patient about short-term postoperative care measures and his role in implementing them. Start with the expected course of his hospital stay—how many days he'll spend in the critical care area, stepdown unit, and regular room before discharge.

Emphasize that his top priority is to relax and rest; stress and anxiety will only hinder his recovery. Encourage him to request pain medication to promote relaxation. When the endotracheal and nasogastric tubes are removed, he'll be able to sit up and swallow liquids. Tell him that solid foods will then gradually be reintroduced to his diet.

To help prevent pulmonary complications, encourage the patient to perform coughing and deep-breathing exercises. Teach him how to splint his incision to minimize pain and how to use an incentive spirometer. Reassure him that coughing won't loosen or damage the graft or reopen his chest incision.

Next, discuss other self-care measures. About 6 days after surgery, the patient will probably be allowed to shower. Instruct him to use warm, not hot, water and to wash all incision sites gently. Explain that complete healing takes time and that he'll always have a scar (although it will fade). Suggest that he wear soft, loose clothing, such as cotton T-shirts, at first for maximum comfort.

Long-term care. As the patient gains strength, begin teaching him about long-term care measures. Review his prescribed exercise program. Emphasize the need to increase his activity level gradually, and encourage him to set realistic goals. Teach him to alternate light and heavy tasks and to rest between tasks. Reinforce the doctor's restrictions on such activities as lifting, working, and driving, as appropriate. Because medications form an important part of postoperative care, make sure the patient understands their administration schedules and possible adverse effects.

INQUIRY

Questions patients ask after valve replacement

How will I know if my new heart valve's working?
You'll feel much better when your valve's working. If it malfunctions, you may have shortness of breath, chest pain, or dizziness. You may also notice that your hands and feet feel cold more frequently. If you experience these symptoms, contact your doctor.

When can I resume my normal activities?
In about 6 weeks. Soon after your surgery, you'll do simple exercises and motions in bed. Within 2 days, you'll be out of bed and sitting in a chair. Next, you'll take short walks and progress to two 10-minute walks a day. Then, you'll either do more walking or you'll get to pedal a stationary bike. When you leave the hospital, you should be able to do light chores.

For the first 3 to 4 weeks at home, try to climb only one flight of stairs once a day.

For the first 5 weeks, don't drive a car; and if you're a passenger, remember to wear a lap and shoulder belt. On long trips, stop hourly to walk and stretch your legs.

For the first 6 weeks (the time it takes your breastbone wound to heal), don't lift, push, or pull anything heavier than 5 lb.

As for work, most patients recuperate at home until their 6-week follow-up examination. Then they return to their work schedule gradually, beginning with half-time and working up to a full day.

Will using my microwave oven or having X-rays affect my new heart valve?
No. The manufacturer designs your valve to operate safely around microwaves and X-rays.

Before discharge, teach the patient the signs and symptoms of valve dysfunction (see *Questions patients ask after valve replacement*). Remind him to notify his other doctors and dentist of the surgery. This is necessary because patients with artificial valves have a higher risk for endocarditis and need antibiotics before, during, and after invasive procedures. Also prepare him for postoperative depression, which may not set in until he's home. Reassure him that depression is usually temporary.

Address the patient's concerns about sex after surgery. Reassure him that once the doctor has given his okay, sex is no more dangerous to his heart than walking up a couple flights of stairs. Point out that a satisfying sex life can help speed his recovery.

Advise him to reduce strain on his heart by avoiding sex right after eating a big meal or drinking alcohol, when he's fatigued or emotionally upset, or when he's in an unfamiliar and stressful situation—in a strange environment or with a new partner, for example. Tell him to choose a position that doesn't restrict his breathing; he should also avoid any position in which he has to support himself or his partner with his arms. Explain that impotence is fairly common but that it's almost always temporary.

Other care measures
If the patient smokes, stress the critical need to quit, especially if he's already experiencing symptoms of valve disease. Explain that because smoking constricts arterioles, it places an extra burden on his already overworked heart and lungs. Refer him to support groups and written materials on how to stop smoking.

Teach the patient to notify his doctor if he experiences the following symptoms of valve disorders: increasing fatigue, dyspnea, irregular heart rate or palpitations, dizziness or syncope, and chest pain.

Source of information and support
American Heart Association
7320 Greenville Avenue, Dallas, Tex. 75231
(214) 373-6300

Further readings

Baas, L., and Kretten, C. "Valvular Heart Disease: Its Causes, Symptoms and Consequences, Part 1," *RN* 50(11):30-36, November 1987.

Cullen, L., and Laxson, C. "Ballooning Open a Stenotic Valve," *American Journal of Nursing* 88(7):987-88, 990, 992, July 1988.

Gortner, S.R., and Zyzanski, S.J. "Values in Choice of Treatment: Replication and Refinement...A Sample of Bypass and Valve Replacement Patients and Families," *Nursing Research* 37(4):240-44, July-August 1988.

Grof, D., et al. "The Homograft: A New Dimension for Cardiac Valve Replacement," *Association of Operating Room Nurses Journal* 48(5):911-13, 915-17, November 1988.

Kretten, C., and Baas L. "Valvular Heart Disease: Surgery and Post-Op Care," *RN* 50(12):38-43, December 1987.

Warshaw, M.P., et al. "Pulmonary Valvuloplasty as an Alternative to Surgery in the Pediatric Patient: Implications for Nursing," *Heart and Lung* 17(5):521-27, September 1988.

Preparing for echocardiography

Dear Patient:

Your doctor has scheduled you for a test called echocardiography to learn about your heart's size, shape, movement, and surrounding structures. The test doesn't hurt. It takes 30 minutes or less to perform, and you don't have to do anything special to prepare for it.

What happens first
Once you reach the test location — usually the echocardiography lab, but elsewhere if the hospital has portable equipment — you'll undress and put on a hospital gown or cover yourself with a large, sheetlike drape. Most likely, you'll see an examining table, some machines, and a TV screen. The lab may be darkened to help the technician view the TV screen.

What happens next
The doctor or a technician will ask you to lie on the table, either on your back or your side. Then he'll rub a gel on your chest and position an instrument called a transducer over your heart. He'll also apply disk-shaped electrodes on your chest and arms. These electrodes will record the electrical activity coming from your heart. (This procedure's called electrocardiography, or ECG.)

How the test works
Because the echocardiography machine generates high-pitched sound waves, you won't be able to hear them,

but the transducer will transmit them toward your heart. The sound waves will bounce off your heart walls, valves, and surrounding structures and will be received by the same transducer that transmitted them.

Then these echoes will be translated electronically into an image of your heart and its structures that the doctor or technician will see on the TV screen (or read on special paper).

Simultaneous ECG tracings will help the doctor interpret the echocardiogram.

Test variations
The doctor or technician may obtain a series of heart images by positioning the transducer at different angles to observe different parts of your heart.

He may ask you to breathe in and out slowly, to hold your breath, or to inhale a sweet-smelling gas (amyl nitrate). Then he'll note changes in the way your heart functions during each task.

You may experience some dizziness, flushing, or rapid heart beats from the gas, but these will subside quickly.

Remember to stay still during the test because movements can distort results.

Test results
The doctor or technician will remove the transducer and electrodes and wipe the gel off your chest. He may give you a preliminary interpretation of the test's results immediately, but usually the lab sends the test results to your doctor who will explain them to you.

Learning about warfarin

Dear Patient:

Your doctor has prescribed warfarin (also called Coumadin or Panwarfin) for you. By reducing your blood's ability to clot, this medicine prevents harmful clots from forming in your blood vessels. Warfarin won't dissolve clots that you already have. But it should stop clots from growing larger and causing complications.

Follow instructions exactly

Take warfarin only as your doctor directs. Don't take more or less, and don't take it more often or longer than he directs. Take it at the same time each day, and take a missed dose as soon as possible. Then go back to your regular schedule.

If you miss a day, don't take the missed dose at all, and never take a double dose. This may cause bleeding.

Report side effects

Call your doctor at once if your gums bleed when you brush your teeth. Also call him if you have bruises or purplish marks on your skin, nosebleeds, heavy bleeding or oozing from cuts or wounds, excessive or unexpected menstrual bleeding, blood in your urine or sputum, bloody or tarry black stools, or vomit that looks like coffee grounds.

Call your doctor if you have unusual pain or swelling in your joints or your stomach, unusual backaches, diarrhea, constipation, dizziness, or a severe or continuing headache.

Watch your diet

Maintain regular eating habits and consume your usual amount of vegetables and fruits. Don't start a weight-loss diet before asking your doctor. If you drink alcoholic beverages, limit yourself to one or two a day.

Ask about other drugs

Check with your doctor before taking any nonprescription medicines. Certain vitamins can reduce warfarin's effectiveness, and aspirin and similar drugs can cause bleeding.

Special instructions

• To reduce your risk of injuring yourself, always wear shoes, place a nonskid mat in your bathtub, shave with an electric razor, and use a soft toothbrush.
• Remember to keep your blood test appointments. If blood tests show that your blood isn't clotting at the right rate, the doctor may decide to adjust your dosage.
• Make sure to let your other doctors and your dentist know you're taking warfarin.
• Wear a Medic Alert tag or card, identifying you as a warfarin user.
• If you're female and considering becoming pregnant, think about delaying pregnancy. That's because warfarin can adversely affect fetal development and cause placental bleeding.
• Check with your doctor before beginning any strenuous programs. And avoid risky activities — for example, roughhousing with children and dogs.

CHAPTER

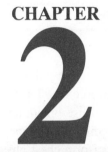

2

Respiratory Conditions

Contents

Chronic obstructive pulmonary disease

The second leading cause of disability in the United States, chronic obstructive pulmonary disease (COPD) will challenge your teaching skills. In acute stages of COPD, the patient's chronic dyspnea, exhaustion, and fear may all interfere with learning. Proceed slowly but steadily with your teaching. Even though you can't halt the progression of this debilitating disease, your teaching can make a tremendous difference in the patient's quality of life.

Much of your time will be devoted to coaching the patient in making necessary life-style changes. For instance, you'll need to convince him to take preventive measures, participate in prescribed exercise regularly, and maintain a proper diet. You may need to persuade him to break entrenched habits, such as smoking. Getting such lessons across effectively will help your patient control his dyspnea and avoid exacerbating his condition.

You'll also need to clarify numerous diagnostic tests and treatments for your patient, including pulmonary function studies, chest X-rays, chest physiotherapy, oxygen therapy, and drug therapy. What's more, you'll need to give him advice on daily disease management: avoiding exposure to toxic inhalants, controlling dyspnea during sexual intercourse, and recognizing early symptoms of peptic ulcer.

Discuss the disorder

The most common forms of COPD are chronic bronchitis, emphysema, and asthma. All share one important characteristic: airway obstruction leading to dyspnea.

In chronic bronchitis, repeated exposure to irritants inflames the airways, causing them to swell and clog with mucus. In emphysema, such inflammation eventually destroys the alveoli and bronchioles, creating air spaces known as blebs or bullae.

Asthma is characterized by episodic bronchospasm and airway obstruction. In extrinsic asthma, external factors (allergens) trigger bronchospasm. In intrinsic asthma, stress, infection, or some other internal factor triggers it. At times, bronchospasm's cause may not be known. Repeated bronchospasm causes bronchial hypertrophy with thickened epithelium and edematous walls. Then, airways become obstructed and secretions trapped.

COPD may also include cystic fibrosis and bronchiectasis. (See *When airways become obstructed,* page 90.)

Sandra Ludwig Nettina, RN,C, MSN, CRNP, who wrote this chapter, is an adult nurse practitioner in the emergency department at Temple University Hospital, Philadelphia.

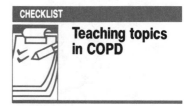

CHECKLIST

Teaching topics in COPD

□ Explanation of COPD, including the patient's specific type
□ Complications
□ Preparation for pulmonary function tests, chest X-rays, and other diagnostic studies
□ Exercise program, activity tips, and breathing exercises to avoid dyspnea
□ Importance of diet, adequate hydration, and combating obesity
□ Drugs and their administration
□ How to use an oral inhaler
□ Chest physiotherapy at home
□ Oxygen therapy at home
□ Importance of avoiding bronchial irritants, such as cigarette smoke, allergens, and adverse weather conditions
□ Warning signs of peptic ulcer
□ Sources of information and support

When airways become obstructed

Explain to your patient with COPD that airway narrowing obstructs flow to and from the lungs. This obstruction markedly increases the work of breathing and resistance to airflow. Air becomes trapped in the bronchioles and alveoli. The trapped air, in turn, hinders normal gas exchange and distends the alveoli. Describe normal breathing; then teach your patient about airway obstruction in his specific form of COPD.

Normal breathing

Inform your patient that during normal breathing, enough air continually moves in and out of the lungs to meet metabolic needs. However, any change in airway size reduces the lungs' ability to provide sufficient air.

NORMAL BRONCHIOLE

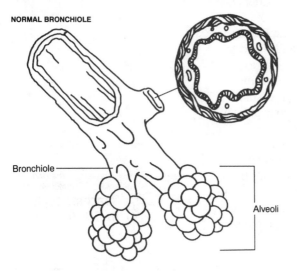

Bronchiole

Alveoli

Emphysema

Tell your patient with emphysema that recurrent inflammation damages and eventually destroys the alveolar walls, thereby creating large air spaces. Alveolar destruction also leads to loss of elastic recoil, causing bronchiolar collapse on expiration and trapping of air within the lungs. However, associated pulmonary capillary destruction usually allows a patient with severe emphysema to match ventilation to perfusion and thus avoid cyanosis.

ALVEOLAR WALL BREAKDOWN

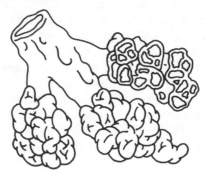

Chronic bronchitis

Explain that in chronic bronchitis repeated exposure to inhaled irritants produces widespread inflammation and increased mucus production, narrowing or blocking the airways. This, in turn, increases airway resistance, causing severe ventilation-perfusion mismatch marked by cyanosis.

MUCOSAL INFLAMMATION AND HYPERTROPHY

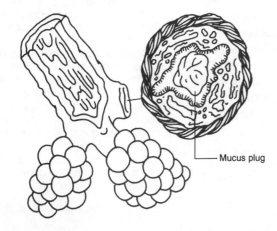

Mucus plug

Asthma

If your patient has bronchial asthma, explain that repeated smooth muscle spasm leads to narrowing of airways. An inflammatory response further narrows airways by engorging blood vessels and swelling mucous glands, forming a mucus plug.

MUSCLE SPASM AND AIRWAY NARROWING

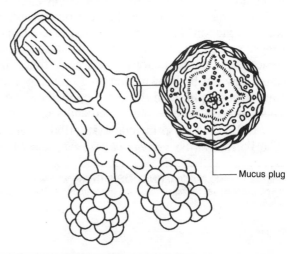

Mucus plug

Pinpoint possible complications

Emphasize to all COPD patients that an untreated respiratory infection can lead to life-threatening acute respiratory failure. Also point out their vulnerability to bronchial occlusion by mucus plugs, leading to atelectasis. Pulmonary vascular involvement may lead to pulmonary hypertension and subsequent cor pulmonale (right side heart failure). Signs of cor pulmonale include increasing dyspnea, dependent edema, and bluish or mottled skin.

Warn the patient with chronic bronchitis that continued exposure to the causative irritant, such as cigarette smoking, may worsen alveolar deterioration, leading to emphysema.

Tell the emphysema patient that he may experience ruptured blebs and bullae, leading to spontaneous pneumothorax or pneumomediastinum. Stress that he must notify his doctor immediately if he feels the major symptom of spontaneous pneumothorax—sudden, sharp pleuritic pain that's exacerbated by chest movement, breathing, or coughing.

Describe the diagnostic workup

Prepare the patient for diagnostic tests to assess respiratory impairment or to deter possible complications. Typically, the doctor relies on pulmonary function tests and chest X-rays, although he may also order thoracic computed tomography, magnetic resonance imaging, or exercise electrocardiography (ECG). Mention that a complete blood count and sputum analysis may be ordered to detect concurrent respiratory infection.

Pulmonary function test

Advise the patient not to smoke for 4 hours before the test and not to eat a large meal or drink copious amounts of fluid. Instruct him to wear loose, comfortable clothing during the test. If he wears dentures, tell him to keep them in to help form a tight seal around the mouthpiece. Just before the test, ask him to void.

Explain that during the test, he will sit upright and need to wear a noseclip. Alternatively, he may sit in a small airtight box called a body plethysmograph. Inside the plethysmograph, he won't need a noseclip but he may experience claustrophobia. Assure him that he won't suffocate and that he can communicate with the technician through the window in the box.

Tell him that he'll be asked to breathe a certain way for each test; for example, to inhale deeply and exhale completely, or to inhale quickly. Explain that he may receive an aerosolized bronchodilator and may then repeat one or two tests to evaluate the drug's effectiveness. He may also undergo arterial puncture for arterial blood gas (ABG) analysis.

Caution the patient that he may experience dyspnea and fatigue, though he'll be allowed to rest periodically. Instruct him to inform the technician if he experiences dizziness, chest pain, palpitations, nausea, severe dyspnea, or wheezing. He should also report swelling or bleeding from the arterial puncture site and any paresthesias or pain in the affected limb.

Emphasize that the test will proceed quickly if the patient follows directions, tries hard, and keeps a tight seal around the mouthpiece or tube to ensure accurate results.

Teaching the COPD patient about life-style changes

How can you help a COPD patient make major life-style changes? Well, you can start with a standard teaching plan and tailor it to the patient's specific needs. Here's one possibility.

Consider your patient's condition
Grace Tyler spent her 67th birthday in the hospital because of respiratory failure. A retired college professor, she has a husband who is in good health. She also has a 10-year history of COPD and hypertension. Three months ago, she quit smoking. She also received medication, though she often failed to take it. While she needed no other medical intervention, a recent respiratory infection aggravated her dyspnea and forced her into the hospital.

Barely breathing, Mrs. Tyler required a tracheostomy and mechanical ventilation. Now weaned from the ventilator, she'll have her tracheostomy tube removed. Then she'll return home with new medications and oxygen therapy to avert another crisis. The memory of the panic she felt at admission motivates her desire to cooperate and learn. You sense she needs to better understand what causes her dyspnea and how to control it.

You decide to review a standard teaching plan for COPD and determine the areas in which Mrs. Tyler needs the most instruction.

What are Mrs. Tyler's learning needs?
Standard teaching plan topics for COPD include:
• normal breathing, lung anatomy, and gas exchange
• COPD causes, pathophysiology, signs and symptoms, and complications
• diagnostic tests, including pulmonary function studies and chest X-rays
• life-style changes, involving activity and exercise, diet, smoking, and avoiding bronchial irritants
• other treatments, such as drug therapy, breathing exercises, oxygen use, and chest physiotherapy.

Mrs. Tyler agrees that her recent breathing crisis made her well aware of COPD's signs and symptoms and the seriousness of its complications. But she needs basic instruction on normal respiratory mechanisms and how COPD caused her breathing to go awry. This will make it easier to explain the diagnostic tests and the need to comply with therapy. Both Mrs. Tyler and her husband appear daunted at learning how to perform chest physiotherapy and to use oxygen at home, so you'll feature these topics. With so much to learn already, adopting major life-style changes may overwhelm Mrs. Tyler. But once she masters oxygen therapy and chest physiotherapy techniques, you can press on, teaching about exercise, energy conservation, bronchial irritants, healthful diet, and breathing exercises.

Setting learning outcomes
Based on Mrs. Tyler's immediate and long-term goals, you list specific learning outcomes. You believe that Mrs. Tyler should be able to:

```
-describe normal lung function
-relate her signs and symptoms to the physio-
logical changes that occur in COPD
-state the purpose of diagnostic tests
-name her medications and the purpose and side
effects of each
-demonstrate proper self-medication techniques,
such as using a hand-held nebulizer
-show (with her husband) how to perform chest
physiotherapy and how to operate oxygen
equipment
-perform pursed-lip and abdominal breathing
-list 10 possible bronchial irritants
-participate in an exercise program, as
tolerated
-complete daily menu plans and demonstrate
energy conservation techniques.
```

Selecting teaching techniques and tools
What techniques and tools are available (and appropriate) for teaching Mrs. Tyler? Because she's well-motivated, you confidently supply her with pamphlets and booklets to read. You decide to ask co-workers to demonstrate the skills Mrs. Tyler will need to survive. You arrange for a respiratory therapist to teach breathing exercises; an occupational therapist to teach energy conservation techniques; a hospital dietitian to discuss menu planning; and a physical therapist to teach chest physiotherapy and initiate an exercise program. You reinforce these lessons with written materials.

Finally, you make it a point to provide a clear explanation of oxygen therapy, backing up your discussion with illustrated handouts.

Evaluating your teaching
Mrs. Tyler's chronic condition requires ongoing assessment. *Discussion* can disclose her comprehension of diagnostic tests, medications, and self-care techniques.

Use *simulation techniques* to assess daily living skills. For example, ask Mrs. Tyler how she would conserve energy while shopping.

Return demonstration will help you assess her new self-care skills. For example, have her perform a breathing exercise or operate oxygen equipment. Or invite her (and her husband) to demonstrate chest physiotherapy.

Chest X-ray

Explain to the patient that this test monitors the progress of his illness. The procedure itself passes quickly, though the technician or doctor will require time to check the quality of the films.

If the X-ray is performed in the radiology department, the patient stands or sits in front of a machine. If the X-ray is performed at bedside, a nurse helps him to a sitting position and places a cold, hard film plate behind his back. The patient must take a deep breath and hold it for a few seconds while the X-ray is taken. Make it clear that he needs to remain still for those few seconds. Reassure him that he'll be exposed to only slight amounts of radiation. Explain that hospital personnel leave the X-ray area because they face exposure to radiation many times a day.

Computed tomography

Inform the patient that a computed tomography (CT) scan uses X-ray images to monitor lung condition. Mention that the test takes 30 to 60 minutes and causes little discomfort, although he may feel chilled because the equipment requires a cool environment. If the test requires use of a dye, instruct the patient to avoid food and fluids for 4 hours beforehand.

Clarify the scanning procedure. A technician positions the patient on an X-ray table. To restrict movement, the technician places a strap across the body part to be scanned. The table then slides into the tubelike opening of the scanner. Instruct the patient to report immediately any discomfort or a feeling of warmth or itching. (Tell him, especially if he experiences claustrophobia, that the technician can see and hear him from an adjacent room.) Describe the noises he'll hear from the scanner as it revolves around him. Remind the patient to lie still; movement may interfere with the results and may make repeat testing necessary.

Permit the patient to resume his usual activities and diet immediately after the test. Urge him to drink additional fluids for the rest of the day to help eliminate the dye, if needed.

Magnetic resonance imaging

Familiarize your patient with this diagnostic tool, which provides cross-sectional images of lung structures and traces blood flow. Point out that magnetic resonance imaging (MRI) allows imaging in regions where blood usually hampers visualization.

Inform the patient that MRI involves no radiation exposure, but requires exposure to a strong magnetic field. Ask if he has any metal objects in his body, such as a pacemaker, aneurysm clip, hip prosthesis, or implanted infusion pump, which could render him ineligible for MRI.

Spell out what the patient can expect during the 1-hour test. A technician will position him on a table that slides into a large cylinder that houses the MRI magnets. His head, chest, and arms will be restrained to help him remain still and thereby avoid blurring images. Tell the patient he'll hear a loud knocking noise while the machine operates. If the noise bothers him, he may be given earplugs or pads for his ears. A radio encased in the machine or earphones may partially block the sound.

Mention also that he may feel some discomfort while enclosed within the large cylinder. Find out if he's claustrophobic. Stress to the patient that during the test, a technician can see and hear him from an adjacent room and that after the test he can resume his normal activities.

Exercise ECG
The doctor may order an exercise ECG (also known as a stress test or a treadmill or graded exercise test) to diagnose the cause of dyspnea, to evaluate the effectiveness of bronchodilator therapy, to assess the degree of pulmonary dysfunction, or to help plan or evaluate an exercise program.

Explain to the patient that he'll walk on a treadmill or pedal a bicycle for about 30 minutes. Instruct him not to eat or smoke for 2 hours beforehand and to wear a loose, lightweight short-sleeved shirt or a patient gown with front closure, since he'll perspire during the test.

Tell the patient that before testing, a technician will clean, shave (if necessary), and abrade sites on his chest and, possibly, his back. Then the technician will attach electrodes at these sites.

Encourage the patient to express his concerns about the procedure. Reassure him that a doctor and a nurse will observe him at all times and that he can stop if he feels chest pain, leg discomfort, breathlessness, or severe fatigue.

Inform the patient that after the test, his blood pressure and ECG will be monitored for 10 to 15 minutes. Advise him to wait at least 1 hour before showering, and then to use warm water.

Teach about treatments
Treatment attempts to relieve symptoms and prevent complications. It may include daily exercise, limits on activity, dietary modifications, drug and oxygen therapy, chest physiotherapy, and other measures.

Activity
After evaluating exercise ECG results, the doctor may prescribe an exercise program to increase the patient's endurance and strength without causing severe dyspnea and to improve his sense of well-being.

Encourage regular participation in such exercise as walking or riding a stationary bicycle. Advise the patient to perform several minutes of warm-up exercises (slow walking, bending, stretching) and finish with cool-down exercises. He should start slowly and gradually increase the pace and duration of activity. If he needs low-flow oxygen during exercise, instruct him and his family on how to use oxygen at home. Also, demonstrate how to take an accurate radial pulse to monitor exercise effects.

Warn the patient to stop exercising immediately and notify

the doctor if he experiences increased dyspnea, heart fluttering, extreme fatigue, nausea, dizziness, or muscle cramps, or develops pale, mottled, or clammy skin. Mention that the doctor will periodically reevaluate exercise tolerance and modify the program, as necessary.

Counsel the patient to plan his daily activities to conserve energy and best cope with dyspnea. Advise him to inhale while resting and exhale when exerting himself, to alternate light and heavy tasks, and to rest frequently. Remind him to use pursed-lip breathing during his activities and give him a copy of the patient-teaching aid *How to overcome shortness of breath,* page 102. Also instruct him to minimize body movements. For example, he should sit instead of stand when talking or dressing. (Tell him that standing requires a 40% greater energy expenditure than sitting.) Instruct him to pull instead of lift and use a cart or wagon to carry groceries and other heavy items.

Diet

Communicate to the patient the importance of a well-balanced, nutritious diet to compensate for the extra calories he expends just to breathe. Because dyspnea and increased sputum production can discourage eating and lead to weight loss, help the patient maintain caloric intake. First, encourage frequent oral hygiene to stimulate his appetite and enjoyment of food. If the patient has severe dyspnea, advise him to chew food slowly and to eat small, frequent meals to reduce fatigue and air swallowing. Advise him to perform breathing exercises 1 hour before meals so secretions won't interfere with eating and to rest for 30 minutes before meals to prevent tiring.

If the patient experiences a bloated feeling at mealtime, advise him to limit his intake of gas-producing foods, such as cabbage, brussels sprouts, beans, onions, apples, and cantaloupe. Recommend nutritious snacks, including fruit juices, or a liquid enteral supplement for added calories between meals. Including fresh fruit, vegetables, and bran in his diet will help prevent constipation.

Unless contraindicated, encourage the patient to drink plenty of water—at least 8 glasses daily—to thin his mucous secretions and make expectoration easier. Adequate fluid intake will also help prevent constipation and avoid breathlessness associated with straining during defecation.

Address any factor that may interfere with the patient's ability to maintain a proper diet. For example, teach him about the basics of good nutrition, if necessary. If limited transportation or financial resources make obtaining food difficult, refer him to an appropriate social service agency or to community programs, such as Meals On Wheels.

Discuss with the overweight patient how obesity interferes with diaphragmatic movement and increases cardiac work load. This, in turn, can increase the work of breathing. Provide a weight-reduction diet if needed.

96 Chronic obstructive pulmonary disease

Tips for using a hand-held nebulizer

When teaching your patient how to use a hand-held nebulizer effectively, instruct him to do the following:
• shake the inhaler, holding it so the canister is above the mouthpiece.
• take a deep breath and exhale completely.
• hold his mouth on or near the mouthpiece, squeeze the canister downward, and inhale the nebulized mist that comes out of the mouthpiece.
• hold his breath a few seconds when inhaling (to enhance placement and action of drug) and to wait 1 minute before taking subsequent puffs.
• be careful not to inhale too early or too late.
• make sure to inhale the mist and not to swallow it.
• rinse mouth with water after each use. Dry nose and throat and an unpleasant taste may occur with inhaled medication.
• be mindful not to use the inhaler more than the prescribed number of times and not to get the spray in his eyes because it may blur his vision.
• take the mouthpiece off the canister and rinse it daily.
• clean the inhaler according to the manufacturer's directions.

Medication

Drug therapy may consist of oral bronchodilators, adrenergic agonists, and corticosteroids. Familiarize patients with prescribed drugs (see *Teaching about drugs for COPD,* pages 98 and 99).

Most patients will tolerate oral bronchodilators, such as theophylline, to manage airway obstruction.

Systemically administered adrenergic agonists—especially selective beta$_2$ agents such as terbutaline and albuterol—may also serve as bronchodilators. However, the patient may experience such adverse effects as tremors, tachycardia, and palpitations. Some beta$_2$-adrenergic agonists (metaproterenol sulfate, for example) may be administered by oral inhalers, hand-bulb nebulizers, propeller-driven nebulizers, or intermittent positive-pressure breathing (IPPB) as an alternative.

Inhaled anticholinergics may act as bronchodilators by blocking vagal influence on the bronchi, resulting in bronchodilation. Anticholinergics can't be given in pill form, however, because of systemic adverse effects.

Corticosteroids may be used, but whether these agents act as bronchodilators or simply prevent airway reactivity to exogenous allergens remains unclear. When used with bronchodilators, parenteral corticosteroids have been shown to improve forced expiratory volume (FEV$_1$) in hospitalized patients with chronic bronchitis. Also, oral corticosteroids used with bronchodilators may improve FEV$_1$ in some stable outpatients. However, long-term corticosteroid use may cause many adverse effects. Often, alternate-day therapy will minimize these effects without diminishing therapeutic value.

If the patient receives an inhaled corticosteroid, such as beclomethasone, explain that this type of administration delivers the drug directly to the bronchial wall. When used in therapeutic doses, aerosol delivery causes fewer systemic adverse effects. However, warn the patient that he may develop thrush.

Caution the patient not to take such widely used drugs as cough suppressants, sedatives, and hypnotic agents. Tell the patient with severe chronic bronchitis that these drugs can actually cause respiratory depression, particularly if he has hypercapnia. Cough suppressants may lead to retention of pulmonary secretions, thereby worsening hypoxia and hypercapnia. This, in turn, may cause central nervous system depression.

Finally, if infection complicates COPD, explain to the patient that he will require antibiotic therapy and may have to undergo culture and sensitivity testing to ensure effective treatment.

Using inhalers. The correct use of inhalers usually will avert severe dyspneic episodes, but it requires a certain degree of psychomotor coordination. You'll want to carefully assess how the patient uses his inhaler and carefully detail each step when correcting his technique. (See *Tips for using a hand-held nebulizer.*)

If a patient cannot fully coordinate all the steps, but still obtains a fairly prompt beneficial effect, his technique is probably adequate. If he doesn't achieve acceptable benefit, a spacer device (such as InspirEase or Aerochamber) may prove useful. Alternatively, the doctor may substitute an oral drug, even though it's slower acting.

Procedures

Teach the patient and his family how to perform chest physiotherapy and manage oxygen therapy.

Chest physiotherapy. Explain to the patient and his family that chest physiotherapy helps mobilize and remove mucus from the lungs. Provide them with a copy of the teaching aid *How to perform chest physiotherapy (for an adult),* pages 106 and 107. Have a family member demonstrate percussion to ensure correct technique. If the family member has limited arm strength, show him how to use a mechanical percussor.

Oxygen therapy. If appropriate, also teach the patient and his family how to use oxygen at home. Acquaint them with the types of oxygen delivery devices available. Before choosing an oxygen supplier, advise the patient to investigate different companies. Encourage him to ask about initial cost of set-up, delivery charge, monthly supply cost, service calls, and insurance coverage.

Compressed oxygen, stored in large tanks or cylinders, accurately delivers 100% oxygen at all liter flows without leakage between uses. When outside his home, the patient can use a portable cylinder mounted on a stroller. Although fairly economical, this system is bulky and unsightly and requires frequent deliveries to sustain continuous oxygen. Warn the patient that high pressure storage of oxygen may present a safety hazard.

An oxygen concentrator increases oxygen concentration from 21% to about 90% and removes other elements from the air. Although this system is less costly and bulky than other delivery systems, the concentrator will increase the patient's electric bill, an expense insurance may not cover. The patient will need a backup system in case of power failure and portable cylinders of oxygen for outside use. (See the patient-teaching aid *Gaining mobility with portable oxygen equipment,* page 108.)

A third delivery system, liquid oxygen, allows for storage of more oxygen at lower pressure than compressed gas. Tell your patient that this system allows him to easily refill reservoirs for ambulatory use. However, it costs the most and small amounts of leakage may occur if he doesn't use it continuously.

The doctor will write a prescription for oxygen therapy specifying the type of system, the liter flow rate, and hours of use. Provide the patient with copies of the teaching aids *Learning to use breathing devices,* page 103, and *Understanding your home oxygen equipment,* pages 104 and 105. Teach the patient to think of oxygen as a medication: He must use it at the liter flow rate and times prescribed. If he feels restless, dyspneic or tired, or if he notices cyanosis, advise him not to turn up the liter flow but to contact his doctor instead. (See *Problems to report when using oxygen.*)

continued on page 100

Problems to report when using oxygen

Warn the patient who's using oxygen that excessive or insufficient oxygen may cause harm. Instruct him to watch for and report these signs and symptoms:

Excessive oxygen
- slow or shallow breathing
- restlessness
- difficulty in waking up (possible CO_2 narcosis)
- headaches
- slurred speech

Insufficient oxygen
- difficult, irregular breathing
- anxiety
- tiredness or drowsiness
- confusion or inability to concentrate
- blue fingernail beds or lips.

If the patient experiences any of these signs and symptoms, he should call the doctor immediately or have someone take him to the emergency room. Warn him not to assume that more—or less—oxygen will make him better. Caution him never to change the oxygen flow rate without first checking with the doctor.

98 Chronic obstructive pulmonary disease

Teaching about drugs for COPD

DRUG	ADVERSE REACTIONS	TEACHING POINTS
Xanthine-derivative bronchodilators		
aminophylline (Aminophyllin, Somophyllin) **dyphylline** (Dilor, Lufyllin) **oxtriphylline** (Choledyl) **theophylline** (Bronkodyl, Elixophyllin, Slo-Phyllin, Theo-Dur)	• Watch for cardiovascular collapse, respiratory arrest, seizures, and ventricular tachycardia. • Other reactions include anorexia, depression, diarrhea, dizziness, epigastric pain, fever, headache, hyperglycemia, hypotension, insomnia, muscle twitching, nausea, palpitations, restlessness, tachypnea, tremors, urine retention, urticaria, and vomiting.	• Tell the patient that if GI symptoms develop, he may take medication with a full glass of water at mealtimes. • Tell him to take medication at regularly scheduled intervals. Tell him to take a missed dose as soon as possible, but not to double-dose. • If he's taking theophylline, inform him that he'll undergo periodic evaluation of serum drug levels and pulmonary function. • Warn him not to combine the drug with over-the-counter (OTC) products, such as cold preparations, because of possible interactions. Caution him to consult his doctor or pharmacist. Also warn against crushing extended-release tablets. • Instruct him to avoid foods and beverages high in caffeine, such as coffee, tea, cola and chocolate. Explain that they may potentiate adverse effects of bronchodilators and cause tremors and palpitations.
Beta₂-adrenergic-agonist bronchodilators		
Oral and inhaled agents: **albuterol** (Proventil, Ventolin) **metaproterenol** (Alupent, Metaprel) **terbutaline** (Brethaire, Brethine, Bricanyl) *Inhaled agents:* **isoetharine** (Bronkosol) **pirbuterol** (Maxair)	• Watch for cardiac arrest with excessive use, hypersensitivity, and paradoxical bronchospasm. • Other reactions include angina, appetite increase, cough, difficult urination, dilated pupils, dizziness, drowsiness, excitement, headache, heartburn, hypertension, hypotension, muscle cramps, nausea, nervousness, palpitations, rash, sweating, tachycardia, tremor, urticaria, vertigo, and vomiting. *Reactions are less likely with inhaled forms.*	• Instruct the patient to take a missed dose within 1 hour. If he doesn't remember until later, he should skip it. • Tell him to notify the doctor of decreased drug effectiveness or signs of toxicity, such as tremors, nausea and vomiting, rapid or irregular pulse. If bronchospasm occurs with repeated use, he should discontinue the drug and notify the doctor. • Instruct him to store his medication away from heat. • Warn him not to take OTC medications, such as cold preparations, because of possible interactions. He should check first with his doctor or pharmacist. • If the patient also takes inhaled corticosteroids, instruct him to inhale the bronchodilator 15 minutes before the corticosteroid.
Inhaled anticholinergics		
atropine sulfate (Dey-dose Atropine Sulfate) **ipratropium bromide** (Atrovent)	• Watch for dry mouth and heart fluttering. • Other reactions include cough, dizziness, GI distress, headache, and nausea.	• Instruct the patient to take a missed dose within 1 hour. If he remembers later, he should skip it. • Tell him to notify the doctor of decreased drug effectiveness or signs of toxicity, such as tremors, nausea and vomiting, rapid or irregular pulse. If bronchospasm occurs with repeated use, he should discontinue the drug and notify his doctor. • Tell him to store his medication away from heat. • Warn him not to take OTC medications, such as cold preparations, because of potential interactions. Tell him to check first with his doctor or pharmacist. • If the patient also takes inhaled corticosteroids, instruct him to inhale the bronchodilator 15 minutes before the corticosteroid.

continued

Teaching about drugs for COPD — *continued*

DRUG	ADVERSE REACTIONS	TEACHING POINTS
Oral corticosteroids		
prednisone (Deltasone)	• Watch for abdominal pain, acne, back or rib pain, easy bruising, fever, hypertension, marked weight gain, melena, menstrual irregularities, psychoses, sore throat, unusual tiredness, and vomiting. • Other reactions include diaphoresis, increased facial and body hair, mild mood swings, and mild nausea.	• Warn the patient not to stop taking the drug abruptly — serious complications could result. • Counsel him to avoid products containing aspirin and alcohol, because they increase the risk of GI ulceration, and to avoid foods or nonprescription medications containing sodium, because they increase the risk of fluid retention. • Suggest taking the drug with food or milk to decrease the risk of gastric irritation. Prophylactic use of low-sodium antacids, such as Maalox, may also help prevent GI distress. • Advise the patient to wear a medical identification tag or to carry a wallet card and to notify any health care provider, such as the dentist or the oral surgeon, about his corticosteroid therapy. Explain that this therapy suppresses the immune system.
Inhaled corticosteroids		
beclomethasone dipropionate (Beclovent, Vanceril) **dexamethasone sodium phosphate** (Decadron Respihaler) **flunisolide** (AeroBid Inhaler) **triamcinolone acetanide** (Azmacort)	• Watch for oral infections (*Candida albicans* or *Aspergillus niger*) in the mouth, pharynx, and, occasionally, the larynx, and worsening of COPD symptoms. • Other reactions include hypothalamic-pituitary axis (HPA) suppression, hypersensitivity reactions, and palpitations.	• Warn the patient to be alert for signs of systemic absorption, including Cushing's syndrome, hyperglycemia, or glucosuria, and to notify the doctor if they occur. • If the patient receives concurrent therapy with antibiotic or antifungal agents and the infection doesn't respond immediately, advise him to check with the doctor who may recommend that the patient discontinue corticosteroid therapy until the infection is controlled. • If the patient also uses inhaled bronchodilators, advise him to inhale the bronchodilator 15 minutes before he inhales the corticosteroid agent. This promotes the corticosteroid benefit. • Tell him to rinse his mouth with water after using the inhaler to reduce the risk of oral fungal infection. Also instruct him to regularly check oral mucous membranes for signs of fungal infection, such as a cracked tongue, pain, and whitish overgrowth. • Warn asthma patients not to increase use of corticosteroid inhaler during a severe asthma attack, but to call the doctor for adjustment of therapy. The doctor may possibly add a systemic steroid. • Tell the patient to contact the doctor if he notices a decreased response to the drug. The doctor may adjust the dosage or discontinue the medicine. • If fever or local irritation develops, advise the patient to discontinue use and report the effect to doctor promptly. • Tell the patient that after the medicine achieves the desired effect, the doctor will reduce the dosage to the smallest amount necessary to control symptoms.

100 Chronic obstructive pulmonary disease

Avoiding respiratory infection

If the COPD patient gets a cold, serious complications could develop—pneumonia or breathing difficulty severe enough to require hospitalization. To help him avoid colds, give him these instructions.
• Avoid contact with people who have colds and stay away from crowds during the cold and flu season. Colds are easily passed through droplets in the air as well as on eating utensils.
• Wash his hands frequently, since cold germs can linger on articles he handles or come from shaking hands with others.
• Eat good, nutritious foods, drink plenty of liquids, and get extra rest to increase resistance to respiratory infections.
• Ask the doctor about getting a flu shot (influenza vaccine) and a pneumonia shot (pneumococcal vaccine) each fall.

Containing a cold
If your patient does catch a cold, effective teaching may keep it from getting worse. Suggest these measures.
• At the first signs of a cold—stuffy or runny nose, sore throat, fatigue or mild achiness—increase intake of liquids and get extra rest to heighten resistance to infection.
• Use a humidifier, making sure to clean the inside of it thoroughly and regularly.
• Consult the doctor before taking any over-the-counter drugs.
• Notify the doctor if cold symptoms last more than 3 days, get worse, or if shortness of breath, wheezing, fever, appetite loss, chest discomfort, or a change in frequency of coughing or quantity of phlegm develop. These symptoms may indicate a worsening infection.
• Follow directions and finish the prescription for antibiotics, if the doctor orders them. Otherwise, the patient could have a relapse.

Other care measures
Every patient with COPD must learn to identify early signs of complications, such as increasing dyspnea, wheezing, fatigue, and a change in cough or in sputum production. Explain that the earlier he performs self-care measures or notifies his doctor, the better his chances of decreasing the length and severity of an attack and the less likely he'll be hospitalized.

Besides, the patient's limited pulmonary reserve makes him susceptible to respiratory infection. Point out the value of following preventive measures and promptly treating infection. (See *Avoiding respiratory infection.*)

When appropriate, give your patient the following advice to help ensure maximum quality of life:

Avoid irritants. Explain to the patient that inhaled pollutants can aggravate his symptoms. Counsel him to avoid heavy traffic and smog, to refrain from using aerosol sprays, and to keep his home and especially his bedroom as dust-free as possible. Encourage him to carefully assess his home and workplace for pollutants and to make changes to minimize exposure to toxic inhalants. If occupational irritant exposure poses a threat, encourage the patient to seek job counseling and retraining.

Teach the asthmatic patient to avoid allergens, such as animal dander, grass, wool, or any others that trigger attacks. Emphasize that in most cases, doing so will slow disease progression or arrest its development and ease the symptoms of cough, dyspnea, and copious mucus production. When appropriate, make him aware that desensitization to specific antigens offers a treatment option, although it rarely brings complete relief from asthma attacks.

Stop smoking. Explain the harmful effects of smoking on respiratory function. Smoking increases mucus production, decreases ciliary motion, and elevates carboxyhemoglobin levels. Tell the patient with chronic bronchitis that his respiratory function may gradually improve if he quits smoking. Unfortunately, the same rarely holds true for the emphysema patient.

Provide the patient with information on stop-smoking programs and refer him to the American Cancer Society or the American Lung Association. Tell him to inform family, friends, and co-workers that he must have a smoke-free environment or his condition will get worse.

Mind the weather. Warn the patient that exposure to blasts of cold or dry air can precipitate bronchospasm. Dry air can also thicken his mucus. Suggest that he avoid cold winds or cover his mouth with a scarf or mask when outdoors in cold weather. On hot days when there's poor air quality, advise the patient to stay indoors, keep the windows closed, and use an air conditioner. Also have him maintain environmental humidity between 40% and 50%, whenever possible. A portable humidifier works well in an enclosed area.

Deal with sexual problems. Because dyspnea may interfere with sexual intercourse, discuss ways the patient and his partner may overcome this hurdle. Advise the patient to use pursed-lip breathing during intercourse and to assume a comfortable position that won't restrict breathing, such as lying on his side. Allowing his partner to take a more active role may also help. Recommend that the patient rest before and after sexual activity and keep oxygen nearby to relieve any dyspnea. Above all, encourage the patient and his partner to communicate openly and to experiment with alternate means of expressing affection.

Recognize signs of peptic ulcer. Describe the signs of peptic ulcer disease, a complication that strikes 20% to 25% of COPD patients. Instruct the patient to check his stool every day for blood and to notify the doctor if he has persistent nausea, vomiting, heartburn, indigestion, constipation, diarrhea, or blood in his stool.

Learn to cope. Help the patient explore the impact of COPD on his life and encourage steps that will help him deal with chronic anxiety and depression. Allow him to express his fears about his illness. If he's anxious, suggest relaxation exercises or biofeedback. Also help family members deal with the added emotional strain in their lives. Encourage the patient and his family to join a support group and to contact the local chapter of the American Lung Association for more information.

Sources of information and support

American Lung Association
1740 Broadway, New York, N.Y. 10019
(212) 315-8700

American Cancer Society (smoking cessation)
1599 Clifton Road, Atlanta, Ga. 30329
(404) 320-3333

Further readings

Baigelman, W. "Exacerbation of Chronic Obstructive Pulmonary Disease," *Emergency Medicine* 19(19):79-80, 82-83, 86, November 15, 1987.
Cerrato, P.L. "The Special Nutritional Needs of a COPD Patient," *RN* 50(11):75-76, November 1987.
"COPD: The Source May Be Treatable," *Emergency Medicine* 20(9):59-60, May 15, 1988.
Hahn, K. "Slow-Teaching the COPD Patient," *Nursing87* 17(4):34-41, April 1987.
Hunter, S.M. "Educating Clients with COPD," *Home Healthcare Nurse* 5(6):41-43, November-December 1987.
Johnson, A.P. "The Elderly and COPD," *Journal of Gerontological Nursing* 14(12):20-24, 35-36, December 1988.

How to overcome shortness of breath

Dear Patient:

When you're having trouble breathing, performing special exercises will help you feel better. Practice these exercises twice a day for 5 to 10 minutes until you get used to doing them.

Abdominal breathing

1 Lie comfortably on your back and place a pillow beneath your head. Bend your knees to relax your stomach.

2 Press one hand on your stomach lightly but with enough force to create slight pressure. Rest the other hand on your chest.

3 Now breathe slowly through your nose, using your stomach muscles. The hand on your stomach should rise during inspiration and fall during expiration. The hand on your chest should remain almost still.

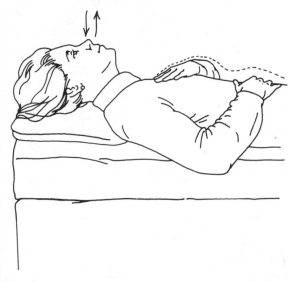

Pursed-lip breathing

1 Breathe in slowly through your nose to avoid gulping air. Hold your breath as you count to yourself: one-1,000; two-1,000; three-1,000.

2 Purse your lips as if you're going to whistle.

3 Now, breathe out slowly through pursed lips as you count to yourself: one-1,000; two-1,000; three-1,000; four-1,000; five-1,000; six-1,000.

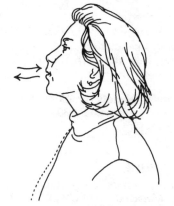

You should make a soft, whistling sound while you breathe out. Exhaling through pursed lips slows down your breathing and helps get rid of the stale air trapped in your lungs.

When performing pursed-lip breathing during activity, inhale before exerting yourself; exhale while performing the activity.

If the recommended counting rhythm feels awkward, find one that feels more comfortable. Keep in mind that you must breathe out longer than you breathe in.

Learning to use breathing devices

Dear Patient:

Your doctor has prescribed a nasal cannula or an oxygen face mask so you can breathe in extra oxygen. Follow these steps for using your breathing device.

Attaching the tubing
Whether you use a nasal cannula or mask, attach one end of the oxygen tubing to the device. Attach the other end to the humidifier nipple.

Setting the flow rate
Next, turn on the oxygen and set the flow rate to the prescribed level. If you're receiving oxygen at a rate of 2 liters per minute or more, you should feel it flowing from the prongs. If you can't, briefly turn up the flow rate. Then turn it back to the prescribed level.

Positioning the device
If you use a nasal cannula, insert the two prongs in your nostrils. Make sure the prongs face upward and follow the curve of your nostrils. Also make sure the flat surface of the tab rests above your upper lip. Position the tubing for the

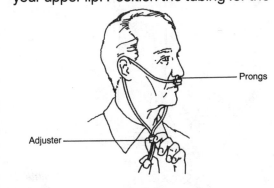

Prongs

Adjuster

nasal cannula behind each ear and adjust it below your chin for a comfortable fit.

If you use an oxygen mask, place the device over your face. Position the elastic strap over your head so that it rests above your ears and the mask fits snugly against your face.

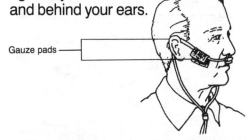

Elastic strap

Preventing skin irritation
To keep the cannula or mask strap from irritating your skin, pad it with 2-inch-square gauze pads, placing them against your cheeks and behind your ears.

Gauze pads

Every 2 hours, check for reddened areas around your nose and ears. If you see redness, rub the area gently, then wash your face and dry it well. Call your doctor if redness continues.

You may moisten your lips and nose with a water-soluble lubricating jelly (such as K-Y Brand Lubricating Jelly), but take care not to get any in the cannula or mask.

Every 8 hours, remove the cannula or mask and wipe it clean with a wet cloth.

Understanding your home oxygen equipment

Dear Patient:

To relieve your shortness of breath, your doctor has ordered oxygen therapy for you to use at home. Your first job is to become familiar with your oxygen delivery equipment.

Oxygen options

You will be using a liquid oxygen container, an oxygen tank, or an oxygen concentrator.

Liquid oxygen is stored at very cold temperatures in thermoslike containers. When released, it's warmed up to breathe as oxygen gas.

Usually, a stationary liquid oxygen unit has a *contents indicator* that shows the amount of oxygen in the unit, a *flow selector* that controls the oxygen flow rate, a *humidifier bottle* that connects to a *humidifier adapter,* and a *filling connector* that attaches to a matching connector on the portable unit.

An *oxygen tank* stores oxygen gas under pressure. It contains a *pressure gauge* that tells you how much oxygen is left, a *flow meter* that tells you the flow rate, and a *humidifier bottle.*

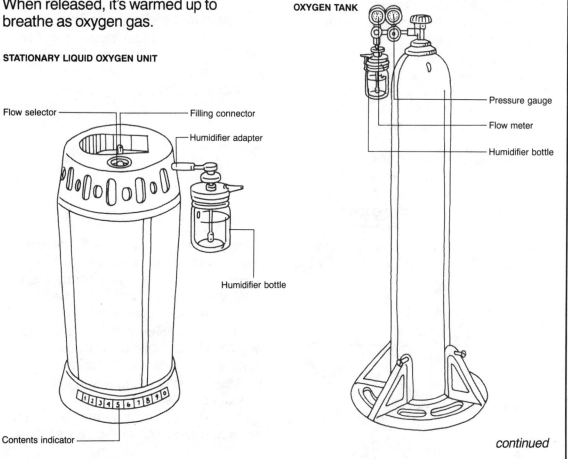

STATIONARY LIQUID OXYGEN UNIT

Flow selector — Filling connector
Humidifier adapter
Humidifier bottle
Contents indicator

OXYGEN TANK

Pressure gauge
Flow meter
Humidifier bottle

continued

Understanding your home oxygen equipment — *continued*

The *oxygen concentrator* removes nitrogen and other components of room air, then concentrates the remaining oxygen and stores it.

Oxygen concentrators come in different models and sizes, but most have the following operating parts: a *power switch and light,* a *flow selector* that regulates the oxygen flow rate, an *alarm buzzer* that warns of power interruptions, and a *humidifier bottle* that attaches to a *threaded outlet.*

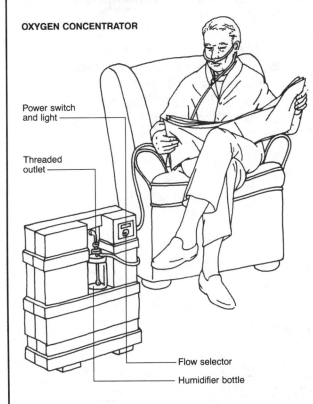

OXYGEN CONCENTRATOR

Power switch and light

Threaded outlet

Flow selector

Humidifier bottle

When using an oxygen concentrator, you must check the *air inlet filter* before operating the unit. If the filter is dirty, wash it with soap and water, rinse, and pat it dry before replacing it. Also push the power switch once to check the alarm buzzer. If the buzzer doesn't sound, use a different oxygen source,

and contact your supplier. If it does sound, push the power switch again to turn it off.

Step-by-step guidelines

When using an oxygen tank, an oxygen concentrator, or liquid oxygen, be sure to follow these important guidelines:

1 Check the level of water in the humidifier bottle. If it's below the correct level, refill the bottle with sterile or distilled water or replace it with a new, prefilled bottle.

2 Attach one end of the oxygen tubing to your breathing device. Attach the other end to the humidifier nipple.

3 Next, set the flow rate using the appropriate method for your device:
● turn the dial to the correct number
● turn the dial until the metal ball rises to the correct level on the scale
● wait for the gauge needle to reach the correct level.

If you're using the liquid oxygen system, set the flow rate to turn on the oxygen. If you're using an oxygen tank, before setting the flow rate, open the tank by turning the valve counter clockwise at the top, until the needle on the pressure gauge moves. If you're using a concentrator, plug the power cord into a grounded electrical outlet and push the power switch before setting the flow rate.

Never increase the flow rate on your equipment without your doctor's permission.

4 Put on your breathing device and breathe the oxygen for as long as your doctor orders.

PATIENT-TEACHING AID

How to perform chest physiotherapy (for an adult)

Dear Patient:

The doctor wants you to perform chest physiotherapy to help make your breathing easier. This treatment has three parts: postural drainage, percussion, and coughing.

You'll be able to perform postural drainage and coughing yourself, but you'll need a family member's or friend's help to percuss your back.

Postural drainage lets the force of gravity drain mucus from the bottom of your lungs. Then percussion helps move thick, sticky mucus from the smaller airways of your lungs into the larger airways. Coughing—the last and most important step—clears mucus from your lungs.

Follow the instructions for each step.

When to perform chest physiotherapy

Unless the doctor tells you differently, perform chest physiotherapy when you get up in the morning and before you have dinner or go to bed. When you have more mucus than usual (for example, during a respiratory infection), increase the number of treatments.

Getting ready

Don't eat for 1 hour before chest physiotherapy to avoid abdominal bloating and the risk of choking on vomited food. If ordered, use your inhaler 10 to 15 minutes before percussion to improve effectiveness.

Avoid wearing tight or restrictive clothing around your chest, neck, or stomach. Wear a light shirt or gown to avoid friction from percussion.

Postural drainage

1 Place a box of tissues within easy reach. Also stack pillows on the floor next to your bed.

2 Next, lie on your stomach over the side of your bed. Support your head, chest, and arms with the pillows you've placed on the floor. Stay in this position for 10 to 20 minutes, as tolerated.

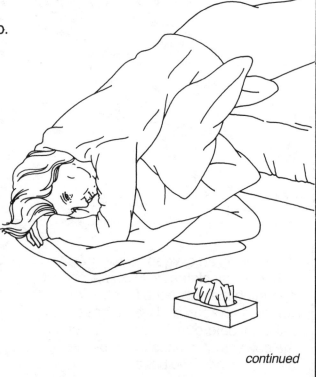

continued

How to perform chest physiotherapy (for an adult) — *continued*

Percussion

1 Remain in the postural drainage position. Have a family member or friend position his hands in a cupped shape, with his fingers flexed and thumbs pressed tightly against the side of his index fingers.

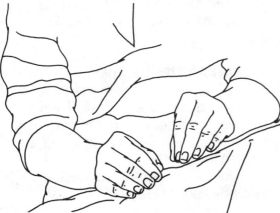

2 Next have him rhythmically pat your back for 3 to 5 minutes, alternating his cupped hands. He can start on one side of the back, just above the waist, and percuss upward, changing sides as he continues. Percussion will feel firm, but shouldn't hurt. You should hear a hollow sound like a horse galloping.

Coughing

1 While remaining in the postural drainage position, take a slow, deep breath through your nose. Hold the breath as you count to yourself: one-1,000; two-1,000; three-1,000.

2 Briefly cough three times through a slightly open mouth as you breathe out. An effective cough sounds deep, low, and hollow; an ineffective one, high-pitched.

3 Next, take a slow, deep breath through your nose and breathe normally for several minutes. Repeat this coughing procedure, as tolerated.

4 After chest physiotherapy, return to an upright position slowly to prevent light-headedness and possible fainting.

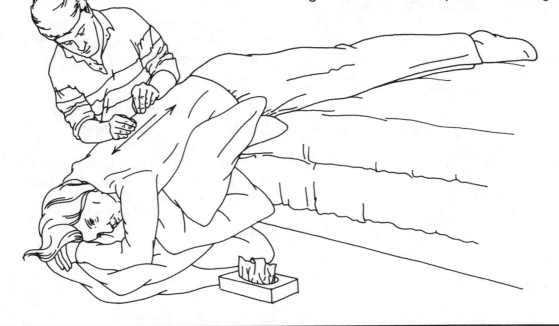

Gaining mobility with portable oxygen equipment

Dear Patient:

Special equipment may offer you greater freedom of movement while you're breathing extra oxygen. For instance, a portable liquid oxygen unit or portable oxygen tank will let you move around freely and leave your home. A wheeled carrier or extension tubing for your regular equipment will allow for a greater range of movement inside your home.

Use these guidelines, along with specific manufacturer's instructions, to operate portable oxygen equipment.

Checking oxygen supply
A portable liquid oxygen unit has a built-in scale that indicates oxygen level each time you hold the unit by its carrying strap. Check the oxygen level often, and refill it when necessary. Your supplier will give you specific instructions for your model.

PORTABLE LIQUID OXYGEN UNIT

Nasal cannula

Oxygen tubing
Oxygen adapter
Flow control knob
Contents scale

Carrying strap

A portable oxygen tank has a contents gauge, a flow meter, and a knob to turn on the oxygen. To check the tank, turn the knob until you see the needle on the flow meter move. Then, turn the knob off.

Attaching the tubing
Connect one end of the oxygen tubing to the nasal cannula or mask. Then connect the other end to the oxygen adapter on the liquid oxygen unit or the oxygen tank.

Make sure the tubing connects securely and isn't kinked.

Setting the flow rate
Now turn the flow meter knob to deliver oxygen at the prescribed rate. You should feel oxygen flowing from the prongs of the cannula or mask. If you don't feel oxygen flowing, briefly turn up the flow rate.

Then, turn the knob back to the prescribed level. Make sure the knob on a liquid oxygen unit clicks into position, or oxygen will not flow.

Carrying the portable tank
Slip the carrying strap over your shoulder and adjust it for a comfortable fit. Try carrying the tank on each side of your body, to determine which is most comfortable. Now, put on the nasal cannula or mask and begin breathing oxygen.

Cystic fibrosis

In cystic fibrosis, you'll concentrate on teaching parents and the patient that early detection and treatment of complications may help the patient survive longer and enjoy a better life. Although no cure exists for cystic fibrosis, improved treatments do offer hope for increased life spans.

You'll need to ensure that parents—and the patient himself, if he's old enough—thoroughly understand cystic fibrosis. Your teaching will cover the pathophysiology of cystic fibrosis, its signs and symptoms, its genetic transmission, and its complications. You'll explain tests to diagnose cystic fibrosis and to determine its severity. You'll also explain treatments, including exercise, diet, medications, chest physiotherapy, aerosol therapy, and ways to avoid dehydration.

Throughout your association with the patient and his parents, you'll provide ongoing encouragement as the patient practices the varied treatments that help him cope with his disease.

Discuss the disorder

Explain that cystic fibrosis is a chronic, progressive, inherited disease affecting the exocrine (mucus-secreting) glands. It's transmitted by an autosomal recessive gene; that is, both parents must contribute the abnormal gene for a child to be born with cystic fibrosis. When both parents are carriers, they have a 25% chance of transmitting the disease with each pregnancy. (See *How the cystic fibrosis gene is transmitted,* page 110.)

Inform the parents that cystic fibrosis affects multiple organ systems with varying degrees of severity and produces diverse symptoms. Sweat gland dysfunction is the most consistent abnormality. The patient has a normal volume of sweat but an abnormally high concentration of sodium chloride. This diminishes the body's sodium and chloride levels and may lead to dehydration, especially during hot weather or when the patient has a fever with profuse sweating.

Explain that bronchial, pancreatic, and other mucus-secreting glands produce a viscous mucus that eventually obstructs the glandular ducts. For example, obstructive changes in the lungs cause the respiratory symptoms associated with cystic fibrosis— wheezing, dyspnea, tachypnea, and a productive cough with thick, tenacious sputum.

Kathleen Boczar, RN,C, MS, and **Cindy Dillon, RN, MS,** wrote this chapter. Ms. Boczar is a certified family nurse practitioner, pulmonary clinical nurse specialist, and coordinator of the adult cystic fibrosis program at Temple University Hospital, Philadelphia. Ms. Dillon is a pediatric pulmonary clinical nurse specialist and coordinator of the Cystic Fibrosis Center at St. Christopher's Hospital, Philadelphia.

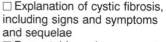

CHECKLIST

Teaching topics in cystic fibrosis

☐ Explanation of cystic fibrosis, including signs and symptoms and sequelae
☐ Preventable and nonpreventable complications
☐ Preparation for and explanation of diagnostic tests, including the sweat test, fecal fat test, sputum culture, chest X-ray, pulmonary function tests, and blood tests
☐ Importance of physical activity to improve overall fitness and lung function and to help dislodge mucus
☐ Necessity for a high-calorie, high-protein diet
☐ Use of pancreatic enzymes to aid digestion
☐ Other medications, including adverse reactions and precautions
☐ Discussion of chest physiotherapy—postural drainage, percussion, vibration, and coughing
☐ Self-care, such as self-percussion (including mechanical percussion mask), positive expiratory pressure, and forced expiratory technique
☐ How to perform aerosol therapy and care for equipment
☐ Other measures, including oxygen therapy, sexual concerns, dehydration prevention, coping techniques, and follow-up care
☐ Source of information and support

How the cystic fibrosis gene is transmitted

Parents of a child with cystic fibrosis will be concerned about how the causative gene is transmitted and what their chances are of having another child with cystic fibrosis. Tell them that cystic fibrosis results from an autosomal recessive gene.

Explain to the parents that genes are either dominant or recessive. The weaker recessive genes manifest themselves only when paired with another recessive gene. At conception, an embryo normally receives two genes — one from each parent. If both parents carry the recessive gene for cystic fibrosis, each offspring has a 25% chance of having the disease. Explain that special laboratories offer prenatal testing for parents of children with cystic fibrosis. Mention that about 75% of cystic fibrosis patients have the cystic fibrosis gene. Researchers are still discovering the other 25% of mutations of the gene. Advise parents to seek up-to-date information from a genetic counselor.

As shown below, C refers to the dominant gene, and c represents the recessive gene. The unaffected noncarrier — CC — has inherited the dominant gene from each parent and won't have cystic fibrosis. C/c and c/C are unaffected carriers; each child has inherited one dominant gene and one recessive gene for cystic fibrosis. Because both genes must be recessive for cystic fibrosis to develop, these children won't have the disease, but they can pass the recessive gene to their offspring.

The affected person — c/c — has inherited the recessive gene from both parents and has cystic fibrosis. He will pass the recessive cystic fibrosis gene on, if he has offspring.

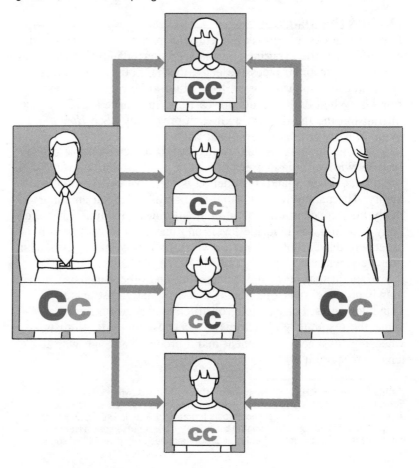

Tell the parents that the lower respiratory tract normally contains a thin lining of mucus that traps bacteria and dust particles. Cilia move the bacteria and particles up to the throat, where they're either coughed up or swallowed. However, in cystic fibrosis, the viscous mucous lining clogs the airways, blocking air flow in and out of the alveoli, interfering with normal gas exchange and preventing the cilia from efficiently removing bacteria and particles. As a result, bacteria proliferate, causing repeated lung infections, especially by *Staphylococcus aureus* and *Pseudomonas aeruginosa*. Eventually, lung infections severely damage the lungs. Unfortunately, the bacteria can't be completely eradicated from the lungs, although medication, chest physiotherapy, and other treatments can control the infections.

Explain that GI effects of cystic fibrosis occur mainly in the pancreas, intestines, and liver. In the pancreas, thick mucus blocks the ducts and prevents the pancreas from secreting its enzymes into the intestines, causing a pancreatic digestive enzyme deficiency. This deficiency blocks the digestion and absorption of food in the intestinal tract and causes bulky, foul-smelling, pale stools with a high fat content.

Malabsorption also results in poor weight gain, poor growth, ravenous appetite, distended abdomen, thin extremities, and poor skin turgor. The degree of blockage in the pancreatic ducts determines the severity of pancreatic digestive enzyme deficiency and malabsorption, and ultimately the patient's nutritional status and the severity of his GI symptoms.

Explain that the thick mucus secreted in cystic fibrosis can cause other pancreatic problems and common bile duct blockage, leading to gallbladder and liver dysfunction. In the pancreas, fibrotic tissue, multiple cysts, thick mucus, and eventually fat replace the acini (small, saclike swellings), producing symptoms of pancreatic insufficiency. Glucose intolerance also can stem from the repeated infections, and as the infection subsides, the glucose level falls. Likewise, thick mucus that blocks the common bile ducts causes fibrotic tissue changes in the liver. Severe biliary cirrhosis and portal hypertension may develop, leading to esophageal varices, episodes of hematemesis, and hepatomegaly.

Complications

Inform the parents and the patient that they can minimize many complications of cystic fibrosis by carefully adhering to the treatment regimen and by calling the doctor at the first sign of a problem. Such complications include bronchiectasis, pneumonia, atelectasis, hemoptysis, dehydration, distal intestinal obstructive syndrome, malnutrition, gastroesophageal reflux, nasal polyps, rectal prolapse, and cor pulmonale.

However, many complications associated with progressive cystic fibrosis aren't preventable. They include liver disease, diabetes, pneumothorax, arthritis, pancreatitis, and cholecystitis. Emphasize, though, that even if these complications develop, early diagnosis and aggressive treatment can enhance the patient's quality of life and sense of well-being.

Describe the diagnostic workup

Prepare the patient and his parents for tests to diagnose cystic fibrosis. Explain that the sweat test confirms the disease. Then subsequent tests—a fecal fat test, chest X-ray, sputum culture with sensitivity, pulmonary function tests, and blood tests—determine the degree of malabsorption and respiratory dysfunction.

Sweat test

Inform the parents and the patient that the sweat test confirms cystic fibrosis by measuring electrolyte concentrations (primarily sodium and chloride) in sweat, using a procedure called pilocarpine iontophoresis.

Explain that you'll clean the patient's forearm (or the right leg in an infant) with distilled water. Then you'll apply two electrodes to the area and secure them with straps. One electrode is covered with a pad saturated with normal saline solution, and the other is covered with a pad saturated with pilocarpine solution (a sweat inducer). You'll attach lead wires to the electrodes, and connect them to an analyzer. Next, you'll administer a mild current (4 milliamperes) over 15 to 20 seconds and continue at 15- to 20-second intervals for 5 minutes. Reassure the patient that the procedure is painless except for a slight tickling sensation.

After iontophoresis, you'll remove the electrodes and again clean the area with distilled water, and then dry it. Describe how you'll place a dry gauze pad or filter paper on the area, cover it with plastic, and seal it with waterproof adhesive tape. After 30 to 40 minutes, you'll remove the dressing and analyze it for electrolyte concentration.

Fecal fat test

Tell the parents and the patient that a fecal fat test evaluates the body's ability to digest fats and confirms malabsorption. Instruct the parents to give the patient a high-fat diet (100 g daily) for 3 days before the test and during the 72-hour collection process. Advise them to record food intake during the 72 hours for fat intake analysis. The doctor will also withhold certain drugs that might interfere with test results. Provide instructions for collecting the stool specimen at home, emphasizing how to prevent contamination with toilet tissue or urine.

Sputum culture with sensitivity

Explain that this test confirms the presence of bacteria in sputum and identifies the type of bacteria and sputum characteristics, such as viscosity or the presence of red blood cells.

Chest X-ray

Inform the parents and the patient that chest X-rays may be used to diagnose respiratory obstruction or monitor its progress. The test takes only minutes, but the technician or doctor will need additional time to check the quality of the films. Mention that the patient will wear a gown and must remove all jewelry from his neck and chest.

Explain that the patient will stand or sit in front of a large, camera-like machine. He'll be asked to take a deep breath, to hold it, and to remain still for a few seconds while the X-ray is taken. Reassure the parents that radiation exposure is minimal.

Pulmonary function tests

Inform the parents and the patient that these tests evaluate lung function and the effectiveness of bronchodilators, chest physiotherapy, and other treatments. Tell the parents to reduce the patient's food and fluid intake for a few hours before testing because a full stomach may constrict the diaphragm and cause vomiting. The patient should also wear loose-fitting clothing and void just before the tests.

Explain that the patient will sit upright and wear a noseclip. Or he may sit in a small, airtight box called a body plethysmograph (then he won't need a noseclip). Warn him that he may feel claustrophobic, but reassure him that he won't suffocate and that he can communicate with the technician through a window in the box. Tell him that he'll breathe through a mouth tube (similar to scuba-diving equipment) and that he may be instructed to breathe in several different ways. For example, he may be asked to inhale deeply and exhale completely or to inhale quickly. He may receive an aerosolized bronchodilator and may then repeat one or two tests to evaluate the drug's effectiveness. An arterial puncture may be performed during the test for arterial blood gas analysis.

Emphasize that the test will proceed quickly if the patient follows directions and keeps a tight seal around the mouthpiece or tube. These measures will also ensure accurate results.

Tell the patient that he may feel short of breath and tired during the test, but he'll be allowed to rest periodically. Instruct him to inform the technician if he experiences dizziness, chest pain, palpitations, nausea, severe dyspnea, or wheezing. If arterial blood was drawn, he should report swelling, bleeding from the puncture site, and any numbness, tingling, or pain in the affected limb.

Blood tests

Explain that blood tests can detect electrolyte disturbances and nutritional deficiencies. Common tests include a chemistry profile, vitamin levels, a complete blood count, and an immunoglobulin test. Clarify that these tests will be done periodically to evaluate the effectiveness of drug and dietary therapy.

Teach about treatments

Emphasize that treatment can improve the patient's quality of life. Point out that treatments vary, depending on the severity of his condition. Discuss special exercises, diet therapy, medications, and pulmonary measures, such as chest physiotherapy and aerosol therapy.

Activity

Stress that exercise improves overall health in a patient with cystic fibrosis. For example, it improves respiratory muscle function and efficiency. By enhancing airflow through the lungs, it improves cardiopulmonary function and improves activity tolerance. It can also help dislodge mucus from the lungs.

Tell the parents and the patient that the doctor will probably prescribe exercises to improve breathing, posture, and chest mobility, as well as aerobic exercises for overall fitness. Outline how to perform these exercises. Give them a copy of the patient-teaching aid *Exercises for healthier lungs and easier breathing,* pages 124 to 127.

Diet

Teach the parents and the patient that a high-calorie, high-protein diet is essential in treating cystic fibrosis. Explain that the patient doesn't digest and absorb his food completely; therefore, many calories are lost through stools. Furthermore, frequent coughing and illnesses such as lung infections increase the patient's need for calories. Instruct the parents and the patient on a proper diet, and reinforce your instruction by providing a copy of the teaching aid *Tips for adding calories to the diet,* page 128.

Encourage eating salty foods to compensate for the sodium chloride lost in sweat, and drinking adequate fluids to maintain good hydration. Also advise including plenty of fats in the patient's diet. Although they're the most difficult foods for a patient with cystic fibrosis to digest, they're nutritionally necessary. Point out that taking pancreatic enzyme capsules can help combat most effects of fat malabsorption.

Medication

Teach about the complex drug regimen used to treat cystic fibrosis. Explain that antibiotics may be prescribed prophylactically to prevent acute respiratory infections or to treat an existing respiratory infection. Aerosol bronchodilators (methylxanthines and sympathomimetics) reverse or control wheezing and airway spasm. Corticosteroids (inhalable and intranasal) reduce the frequency and severity of airway spasm and dyspnea, as do mast cell stabilizers, such as cromolyn sodium. Other prescribed drugs include vitamin supplements and digestant pancreatic enzymes, which are used to treat malabsorption. Provide a copy of the patient-teaching aid *Improving digestion with pancreatic enzymes,* page 129. Discuss possible adverse effects of each prescribed drug and any necessary precautions. (See *Teaching about drugs for cystic fibrosis,* pages 116 to 121.)

Procedures

Inform the parents and the patient that two types of treatments—chest physiotherapy and aerosol therapy—help loosen and remove mucus from the respiratory tract.

Chest physiotherapy. Explain that this treatment is usually performed with a partner. It uses four techniques—postural drainage, percussion, vibration, and coughing. Outline these techniques with the help of the patient-teaching aid *How to perform chest physiotherapy in cystic fibrosis,* pages 130 to 133.

Point out that as the child with cystic fibrosis matures and strives for independence, he'll want more control over his treatments. He can learn to perform some treatments himself, using three techniques—self-percussion, positive expiratory pressure (PEP), and forced expiratory technique (FET).

Explain that in *self-percussion,* the patient assumes various postural drainage positions and percusses his own chest, either with his cupped hand or with a mechanical percussor. Caution, though, that this technique can be very tiring and that some parts of the back are hard to reach. Before the parents buy a percussor, suggest renting several different models for a week each to determine which machine works best.

Explain that in using the *PEP mask,* the patient takes a deep breath and then blows forcefully into the mouthpiece of a special device that resists airflow. The treatment takes 15 to 20 minutes. Although this technique requires cooperation and concentration, most children can perform it by age 10. Because the device is portable, PEP can be done anywhere. The PEP mask is not FDA-approved, so it is not widely available.

Describe another self-care technique, *FET,* which couples deep breathing and normal breathing with long, controlled exhalation. (See *How to perform forced expiratory technique,* page 134.)

Aerosol therapy. Explain that several aerosol delivery systems are available. Nebulizer treatments using a compressed air machine or a metered dose inhaler, or both, are usually used in cystic fibrosis. Teach the parents and the patient how to use the prescribed system. Give them a copy of the patient-teaching aid *How to use an oral inhaler with a holding chamber,* page 135. Instruct them how to care for the aerosol equipment, providing a copy of the patient-teaching aid *Caring for aerosol equipment,* page 136. Also discuss ways to elicit cooperation from young patients during breathing treatments. (See *Promoting cooperation with treatments,* page 122.)

Describe how the patient should sit upright during aerosol treatments to help the medication penetrate deeper into the lungs. If he's using a nebulizer, he should breathe the mist through his mouth. He should continue treatment for 15 minutes or until the medication stops making a mist. Instruct him to perform aerosol treatments before chest physiotherapy so that the medication can help open the airways and thin the mucus before it's expelled from the lungs.

Other care measures
Discuss any special concerns associated with cystic fibrosis, including oxygen therapy, sexuality, dehydration, general coping measures, and follow-up care.

continued on page 121

Teaching about drugs for cystic fibrosis

DRUG	ADVERSE REACTIONS	TEACHING POINTS
Antibiotics		
Aminoglycosides **aerosolized tobramycin sulfate** (Nebcin) **gentamicin sulfate** (Garamycin) **amikacin sulfate** (Amikin)	• Watch for fever, headache, lethargy, nausea, pruritus, rash, superinfection, urticaria, and vomiting. • Other reactions include hematuria, neurotoxicity (balance problems) and ototoxicity (such as ringing in the ears).	• If appropriate, teach the parents to have the child use his regular aerosol nebulizer or inhaler followed by airway clearing, then to administer inhalable form of the drug. • Teach signs and symptoms of superinfections and of unusual reactions. Instruct the parents to notify the doctor of any of these at once. • If appropriate, instruct the parents or the patient how to administer the I.V. form of the drug. Emphasize giving the drug slowly over at least 40 minutes to prevent tinnitus.
Cephalosporins **cefaclor** (Ceclor) **ceftazidime** (Fortax, Tazicef Tazidime) **cefuroxime** (Kufurox, Zinacef) **cefuroxime axetil** (Ceftin) **cephalexin** (Keflex) **cephalothin** (Keflin)	• Watch for abdominal pain and distention, diarrhea (severe, watery, perhaps bloody), fever, hives, itching, local irritation at I.V. site (if appropriate), nausea, rash, unusual fatigue, thirst, weakness, weight loss, vomiting, and wheezing. • Other reactions include mild diarrhea, mild GI upset, and sore mouth or tongue.	• Teach parents the signs and symptoms of hypersensitivity, bacterial and fungal superinfection, and other adverse reactions; urge them to report any unusual reactions. • Warn them that the patient shouldn't ingest alcohol in any form (even in liquid acetaminophen) within 72 hours of the drug dose. • Recommend adding live-culture yogurt or buttermilk to patient's diet to prevent intestinal superinfection. • If oral form prescribed, advise taking the drug with food if GI irritation occurs. • Inform parents of infants about potential for yeast infections, especially in the diaper area. Instruct them to keep the diaper area clean and dry and to avoid use of plastic pants. • Urge parents to comply with instructions and to keep follow-up appointments. Advise them to discard unused or expired drug. • If prescribed I.V., advise parents or the patient to report any signs of vein irritation immediately.
Penicillins **azlocillin** (Azlin) **carbenicillin** (Geopen) **cloxacillin** (Tegopen) **dicloxacillin** (Dynapen) **methicillin** (Staphcillin) **mezlocillin** (Mezlin) **nafcillin** (Nafcil, Nallpen, Unipen) **oxacillin** (Bactocill, Prostaphilin) **piperacillin** (Viaflex) **ticarcillin** (Timentin)	• Watch for diarrhea, signs of hypersensitivity (hives, itching, rash, wheezing), and local irritation at I.V. site. • Other reactions include bleeding episodes, mild nausea and vomiting.	• Explain that the oral form should not be taken with acidic beverages, such as fruit juices. • Teach the signs and symptoms of adverse reactions, and emphasize the need to report any unusual reactions. Teach how to differentiate a rash from an allergic reaction. • Encourage parents to report diarrhea and bleeding promptly. • Be sure the parents and the patient understand how and when to administer the drug; urge them to keep follow-up appointments. • Counsel them to check the expiration date of the drug and discard unused drug. • If drug is given I.V., advise parents or the patient to report any signs of vein irritation immediately.

continued

Teaching about drugs for cystic fibrosis — *continued*

DRUG	ADVERSE REACTIONS	TEACHING POINTS
Quinolone **ciprofloxacin** (Cipro)	• Watch for dizziness, drowsiness, light-headedness, nausea, photosensitivity, rash, and vomiting. • Other reactions include blurred or disturbed vision, diplopia, tinnitus, and unpleasant taste.	• Inform the parents and the patient that this drug may be taken with or without meals. • Instruct the patient to avoid activities that require mental alertness until the central nervous system (CNS) reaction to the drug is determined. • Advise him to avoid taking antacids and to drink plenty of fluids during drug therapy.
Sulfonamide **cotrimoxazole** (Bactrim, Septra)	• Watch for aching joints and muscles; difficulty swallowing; itching; pale skin; rash; redness; skin blistering, peeling, or loosening; sore throat and fever; unusual bleeding or bruising; unusual tiredness or weakness; and yellow eyes or skin. • Other reactions include appetite loss, diarrhea, dizziness, headache, nausea, photosensitivity, and vomiting.	• Instruct the patient to take the drug with a full glass of water and to drink plenty of fluids. • Emphasize the importance of continuing the drug even after symptoms subside. • Caution against performing activities that require alertness until the drug's effect on the CNS is known. • Advise the patient to stay out of the sun to prevent a reaction. • Teach the parents or the patient to tell the patient's dentist and other doctors of sulfonamide therapy. Advise them to check the drug's expiration date.
Miscellaneous **chloramphenicol** (Chloromycetin)	• Watch for blurred vision, eye pain; fever; numbness, tingling, burning pain, or weakness in hands or feet; pallor; sore throat; unusual bleeding or bruising, and fatigue. *Also watch for in children:* abdominal distention, drowsiness, gray skin, subnormal temperature, and uneven breathing. • Other reactions include diarrhea and nausea.	• Instruct the patient to take this drug on an empty stomach — 1 hour before or 2 hours after meals. • Emphasize that the patient complete the entire prescribed course of therapy — including every dose. • Explain that the patient will have regular blood tests during therapy.

Bronchodilators

DRUG	ADVERSE REACTIONS	TEACHING POINTS
Methylxanthines **aminophylline** (Aminophyllin, Phyllocontin, Somophyllin) **oxtriphylline** (Choledyl) **theophylline** (Bronkodyl, Elixophyllin, Theo-Dur, Theolair, Theospan SR, Theostat)	• Watch for anorexia, diarrhea, dizziness, flushing, headache, insomnia, irritability, light-headedness, nausea, palpitations, pulse rate or rhythm changes, restlessness, seizures, tachypnea, tremor, and vomiting. • Other reactions include mild dyspepsia and bitter taste.	• Emphasize that the patient must take the drug exactly as ordered even if he feels fine. • Instruct the parents to notify the doctor if the patient comes down with the flu or develops a high fever. • Teach parents how to take the patient's pulse. Advise them to notify the doctor if his pulse rhythm changes or pulse rate decreases or increases 20 beats or more per minute. • Inform parents that it may take some time to regulate the drug so that it works without causing adverse reactions. • Tell them not to give the patient over-the-counter drugs containing CNS stimulants, such as ephedrine or epinephrine, to avoid increased CNS stimulation. • Advise that beverages containing xanthines, such as coffee and tea, and colas that contain caffeine can magnify the drug's effects. • Instruct parents to give this drug on an empty stomach or 1 hour before or 3 hours after meals. If the patient experiences mild dyspepsia, advise the parents to give the drug with food.

continued

118 Cystic fibrosis

Teaching about drugs for cystic fibrosis — *continued*

DRUG	ADVERSE REACTIONS	TEACHING POINTS
Sympathomimetics **albuterol** (Proventil, Ventolin) **bitolterol** (Tornalate) **epinephrine** (Medihaler-Epi, Primatene Mist) **isoetharine** (Bronkometer, Bronkosol) **isoproterenol** (Isuprel, Medihaler-Iso) **metaproterenol** (Alupent, Metaprel) **terbutaline** (Brethine, Bricanyl)	• Watch for chest pain, diaphoresis, dizziness, dyspnea, flushing, headache, pallor, pounding heartbeat, and vomiting. • Other reactions include anxiety, bad taste, fear, heartburn, insomnia, mild tachycardia, nausea, nervousness, palpitations, restlessness, throat irritation, and tremor.	• Tell parents to notify the doctor if the patient gets minimal or no relief from wheezing and airway spasm. • Warn that increasing the prescribed dosage can cause serious complications, such as severe wheezing, stroke, myocardial infarction, and perhaps even death. • Advise against taking the prescribed dosage more frequently than ordered. Excessive use can cause respiratory distress or reduce the drug's effectiveness. • Tell the parents to stop giving the drug and notify the doctor immediately if the patient develops any signs or symptoms of serious complications. • Instruct the parents not to administer more than one bronchodilator at a time. The patient should wait at least 4 hours between doses of separate drugs. • Advise parents to discard the inhalation solution if it turns brown or contains a precipitate. Tell them to store the drug in its original container and to refrigerate it if the label directs. • Instruct the patient to rinse his mouth with water or gargle after using an oral inhaler to minimize the bitter taste. • Tell the parents not to give over-the-counter drugs containing CNS stimulants, such as ephedrine and epinephrine. Such medications may trigger increased adverse reactions and drug toxicity.
Corticosteroids		
Inhalable and intranasal **beclomethasone** (Beclovent Oral Inhaler, Beconase Nasal Inhaler, Vancenase Nasal Inhaler, Vanceril Inhaler) **dexamethasone** (Decadron Phosphate Respihaler) **flunisolide** (AeroBid Inhaler, Nasalide) **triamcinolone** (Azmacort)	• Watch for bleeding from or ulceration of nasal passages, chest tightness, confusion, depression, dizziness, dyspnea, fainting, fatigue, fever, gastric distress, insomnia, itching, mouth and throat lesions, weakness, and wheezing. • Other reactions include altered perception, dry mouth and throat, hoarseness, increased appetite, and nasal burning.	• Warn that the inhalable dosage won't relieve airway spasm immediately; and caution the parents and the patient never to increase the dose in the hope that more medicine will work favorably and faster. • Tell the parents to call the doctor immediately if wheezing, chest tightness, or dyspnea develops after taking the dose. • Advise the patient to rinse his mouth and gargle with water after inhalation to remove drug deposits from his mouth and pharynx. This will help to eliminate any annoying aftertaste. • If the patient is taking inhalation bronchodilators, instruct the parents to give the bronchodilator before the steroid. That way, the bronchodilator can fully dilate the patient's airways, thereby improving deposition of the steroid. Because both drugs contain fluorocarbon propellants, advise waiting 5 minutes between treatments to avoid potential toxicity. • Remind the parents that up to a month may pass before they notice an improvement in the patient's condition. • Warn that inhalation cartridges are flammable and shouldn't be used or stored near heat.

continued

Teaching about drugs for cystic fibrosis — *continued*

DRUG	ADVERSE REACTIONS	TEACHING POINTS
Digestant pancreatic enzymes		
pancreatin (Dizymes, Hi-Vegi-Lip, Pancreatin Enseals, Pancreatin Tablets)	• Watch for allergic reaction (difficulty breathing, skin rash, wheezing). • Other reactions include diarrhea, nausea, stomach cramps, and vomiting.	• Advise storing the drug away from heat and light. • Be sure parents understand special dietary instructions. • Inform parents and the patient that adequate replacement of enzymes decreases the number of bowel movements and improves stool consistency. • Inform them that preparations are coated to protect the enzymes from gastric juices; the patient shouldn't crush or chew them to prevent inactivating the enzymes. • Inform them that there are usually no reactions to standard doses. • Review the signs and symptoms of an allergic reaction. And instruct the parents to notify the doctor if an allergic reaction occurs. The doctor will probably discontinue the drug.
pancrelipase (Cotazym, Cotazym-S, Creon, Entolase, Entolase HP, Festal II, Ilozyme, Ku-Zyme HP, Pancrease, Pancrease MT 4, Pancrease MT 10, Pancrease MT 16, Zymase)	• Watch for allergic reactions (difficulty breathing, skin rash, wheezing). • Other reactions include diarrhea, gout, kidney stones, nausea, occult bleeding (with high doses), stomach cramps, and vomiting.	• Teach parents and the patient the proper use of the drug, and advise storing it away from heat and light. • Be sure parents understand special dietary instructions. • Advise parents to keep a record of the patient's weight, the number of fatty stools, and any stomach problems. Then they should discuss this record with the nurse, doctor, or nutritionist to help determine the patient's fat tolerance and enzyme needs. • Instruct parents to mix powders (including content of capsules) with applesauce and give to young children at mealtime. • Tell the parents or the patient to avoid inhaling the powder because doing so may trigger an allergy. • Advise older children or their parents that capsules may be swallowed with food. • Tell parents that capsules may be opened to facilitate swallowing. The contents may be sprinkled on food, such as applesauce, but a pH of 5.5 or less is necessary to prevent dissolving the enteric coating on the microspheres within the capsule. • Advise parents and the patient that adequate replacement of enzymes decreases the number of bowel movements and improves stool consistency. • Inform them that preparations are coated to protect the enzymes from gastric juices; the patient shouldn't crush or chew the medication because doing so is likely to inactivate the enzymes. • Mention that there are usually no reactions to standard doses. • Review the signs and symptoms of an allergic reaction. And instruct the parents to notify the doctor if an allergic reaction occurs. The doctor will probably discontinue the drug.

continued

120   Cystic fibrosis

Teaching about drugs for cystic fibrosis — *continued*

DRUG	ADVERSE REACTIONS	TEACHING POINTS
Mast cell stabilizers		
cromolyn (Intal [inhaler], Intal Capsules for use with Spinhaler, Intal Nebulizer Solution)	• Watch for anaphylaxis (angioedema, chest tightness, urticaria, and increased wheezing), epistaxis, severe headache, nausea, painful urination, and vomiting. • Other reactions include bad taste, coughing, mild headache, nasal burning, nasal congestion, and sneezing.	• When the doctor prescribes oral inhalable cromolyn sodium, explain that this drug helps prevent airway spasm and wheezing, but it doesn't reverse acute airway spasm; the parents shouldn't increase the dose to treat acute airway spasm. • Remind them that up to a month may pass before the patient improves. • If the patient is also taking an inhaled bronchodilator, advise the parents to give the bronchodilator before the cromolyn sodium. That way, the bronchodilator can dilate the patient's airways, thereby improving deposition of the cromolyn sodium. • Warn against reducing the prescribed dosage or discontinuing the drug. Tell parents to notify the doctor if the patient experiences airway spasm and wheezing after taking an inhalable dose. • Suggest that the patient rinse his mouth after taking the drug to minimize any bad taste. • Before administering the nasal solution, the parents should tell the patient to clear his nasal passage. During drug administration, he should inhale through his nose. • Instruct parents to store this drug in a closed container away from moisture and light.
mucolytic **acetylcysteine** (Mucomyst)	• Watch for burning sensation in upper passages, difficulty breathing, runny nose, and wheezing. • Other reactions include chills, fever, and nausea.	• Stress the importance of always administering this drug via a nebulizer. • Tell the parents that intermittent aerosol treatments are commonly administered when the patient arises, before meals, and before going to bed at night. • For maximum effect, instruct the patient to clear his airway, if possible, by coughing productively before aerosol administration. • Instruct parents and the patient not to place the drug into the chamber of a heated (hot pot) nebulizer. • An unpleasant drug odor (rotten egg odor of hydrogen sulfide) and excess volume of liquefied bronchial secretions may cause nausea and possibly vomiting, particularly when using a face mask. Assure patient that the odor becomes less noticeable with continued inhalation. • Advise parents to store vial (once opened) in refrigerator to retard oxidation, and use within 96 hours. A light purple color apparently doesn't significantly impair its mucolytic effectiveness. • Unopened vial should be stored at room temperature, preferably between 59° and 86° F. (15° and 30° C.), unless otherwise directed by manufacturer. • Drug can cause bronchospasm. Many cystic fibrosis centers no longer prescribe it.

continued

Teaching about drugs for cystic fibrosis — *continued*

DRUG	ADVERSE REACTIONS	TEACHING POINTS
Vitamins		
multivitamins	• Watch for diarrhea, fatigue, headache, itching, loss of appetite, nausea, skin rash, vomiting, and weakness. • No other reactions.	• Explain that this drug supplements dietary vitamins that may not be properly absorbed because of the disease. • Tell parents to store vitamins away from heat and light and out of small children's reach. • Warn that vitamins with iron may cause constipation and black tarry stools. • Tell parents to read all label directions. Warn them not to give the patient large doses unless prescribed. • Tell them that liquid vitamins may be mixed with food or juice. • Advise them not to refer to vitamins or other drugs as candy. Children should be taught that vitamins and other drugs cannot be taken indiscriminately.
vitamin E (alpha tocopherol) (Aquasol E, Ferol, Eprolin, Epsilan-M, Tocopher-Caps, Vita-Plus E, Viterra E)	• None	• Inform parents and the patient about dietary sources of vitamin E, such as vegetable oil, green leafy vegetables, nuts, wheat germ, eggs, meat, liver, dairy products, and cereals. • Tell the parents to store vitamin E in a tight, light-resistant container.
vitamin K derivatives **menadiol** (Synkayvite) **phytonadione** (AquaMEPHYTON, Konakion, Mephyton)	• Watch for allergic signs (difficulty breathing, flushing, itching, rash, and wheezing) and dysrhythmias. • Other reactions include bruising, pain, and swelling at injection site, convulsions, dizziness, headache, nausea, pain, rapid weak pulse, stomach cramps, and vomiting.	• Stress the importance of complying with the prescribed regimen and keeping follow-up appointments. Tell parents to give a missed dose as soon as possible, but not if it is almost time for the next dose, and to report missed doses. • Instruct parents to tell every doctor and dentist that the child is taking this drug.

Oxygen therapy. Explain that the patient may occasionally need oxygen therapy at home. Teach the parents how to administer oxygen safely and effectively.

Sexuality. Inform the patient that the reproductive system in a patient with cystic fibrosis is basically normal; however, the vas deferens (the tube that carries sperm from the testicles to the penis) is incompletely formed or totally blocked with mucus in 98% of male patients. Consequently, most men with cystic fibrosis are infertile.

Explain that women with cystic fibrosis may have thick, sticky cervical mucus, which can also lead to infertility.

Emphasize, though, that men and women with cystic fibrosis have normal sexual function, and that women with cystic fibrosis can become pregnant. Forewarn a female patient that her pregnancy will be considered high risk and that it may cause her con-

122   Cystic fibrosis

Promoting cooperation with treatments

Parents may worry that their children won't cooperate with chest physiotherapy or aerosol therapy—and this is a legitimate concern. Young children often become bored, restless, or cranky during treatments; some might even be frightened at first.

Tell parents that persistence, patience, and creativity help encourage cooperation and maximize the benefits of therapy. Offer these suggestions:
• Encourage the child to participate in self-care. Even a young child can be taught to cough and move to the next postural drainage position. Or he can help by taking deep breaths and exhaling when you do vibrations.

A young child can also hold the mask during aerosol treatments, and an older child can inject the medicine or even learn to draw it up.
• Distract the child with a fun activity during treatments. For example, read to him, talk about what he did during the day, or have him watch TV or listen to music. Let an older child choose an activity; offer a preschooler two choices. This will help him feel more in control.
• Praise your child for his help and cooperation.

---

dition to deteriorate. Caution her to consult her pulmonologist and to seek genetic counseling before becoming pregnant.

Dehydration. Discuss the risk for dehydration associated with abnormally high concentrations of sodium and chloride lost in the patient's sweat. Warn that dehydration is most likely to occur in an infant or a young child. Dehydration may occur if the patient:
• experiences prolonged exposure to temperatures above 80° F. (26.6° C.)
• experiences fever, vomiting, or diarrhea
• exercises vigorously in hot weather, especially in areas without shade
• has an increased respiratory rate
• fails to drink adequate fluids or fluids high in sodium chloride.

Describe the signs and symptoms of dehydration: headache, muscle cramping, dizziness, irritability, lack of energy, decreased urine volume, or urine with a strong odor. If any of these conditions develop, advise drinking plenty of fluids, eating salty foods, resting in an air-conditioned room or in front of a fan, and dressing in lightweight clothing (diaper only for infants). Tell the parents to notify the doctor if the patient refuses to eat or drink for several hours or if his symptoms don't improve.

Coping. Help the patient and his parents cope with the realization that cystic fibrosis can mean a shortened life span. Encourage the whole family to use the resources available in their cystic fibrosis center, and help them find appropriate support groups. Advise the parents not to be overly protective; instead they should explore ways to enhance the patient's quality of life. Help the parents foster responsibility and independence in their child from an early age. Stress the importance of good communication so that the patient may express his fears and frustrations. If the patient is in his end stage, help the patient and family deal with approaching death.

Follow-up care. Discuss lifelong follow-up care. Stress the importance of keeping all regular doctor's appointments and notifying the doctor of signs of infection or any other sudden changes in the patient's condition. For example, the patient should contact the doctor if his cough increases, his appetite decreases, sputum becomes thicker and contains blood, or if he becomes short of breath or chest pain develops. Mention that medications will be adjusted as the patient grows. Also give instructions for obtaining emergency help if needed. Inform the family of the network of cystic fibrosis centers for expert, up-to-date care.

Source of information and support
Cystic Fibrosis Foundation
6931 Arlington Road, Bethesda, Md. 20814
(301) 951-4422, (800) FIGHT CF

Further readings
Bartholomew, L.K., et al. "Planning Patient Education for Cystic Fibrosis: Application of a Diagnostic Framework," *Patient Education Counsel* 13(1):57-68, February 1989.

Dankert-Roelse, J.E., et al. "Survival and Clinical Outcome in Patients with Cystic Fibrosis, With or Without Neonatal Screening," *Journal of Pediatrics* 114(3):362-67, March 1989.

Hayward, J. "Extending the Good Life...Cystic Fibrosis," *Nursing Times* 84(35):55-58, August 31-September 6, 1988.

LeGrys, V., and Silverman, L. "DNA Studies in Cystic Fibrosis," *Emergency Medicine* 19(16):57-58, 63-64, 67, September 30, 1987.

Lotfus, T. "Reclaiming Their Childhood: Helping Cystic Fibrosis Patients with High-Tech Home Care," *Caring* 7(6):22-27, June 1988.

Ries, A.L., et al. "Restricted Pulmonary Function in Cystic Fibrosis," *Chest* 94(3):575-79, September 1988.

Rose, J., and Jay, S. "A Comprehensive Exercise Program for Persons with Cystic Fibrosis," *Journal of Pediatric Nursing* 1(5): 323-34, October 1986.

Walker, C.L. "The Clinical Challenge of Cystic Fibrosis," *Journal of Intravenous Nursing* 11(6):373-81, November-December 1988.

Wells, P.W., and Meghadpour, S. "Research Yields New Clues to Cystic Fibrosis," *American Journal of Maternal Child Nursing* 13(3):187-90, May-June 1988.

Zach, M.S., and Oberwaldner, B. "Chest Physiotherapy—The Mechanical Approach to Anti-infective Therapy in Cystic Fibrosis," *Infection* 15(5):381-84, 1987.

Exercises for healthier lungs and easier breathing

Dear Caregiver:

The doctor has prescribed special exercises for the patient. Encourage him to perform them correctly and regularly. By improving the airflow through his lungs, exercise will help him feel like being more active.

Keep in mind that these exercises are performed in addition to chest physiotherapy — not in place of it.

Breathing exercises

Diaphragmatic breathing. This exercise can help the patient breathe more efficiently. He should perform it while he's resting or performing activities that don't make him breathless. Have him practice until it becomes second nature. Give the patient these instructions:

Rest your hands lightly over your abdomen. Breathe in slowly, expanding only your lower chest and abdomen. You should see your hands rise with your abdomen as air fills your lungs.

As you breathe out slowly, your hands should move in. Make sure to relax your shoulders and upper chest.

Breath control. This exercise can help the patient combat breathlessness during physical activity. Instruct the patient to follow these steps:

Inhale when reaching up and expanding the chest, and exhale when bending down and compressing the chest. Also inhale during the relaxation phase of an exercise, and exhale during the exertion phase.

Try to establish a normal breathing ratio: that is, taking slightly longer when exhaling than inhaling. For example, when climbing stairs, take three steps per inhalation and four steps per exhalation.

Posture exercises

Good posture promotes efficient breathing and prevents back pain. Tell the patient how to check his posture:

Stand sideways in front of a full-length mirror. Lift your shoulders up and back, hold your head erect, and keep your lower back slightly arched. Don't flex your back, contract your abdomen, or round your shoulders.

continued

Exercises for healthier lungs and easier breathing — *continued*

The following exercises will improve the posture, strengthen the back muscles, and stretch breathing muscles. Encourage the patient to do them 3 times a week in twin sessions of 10 times each (10 exercises, pause, 10 more exercises). Give him these instructions:

Shoulder pinch. Sit with your back straight and your elbows raised to about shoulder level.

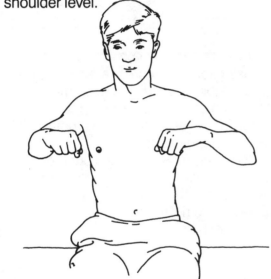

Pull your elbows back, and pinch your shoulder blades together.

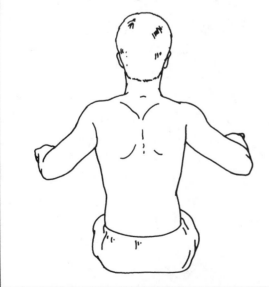

Shoulder depression. Sit with your back straight. Tilt your head to the right while pulling your left shoulder down.

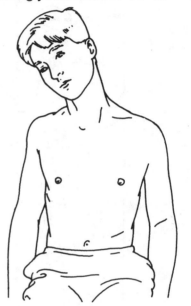

Then tilt your head to the left while pulling your right shoulder down.

Back arch. Lie facedown in bed with your elbows pointing to the sides. Inhale, lifting your back, shoulders, and head off the bed.

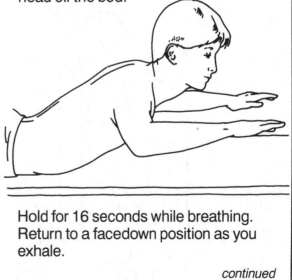

Hold for 16 seconds while breathing. Return to a facedown position as you exhale.

continued

Exercises for healthier lungs and easier breathing — *continued*

Pectoral stretch. Stand in a doorway or a corner. Place your palms or your forearms on the wall, rotating your shoulders about 90 degrees backward.

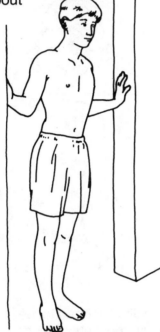

Then lean into the corner or doorway, keeping your back straight and flexing only at the ankles for a count of 60.

Abdominal stretch. Lie on your back with a pillow underneath your shoulder blades and your upper and lower back. Relax your abdominal muscles, and stretch them over the pillow for about 5 minutes.

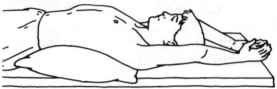

Chest mobility exercises

These exercises increase the strength and flexibility of the chest wall muscles. Have the patient do them 3 times a week in twin sessions of 10 times each. Give him these directions:

Side bends. Stand with your feet about 12 inches apart and your arms extended to the sides. Bend to the right side as you exhale,

continued

Exercises for healthier lungs and easier breathing — *continued*

and return to the center while inhaling.

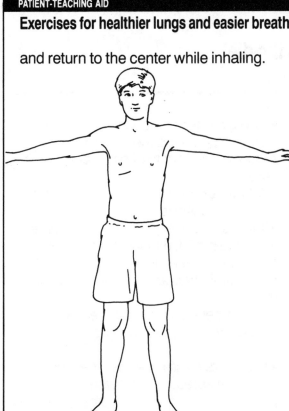

Bend to the left side as you exhale, then return to the center as you inhale.

Trunk rotation. Sit with your arms raised to about shoulder level and your elbows bent. Twist to the right while exhaling,

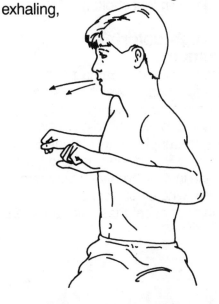

then return to the center as you inhale.

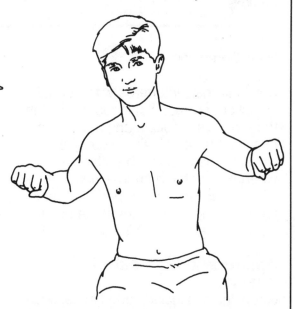

Twist to the left while exhaling, and return to the center while inhaling. Keep your hips facing forward.

Aerobic exercises

This form of exercise helps lower the heart rate (because the heart muscles work more efficiently), helps clear mucus from the lungs, and can increase the patient's activity level. It can also be lots of fun.

Keep in mind that any moderate exercise performed continuously for at least 20 minutes is considered aerobic — for example, walking, swimming, jogging, bicycling, dancing, basketball, soccer, or jumping rope.

Encourage the patient to increase the duration of his exercise gradually.

For maximum benefit, he should exercise at least three times a week at his target heart rate. (The doctor or physical therapist can give him an ideal heart rate to strive for).

Tips for adding calories to the diet

Dear Caregiver:

Cystic fibrosis interferes with normal digestion, so many calories are lost in the patient's stools. Many more calories are burned when he coughs, when he has trouble breathing, or when he's fighting an infection.

Because of this, the patient needs more calories. Here are some tips to help add calories to his diet:

Encourage high-calorie snacks

Good choices include dried fruits, such as raisins and apricots; peanut butter or cheese spread on crackers, bread, fresh fruit, or raw vegetables; milk shakes made with ice cream, cream, powdered milk, or instant breakfast powders; and breakfast bars.

Add extra fats and sugar to food

Fats are a great source of calories. But fat is difficult for patients with cystic fibrosis to digest, so watch for signs of malabsorption to see if more enzymes are needed. Try the following suggestions:

• Put margarine or butter on bread, rice, noodles, potatoes, and vegetables. Use mayonnaise or margarine on sandwiches.
• Add sour cream to casseroles, or serve it with potatoes, vegetables, meat, and fruit.

• Serve meat, vegetables, and casseroles with cream sauces or gravy.
• Mix extra amounts of salad dressing in salads.
• Add whipped cream to hot chocolate, fruit, and desserts.
• Top ice cream with syrup or preserves.
• Spread bread, muffins, biscuits, or crackers with jam, jelly, or honey.
• Substitute half-and-half or cream for milk.
• Add cheese to scrambled eggs, sauces, vegetables, casseroles, and salads.
• Use extra eggs in sauces, casseroles, sandwich spreads, and salads. Add powdered eggs to milk shakes. (Don't use raw eggs—they can cause food poisoning.)
• Sprinkle chopped or ground nuts on ice cream, yogurt, frozen yogurt, pudding, breads, and desserts. (Children under age 4 shouldn't eat whole nuts because they might choke.)

Serve high-calorie supplements

If the patient has lung damage, repeated infections, or weight loss, try adding commercial, high-protein calorie supplements to his daily diet. Typical commercial supplements include Ensure, Ensure Plus, Meritene, and Sustacal. Or use instant breakfast powders mixed with whole milk for about the same number of calories and nutritional value.

Improving digestion with pancreatic enzymes

Dear Caregiver:

The doctor has prescribed pancreatic enzymes to aid the patient's digestion. Pancreatic enzymes may reduce the patient's symptoms of malabsorption.

What is malabsorption?
This condition develops in many patients with cystic fibrosis because thick mucus blocks the pancreatic ducts. This prevents the digestive enzymes (lipase, amylase, and protease) from reaching the small intestine where they're needed to help absorb nutrients.

Malabsorption can interfere with the patient's normal weight gain and growth. He may have other symptoms too, such as frequent, loose, fatty stools and stomach pains from bloating and gas.

How to take pancreatic enzymes
● Give enzymes to the patient with a meal or a snack. Skip them when he eats *small* amounts of simple carbohydrates, such as fruit, juices, and soft drinks. But when in doubt, give them anyway — taking an enzyme won't harm him. Older patients should carry enzymes with them at all times.
● Instruct the patient to swallow the capsules whole with liquid. They should never be chewed or crushed because the tiny particles inside will rupture, and stomach acid will inactivate the enzymes.

● For an infant or a young child, place the capsule contents (particles) on his tongue before giving milk or formula. Or open the capsules and sprinkle the contents on fruit.

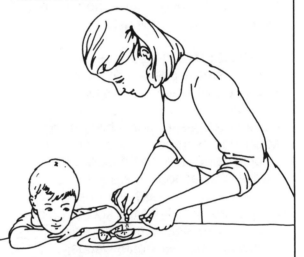

● If digestive problems continue, increase the number of enzymes by one or two capsules when eating.
● Remember that everyone's digestive system is different. Some patients need only one enzyme capsule per meal or snack. Others may need eight.

Some may find that even while taking enzymes they still have symptoms of malabsorption.

To determine the patient's fat tolerance and enzyme needs, keep a record of his weight, the number of fatty stools, and any stomach problems.

Discuss the record with the nurse, doctor, or nutritionist.

How to perform chest physiotherapy in cystic fibrosis

Dear Caregiver:

The doctor has prescribed chest physiotherapy to help remove mucus from the patient's lungs. This treatment consists of postural drainage, percussion, vibration, and coughing.

Postural drainage

The first step is positioning the patient so that gravity can drain his lungs of mucus. Infants and toddlers can sit on your lap or lie across it. Older children and adults can assume various drainage positions, using slant boards, pillows, and wedge-shaped foam supports.

Some slant boards have legs. Others are placed directly on the floor or on a bed. They're available from medical supply companies. Foam wedges can be purchased at department stores. Try various supports to see which type works best.

Percussion

Once the patient has assumed a drainage position, the next step is percussion. This gentle force travels throughout the lungs, loosening mucus.

Although percussion isn't painful if it's done correctly, the patient may want to wear a thin shirt, or you may cover the area with a sheet during treatment.

Percussion involves cupping your hand to create an air pocket and using your cupped hand to clap the patient's chest or back. Remember to keep your fingers flexed and thumbs pressed

tightly against the sides of your index fingers. Your hand should clap the chest with a hollow sound (like a horse galloping).

Rhythmically percuss each area for 3 to 5 minutes, alternating your cupped hands.

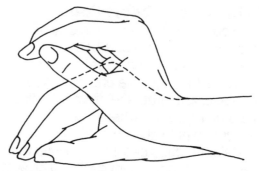

Vibration

After percussing an area, use vibration to help move mucus into the larger airways. First ask the patient to take a deep breath. Then as he exhales, gently press down on the area with your hand, using a quivering motion. Repeat three to five times in each area.

If you're performing chest physiotherapy on an infant, watch him breathe and try to vibrate about every third exhalation.

Coughing

After percussing and vibrating an area, help the patient sit up with his body bent slightly forward. If coughing doesn't occur reflexively, ask him to cough two or three times. This helps clear the mucus

continued

How to perform chest physiotherapy in cystic fibrosis — *continued*

from the airways even if none is expelled.

To maximize the effectiveness of coughing, have the patient breathe once, quietly and deeply. Advise him to cough deeply (not in his throat) two or three times with his mouth slightly open, tightening his stomach muscles each time.

If breathing deeply irritates his airways and causes uncontrolled coughing, tell him that taking several shallow breaths may help relieve the coughing.

Procedure for chest physiotherapy

Chest physiotherapy is time-consuming — it takes at least 30 minutes, and you may need to do it several times a day. Just remember that it's essential for the patient's health and comfort.

Make sure to wait 1 to 2 hours after a meal to prevent vomiting and discomfort.

Perform chest physiotherapy, using percussion, vibration, and coughing, in the following nine positions. Each position drains a different lobe of the lungs. Start with the lower lung lobes and work toward the upper ones or as the doctor directs.

Lower lobes (posterior basal segments)

1 Help the patient lie on his stomach, and place a pillow under his hips. Elevate his lower body 18 inches, with his hips higher than his chest and his head pointing down (see above, right).

Percuss and vibrate over the lower ribs near the spine on each side of the chest.

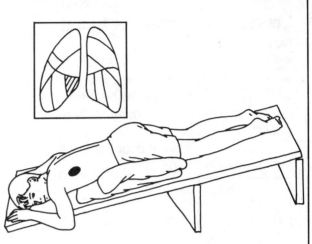

Lower lobes (lateral basal segments)

2 Help the patient lie on his stomach with his body rotated ¼ turn to the left and his upper leg bent over a pillow. Elevate his lower body as described in position 1.

Percuss and vibrate over the upper part of the lower ribs.

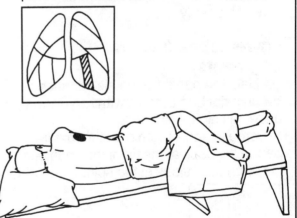

Then help him turn to his right side, and repeat the treatment on the opposite side of his back.

continued

PATIENT-TEACHING AID

PATIENT-TEACHING AID

How to perform chest physiotherapy in cystic fibrosis — *continued*

Lower lobes (anterior basal segments)

3 Help the patient lie on his right side with his left arm overhead and his left leg bent. Place a pillow between his knees, and elevate his lower body as described in position 1.

Percuss and vibrate over the lower ribs just beneath the armpit.

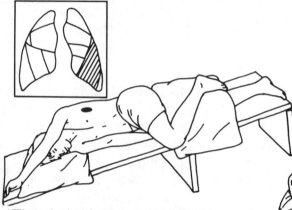

Then help him lie on his left side, and repeat the treatment on the opposite side of his body.

Lower lobes (superior segments)

4 Help the patient lie on his stomach on a flat bed or table with two pillows under his hips.

Percuss and vibrate over the middle part of his back at the tip of the shoulder blade on both sides of the spine.

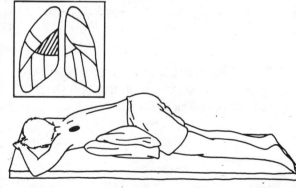

Left upper lobe (superior and inferior lingular segments)

5 Help the patient lie on his right side with his body rotated ¼ turn backwards. Elevate his lower body 14 inches, keeping his hips slightly higher than his chest and his head pointing down.

Percuss and vibrate over the left nipple.

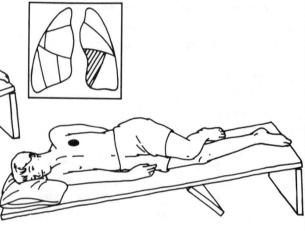

Right middle lobe (lateral and medial segments)

6 Help the patient lie on his left side with his body rotated ¼ turn backwards. Place a pillow behind him from shoulder to hip, and have him bend his knees. Elevate his lower body as described in position 5 and as illustrated (top, left) on page 91.

Percuss and vibrate over the right nipple. In female children with breast development or tenderness, percuss and vibrate by placing the heel of your hand under the armpit with your fingers extending beneath the breast.

continued

How to perform chest physiotherapy in cystic fibrosis — *continued*

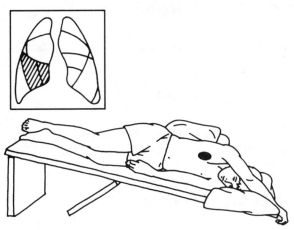

Upper lobes (posterior and apical-posterior segments)

7 Help the patient sit up with his legs dangling. Have him lean forward over a folded pillow at a 30-degree angle.

Stand behind him and percuss and vibrate both sides of the upper back under the shoulders.

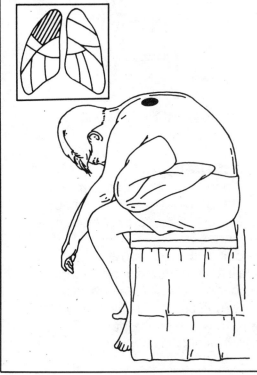

Upper lobes (anterior segments)

8 Help the patient lie on his back with a pillow under his knees. Keep his body flat.

Percuss and vibrate between the collarbone and nipple on each side of the chest.

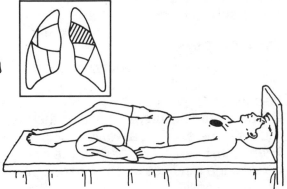

Upper lobes (apical segments)

9 Help the patient sit up. Then place a pillow against his back and lean him against you at a 30-degree angle.

Percuss and vibrate over the area between the collarbone and the top of the shoulder blade on each side.

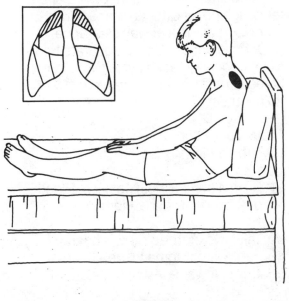

How to perform forced expiratory technique

Dear Caregiver:

The doctor has ordered a type of chest physiotherapy for the patient called forced expiratory technique (FET) to help clear her lungs.

How FET works
FET combines deep breathing and normal breathing with long, controlled exhalations (breathing out).

This treatment forces air behind the mucus in the patient's airways to help keep them open. It also helps move mucus into the windpipe so she can cough it up more easily.

FET isn't hard to learn. Just remember, the patient must concentrate during the long exhalations. Otherwise, the mucus won't move.

When to perform FET
Have the patient perform FET after each postural drainage position, before or after coughing, or after an aerosol treatment to maximize airway clearance.

Or have her use it as a separate treatment, repeating each cycle five to six times or until her lungs are clear (15 to 20 minutes).

How to perform FET
Give the patient these directions:

1 Sit in a comfortable position. Place one hand on your abdomen.

2 Take two or three slow, moderately deep diaphragmatic breaths (expand your lower chest and abdomen).

Try to breathe in through your nose and out through your mouth.

3 Then inhale gently and slowly, expanding your lungs about halfway. Pause.

4 Keep your mouth in an 0-shape and the back of your throat open. Then force the air out, using your stomach muscles. But don't force it out too hard. Repeat until you cough up some mucus.

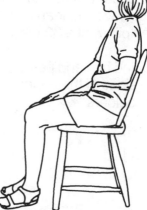

5 Repeat steps 2 through 4 until your lungs are clear.

Did I do it right?
If FET is done correctly, the patient will make a "ha" sound when coughing, or she'll hear a crackling sound before mucus is coughed up.

If she does FET too hard or for too long, she'll have a hacking, dry, nonproductive cough, or she'll hear a hiss, wheeze, grunt, or a catch. She may also get a sore throat. If she performs FET too gently, nothing will happen.

How to use an oral inhaler with a holding chamber

Dear Caregiver:

The doctor has prescribed an oral inhaler to dilate the patient's bronchial tubes. This treatment involves inhaling medicine called a bronchodilator through a small appliance placed in the mouth. A holding chamber attached to the inhaler allows the medicine to penetrate deep into the lungs.

The two most common spacer devices are the InspirEase System and the Aerochamber. Here are instructions for using an inhaler with these holding chambers.

InspirEase System

This system consists of a holding chamber that collapses and inflates during inhaling and exhaling. To use the inhaler with this device, tell the patient to follow these steps:

1 Insert the inhaler into the mouthpiece and shake the inhaler. Then place the mouthpiece into the opening of the holding device, and twist the mouthpiece to lock it in place.

2 Extend the holding device, exhale, and place the mouthpiece in your mouth.

3 Firmly press down on the inhaler once. Then inhale slowly and deeply, collapsing the bag completely. If you breathe incorrectly, the bag will whistle. Hold your breath for 5 to 10 seconds, then exhale into the bag slowly. Repeat the inhaling and exhaling steps.

4 Wait 5 minutes. Then shake the inhaler again and repeat the dose, following steps 2 and 3.

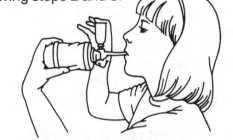

Aerochamber system

This system uses a small cylinder called an aerochamber to trap medication. To use the inhaler with this spacer device, tell the patient to follow these steps:

1 Remove the caps from the inhaler and from the mouthpiece of the aerochamber. Then insert the inhaler mouthpiece into the wider rubber-sealed end of the aerochamber. Shake the entire system for 2 seconds.

2 Exhale. Place the aerochamber in your mouth and close your lips. Depress the inhaler once. Inhale slowly and deeply. Hold your breath and count to 10.

Wait 5 minutes, then shake the entire system again, and repeat the dose.

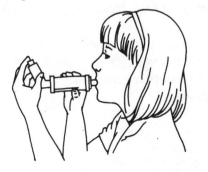

Caring for aerosol equipment

Dear Caregiver:

The patient's aerosol equipment consists of a compressed air machine and disposable plastic parts (mouthpiece, mask, syringes, and medicine cups). The equipment must be kept scrupulously clean. If it isn't, bacteria can enter the patient's lungs along with the mist.

Be sure to clean the plastic parts after each treatment, replace them every month, and perform periodic maintenance on the air compressor. Here's how:

Cleaning the plastic parts
You don't need to clean the parts every time they're used, but you should rinse them in warm or cool water after each treatment.

Allow them to air-dry before storing them in a clean plastic bag or other clean container.

Clean the parts *daily,* following the doctor's recommendations or those of the equipment manufacturer. Or use the following procedure:
• Wash the plastic parts daily in warm water and a mild dishwashing detergent, then rinse. The air compressor doesn't require cleaning. *Never* submerge it in water.
• After rinsing, soak the parts for 30 minutes in a solution of 1 cup white vinegar and 3 cups warm water. Rinse well in cool water.

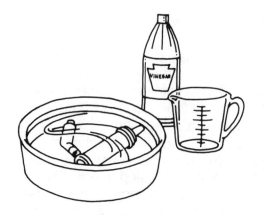

• Let the parts air-dry before placing them in a clean storage container.

Maintaining the air compressor
Keeping the compressor in perfect working order promotes better treatments and extends the life of the compressor. How often should you have the compressor serviced? That depends on the type of compressor and the manufacturer's recommendations.

Troubleshooting problems
If the machine isn't producing enough mist, the problem may be a simple one that you can solve yourself. For example, you might need to:
• change the air filter
• tighten the connections
• try a new aerosol cup.

If these measures fail, take the compressor to your medical equipment supplier for checking. It may need internal cleaning, but if the compressor is 8 to 10 years old, you'll probably need to replace it.

Asthma

In this chronic respiratory disorder, your teaching will focus on helping the patient prevent and control asthma attacks. A host of factors can trigger an attack—from eggs and aspirin to infection and emotional stress. Helping the patient identify and avoid such triggers marks the first step toward preventing attacks.

Because the patient usually remains asymptomatic between attacks, he may forget to take prescribed medications—or mistakenly believe he no longer needs them—so you'll stress the need for complying with drug therapy. To help him control an asthma attack once it starts, you'll teach him how to use an oral inhaler to take prescribed medications and how to perform breathing exercises and relaxation techniques.

Helping the patient learn about his condition and achieve some control over it can relieve much of the anxiety associated with asthma attacks. More important, a thoughtful and carefully implemented teaching plan can ensure that asthma doesn't prevent the patient from leading a normal life (see *Teaching a difficult asthma patient,* pages 138 and 139).

Discuss the disorder

Explain to the patient that asthma is a chronic, episodic disorder in which the respiratory system overreacts to allergy-producing substances (allergens), infection, emotional stress, or some combination of these. An asthma attack may begin dramatically, with simultaneous onset of severe, multiple symptoms, or insidiously, with gradually increasing respiratory distress. An attack can cause acute dyspnea, wheezing, chest pressure or tightness, and, usually, a productive cough with thick, clear sputum. It may last from minutes to hours and subside spontaneously or in response to drug therapy.

Explain that during an asthma attack, the muscles of the smaller bronchi and bronchioles contract (bronchospasm), narrowing the airways and making it difficult for air to pass in and out of the lungs. The airway linings become congested and swollen and secrete excess mucus, which further obstructs airflow (see *What happens in asthma,* page 140). In fact, some patients can't speak more than a few words without pausing for breath.

Complications

Warn the patient about complications that may occur if he doesn't adhere strictly to the treatment plan. A potentially fatal complication is status asthmaticus—a prolonged, severe attack that fails to respond to drug therapy. In status asthmaticus, mucus plugs may

Sandra K. Crabtree Goodnough, BSN, MSN, wrote this chapter. Formerly, Ms. Goodnough was director, Research Support Services, Hermann Hospital, Houston.

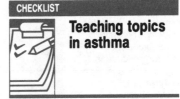

CHECKLIST

Teaching topics in asthma

☐ An explanation of how asthma triggers cause bronchospasm, airway edema, and mucus production
☐ Complications, such as status asthmaticus
☐ Preparation for arterial blood gas analysis, pulmonary function tests, and other diagnostic studies
☐ Importance of diet and adequate hydration
☐ Warning signs and prevention of respiratory infection
☐ Drugs and their administration
☐ How to use an oral inhaler or, if appropriate, a turbo-inhaler
☐ Identification and avoidance of asthma triggers
☐ How to control an asthma attack
☐ Sources of information and support

138 Asthma

Teaching a difficult asthma patient

Your patient, Bobby Keel, is a 19-year-old construction worker who's engaged to be married. He's been hospitalized with severe dyspnea, chest tightness, wheezing, and coughing that developed after a bout with the flu. The doctor diagnosed this episode as asthma. Bobby says that until now he's been healthy.

During your initial assessment, you find Bobby angry about the diagnosis of asthma. He's afraid he'll lose his job and his fiancée. Besides, he doesn't believe the diagnosis. He thinks he still has the flu. He shows little interest in learning about asthma and its treatment.

What are Bobby's learning needs? What, if anything, can you teach him today? What activities will you choose?

Using the standard teaching plan as your guide, formulate a modified plan to address Bobby's immediate needs. Draw up individualized learning goals for him (see next page) and then determine teaching priorities. Clearly, Bobby's inability to accept his disorder poses a barrier to learning. Thinking that background reading might make him more receptive to teaching later on, you give him some American Lung Association pamphlets about asthma. Then you decide that he'll probably want to learn about symptomatic relief, so you teach Bobby relaxation techniques and breathing exercises to relieve dyspnea. Inform him that he can use these techniques any time he feels short of breath. However, at this time, you decide to address your teaching primarily to Bobby's fiancée. Perhaps her interest will spur his.

Reluctantly, Bobby agrees to have the three of you meet when his fiancée visits later this afternoon. You'll discuss life-style changes that asthma may require, emphasizing that it's controllable and usually doesn't preclude a productive, full life. Then you'll evaluate Bobby's response to see what else you may want to use from the standard teaching plan.

Standard teaching plan for asthma

CONTENT	TOOLS AND ACTIVITIES	EVALUATION METHODS
Respiratory function • Airway anatomy • Gas exchange • Mucus production	Discussion, model or drawing of airways, charts, diagrams	• Question and answer • Discussion • Patient drawing of normal airway
Asthma • Pathophysiology • Signs of asthma attack • Complications • Signs of complications • Asthma triggers	Discussion, charts, diagrams, trigger list	• Question and answer • Discussion • Patient drawing of airways during asthma attack • Trigger list recitation
Diagnostic tests • Blood studies, including theophylline levels and eosinophil count • Sputum studies • Arterial blood gas (ABG) analysis • Radiographic studies • Pulmonary function studies	Discussion, spirometry demonstration	• Question and answer • Discussion • Return spirometry demonstration
Treatments • Activity • Diet • Medication • Relaxation techniques • Breathing exercises • Chest physiotherapy	Discussion of activity modifications and coordination with medication; medication cards for each drug; medication reaction log; demonstration of oral inhaler, relaxation techniques, breathing exercises, and chest physiotherapy	• Question and answer • Discussion • Return demonstrations • Medication management demonstration
Prevention • Smoking cessation • Trigger avoidance • Avoidance of respiratory infection • Support groups	Discussion, American Lung Association information	• Question and answer • Discussion

Teaching a difficult asthma patient—*continued*

Bobby Keel's learning outcomes:
Bobby and his fiancée will be able to:
- discuss potential life-style changes, if any, that Bobby's asthma may require
- show they understand the airway changes that occur during an asthma attack by drawing a normal airway and one affected by asthma, then comparing the two
- describe the early signs of an asthma attack
- list at least 10 possible asthma triggers
- state the reasons for diagnostic tests (ABG analysis and other blood studies, chest X-rays, and pulmonary function studies) and describe the sensations Bobby may experience during the tests
- demonstrate effective relaxation techniques
- correctly demonstrate pursed-lip and abdominal breathing exercises
- correctly demonstrate chest physiotherapy
- correctly demonstrate how to use an oral inhaler (Bobby only)
- create a medication reaction log
- list reportable adverse reactions to medications
- discuss and demonstrate how to control an asthma attack.

constrict or block the airways, which leads to impaired gas exchange and respiratory arrest (see *How status asthmaticus progresses,* page 141).

Describe the diagnostic workup

Before testing for asthma, other causes of airway obstruction and wheezing must be ruled out. In children, such causes may include cystic fibrosis, aspiration, congenital anomaly, acute viral bronchitis, and benign or cancerous tumors of the bronchi, thyroid gland, thymus, or mediastinum. In adults, causes may include obstructive pulmonary disease and congestive heart failure.

If other causes of airway obstruction have been eliminated, prepare the patient for diagnostic tests. Explain that no one test can conclusively diagnose asthma. Instead, he'll usually undergo a battery of tests. Be sure to tell the patient who will perform each test and when and where it will be done.

Venous and arterial blood tests

Inform the patient that blood tests can help confirm a diagnosis of asthma and monitor its treatment.

Venous blood tests. Tell the patient that the doctor will order blood samples, to detect increased serum IgE levels from an allergic reaction. (He'll also order a sputum culture, to check for increased eosinophil levels.)

Inform the patient that he may require daily venous blood studies to monitor the effectiveness of drug therapy (commonly

What happens in asthma

In susceptible patients, asthma results from exposure to an allergen, such as pollen. With initial exposure to an allergen, IgE antibodies form and bind with basophils or, as shown here, mast cells. These cells are now sensitized but remain inactive until a second exposure to the allergen.

When the allergen reappears, it interacts with the bound IgE antibodies, activating cell degranulation and the release of powerful chemical mediators.

These mediators—slow-reacting substance of anaphylaxis (SRS-A), histamine, prostaglandin, and eosinophil chemotactic factor of anaphylaxis (ECF-A)—produce the bronchoconstriction and edema of an asthma attack.

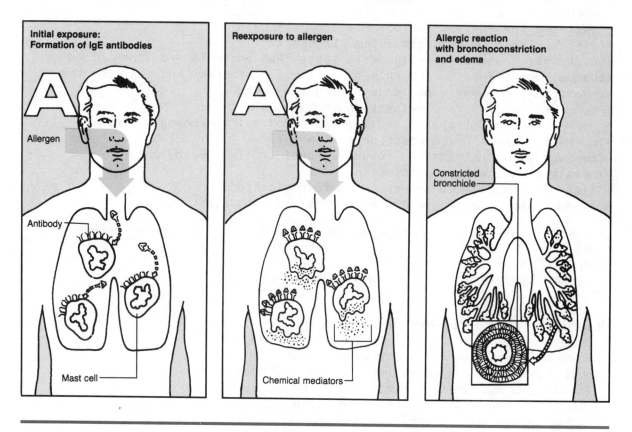

when theophylline is used). Reassure him that when drug levels reach the desired therapeutic range (10 to 20 mcg/ml), he won't need this test anymore.

Arterial blood gas (ABG) analysis. If the doctor orders ABG analysis to detect hypoxemia, explain to the patient that this test evaluates how well his lungs deliver oxygen to blood and eliminate carbon dioxide. Tell him which puncture site will be used (radial, brachial, or femoral artery) and, if appropriate, whether he should continue oxygen therapy during the test. Instruct him to breathe normally during the test. Warn him that he may experience a brief cramping or throbbing pain at the puncture site.

Allergy tests
Teach the patient about tests to confirm an allergy.

Skin tests. If the patient has asthma symptoms but no allergy history, he may undergo skin tests. Describe the procedure the doctor uses to identify specific allergens. He'll apply the suspected allergen to the patient's forearm, using paper backed by a layer of material that the allergen can't penetrate, or he'll inject small doses of the allergen, usually into the forearm. Test results are read after 1 or 2 days to reveal an early reaction and again after 4 or 5 days to reveal a late reaction.

Bronchial challenge testing. Inform the patient that, depending on the allergy test results, the doctor may order a bronchial challenge test. In this test, the doctor will ask him to breathe in an identified allergen, such as pollen, through a hand-held inhaler. Explain that the patient's reaction to this test helps determine drug therapy and life-style changes, if any.

Chest X-rays

Explain that chest X-rays may be used to diagnose asthma or monitor its progress. The test takes only minutes, but the technician or doctor will need additional time to check the quality of the films. Tell the patient that he'll wear a gown without snaps but may keep his pants, socks, and shoes on. Instruct him to remove all jewelry from his neck and chest.

Assure the patient that X-rays don't hurt. Explain that if the test is performed in the radiology department, he'll stand or sit in front of a large, camera-like machine. If it's performed at bedside, someone will help him to a sitting position and place a cold, hard film plate behind his back. He'll be asked to take a deep breath, to hold it, and to remain still for a few seconds while the X-ray is taken. Reassure him that radiation exposure is minimal for him, but that hospital personnel will leave the area during the test because they're potentially exposed to radiation many times a day.

Pulmonary function tests

Explain to the patient that pulmonary function tests evaluate lung function and the effectiveness of therapy, such as the use of bronchodilators or corticosteroids. If appropriate, advise him not to smoke for 4 hours before the test because smoking alters normal blood oxygen levels. Tell him not to eat a large meal or drink a lot of fluid before the test because a full stomach may restrict the diaphragm and cause vomiting. Also tell him to wear loose, comfortable clothing. If he has dentures, advise him to wear them to help form a tight seal around the mouthpiece of the breathing tube (spirometer) he'll use. Just before the test, instruct him to void.

Explain that during the test, the patient will sit upright and wear a noseclip. Or, he may sit in a small airtight box called a body plethysmograph, in which case he won't need a noseclip (but he might experience claustrophobia). Assure him that he won't suffocate and that he can communicate with the technician through the window in the box. Tell him that he'll breathe through a mouth tube (similar to scuba-diving equipment) for each test and that he may be instructed to breathe in several ways; for example, to inhale deeply and exhale completely or to inhale quickly. Explain that he may receive an aerosolized bronchodilator

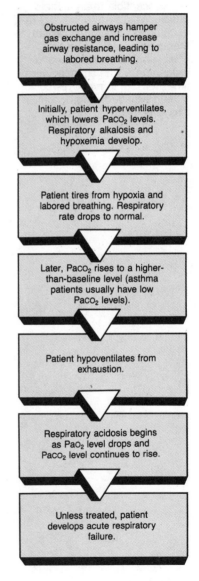

How status asthmaticus progresses

A potentially fatal complication, status asthmaticus arises when impaired gas exchange and heightened airway resistance increase the work of breathing. The flowchart below shows the stages of status asthmaticus.

Obstructed airways hamper gas exchange and increase airway resistance, leading to labored breathing.

Initially, patient hyperventilates, which lowers $PaCO_2$ levels. Respiratory alkalosis and hypoxemia develop.

Patient tires from hypoxia and labored breathing. Respiratory rate drops to normal.

Later, $PaCO_2$ rises to a higher-than-baseline level (asthma patients usually have low $PaCO_2$ levels).

Patient hypoventilates from exhaustion.

Respiratory acidosis begins as PaO_2 level drops and $PaCO_2$ level continues to rise.

Unless treated, patient develops acute respiratory failure.

Teaching tips
for asthma drugs

Regardless of what drug your patient's taking for his asthma, be sure to:
• Emphasize that he must take the drug even when he feels well.
• Stress that stopping the drug or changing the dose can make him susceptible to an asthma attack. What's more, he may require hospitalization to restore therapeutic levels of the drug.
• Explain that his response to drug therapy can change over time. Tell him to notify his doctor if the prescribed drug becomes less effective.

and may then repeat one or two tests to evaluate the drug's effectiveness. An arterial puncture may be performed during the test for ABG analysis.

Emphasize that the test will proceed quickly if the patient follows directions and keeps a tight seal around the mouthpiece or tube. These measures will also ensure accurate results.

Tell the patient that he may experience shortness of breath and fatigue during the test, but he'll be allowed to rest periodically. Instruct him to inform the technician if he experiences dizziness, chest pain, palpitations, nausea, severe dyspnea, or wheezing. If arterial blood was drawn, he should report swelling, bleeding from the puncture site, and any numbness, tingling, or pain in the affected limb.

Teach about treatments

Explain that treatment consists mainly of drug therapy. Other measures include appropriate exercise, a well-balanced diet, and avoidance of asthma triggers.

Activity

Explain to the patient that exercise generally promotes good health, but emphasize that he may need to avoid or curtail certain forms of exercise—especially if they trigger an attack. Encourage him to use trial and error to find the exercise that's right for him. For example, if he starts wheezing when he jogs, suggest that he slow his pace or try a different exercise, such as bicycling. Advise him to consult his doctor about taking his prescribed medication before exercise to prevent an attack.

Diet

Stress the importance of a nutritious, well-balanced diet to help prevent respiratory infection and fatigue. Tell the patient to drink plenty of fluids (48 to 64 oz) daily to maintain adequate hydration and to keep his mucus thin, which helps reduce bronchospasm. Encourage him to try to associate what he eats with his asthma attacks. Recommend compiling a list of attack-triggering foods—such as egg yolks, chocolate, and shellfish—for his doctor's information. Make sure he knows and avoids these foods.

Medication

Teach the patient about inhalable and oral forms of asthma drugs. Inhalable forms include the adrenergics, some corticosteroids, and cromolyn sodium. (See *Inhalation drug therapy for asthma.*) Teach the patient how to use an oral inhaler or a turbo-inhaler, and give him a copy of the patient-teaching aid *How to use an oral inhaler*, pages 146 and 147, or *How to use an oral turbo-inhaler*, pages 148 and 149, for reference.

If appropriate, teach the patient about the methylxanthines or the oral corticosteroid prednisone (Orasone).

Methylxanthines. Tell the patient taking a methylxanthine, such as aminophylline (Amoline, Phyllocontin), oxtriphylline

Inhalation drug therapy for asthma

DRUG	ADVERSE REACTIONS	TEACHING POINTS
Anti-inflammatories		
Inhalable and intranasal **beclomethasone** (Beclovent Oral Inhaler, Beconase Nasal Inhaler, Vancenase Nasal Inhaler, Vanceril Inhaler) **dexamethasone** (Decadron Phosphate Respihaler) **flunisolide** (AeroBid Inhaler, Nasalide) **triamcinolone** (Azmacort)	• Watch for bleeding from or ulceration of nasal passages, chest tightness, confusion, depression, dizziness, dyspnea, fainting, fatigue, fever, gastric distress, insomnia, itching, mouth and throat lesions, weakness, and wheezing. • Other reactions include increased appetite, nasal burning, dry mouth and throat, hoarseness, and altered taste perception.	• Explain to the patient that the prescribed drug should reduce the frequency and severity of his airway spasms and dyspnea. • Warn him that the inhalable dosage won't relieve airway spasm immediately; he mustn't increase the dose in response. Tell him to call his doctor immediately if he develops wheezing, chest tightness, or dyspnea after taking the dose. • Emphasize that he follow his doctor's orders when initiating, terminating, or tapering the use of oral steroids in conjunction with inhalable steroids to avoid acute adrenal insufficiency. Sudden withdrawal of oral steroids may be fatal. • If the patient is taking or has recently discontinued taking systemic corticosteroids, explain the need for additional steroids when coping with stress. He should call his doctor for instructions during stressful periods. • Advise him to rinse his mouth and gargle with water after inhalation to remove drug deposits from his mouth and pharynx. • If the patient is taking inhalation bronchodilators, instruct him to take the bronchodilator before the steroid. That way, the bronchodilator can fully dilate his airways, thereby improving deposition of the steroid. Since both drugs contain fluorocarbon propellants, tell him to wait 5 minutes between treatments to avoid potential toxicity. • Remind him that up to a month may pass before he improves. • Warn him that inhalation cartridges are flammable and should not be used or stored near heat.
Prophylaxis agent		
cromolyn sodium (Intal [inhaler], Intal Capsules for use with Spinhaler, Intal Nebulizer Solution)	• Be alert for anaphylaxis (angioedema, chest tightness, urticaria, and increased wheezing), epistaxis, severe headache, nausea, painful urination, and vomiting. • Other reactions include coughing, mild headache, nasal burning, nasal congestion, sneezing, and bad taste.	• When the doctor prescribes oral inhalable cromolyn sodium, explain to the patient that this drug helps prevent airway spasm and wheezing associated with asthma. Emphasize that it doesn't reverse acute airway spasm; he shouldn't increase the dose to treat acute airway spasm. • Remind the patient that up to a month may pass before he improves. • If the patient is also taking an inhaled bronchodilator, advise him to take the bronchodilator before the cromolyn sodium. That way, the bronchodilator can dilate his airways, thereby improving deposition of the cromolyn sodium. • Warn him that asthmatic symptoms may recur if he reduces the prescribed dosage or discontinues the drug. Tell him to notify his doctor if he experiences airway spasm and wheezing after taking an inhalable dose. • Instruct him to store this drug in a closed container away from moisture and light. • Suggest that he rinse his mouth after taking the drug to minimize taste. • Before administering the nasal solution, tell the patient to clear his nasal passage. During drug administration, he should inhale through his nose.
Bronchodilators		
albuterol (Proventil, Ventolin) **bitolterol** (Tornalate) **isoetharine** (Bronkometer, Bronkosol) **isoproterenol** (Isuprel, Medihaler-Iso) **metaproterenol** (Alupent, Metaprel) **terbutaline** (Brethine, Bricanyl)	• Watch for chest pain, diaphoresis, dizziness, dyspnea, flushing, headache, pallor, pounding heartbeat, and vomiting. • Other reactions include anxiety, fear, heartburn, insomnia, nausea, nervousness, restlessness, mild tachycardia, bad taste, tremors, and throat irritation.	• Explain to the patient that this drug should reverse or control wheezing and airway spasm. Tell him to notify his doctor if he gets minimal or no relief. • Warn him that increasing the prescribed dosage can cause serious complications, such as severe wheezing, stroke, myocardial infarction, and perhaps even death. Also advise against taking the prescribed dosage more frequently than ordered. Excessive use can cause respiratory distress or reduce the drug's effectiveness. Tell him to immediately stop using the drug and notify his doctor if he develops any signs or symptoms of serious complications. • Instruct him not to take more than one bronchodilator at a time. He should wait at least 4 hours between doses of separate drugs. • Advise him to discard the inhalation solution if it turns brown or contains a precipitate. Tell him to store the drug in its original container and to refrigerate it if the label directs. • Instruct him to rinse his mouth with water or gargle after using an oral inhaler to minimize the bitter taste. • Tell the patient not to take over-the-counter drugs containing central nervous system stimulants, such as ephedrine and epinephrine, to avoid increased adverse reactions and drug toxicity.

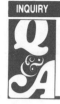

INQUIRY

Questions patients ask about asthma

Because I have asthma, are my children going to have it too?
They might. Sometimes asthma runs in families. In fact, about one-third of all people with asthma share the disorder with at least one member of their immediate family. If both parents have asthma, about three-fourths of their children have asthma too.

Can I prevent asthma attacks?
You can help prevent an attack by knowing and avoiding what triggers your asthma. What's more, recognizing the early warning signs of an attack—chest tightness, coughing, wheezing, and awareness of your breathing—and following your treatment plan can also help you prevent an attack.

Can asthma be cured?
No, but it can be controlled. Keep in mind that asthma doesn't cause permanent lung damage. And death from asthma is rare and usually related to lack of medical care or noncompliance with treatment. Asthma won't prevent you from living a full life if you accept it and work closely with your doctor, nurse, and pharmacist.

(Choledyl), or theophylline (Bronkodyl, Slo-bid), that the drug will control his wheezing and prevent airway spasm. Mention that it may cause mild GI upset or a bitter taste. If he experiences GI upset, advise him to take the drug with food.

Instruct him to report adverse reactions—such as anorexia, diarrhea, dizziness, flushing, headache, insomnia, irritability, light-headedness, nausea, palpitations, pulse rate or rhythm changes, restlessness, seizures, tachypnea, tremulousness, and vomiting—to his doctor. Teach him how to take his pulse, and tell him to check it daily and to notify the doctor if the rhythm changes or the rate rises or falls 20 or more beats per minute.

Inform the patient that it may take time to adjust the dosage so that the drug works without causing adverse reactions. Instruct him to notify the doctor if he comes down with the flu or develops a high fever; these may influence the drug's effectiveness.

Oral prednisone. Explain that therapy may continue for up to a month before improvement is apparent. Tell the patient to report abdominal pain, acne, back or rib pain, bloody or tarry stools, easy bruising, unusual fatigue, fever, hypertension, leg swelling, menstrual irregularity, extreme personality changes, purple striae, sore throat, vomiting, weakness, weight gain, and wounds that don't heal. Other reactions include unusual appetite, diaphoresis, dizziness, euphoria or feeling of well-being, headache, indigestion, insomnia, mild mood swings, mild nausea, nervousness, and restlessness.

Emphasize that the patient must strictly follow his doctor's orders when starting, ending, or tapering the use of prednisone in conjunction with inhalable steroids to avoid acute adrenal insufficiency. Warn him that sudden withdrawal of prednisone may be fatal. If the patient's on long-term (longer than 2 weeks) or high-dose (greater than 40 mg daily) prednisone therapy, teach him the early signs of adrenal insufficiency: fatigue, weakness, joint pain, fever, anorexia, nausea, dyspnea, dizziness, fainting, and weight loss. Also warn the patient on long-term therapy about cushingoid effects, such as acne, moonface, hirsutism, buffalo hump, truncal obesity, thinning of the limbs, and high blood pressure. Instruct the patient on long-term therapy to wear a medical identification bracelet. Explain the need for additional steroids when coping with physical stress, such as illness or surgery.

Because prednisone affects protein metabolism and water retention, instruct the patient to eat a salt-restricted diet high in protein and potassium. Advise him to take the drug with food to reduce GI irritation. To avoid GI ulceration, he shouldn't take this drug with alcohol. Also, instruct him not to take over-the-counter drugs containing aspirin or sodium. Aspirin may increase the risk of GI ulcers, and sodium may heighten the risk of fluid retention.

Other care measures
Teach the patient to eliminate or reduce his exposure to known asthma triggers whenever possible. For example, if he's sensitive

to aspirin, suggest that he substitute acetaminophen (Tylenol) or sodium salicylate (Uracel). Give him a copy of the patient-teaching aid *Avoiding asthma triggers,* pages 150 and 151.

Review how to prevent respiratory infection, another common asthma trigger. But if a respiratory infection does develop, tell the patient to notify the doctor. Also, teach him and a family member how to perform chest physiotherapy and recommend that it be done at least twice daily to clear mucus from the lungs.

Because emotions can trigger or worsen an asthma attack, the patient may need additional medication when he's upset for a prolonged period. To help prevent an attack, show him how to practice breathing exercises and relaxation techniques when he becomes fearful, angry, sad, or excited. Give him a copy of the patient-teaching aid *How to control an asthma attack,* page 152.

If appropriate, discuss the link between tobacco use and asthma attacks. Explain other harmful effects of smoking and refer the patient to a local stop-smoking program.

Explain that the doctor may try desensitization treatment when the patient can't avoid an airborne allergen. Explain that he'll inject tiny amounts of the offending substance under the skin at regular intervals. He'll inject only as much as the patient can tolerate without producing symptoms. Over several years, doses are increased until the body learns not to react to the substance with bronchospasm.

Most patients with asthma learn to live with it without the immediate aid of a doctor. However, teach the patient to notify the doctor if he develops a fever over 100° F. (37.8° C.) during an asthma attack, chest pain, shortness of breath without coughing or exercising, or uncontrollable coughing. Advise him to get medical help right away if he experiences a severe, uncontrollable asthma attack. He shouldn't wait for the attack to subside. Without prompt treatment, he could develop respiratory failure.

Sources of information and support

American Lung Association
1740 Broadway, New York, N.Y. 10019
(212) 315-8700

Asthma Hotline
(800) 222-LUNG

National Institute of Allergy and Infectious Diseases
9000 Rockville Pike, Building 31, Room 7A-03, Bethesda, Md. 20205
(301) 496-4000

Further readings

Cherniack, R. "Continuity of Care in Asthma Management," *Hospital Practice* 22(9):119, September 15, 1987.
Desmond, M. "When Asthma Is Work Related," *Patient Care* 21(9):42, May 15, 1987.
Fishman, A., ed. *Pulmonary Diseases and Disorders,* 2nd ed. New York: McGraw-Hill Book Co., 1988.
Kunkel, D. "Occupational Asthma: Some Basics . . . Some Puzzles," *Emergency Medicine* 18(19):91, November 15, 1986.
Loomis, C. "Childhood Asthma: What You Should Know," *Parents* 62(5): 227, May 1987.

PATIENT-TEACHING AID

How to use an oral inhaler

Dear Patient:

Inhaling your medication through this metered-dose nebulizer will help you breathe more easily. Use it exactly as your doctor has directed at these times: _____ .
Here's how:

1 Remove the mouthpiece and cap from the bottle. Then remove the cap from the mouthpiece.

Nebulizer bottle ——

Cap ——

Mouthpiece ——

2 Turn the mouthpiece sideways. On one side of the flattened tip you'll

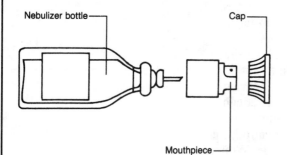

see a small hole. Fit the metal stem on the bottle into the hole to assemble the nebulizer.

3 Exhale fully through pursed lips. Hold the nebulizer upside down, as you see here. Close your lips and teeth loosely around the mouthpiece.

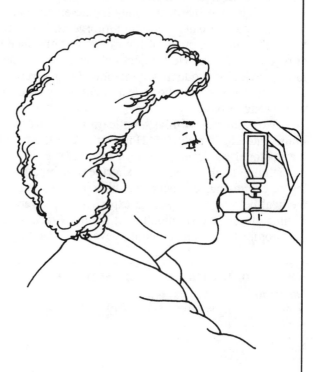

4 Tilt your head back slightly. Take a slow, deep breath. As you do, firmly push the bottle against the

continued

How to use an oral inhaler—*continued*

mouthpiece—one time only—to release one dose of medication. Continue inhaling until your lungs feel full.

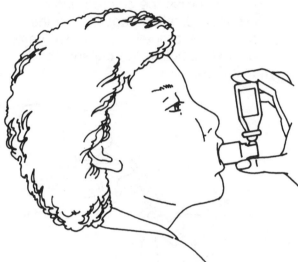

6 Purse your lips and exhale slowly. If your doctor wants you to take more than one dose, wait a few minutes and then repeat steps 3 through 6. Now, rinse your mouth, gargle, and drink a few sips of fluid.

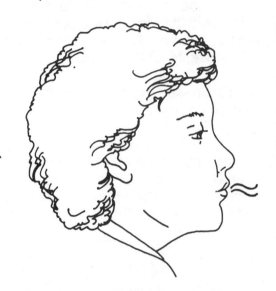

5 Take the mouthpiece away from your mouth, and hold your breath for several seconds.

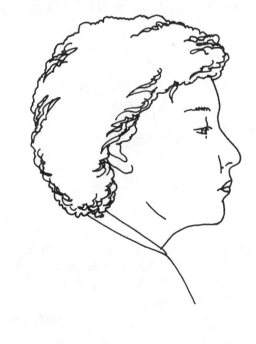

7 Remember to clean the inhaler once a day by taking it apart and rinsing the mouthpiece and cap under warm running water for 1 minute (or immerse in alcohol). Shake off the excess fluid, allow the parts to dry, and then reassemble them. This prevents clogging and also sanitizes the mouthpiece.

Precautions

Remember to discard the inhalation solution if it turns brown or contains solid particles. Store your medicine in its original container and put it in the refrigerator, if the label directs.
Important: Never overuse your oral inhaler. Follow your doctor's instructions exactly.

PATIENT-TEACHING AID

How to use an oral turbo-inhaler

Dear Patient:

Inhaling your medication through this "whirlybird" device will help prevent asthma attacks. Use it exactly as your doctor directs, at these times: _____

_____ .

Caution: Never use more than four capsules a day.

1 Wash and dry your hands. Unwrap one capsule so it's ready to use. Then hold the inhaler so the mouthpiece is on the bottom, as shown here. Slide the sleeve all the way to the top.

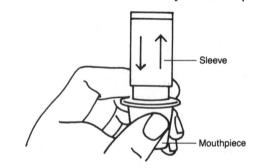

2 Open the mouthpiece by unscrewing its tip counterclockwise. Inside you'll see a small propeller on a stem.

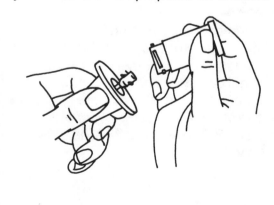

3 Firmly press the colored end of your medication capsule into the center of the propeller, as shown here. Avoid overhandling the capsule, or it may soften.

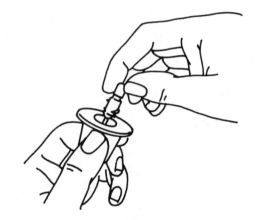

4 Now screw the device together securely, and hold it with the mouthpiece at the bottom, as shown here.

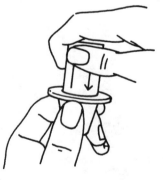

To puncture the capsule and release the medication, slide the sleeve all the way down. Then slide it up again. Do this step only once.

continued

How to use an oral turbo-inhaler—*continued*

5 Make sure everything is secure. Then hold the device away from your mouth, and exhale as much air as you can.

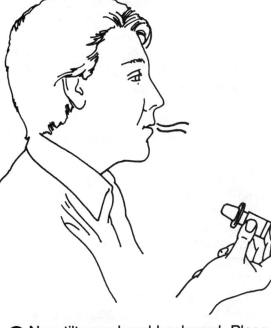

6 Now tilt your head backward. Place the mouthpiece in your mouth and close your lips around it, as shown here.

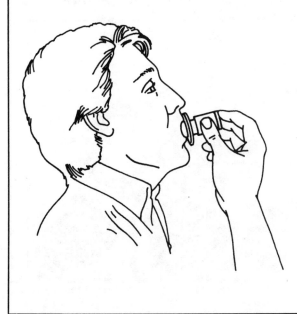

Quickly inhale once to fill your lungs. Inhaling through the mouthpiece spins the propeller, releasing the medicine, which will then reach your airways.

7 Hold your breath for several seconds. Then remove the device from your mouth, and exhale as much air as you can. Repeat steps 6 and 7 several times, until all the medication in the device is gone. Never exhale through the mouthpiece.

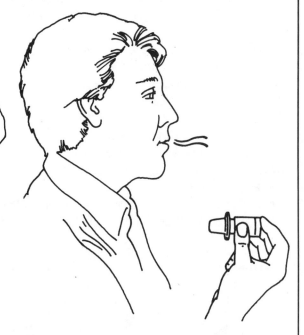

8 Discard the empty medication capsule. Then place the entire turbo-inhaler in its metal can, and screw on the lid.
　At least once a week, remove the device from the can, take it apart, and rinse it thoroughly with warm water. Make sure it's completely dry before reassembling it. Keep the capsules from deteriorating too rapidly by leaving them wrapped until needed.

PATIENT-TEACHING AID

Avoiding asthma triggers

Dear Patient:

To make it easier for you to live with asthma, try to avoid the following common asthma triggers:

At home
• Such foods as nuts, chocolate, eggs, shellfish, and peanut butter
• Such beverages as orange juice, wine, beer, and milk
• Mold spores; pollens from flowers, trees, grasses, hay, and ragweed. If pollen is the offender, install a bedroom air conditioner with a filter, and avoid long walks when pollen counts are high.
• Dander from rabbits, cats, dogs, hamsters, gerbils, and chickens. Consider finding a new home for the family pet, if necessary.
• Feather or hair-stuffed pillows, down comforters, wool clothing, and stuffed toys. Use smooth (not fuzzy), washable blankets on your bed.
• Insect parts, such as those from dead cockroaches
• Medicines, such as aspirin
• Vapors from cleaning solvents, paint, paint thinners, and liquid chlorine bleach
• Fluorocarbon spray products, such as furniture polish, starch, cleaners, and room deodorizers
• Scents from spray deodorants, perfumes, hair sprays, talcum powder, and cosmetics
• Cloth-upholstered furniture, carpets, and draperies that collect dust. Hang lightweight, washable cotton or synthetic-fiber curtains, and use washable, cotton throw rugs on bare floors.
• Brooms and dusters that raise dust. Instead, clean your bedroom daily by damp dusting and damp mopping. Keep the door closed.

continued

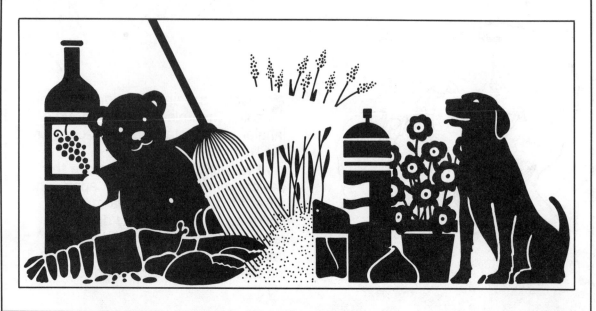

Avoiding asthma triggers—*continued*

• Dirty filters on hot-air furnaces and air conditioners that blow dust into the air
• Dust from vacuum cleaner exhaust.

In the workplace
• Dusts, vapors, or fumes from wood products (western red cedar, some pine and birch woods, mahogany); flour, cereals, and other grains; coffee, tea, or papain; metals (platinum, chromium, nickel sulfate, soldering fumes); and cotton, flax, and hemp
• Mold from decaying hay

Outdoors
• Cold air, hot air, or sudden temperature changes (when you go in and out of air-conditioned stores in the summer)
• Excessive humidity or dryness
• Changes in seasons
• Smog
• Automobile exhaust

Anyplace
• Overexertion, which may cause wheezing

• Common cold, flu, and other viruses
• Fear, anger, frustration, laughing too hard, crying, or any emotionally upsetting situation
• Smoke from cigarettes, cigars, and pipes. Don't smoke and don't stay in a room with people who do.

Preventive measures
Remember to:
• drink enough fluids—six to eight glasses daily
• take all prescribed medications exactly as directed
• tell your doctor about any and all medications you take—even nonprescription ones
• avoid sleeping pills or sedatives to help you sleep because of a mild asthma attack. These medications may slow down your breathing and make it more difficult. Instead, try propping yourself up on extra pillows while waiting for your antianxiety medication to work.
• schedule only as much activity as you can tolerate. Take frequent rests on busy days.

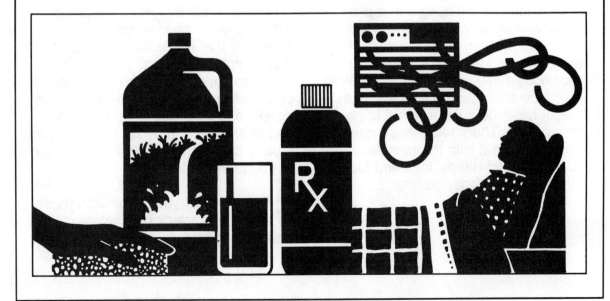

How to control an asthma attack

Dear Patient:

Usually, an asthma attack is preceded by warning signs that give you time to take action. Be alert for:
- chest tightness
- coughing
- awareness of your breathing
- wheezing.

Once you've had a few asthma attacks, you'll have no trouble recognizing these early warning signs. Above all, *do not ignore them*. Instead, follow these steps:

1 Take your prescribed medicine with an oral inhaler, if directed, to prevent the attack from getting worse.

2 As your medicine goes to work, try to relax. Although you may be understandably nervous or afraid, remember that these feelings only increase your shortness of breath.

To help relax, sit upright in a chair, close your eyes, and breathe slowly and evenly. Then, begin consciously tightening and relaxing the muscles in your body. First, tighten the muscles in your face and count to yourself: one-1,000; two-1,000. Be sure not to hold your breath. Then, relax these muscles and repeat with the muscles in your arms and hands, legs and feet. Finally, let your body go limp.

3 Regain control of your breathing by doing the pursed-lip breathing exercises you've been taught. *Don't gasp for air.* Continue pursed-lip breathing until you no longer feel breathless.

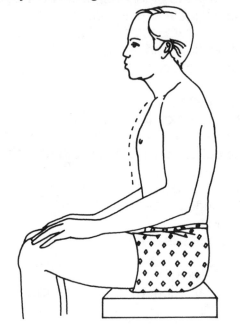

4 If the attack triggers a coughing spell, you'll need to control your cough so that it effectively brings up mucus and helps clear your airways. To do so, lean forward slightly, keeping your feet on the floor. Next, breathe in deeply and hold that breath for a second or two. Cough twice, first to loosen mucus and then to bring it up. Be sure to cough into a tissue.

5 If, even after you've followed these steps, the attack gets worse, call your doctor right away.

Occupational respiratory diseases

Airborne pollutants in the workplace can cause a host of respiratory diseases, ranging from acute problems to chronic pulmonary fibrosis. Unfortunately, many patients already have irreversible lung damage by the time they seek treatment. The reason: Occupational respiratory diseases usually develop gradually from repeated exposure to an inhaled pollutant.

Once the patient seeks treatment, you'll need to prepare him for chest X-rays and other tests to evaluate pulmonary function and identify the causative pollutant. Later, you'll review how to prevent or forestall further lung damage and how to relieve discomfort by following a prescribed exercise program and a well-balanced diet. As appropriate, you'll also discuss medications, oxygen therapy, and chest physiotherapy.

As a nurse, you're in an ideal position to identify patients at high risk for occupational respiratory diseases and to teach them how to recognize and avoid hazards at work. Teaching about ways to prevent these potentially life-threatening diseases may be your most satisfying teaching contribution.

Discuss the disorder

Inform the patient that these respiratory diseases typically result from inhaling air pollutants on the job. These diseases are characterized by alveolitis—inflammation of the tiny air sacs in the lungs where gas exchange occurs—and progressive fibrosis—either permanent scarring or scar tissue formation that prevents the lungs from expanding fully.

Identify the three main occupational respiratory disease categories: pneumoconiosis, hypersensitivity diseases, and toxic lung injury. Elaborate on the patient's specific disease.

Pneumoconiosis

Tell the patient with pneumoconiosis that the disease results from inhaling inorganic particles—for example, the fibers produced by manufacturing asbestos-containing materials or the dust produced by coal mining (see *Reviewing causes of pneumoconiosis,* page 154). Gradually, stiff scar tissue replaces the lungs' normally elastic tissue. As this process—called pulmonary fibrosis—advances, the spreading scar tissue limits the lungs' ability to expand and contract and destroys capillary units in the alveoli. This, in turn, impairs gas exchange. Like pneumoconiosis, a disease called idiopathic pulmonary fibrosis is also characterized by replacement of healthy lung tissue with inelastic scar tissue. This disease results from unknown pollutants or abnormalities.

Karen A. Landis, RN, MS, CCRN, who wrote this chapter, is a pulmonary clinical nurse specialist at the Allentown Hospital–Lehigh Valley Hospital Center, in Allentown, Pa.

CHECKLIST

Teaching topics in occupational respiratory diseases

☐ How air pollutants cause lung damage, such as chronic alveolitis and fibrosis
☐ Occupational respiratory disease categories: pneumoconiosis, hypersensitivity diseases, and toxic lung injury
☐ Preparation for diagnostic procedures, such as pulmonary function testing, magnetic resonance imaging, computed tomography, or mediastinoscopy
☐ Importance of an exercise program and a well-balanced diet with increased caloric intake, if appropriate
☐ Medications to relieve symptoms
☐ Using oxygen therapy and chest physiotherapy
☐ Avoiding respiratory infection
☐ Preventing job-related exposure to breathing hazards
☐ Sources of information and support

Reviewing causes of pneumoconiosis

If your patient works in a mine or processes inorganic materials, his job may be hazardous to his health. Review this chart to determine whether he's at high risk for pneumoconiosis.

DISEASE	CAUSATIVE POLLUTANT	HIGH-RISK OCCUPATIONS
Anthracosilicosis	Coal	• Mining and handling coal
Antimony pneumoconiosis	Antimony	• Mining and crushing antimony ore • Cleaning extraction chambers
Asbestosis	Asbestos	• Mining asbestos • Manufacturing asbestos cement products (tiles and roofing) • Manufacturing and installing insulating and fireproofing materials • Maintaining equipment in asbestos-processing factories
Baritosis	Barium	• Mining crude barium ore • Drying and bagging ground ore
Carbon pneumoconiosis	Carbon, carbon black, graphite	• Handling carbon black • Manufacturing carbon electrodes and carbon paper • Mining and handling graphite • Manufacturing refractory ceramics and crucibles, pencils, lubricants, electrodes, and neutron moderators in atomic reactors
Diatomite silicosis	Diatomite	• Mining, processing, and handling diatomite • Manufacturing filters for inorganic and organic liquids • Manufacturing bricks and cement used for heat and sound insulation
Fuller's earth lung	Fuller's earth (type of clay)	• Mining and processing fuller's earth • Clarifying mineral, animal, or vegetable oils • Manufacturing herbicides, insecticides, paints, and cosmetics • Refining mineral oils
Kaolin pneumoconiosis	Kaolin (China clay)	• Processing kaolin • Manufacturing paper, rubber, or plastics
Siderosis	Iron	• Iron and steel rolling and steel grinding • Electric arc and steel welding • Silver and steel polishing with iron oxide • Scouring, chipping, and dressing castings in iron foundries • Boiler scaling (cleaning fireboxes) • Mining and crushing iron ore • Mining, milling, and mixing emery
Silicosis	Free silica	• Mining gold, tin, copper, platinum, and mica • Quarrying granite, slate, and pumice • Tunneling for sewers and roads; excavating sandstone • Stonecutting and polishing, cleaning, and carving of masonry • Manufacturing abrasives using crushed sand, sandstone, or quartzite; abrasive blasting • Manufacturing glass and enameling • Processing products that use rock-containing quartz • Working in iron and steel foundries • Manufacturing china, porcelain, stoneware, and earthenware • Building and dismantling kilns, steel furnaces, ovens in gas-making plants, and boiler houses • Cleaning and scaling boiler flues and fireboxes
Stannosis	Tin	• Milling, grinding, and handling tin ore • Tipping ore into, and raking out, refinery furnaces
Talc pneumoconiosis	Talc	• Mining and processing talc • Manufacturing cosmetic powders or paints

What causes hypersensitivity diseases?

If your patient tells you he's allergic to work, he may not be joking. As this chart shows, occupational exposure to various organic pollutants may cause hypersensitivity diseases in susceptible workers.

DISEASE	ORGANIC PATHOGEN	ENVIRONMENTAL SOURCE
Air-conditioner (or humidifier) lung	*T. candidus* and *vulgaris*	Fungal spores
Bird-fancier's lung	Avian dust, excrement, or serum	Birds
Byssinosis (brown lung)	Flax, hemp, or cotton dust	Textiles
Cheesewasher's lung	*Penicillium, Aspergillus clavatus*	Moldy cheese
Farmer's lung	*Micropolyspora faeni, Thermoactinomyces vulgaris, candidus,* and *virdis*	Moldy hay
Furrier's lung	Unknown	Hair and dander
Hen worker's lung	Feathers, serum	Hens
Malt worker's lung	*A. clavatus* and *fumigatus*	Malt and barley dusts
Maple bark disease	*Cryptostroma corticale*	Moldy maple bark
Mushroom worker's lung	*M. faeni, T. vulgaris*	Mushroom compost
Sauna taker's lung	*Pullularia* species	Moldy water and container
Sequoiosis	*Graphium aureobasidium pullulans*	Moldy redwood sawdust
Wheat weevil disease	*Sitophilus granarius*	Wheat flour
Wood pulp worker's disease	*Alternaria tenuis*	Moldy logs

Hypersensitivity diseases

Explain that hypersensitivity diseases result from inhaling *organic particles,* such as mushroom compost or chicken feather dust. (For more information, see *What causes hypersensitivity diseases?*) The organic particles trigger an antibody response, which may be immediate or delayed, depending on where the particles lodge. For example, inhaled larger particles that lodge in the bronchi and bronchioles usually trigger an immediate antibody response and may lead to the condition called occupational asthma. Signs and symptoms include bronchospasms, dyspnea, and increased mucus production.

In contrast, inhaled smaller particles may lodge in the alveoli, generating a delayed antibody response called allergic alveolitis (or hypersensitivity pneumonitis). Localized alveolar inflammation, increased white blood cell production, and, possibly, accumulated fluid in the alveoli characterize allergic alveolitis. Caution the patient that long-term exposure to the harmful pathogens may cause chronic inflammation of the alveoli and surrounding tissue and, eventually, fibrosis.

How smoke damages lung tissue

Most occupational respiratory damage occurs over time. The exception is lung damage caused by smoke inhalation. Smoke—from a chemical explosion, for instance—can destroy lung tissue in minutes. The outline below lists the body's typical responses to this life-threatening situation.

Initial response
- The bronchioles constrict and impair ventilation.
- Increased carboxyhemoglobin saturation causes systemic toxicity and damage.
- Laryngeal edema obstructs the airway.
- Signs and symptoms: cough, cherry red mucosa, stridor.

Delayed response
- Increased pulmonary capillary permeability permits absorption of toxins.
- Destruction of lung parenchyma occurs.
- Signs and symptoms: dyspnea and crackles, increased sputum production, hyperinflation of lungs, rhonchi.

Toxic lung injury

Inform the patient that toxic lung injury results from inhaling noxious chemical fumes or smoke or both. For example, acute airway injury results from inhaling such toxic gases as ammonia, acetylene, chlorine, and formaldehyde. Those at high risk include farmers, chemical workers, and welders. Explain that the type of lung damage depends on whether the worker inhales the noxious chemicals in smoke or gas form and whether the inhaled gas is water-soluble. (For more information, see *How smoke damages lung tissue*.) For example, water-soluble gases, such as ammonia or sulfur dioxide, cause immediate and extreme irritation of the upper airways. Coughing and expectoration follow. Typically a person who inhales such a gas flees the contaminated area. And his flight saves him from further lung damage. If he's trapped, however, he'll inhale a greater volume of the gas. This allows the gas to penetrate the lower airway cells, causing acute respiratory dysfunction, damaging the bronchial mucosa and alveolar membranes, and leading, possibly, to chronic disease.

If the patient inhales an insoluble gas, his initial discomfort will be minimal because his upper airway symptoms, if any, will remain mild. As the gas enters the lower airways, however, severe impairment occurs, including alveolar membrane damage, pulmonary edema with crackles and dyspnea, pneumonia, emphysematous changes, and fibrosis.

Inform the patient that most occupational respiratory diseases develop over time (except for toxic lung injury, which is known for its rapid onset). Early signs and symptoms—typically, a chronic cough—may be easily overlooked or dismissed. As the disease progresses, though, the chronic cough may become spasmodic, producing copious sputum and mucus. Other symptoms include severe dyspnea and chest pain. In later disease stages, persistent hypoxemia and hypercapnia may cause cyanosis, headaches, insomnia or somnolence, and personality changes.

Complications

Tell the patient that limited pulmonary reserve may leave him susceptible to respiratory infection. However, by adhering to his treatment plan, he can reduce the risk for infection. Note that untreated respiratory infection can lead to life-threatening acute respiratory failure.

Describe the diagnostic workup

Emphasize that a detailed occupational history can help determine what, if any, breathing hazards the patient encounters at work. Then prepare him for tests to assess lung function, to determine what causes his signs and symptoms, and to identify causative pollutants. Explain that a typical diagnostic workup may include pulmonary function tests, chest X-rays, magnetic resonance imaging (MRI), computed tomography (CT), arterial blood gas (ABG) analysis, and sputum analysis. Additional procedures may include bronchoscopy, mediastinoscopy, thoracentesis, and exercise electrocardiography (ECG).

Pulmonary function tests

Teach the patient that this test evaluates ventilatory function. Before the test, give him a copy of the patient-teaching aid *Preparing for pulmonary function tests*, page 167. Also show him how to use a spirometer.

Chest X-ray

Inform the patient that chest X-rays can detect or monitor the progress of occupational respiratory disease. Mention that the test takes only minutes. Tell him that he'll wear a hospital gown or drape to cover his chest area. Instruct him to remove all jewelry from his neck and chest.

If he has the test in the radiology department, tell him that he'll stand or sit in front of the X-ray machine. If the test's performed at bedside, someone will help him to a sitting position and place a cold, hard film plate behind his back. He'll be asked to take a deep breath and to hold it for a few seconds while the X-ray is taken. Instruct him to remain still for those few seconds to ensure a clear and well-focused X-ray image. Reassure him that he'll be exposed to minimal radiation.

Magnetic resonance imaging

Explain that this painless, noninvasive test relies on a powerful magnet, radio waves, and a computer to produce clear cross-sectional images of the chest. Mention that it will be done in a special room that shields the MRI scanner's powerful magnetic field. Ask the patient to remove all jewelry and take everything out of his pockets. Emphasize that there must be no metal in the test room. Make sure he has notified the doctor if he has any metal inside his body, such as shrapnel, a pacemaker, an artificial hip, or orthopedic pins.

During the test, he'll lie on a table that slides into a hollow cylinder. Tell him to breathe normally but not to talk or move because motion may distort the test results. Forewarn him that the machine will be noisy and that his position within the scanner may make him feel confined. Reassure him that he and the examiner can talk to each other at all times. Although he can't see the examiner, the examiner can see him. Encourage the patient to relax and concentrate on a favorite subject or image or on his breathing.

CT scan

Inform the patient that this test uses computer technology to help diagnose or evaluate occupational respiratory diseases. If the examiner orders a radiopaque contrast medium to enhance the cross-sectional chest images, instruct the patient to fast for 4 hours before the test. Just before the test, have him remove all jewelry.

Explain that during the test he'll lie supine on a cold, hard X-ray table that will move into the center of a large, noisy, tunnel-shaped machine. If the examiner injects the radiopaque contrast medium into the patient's arm vein, the patient may experience transient nausea, flushing, warmth, and a salty taste.

Caution him not to move during the test but to relax and breathe normally. Movement may invalidate the results and require repeated testing. Reassure him that his exposure to radiation will be minimal.

ABG analysis

Explain that the doctor will order these blood studies to evaluate hypoxemia—or how well his lungs deliver oxygen to his blood. Prepare him for arterial puncture, and tell him from which artery—radial, brachial, or femoral—he'll have blood drawn. Remind him to breathe normally during the test. Warn him that he may feel a cramping or throbbing pain at the puncture site, but reassure him that the sensation will subside quickly.

Sputum analysis

Tell the patient that a sputum analysis isolates and identifies the cause of infection. Inform him that the best time to collect the specimen is early morning after secretions have accumulated overnight. Remind him to drink plenty of fluids the night before and to avoid brushing his teeth before collection.

Outline the technique for sputum collection. Instruct him first to take several deep abdominal breaths. When he's ready to cough, he should take one more deep abdominal breath, bend forward, and make a soft, staged, shortened cough into the container. Finally, describe the procedure for preparing the specimen container and avoiding contamination.

Exercise ECG

Point out that an exercise ECG, also known as a stress test, may be ordered to monitor how the patient's heart responds to occupational respiratory disease. The examination usually takes about 30 minutes.

Inform the patient that he'll ride a stationary bicycle or walk or run on a treadmill. Advise him not to eat for 2 hours before the test, and suggest he wear loose, lightweight clothing and snug shoes.

Describe how the examiner will cleanse sites on the patient's chest and, possibly, his back before attaching electrodes to these sites. Reassure the patient that an assistant will be present throughout the test. Urge him to report immediately any chest pain, leg discomfort, breathlessness, or severe fatigue. Explain that after the test his blood pressure, oxygen level, and heart activity (ECG) will be monitored for 10 to 15 minutes.

Bronchoscopy

Tell the patient that this test allows direct examination of his airways. Mention that it takes 45 to 60 minutes. Instruct him not to eat or drink for 6 hours before the test. However, he should continue taking any prescribed drugs unless the doctor orders otherwise. If the test is being done under a local anesthetic, tell him that he may receive a sedative to help him relax. Prepare him for the unpleasant taste and coolness of the anesthetic throat spray used to suppress the gag reflex.

During the test, the patient may be asked to lie supine on a table or bed, or he may be asked to sit upright in a chair. Tell him to concentrate on relaxing, with his arms at his sides, and to breathe through his nose during the test. The doctor will insert the bronchoscopic tube through the patient's nose or mouth into the airway. Then small amounts of anesthetic will be flushed through the tube to suppress coughing and wheezing. Alert the patient that he may experience dyspnea during the test. Reassure him that he won't suffocate and that oxygen will be administered through the bronchoscope.

Mention that after the test his blood pressure, heart activity, and breathing will be monitored for about 15 minutes. Instruct him to lie on his side or to elevate his head at least 30 degrees until his gag reflex returns. Reassure him that hoarseness or a sore throat is temporary and that he can have throat lozenges or a soothing gargle when his gag reflex returns. Tell him to report bloody mucus, dyspnea, wheezing, or chest pain immediately. Also inform him that a chest X-ray will be taken after the test and that he may receive an aerosolized bronchodilator treatment.

Mediastinoscopy
Explain that mediastinoscopy allows the doctor to visualize and obtain a biopsy of the mediastinal area and thereby confirm the diagnosis. Instruct the patient not to eat or drink for 8 hours before the test. Tell him that he'll receive an I.V. sedative before the test and then a general anesthetic.

Describe how the doctor will first insert an endotracheal tube and then make a small transverse suprasternal incision. He'll insert a mediastinoscope through this incision and obtain tissue specimens for analysis. After the test, the patient may remain intubated for several hours or overnight. Mention that his vital signs and dressing will be checked frequently for the first 4 hours.

Warn him that he may experience pain or tenderness at the incisional site, a sore throat, and hoarseness. He may also experience nausea, vomiting, and a sense of unreality from the anesthetic. Reassure him that these effects soon subside. Advise him to request analgesics for pain.

Thoracentesis
Inform the patient that through thoracentesis the doctor can obtain respiratory tissue or fluid samples for analysis. This will help diagnose the patient's disease and determine effective treatment. Explain that before the test the patient will put on a hospital gown, the nurse will assess his vital signs, and then the area around the needle insertion site will be shaved.

During the test the patient will be comfortably positioned—either sitting with his arms on pillows or lying partially on his side in bed. The doctor will cleanse the needle insertion site with a cold antiseptic solution and then inject a local anesthetic, which may cause a burning sensation. After numbing the skin, the doctor will insert the needle. Warn the patient that he will feel pressure during needle insertion and withdrawal.

Encourage the patient to relax and breathe normally, and

Warning: Cigarette smoking and working don't mix

Your patient already knows that smoking is bad for his health. But does he know that smoking on the job compounds the harmful health effects? Here's what the American Lung Association says:

• Cigarette smoke combined with workplace chemicals increases lung damage. Explain that the effect is synergistic — making health problems far greater than would be expected from simply adding together the damage caused by each factor. For example, asbestos workers who smoke more than a pack a day have up to 90 times the chance of dying of lung cancer as workers who don't smoke and who don't work with asbestos.

• Cigarette smoke increases a person's total exposure to some pollutants. Explain that cigarette smoke contains such harmful agents as acetone, arsenic, and carbon monoxide, which also may be in the workplace.

• Cigarettes carry harmful chemicals from the workplace into the body. For instance, cigarettes absorb toxic substances, such as lead or mercury, from the environment. Then when the worker smokes or handles the contaminated cigarettes, the body absorbs the toxic agents.

• A lit cigarette can transform a workplace chemical into a more dangerous substance. Explain that burning tobacco generates heat, which can change workplace chemicals into highly toxic substances.

• Smokers are twice as likely as nonsmokers to have on-the-job accidents. Warn the patient that a smoking-related accident near flammable chemicals could trigger a fire or explosion.

warn him not to cough and to remain still during the test. Tell him to notify the doctor if he experiences dyspnea, palpitations, wheezing, dizziness, weakness, or diaphoresis, which may indicate respiratory distress.

After withdrawing the needle, the doctor will apply slight pressure and then an adhesive bandage. Tell the patient that his vital signs will be monitored frequently for the first few hours after the test. Instruct him to report any fluid or blood leakage from the needle insertion site and any signs of respiratory distress. Explain that a chest X-ray will be taken later to detect any posttest complications.

Teach about treatments

Although occupational respiratory diseases can't be cured, treatment can prevent further lung damage and relieve signs and symptoms. The patient's treatment program may include exercise, a balanced and nutritious diet, medications, oxygen therapy, and chest physiotherapy. Discuss measures he can take to prevent respiratory infections and avoid further exposure to the causative pollutant (if known) or intensification of its effects. (See *Warning: Cigarette smoking and working don't mix.*)

Activity

After evaluating the patient's exercise ECG, the doctor may prescribe an individual exercise program. Emphasize that this program is designed to increase endurance and strength without causing severe dyspnea. Teach the patient and a family member or other caregiver how to take an accurate radial pulse to monitor the effects of the exercise program. Teach the patient to organize his daily activities to conserve energy. Suggest that he alternate light and heavy tasks and rest frequently between tasks.

Diet

Discuss how a well-balanced, nutritious diet can compensate for the extra calories the patient expends just to breathe. Because dyspnea can discourage eating and lead to weight loss, teach the patient how to maintain his caloric intake.

First, encourage frequent oral hygiene to stimulate the appetite. If the patient has severe dyspnea, advise him to eat small, frequent meals to reduce fatigue and air swallowing during eating. Also encourage him to chew his food slowly. Finally, recommend that he eat nutritious snacks (including fluids like fruit juices) or drink a liquid enteral supplement for additional calories between meals.

Unless contraindicated, encourage the patient to drink plenty of water—at least six glasses daily—to thin his mucus. Adequate fluid intake will also help prevent constipation and avoid breathlessness associated with straining during defecation. Tell him to include fresh fruits, vegetables, and bran in his diet to help prevent constipation. If the patient is obese, explain how obesity interferes with diaphragmatic movement and increases cardiac work load. This, in turn, can make breathing even more difficult. Suggest a weight-reduction program, if appropriate.

Medication

Tell the patient that drug therapy will help to relieve his symptoms and make him more comfortable. Inform him that his drug regimen may include:
• short-term corticosteroids to relieve an acute episode of respiratory distress
• long-term corticosteroids to diminish airway spasms and dyspnea if he has asthma, bronchitis, or pulmonary fibrosis
• antihistamines to relieve symptoms associated with hypersensitivity diseases
• antitussives or expectorants to control a nonproductive cough
• mast cell stabilizers, methylxanthines, or sympathomimetics to prevent airway spasm and wheezing associated with asthma
• aminoglycosides to prevent respiratory infections
• cytotoxic drugs to improve respiratory function in cases of severe pulmonary fibrosis.

For specific teaching points, see *Teaching about drugs for occupational respiratory diseases*, pages 162 to 165. Show how to use an oral inhaler, if ordered. Give the patient a copy of the teaching aid *How to use an oral inhaler*, pages 146 and 147.

Procedures

If appropriate, teach the patient and a family member or another caregiver how to use portable oxygen. As appropriate, offer safety information for traveling with oxygen. For example, advise the patient to obtain guidelines regarding oxygen regulations on an airplane, train, or bus. Suggest that he call the airline to ensure that enough oxygen will be aboard to make the trip and to circle in a holding pattern. Before takeoff, he should double-check the availability of sufficient oxygen. Make sure he understands that he'll experience the effects of high altitude even in the pressurized cabin of a commercial airliner, and instruct him to use breathing exercises to help minimize dyspnea. Also, advise him to contact a medical equipment supplier at his destination so that the necessary equipment will be ready upon his arrival.

Chest physiotherapy. If appropriate, teach about chest physiotherapy to help mobilize and remove pulmonary mucus. Show the patient and a family member how to perform this procedure, and supply a copy of the patient-teaching aid *How to perform chest physiotherapy (for an adult)*, pages 106 and 107. Instruct the patient to perform physiotherapy (waiting 1 to 2 hours after meals) and to take aerosol medication before the procedure—or as instructed by his doctor.

Other care measures

Advise the patient to avoid inhaled pollutants—such as cigarette smoke, aerosol sprays, and industrial fumes—which may aggravate his dyspnea. Give him a copy of the patient-teaching aid *Breathing easily—and safely—at work*, page 168. If the patient smokes, urge him to quit. Also show him how to do abdominal breathing exercises and how to use them when he performs strenuous tasks. Offer him the patient-teaching aid *How to overcome*

continued on page 165

Teaching about drugs for occupational respiratory diseases

DRUG	ADVERSE REACTIONS	TEACHING POINTS
Aminoglycosides		
gentamicin sulfate (Garamycin) **tobramycin sulfate (aerosolized)** (Nebcin)	• Watch for fever, headache, lethargy, nausea, pruritus, rash, superinfection, urticaria, and vomiting. • Other reactions include neurotoxicity and ototoxicity.	• Teach the patient to use an aerosolized nebulizer or inhaler, to perform airway clearing techniques, and then to administer this drug. • Review the signs and symptoms of bacterial or fungal superinfections and advise notifying the doctor immediately if the patient suspects he has an infection. • Instruct him to notify the doctor if he experiences any unusual effects, such as ringing in the ears.
Antihistamines		
azatadine (Optimine) **brompheniramine** (Dimetane) **chlorpheniramine** (Chlor-Trimeton, Teldrin) **clemastine** (Tavist) **dexchlorpheniramine** (Polaramine)	• Watch for fever, hallucinations, severe drowsiness, severe dry mouth or throat, unusual fatigue or weakness, sore throat, and unusual bleeding or bruising. • Other reactions include anorexia; blurred vision; mild drowsiness; mild dry nose, mouth, or throat; insomnia; irritability; thickened bronchial secretions; and tremor.	• Inform the patient that antihistamines may cause drowsiness so he should use caution when performing activities that require alertness. • Advise taking the drug with food or milk to avoid gastric upset. • Suggest using sugarless gum, ice chips, or hard candy to help relieve dry mouth and throat. Instruct the patient to drink extra fluids to help thin bronchial secretions. • Urge him to keep appointments for periodic blood tests because long-term antihistamine use can cause blood dyscrasias. • Tell him that antihistamines interfere with the skin-test response in a desensitization program for allergy. Therefore, for testing purposes, the doctor may temporarily discontinue the drug. • Advise against taking this drug with alcohol. The combination can increase central nervous system (CNS) depression. • Urge the patient to avoid over-the-counter cough and cold medicines that contain additional antihistamines or alcohol, which may increase CNS depression.
astemizole (Hismanal) **terfenadine** (Seldane)	• Watch for dizziness. • Other reactions include abdominal distress, appetite increase, arthralgia, conjunctivitis, diarrhea, dry mouth and throat, fatigue, headache, nasal stuffiness, nausea, nervousness, and weight increase.	• Tell the patient that this drug usually causes less drowsiness than other antihistamines because it doesn't enter the CNS. • Advise taking the drug with food or milk to avoid gastric upset. • Suggest using sugarless gum, ice chips, or hard candy to help relieve dry mouth and throat.
Antitussives and expectorants		
codeine	• Watch for confusion, dizziness, respiratory difficulty, and sedation. • Other reactions include constipation, drowsiness, dry mouth, and nausea.	• If the patient's cough changes to a productive cough, instruct him to consult the doctor. • Warn that prolonged codeine use generates drug tolerance and dependence. • Tell the patient to use caution when performing activities that require alertness because this drug can impair mental and physical functioning. • Suggest using sugarless gum, ice chips, or hard candy to relieve dry mouth and throat. • Advise that taking this drug with alcohol increases CNS depression.

continued

Teaching about drugs for occupational respiratory diseases — *continued*

DRUG	ADVERSE REACTIONS	TEACHING POINTS
Antitussives and expectorants — *continued*		
dextromethorphan (Benylin DM, Congespirin for Children, Delsym, Cremacoat 1, DM Cough, Hold, Mediquell, Pertussin, PediaCare 1, St. Joseph's Cough, Sucrets Cough Control)	• Watch for insomnia, irritability, nervousness, and unusual excitement. • Other reactions include dizziness, drowsiness, and gastric upset.	• Urge the patient to check with the doctor or pharmacist before taking any other cough or cold formulas because manufacturers typically add dextromethorphan to antihistamine, sympathomimetic, or other drug combinations. • Instruct the patient to avoid activities that require alertness if the drug makes him feel drowsy. • Suggest using sugarless gum, ice chips, or hard candy to relieve dry mouth. • Warn that taking this drug with alcohol increases CNS depression.
guaifenesin (Gee Gee, Glycotuss, Hytuss, Robitussin)	• Watch for nausea and vomiting. • Other reactions include diarrhea, drowsiness, and mild gastric upset.	• If not contraindicated, encourage the patient to drink as much water as possible to help liquefy his mucus. • Advise him to check with the doctor before taking an expectorant because most products containing guaifenesin also contain other drugs, such as antihistamines and decongestants.
Corticosteroids		
Inhalable and intranasal **beclomethasone** (Beclovent Oral Inhaler, Beconase Nasal Inhaler, Vancenase Nasal Inhaler, Vanceril Inhaler) **dexamethasone sodium phosphate** (Decadron Phosphate Respihaler) **flunisolide** (AeroBid Inhaler, Nasalide) **triamcinolone acetonide** (Azmacort Inhaler)	• Watch for bleeding from or ulceration of nasal passages, chest tightness, confusion, depression, dizziness, dyspnea, fainting, fatigue, fever, gastric distress, insomnia, itching, mouth and throat lesions, oral infections, weakness, and wheezing. • Other reactions include altered taste perception, dry mouth and throat, hoarseness, hypersensitivity reactions, increased appetite, inflamed nasal passages, and palpitations.	• As appropriate, tell the patient that the doctor has prescribed an inhalable dosage to relieve the patient's symptoms. • Caution him not to increase the prescribed dose if the inhalable medicine doesn't relieve airway spasm immediately. • Tell him to call the doctor immediately if he experiences wheezing, chest tightness, or dyspnea after taking the medicine. • Instruct the patient to avoid triggering acute adrenal insufficiency by strictly following the doctor's orders when initiating, terminating, or tapering any oral corticosteroids if he also uses inhalable corticosteroids. Caution him not to withdraw abruptly from long-term corticosteroid therapy because the effects triggered may be fatal. • Discuss medication and stress. If the patient now takes or has recently discontinued systemic corticosteroids, explain that he'll need additional corticosteroids to cope with stress. Advise him to consult the doctor for instructions. • Recommend rinsing the mouth and gargling with water after inhaling medicine to remove drug deposits from his mouth and pharynx. • If the patient is taking an inhalable bronchodilator, instruct him to take the bronchodilator before the steroid. That way, the bronchodilator can fully dilate the airways, and thereby improve deposition of the corticosteroid. Because both drugs use fluorocarbon propellants, tell him to wait 5 minutes between treatments to avoid potential toxicity. • Remind him that he may not notice an improvement from the steroid therapy for about 1 month. • Warn him not to use or store flammable inhalation cartridges near heat.

continued

Teaching about drugs for occupational respiratory diseases — *continued*

DRUG	ADVERSE REACTIONS	TEACHING POINTS
Corticosteroids — *continued*		
Oral systemic **prednisone** (Orasone)	• Watch for abdominal pain, acne, back or rib pain, bloody or tarry stools, easy bruising, extreme or unusual fatigue, fever, hypertension, leg swelling, menstrual irregularity, personality changes, purple striae, sore throat, vomiting, weakness, significant weight gain, and wounds that won't heal. • Other reactions include unusual appetite, diaphoresis, dizziness, euphoria, headache, hirsutism, indigestion, insomnia, mild mood swings, mild nausea, nervousness, restlessness, and slight weight gain.	• Review the early signs of adrenal insufficiency — fatigue, weakness, joint pain, fever, anorexia, nausea, dyspnea, dizziness, fainting, and weight loss — if the patient's on long-term (longer than 2 weeks) or high-dose (more than 40 mg daily) prednisone therapy. • Emphasize that the patient must strictly follow his doctor's orders to avoid triggering acute adrenal insufficiency when initiating, terminating, or tapering prednisone if he also uses inhalable corticosteroids. (Abrupt withdrawal from prednisone may be fatal.) • Forewarn the patient about possible cushingoid effects if he's on long-term therapy. • Tell him to follow a salt-restricted, high-protein, high-potassium diet because this drug affects protein metabolism and water retention. • Instruct him to take this drug with food to reduce gastric irritation. • Urge him to wear medical identification if he's on long-term therapy. • Instruct him to call the doctor about using additional inhalational corticosteroids during stressful times. • Remind him that he may not notice an improvement in his condition for about 1 month. • Explain that using alcohol with this drug may promote GI ulceration. • Warn against taking over-the-counter drugs containing aspirin, which increases the risk of GI ulceration, unless the doctor recommends otherwise. • Caution him to avoid over-the-counter drugs, foods, and beverages containing sodium, which increases the risk of fluid retention.
Mast cell stabilizer		
cromolyn sodium (Intal [inhaler], Intal Capsules for use with Spinhaler, Intal Nebulizer Solution)	• Watch for anaphylaxis (chest tightness, hives, and increased wheezing), epistaxis, extreme headache, nausea, painful urination, and vomiting. • Other reactions include cough, mild headache, nasal burning and congestion, sneezing, and unpleasant taste sensation.	• Caution the patient not to change the dosage without consulting the doctor. • Remind him that it may take up to 1 month before he notices improvement with drug therapy. • If he also uses an inhaled bronchodilator, advise him to take the bronchodilator before the cromolyn sodium. That way, the bronchodilator can dilate his airways and improve deposition of the cromolyn sodium. • Warn that symptoms may recur if he reduces the prescribed dosage or discontinues the drug. Tell him to notify the doctor if he experiences airway spasm and wheezing after taking an inhalable dose. • Instruct him to store this drug in a closed container away from moisture and light. • Suggest that he rinse his mouth after taking the drug to minimize unpleasant taste. • Tell him to clear his nasal passages before using the nasal solution. Advise him to inhale the drug through his nose.

continued

Teaching about drugs for occupational respiratory diseases — *continued*

DRUG	ADVERSE REACTIONS	TEACHING POINTS
Methylxanthines		
aminophylline (Aminophyllin, Phyllocontin, Somophyllin) **oxtriphylline** (Choledyl) **theophylline** (Bronkodyl, Elixophyllin, Theo-Dur, Theolair, Theospan-SR, Theostat)	• Watch for anorexia, diarrhea, dizziness, flushing, headache, insomnia, irritability, lightheadedness, nausea, palpitations, pulse rate or rhythm changes, restlessness, seizures, tachypnea, tremulousness, and vomiting. • Other reactions include mild dyspepsia and bitter taste sensation.	• Urge the patient to take the drug exactly as ordered, even if he feels fine. • Instruct him to notify the doctor if he comes down with the flu or a high fever; these may influence the drug's effectiveness. • Show him how to take his pulse daily. Tell him to notify the doctor if his pulse rhythm changes or if his pulse rate decreases or increases 20 beats or more a minute. • Advise him to take the drug with food to relieve mild dyspepsia. • Caution him that taking over-the-counter drugs containing CNS stimulants, such as ephedrine or epinephrine, may increase CNS stimulation. • Advise him that beverages containing xanthines, such as coffee and tea, can intensify the drug's effects. • Warn him, if appropriate, not to stop smoking abruptly. Abrupt withdrawal from cigarette smoking could trigger drug toxicity. • Instruct him to take this drug on an empty stomach or 1 hour before or 3 hours after meals for best absorption.
Sympathomimetics		
albuterol (Proventil, Ventolin) **bitolterol** (Tornalate) **epinephrine** (Medihaler-Epi, Primatene Mist) **epinephrine, racemic** (microNefrin, Vaponefrin) **isoetharine** (Bronkometer, Bronkosol) **isoproterenol** (Isuprel, Medihaler-Iso) **metaproterenol** (Alupent, Metaprel) **terbutaline** (Brethine, Bricanyl)	• Watch for chest pain, diaphoresis, dizziness, dyspnea, flushing, headache, pallor, pounding heartbeat, and vomiting. • Other reactions include anxiety, fear, heartburn, insomnia, nausea, nervousness, palpitations, restlessness, mild tachycardia, unpleasant taste sensation, throat irritation, and tremor.	• Tell the patient to notify the doctor if he gets minimal or no relief from the prescribed drug dosage. • Warn him that increasing the prescribed dosage can cause serious complications, such as severe wheezing, stroke, myocardial infarction, and even death. Also advise against taking the drug more frequently than ordered because this can cause respiratory distress or reduced drug effectiveness. Advise him to immediately stop using the drug and notify the doctor if symptoms of serious complications develop. • Instruct him not to take more than one sympathomimetic at a time. He should wait at least 4 hours between doses of separate drugs. • Teach him how to use an inhaler and how to clean the mouthpiece. • Advise him to discard any inhalation solution that turns brown or contains a precipitate. Tell him to store the drug in its original container and to refrigerate it if the label directs. • Suggest he rinse his mouth with water or gargle after using an oral inhaler to minimize the bitter taste. • Tell him to avoid increased adverse reactions and drug toxicity by avoiding over-the-counter drugs containing CNS stimulants, such as ephedrine.

shortness of breath, page 102. As appropriate, suggest that he wear nonrestrictive clothing to facilitate breathing.

Adapt sexual intercourse. Because dyspnea may interfere with sexual intercourse, discuss ways to overcome this problem. Advise the patient to assume a comfortable position (sidelying, for example) that doesn't restrict breathing. Allowing the healthier partner to take the more active role may also help. Above all, encourage the partners to communicate with each other and to try alternate ways of showing affection.

Avoid infection. Warn the patient that untreated respiratory infection can lead to life-threatening respiratory failure. Discuss how to detect and report early signs of infection. Also instruct him to report symptoms of spontaneous pneumothorax, including a sudden, sharp, pleuritic pain that's exacerbated by movement, breathing, or coughing; and shortness of breath. Finally, instruct him to report warning symptoms of cor pulmonale, a chronic complication of pulmonary fibrosis, marked by progressively worsening dyspnea, leg edema, fatigue, and weakness.

Learn to cope. Be sure to explore with the patient and his family the impact of occupational respiratory disease on their lives. Help them identify coping mechanisms to deal with chronic anxiety and depression. Encourage them to contact the local chapter of the American Lung Association for more information, or if appropriate, recommend joining a local support group.

Sources of information and support

American Lung Association
1740 Broadway, New York, N.Y. 10019
(212) 315-8700

National Institute for Occupational Safety and Health (NIOSH)
1600 Clifton Road, NE, Atlanta, Ga. 30333
(404) 639-3771

National Jewish Center for Immunology and Respiratory Medicine
1400 Jackson Street, Denver, Colo. 80206
(303) 388-4461

Occupational Safety and Health Administration (OSHA)
U.S. Department of Labor, 200 Constitution Avenue, NW, Washington, D.C. 20210
(202) 523-7162

Further readings

Chung, F., and Dean, E. "Pathophysiology and Cardiorespiratory Consequences of Interstitial Lung Disease—Review and Clinical Implications: A Special Communication," *Physical Therapy* 69(11):956-66, November 1989.

Garbo, M.J., et al. "OSHA Hazard Communication Standard: Helping Prevent Chemical Hazards," *American Association of Occupational Health Nurses Journal* 36(9):366-71, 394-96, September 1988.

Kane, K. "The Killing Fields....Farmer's Lung Disease," *Nursing Times* 85(8):40-42, 44, February 22-28, 1989.

Kronenberg, R.S. "Asbestos Inhalation and Cigarette Smoking Make a Lethal Combination," *Occupational Health SAF* 58(3):50-53, 55-56, 68, March 1989.

Mandel, J.H., and Baker, B.A. "Recognizing Occupational Lung Disease," *Hospital Practice* 24(1A):21-22, 24, 27-30, January 30, 1989.

Preparing for pulmonary function tests

Dear Patient:

The doctor has ordered pulmonary (or lung) function tests for you. These tests measure how well your lungs work. Here's what to expect.

How the tests work
You will be asked to breathe as deeply as possible into a mouthpiece that is connected to a machine called a *spirometer*. This measures and records the rate and amount of air inhaled and exhaled.

Or you may sit in a small, telephone booth-like enclosure for a test called *body plethysmography*. Again, you'll be asked to breathe in and out, and the measurements will be recorded.

Before the tests
Avoid smoking for at least 4 hours before the tests. Eat lightly, and don't drink a lot of fluid. Wear loose, comfortable clothing. Remember to use the bathroom.

To make the tests go quickly, give them your full cooperation. Tell the technician if you don't understand the instructions. If you wear dentures, keep them in—they'll help you keep a tight seal around the spirometer's mouthpiece.

During the tests
During spirometry, you'll sit upright, and you'll wear a noseclip to make sure you breathe only through your mouth. During body plethysmography, you won't need a noseclip.

If you feel too confined in the small chamber, keep in mind that you can't suffocate. You can talk to the nurse or technician through a window.

The tests have several parts. For each test, you'll be asked to breathe a certain way—for example, to inhale deeply and exhale completely or to inhale quickly. You may need to repeat some tests after inhaling a bronchodilator medicine to expand the airways in your lungs. Also the nurse may take a sample of blood from an artery in your arm. This sample will be used to measure how well your body uses the air you breathe.

How will you feel?
During the tests, you may feel tired or short of breath. However, you'll be able to take rest breaks between measurements.

Tell the technician right away if you feel dizzy, begin wheezing, or have chest pain, a racing or pounding heart, an upset stomach, or severe shortness of breath.

Also tell him if your arm swells or you're bleeding from the spot where a blood sample was taken or if you experience weakness or pain in that arm.

After the tests
When the tests are over, rest if you feel like it. Then plan to resume your usual activities when you regain your energy.

Breathing easily – and safely – at work

Dear Patient:

Breathing dirty air on the job can damage your lungs. To protect yourself, try to reduce or eliminate your exposure to breathing hazards. Here are some tips.

Identify breathing hazards
Keep alert for air pollution signs at work, including:
- *Dust clouds.* Inhaling dust particles can irritate your lungs. Repeated exposure over months or years can cause serious disease.
- *Unusual fumes.* The first warning of a breathing hazard may be a strange odor as you enter your work area.
- *Burning eyes, throat, and lungs.* If your eyes start to smart and your throat and chest feel tight as soon as you enter the workplace, suspect a breathing hazard.
- *Chronic cough or shortness of breath.* See your doctor if you have these symptoms. They may be job-related if they occur or get worse when you're at work or if your co-workers have the same symptoms.

Safeguard your lungs
Follow these tips to avoid inhaling dust, smoke, and noxious gases:
- Stay away from unnecessary dust, fumes, and vapors if possible.
- Wash your skin thoroughly after working with hazardous materials — especially before you eat or drink. Also change into clean clothing. Wash contaminated clothes separately from other laundry.
- Insist on good ventilation at work. An open window or cooling fan may not be enough to remove air pollutants. If your work area has an exhaust system to remove contaminated air, make sure the system works. If you're given a respirator, wear it properly. Also insist on and use other protective equipment for the job.
- Don't smoke. Cigarette smoke injures lungs and contains carbon monoxide. By smoking, you also breathe in other airborne pollutants.

Work safely with chemicals
Your employer's responsible for providing training and equipment to do your job safely. But you can help too.
- Read label warnings on chemical containers before you open them. Then heed them.
- Ask for and follow your employer's instructions on how to use chemicals safely to avoid illness and injury.
- Make sure to read the Material Safety Data Sheet that the law says your employer must keep on file (or post) for all hazardous chemicals. This sheet identifies the chemical's physical properties and health effects. It tells how to use, store, and handle the chemical safely on the job and in emergencies.
- Ask your employer to set up a workplace safety and health training program for employees if you don't have one yet.

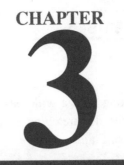

Neurologic Conditions

Contents

Parkinson's disease

Your teaching can help the Parkinson's patient retain control over his life for as long as possible. It can, for instance, help him learn to perform daily activities despite motor deficits that disrupt his coordination and movement.

To keep the patient active and independent, you'll need to emphasize the importance of complying with long-term drug therapy and supportive treatments, such as a diet and exercise program. As the patient's symptoms change, you'll need to modify your teaching to fit the patient's needs (see *Teaching the Parkinson's patient,* page 172). For instance, if drug therapy fails to control tremors, you may need to teach him about stereotaxic thalamotomy.

Discuss the disorder

Explain that this chronic, progressive disorder results from a deficiency of dopamine, a chemical that relays messages across the nerve pathways. This deficiency involves the area of the brain responsible for control of voluntary muscle movements and posture (the basal ganglia, particularly the substantia nigra and corpus striatum). As a result, most symptoms relate to difficulty with posture and movement.

Inform the patient that the characteristic signs—tremors, slow movement (bradykinesia), and rigidity—may vary in severity from one patient to another. Also tell him that the disorder initially affects one side of the body but will eventually involve both sides. Explain that tremors begin in the fingers, increase during stress or anxiety, and decrease with purposeful movement and sleep. Describe how bradykinesia changes his gait so that his body tilts forward while his arms remain at his sides (instead of swinging with walking). He may also notice muscle rigidity or widespread stiffness when performing any activity.

If the patient complains of other symptoms, such as oily skin, increased perspiration, insomnia, or mood changes, inform him that these are also part of the disorder. (See *Reviewing clinical features of Parkinson's disease,* page 173.)

Complications

Emphasize that noncompliance with drug therapy and other treatments can lead to poorly controlled symptoms and injury. For example, postural and coordination difficulties may lead to falls if the patient's unable to stop or start walking. Also, if he doesn't

Janette R. Yanko, RN, MN, CNRN, who wrote this chapter, is a neuroscience clinical nurse specialist at Allegheny General Hospital, Pittsburgh.

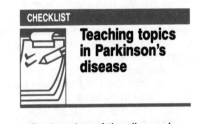

CHECKLIST

Teaching topics in Parkinson's disease

☐ Explanation of the disease's progressive course
☐ Preparation for tests, such as cerebrospinal fluid analysis
☐ Exercise program and precautions
☐ Dietary modifications
☐ Drug therapy
☐ Stereotaxic thalamotomy, if appropriate
☐ Home modifications for safety
☐ Self-help aids for dressing and walking
☐ Availability of information and support groups

Teaching the Parkinson's patient

You'll probably find a standard teaching plan to be a useful starting point when teaching the Parkinson's patient. After you assess him, though, you'll modify this plan to meet his distinct needs. Let's look at an example of how to modify a standard plan.

Assessment

Suppose you're caring for 60-year-old Stan Hamilton. For 6 years Mr. Hamilton has undergone treatment for Parkinson's disease. He was recently forced into early retirement because his symptoms worsened.

You observe that Mr. Hamilton suffers from bilateral hand tremors, worse on the right side than on the left. He also has bradykinesia and rigidity, periodic drooling and eye incoordination, and oily skin. He tells you that "things look blurry sometimes" and that he feels light-headed when getting out of bed.

Mr. Hamilton speaks softly, making it difficult to hear him. Expressionless, he hardly converses except to answer questions. Although his behavior may be a sign of illness or fatigue, you suspect that depression may be a contributing factor.

Despite his tendency to withdraw, Mr. Hamilton is well versed in the pathophysiology of Parkinson's disease, and he's aware of the importance of drug therapy. Similarly, his family seem knowledgeable about the disease.

What are Mr. Hamilton's learning needs?

To find out what you'll teach Mr. Hamilton, compare what he knows about Parkinson's disease with the content of a standard teaching plan. This will tell you what points to include or modify.

A standard teaching plan covers:
• pathophysiology of Parkinson's disease
• signs and symptoms
• diagnostic tests, such as radiographic studies and cerebrospinal fluid analysis
• treatment, including drug therapy, exercise, modifications for activities of daily living, and, if appropriate, surgery.

Your assessment leads you to decide that Mr. Hamilton doesn't need a review of Parkinson's pathophysiology or diagnostic tests. Instead, you plan to reinforce self-care skills, such as exercise and communication techniques. Your goal? Improving Mr. Hamilton's self-image. And because patient self-care is often related to medication compliance, you'll review medications as well.

Encourage Mr. Hamilton to remain as independent as possible in his daily activities. A retired businessman used to directing others, Mr. Hamilton needs to maintain a sense of control over his own life to curb his depression. Introducing assistive devices at the appropriate time will support this goal.

Using the standard teaching plan as a foundation, establish learning outcomes suited to the patient's individual needs. Specifically, Mr. Hamilton will be able to:

- express his feelings about Parkinson's disease.
- participate in forming learning outcomes.
- perform a return demonstration of his exercise routine.
- correctly use personal assistance equipment.
- practice effective communication techniques.
- select foods from the menu that don't interfere with his medications and that he can swallow without aspirating.
- list the side effects of medications that should be reported to his doctor.
- list over-the-counter medications that he should avoid ingesting.

What teaching techniques and tools will you use?

To teach about Parkinson's disease, choose such techniques as *discussion* and *explanation* of dopamine function in the brain (and what happens in dopamine deficiency), nutrition, and surgery, and *demonstration* of exercise, assistive devices, and communication techniques. Teaching tools may include *booklets* on Parkinson's disease and *visual aids,* such as posters, flip-charts, or models of the human brain.

Mr. Hamilton's depression will influence your teaching strategy. Plan to communicate small pieces of information at each lesson. Encourage him to participate in establishing realistic learning goals, and acknowledge his feelings of fatigue and sadness.

How will you evaluate your teaching?

Appropriate evaluation methods include *direct observation, discussion* (sometimes using questions and answers), and *simulation* of the medication regimen or of typical problems the patient may encounter. *Return demonstration* can help you to evaluate exercise, assistive devices, menu selection, and performance of daily activities.

Reviewing clinical features of Parkinson's disease

When a loved one develops Parkinson's disease, family members need to know what to expect. By describing what will happen at each stage of the disease, you may lessen their anxiety.

Early unilateral features
Initially, the family may notice changes in the patient's posture, gait, facial expression, or speech. Early signs usually affect only one side of the body. A tremor in the arm, the most common sign, usually occurs at rest. Also, the patient may lean slightly toward the unaffected side. Other early signs include a blank facial expression and slight muscle rigidity that increases in resistance to passive muscle stretching. Muscle rigidity and tremors may also occur in the leg on the affected side, along with mild edema of the foot and ankle.

Later bilateral involvement
As signs of Parkinson's disease gradually spread from one side of the body to the other, the patient assumes a stooped posture. He may complain of fatigue and weakness as bradykinesia progressively affects all his body movements. Gradually, his movements lose their spontaneity, becoming carefully executed. Eye blinking, arm swinging while walking, and expressive facial and hand gestures disappear. This loss of motor function may force the patient to stop working. Although still able to care for himself, he may become depressed and withdrawn.

During this period, encourage family members to include the patient in their activities to maintain his sense of value and belonging. To preserve independence, encourage them to allow the patient to do as much for himself as possible.

Gait problems and disability
The hallmarks of this stage include progressively pronounced gait disturbances. The patient walks more slowly in small, mincing steps and may unexpectedly find himself locked in a position, unable to move.

As his disability increases, the patient will require assistance for all activities of daily living. Tremors may not increase, but muscle rigidity and bradykinesia affect every aspect of his life, from rolling out of bed in the morning to eating.

Eventually motionless and unable to stand, the patient is left with little remaining voluntary motor function. Bradykinesia causes soft, monotonous speech, a masklike facial expression, and constant drooling. Neurogenic bladder and diminished thoracic excursion leave the patient susceptible to infection.

EARLY FEATURES

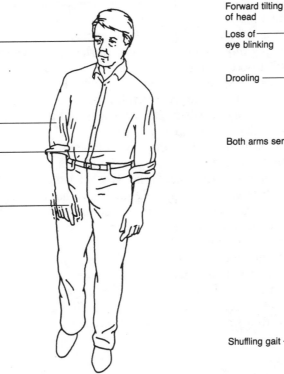

Loss of facial expression

Semiflexed arm

Leaning to unaffected side

Tremors

LATER FEATURES

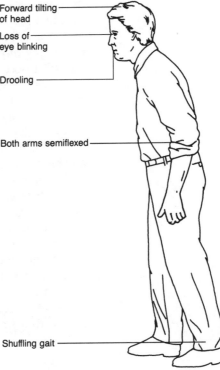

Forward tilting of head

Loss of eye blinking

Drooling

Both arms semiflexed

Shuffling gait

rise slowly from a sitting or recumbent position, orthostatic hypotension, a common symptom, may also lead to falls and injuries.

Point out that failure to follow an exercise program may lead to decreased mobility and such complications as pneumonia, pulmonary emboli, and urinary tract infections. Does the patient faithfully perform his facial exercises? If the answer is no, explain that he may develop or intensify dysphagia, leading to weight loss and aspiration pneumonia. Lack of facial mobility may hamper communication, contributing to social isolation and depression.

Describe the diagnostic workup

Although diagnosis of Parkinson's disease relies on clinical symptoms, you may need to prepare the patient for a computed tomography scan or magnetic resonance imaging to rule out such abnormalities as tumors. The patient may also undergo positron emission tomography or single-photon-emission computed tomography (SPECT). These tests help detect tumors and disorders that alter cerebral metabolism.

More likely, though, you'll need to prepare the patient for cerebrospinal fluid (CSF) analysis.

CSF analysis

Explain to the patient that this test involves the removal and laboratory analysis of spinal fluid and takes about 15 minutes. The doctor will obtain a sample of CSF by lumbar or cisternal puncture. With either procedure, warn the patient that he may feel pressure upon needle insertion.

To prepare the patient for a *lumbar puncture,* tell him that he'll be seated with his head bent toward his knees, or he'll lie on the edge of a bed or table, with his knees drawn up to his abdomen and his chin resting on his chest. After cleansing the lumbar area, the doctor will inject a local anesthetic. Tell the patient to report any tingling or sharp pain. During the procedure, the doctor will insert a hollow needle into the subarachnoid space surrounding the spinal cord. Tell the patient to hold still to avoid dislodging the needle. Also tell him that he may be asked to breathe deeply or to straighten his legs and that the doctor may apply pressure to the jugular veins.

After lumbar puncture, the doctor will remove the needle and apply an adhesive bandage. The patient must lie flat for 4 to 24 hours to prevent a headache. His head should be even with or below the level of his hips. Remind him that although he mustn't raise his head, he can turn from side to side. Also tell him to increase fluid intake for the rest of the day to help replenish CSF and to prevent a headache.

To prepare the patient for a *cisternal puncture,* instruct him to restrict food and fluids for 4 hours before the test, as ordered. Explain that he'll assume a sitting position with his chin resting on his chest, or he'll be positioned on his side at the edge of the bed, with a small pillow placed beneath his forward-bending head. After cleansing and possibly shaving the upper neck area, the doctor will inject a local anesthetic. During the test, the patient should remain still as the doctor inserts a hollow needle into the midline of the vertebral column below the occipital bone.

After cisternal puncture, the doctor will remove the needle and apply an adhesive bandage. The patient must briefly lie flat on his abdomen while the puncture site seals. Then he can resume his usual activities.

Teach about treatments

Because Parkinson's disease has no cure, treatment aims to relieve symptoms and keep the patient functional as long as possible. To achieve this goal, the patient may participate in daily exercise, modify his diet, take medications, and if necessary, undergo surgery.

Activity

Inform the patient that moderate daily exercise will help him improve mobility, reduce the risk of contractures, improve respiration and circulation, promote bowel function, lessen rigidity, and increase strength. If possible, encourage him to perform active range-of-motion exercises. Otherwise, teach a caregiver how to perform passive range-of-motion exercises. Tell the patient to exercise when he feels rested and movement seems easiest, such as in the late morning or soon after taking medication.

Review specific exercises, using pictures when helpful. Provide a checklist to help structure an exercise routine. (See *How to do stretching exercises,* pages 182 and 183.) Caution him not to exercise excessively, as fatigue will interfere with daily activities. Instruct him to start his program slowly, and build up gradually. Enlist the family's help in encouraging exercise.

Diet

Instruct the patient about the importance of maintaining a stable protein level. Excessive dietary protein can affect the action of levodopa, an amino acid used to treat Parkinson's disease. Insufficient protein may cause nutritional imbalance.

Tell the patient to avoid caffeine, which may worsen his symptoms. Because intestinal motility may decrease, advise him to drink adequate amounts of fluid and to eat more high-fiber foods, especially if he's troubled by constipation.

If the patient has difficulty chewing or swallowing, recommend semisoft foods (applesauce, mashed potatoes, solid foods prepared in a blender) to help ensure adequate nutrition and minimize the risk of aspiration. To prevent choking, suggest freezing liquids to a slush or mixing them with other foods, such as cereals. Instruct the patient to sit up straight, move food to the back of his mouth, tilt his head slightly forward, and then swallow. (For more tips, see *Making eating more enjoyable*.)

If the patient eats slowly, advise eating small, frequent

Making eating more enjoyable

Recommend that the patient use the following aids to overcome problems related to eating:
• a warming tray, especially if he eats slowly
• an extra supply of napkins to absorb excess saliva
• an arm brace for steadiness in case of severe tremors
• flexible straws or cups with lid spouts, such as travel cups
• utensils with built-up handles that provide a better grip.

meals. Instruct an obese patient in a weight-reduction diet. Explain that his weight affects his mobility and the absorption of his medications.

Medication

Explain to the patient that drug therapy aims to control his symptoms. It may include:
• levodopa or levodopa-carbidopa to replace the neurotransmitter dopamine.
• anticholinergics, such as trihexyphenidyl or benztropine, and antihistamines, such as diphenhydramine. These drugs increase the inhibition of central motor neurons.
• bromocriptine, an ergot derivative, which acts as a dopamine agonist.
• the antiviral agent amantadine, which promotes dopamine synthesis and release.

For specific patient-teaching points, see *Drug therapy for Parkinson's disease*.

Stress that the patient should never abruptly discontinue his medication. Doing so may precipitate a parkinsonian crisis, intensifying his symptoms. As the disease progresses, the doctor may increase the dosage. Caution the patient against increasing it on his own, since this may lead to toxicity.

Initially, drug therapy may cause nausea and vomiting. Reassure the patient that such reactions will disappear in a few months. Suggest that taking medications after meals may help to decrease nausea.

If the patient has an intellectual impairment or memory difficulties, instruct him and his family to premeasure his medication doses for the day in separate containers, each marked with the scheduled administration time. If the patient has difficulty swallowing, tell him that he can crush pills or open capsules (unless he's taking an experimental sustained-release form of medication) and mix the medication with a food that's easy to swallow, such as applesauce.

Surgery

If medication fails to relieve unilateral tremors, stereotaxic thalamotomy may be performed. Tell the patient who will undergo this surgery that first his head will be shaved and cleansed. Then a metal frame will be attached to his head to hold it still and to guide the surgeon.

Inform the patient that after he's given a local anesthetic, the surgeon will make a burr hole in his skull and create a surgical lesion in the thalamus on the side *opposite* the tremors. This lesion will block the transmission of nerve impulses that cause the tremors. To clarify the procedure, discuss how the right side of the brain controls the left side of the body, and vice versa.

Tell the patient that he'll experience some pressure and discomfort when the doctor applies the head frame. During surgery,

Drug therapy for Parkinson's disease

DRUG	ADVERSE REACTIONS	TEACHING POINTS
amantadine (Symmetrel)	• Watch for confusion, depression, edema, fainting, hallucinations, insomnia, nystagmus, orthostatic hypotension, shortness of breath, slurred speech, sore throat, and urine retention. • Other reactions include anorexia, difficulty concentrating, dizziness, dry mouth, indigestion, irritability, lethargy, nightmares, and rose-colored skin mottling.	• Explain to the patient that this drug helps relieve symptoms of Parkinson's disease. • Tell him to avoid alcohol (which may worsen dizziness and confusion) and decongestants that contain central nervous system (CNS) stimulants (which may increase irritability). • If he misses a dose, tell him to take it when he remembers, unless his next scheduled dose is within 4 hours. He should never double-dose. • Tell him to schedule his last daily dose at least 3 hours before bedtime to help prevent insomnia. • Warn him that stopping the drug could cause a parkinsonian crisis. • If he experiences dry mouth, tell him to suck on ice chips or sugarless candy or to chew sugarless gum. • Warn him to operate machinery cautiously and to avoid driving if he feels dizzy or (rarely) has blurred vision. • To reduce the risk of orthostatic hypotension, tell him to rise slowly from a sitting or lying position. • Caution against overexertion when his symptoms subside.
benztropine mesylate (Cogentin) **trihexyphenidyl** (Artane, Tremin)	• Watch for abdominal cramps, ataxia, blurred vision, confusion, decreased sweating, dizziness, dry mouth, dyspnea, eye pain, hallucinations, insomnia, muscle weakness, nausea, photosensitivity, rash, tachycardia, and vomiting. • Other reactions include mild constipation, orthostatic hypotension, and sore mouth or tongue.	• Explain to the patient that this drug improves muscle control and relieves muscle spasms. • Tell him to avoid alcohol and drugs that contain CNS depressants, such as antihistamines, including cold and cough preparations and allergy and sleeping medications. • Instruct him to take antacids or antidiarrheals at least 1 hour before or after taking this drug. Antacids and antidiarrheals may decrease absorption of this drug. • If he misses a dose, tell him to take it as soon as he remembers. But if his next scheduled dose is within 8 hours, tell him not to take the missed dose. He should never double-dose. • Tell the patient to take this drug with or immediately after meals to help prevent GI distress. • Warn him that stopping the drug could trigger a parkinsonian crisis. • To minimize orthostatic hypotension, tell him to rise slowly from a sitting or lying position. • Warn him to operate machinery cautiously and to avoid driving if he feels dizzy or has blurred vision. • Tell him that this drug may cause heat intolerance. As a result, he should avoid overexertion in warm temperatures. • Also tell him that his eyes may be sensitive to sunlight; wearing sunglasses should help. • If he experiences dry mouth, tell him to suck on ice chips or sugarless candy or to chew sugarless gum.
bromocriptine mesylate (Parlodel)	• Watch for abdominal pain, anorexia, confusion, diarrhea, fainting, hallucinations, hematemesis, melena, nausea, orthostatic hypotension, persistent constipation, twitching, and vomiting. • Other reactions include constipation, drowsiness, headache, leg cramps, stuffy nose, and tingling fingers and toes when cold.	• Explain to the patient that this drug helps relieve symptoms of Parkinson's disease. • If he misses a dose, tell him to take it as soon as he remembers. But if his next scheduled dose is within 4 hours, tell him not to take the missed dose. He should never double-dose. • Tell him to take this drug with or immediately after meals to reduce GI distress. • To minimize orthostatic hypotension, advise him to rise slowly from a sitting or lying position. • Warn him to operate machinery cautiously and to avoid driving if he feels drowsy.

continued

Drug therapy for Parkinson's disease —*continued*

DRUG	ADVERSE REACTIONS	TEACHING POINTS
diphenhydramine (Benadryl)	• Watch for disturbed coordination, dizziness, drowsiness, epigastric distress, sedation, and thickening of bronchial secretions. • Other reactions include anorexia; blurred vision; chest tightness; chills; confusion; constipation; diarrhea; difficult breathing; difficult urination; diplopia; dry mouth, nose, and throat; early menses; easy bruising; euphoria; excessive perspiration; fatigue; headache; insomnia; irritability; nasal stuffiness; nausea; nervousness; neuritis; palpitations; paresthesia; photosensitivity; rash; restlessness; seizures; tinnitus; tremors; urinary frequency; urine retention; vertigo; vomiting; and wheezing.	• Inform the patient that this drug helps relieve symptoms of Parkinson's disease. • Warn him against drinking alcohol during therapy and against driving or engaging in other activities that require mental alertness until CNS response is determined. • Tell him that he can reduce GI distress by taking the drug with food or milk. • Tell him that coffee or tea may reduce drowsiness, and sugarless gum, sour hard candy, or ice chips may relieve dry mouth. • Warn him of possible photosensitivity. Advise use of a sunscreen.
levodopa (Dopar, Larodopa, Levopa) **levodopa-carbidopa** (Sinemet)	• Watch for depression, diarrhea, dry mouth, dysuria, frequent blinking, mood changes, mouth ulcers, nausea, nightmares, orthostatic hypotension, sore throat, tachycardia, tremors, twitching, urine discoloration, vomiting, and weakness. • Other reactions include blurred vision, constipation, and mild dizziness.	• Explain to the patient that this drug helps relieve symptoms of Parkinson's disease, including tremors, stiffness, and slow movements. • Tell the patient taking levodopa to avoid vitamin preparations containing vitamin B_6 and foods high in vitamin B_6, such as avocados, bacon, beans, beef liver, powdered milk, oatmeal, peas, pork, sweet potatoes, and tuna. • Tell him to avoid cough, cold, sinus, or allergy medications that contain sympathomimetics or CNS stimulants. • For best absorption, tell him to take this drug at least 1 hour before meals. Also, tell him to avoid high-protein foods (organ meats, cheese, milk, sardines, mussels) that will block the effect of levodopa. • Instruct him to take a missed dose as soon as he remembers, but to skip it if the next scheduled dose is within 2 hours. He must never double-dose. • Warn him that he could trigger a parkinsonian crisis by abruptly stopping the drug. • Tell him to take the drug with or immediately after meals if he experiences GI distress. If he experiences a dry mouth, tell him to suck on ice chips or sugarless candy or to chew sugarless gum. • Warn him to operate machinery cautiously and to avoid driving if he feels dizzy or has blurred vision. • Caution against overexertion when his symptoms subside. • To reduce the risk of orthostatic hypotension, instruct him to rise slowly from a sitting or lying position. Also tell him to avoid hot baths or showers if they cause dizziness. • Explain that his urine may turn red or dark brown. Also tell him that his urine may change the color of some sanitation products, such as toilet bowl cleaners. • Warn the diabetic patient that this drug may interfere with urine glucose and ketone tests. • Advise him that before any surgery, he should inform his doctor or dentist that he's taking this drug.

he'll be asked to follow commands, such as raising an arm, and to answer questions, as a test of memory and speech. Explain that he may have a headache after surgery, in part because of the prolonged immobility of his neck and shoulder muscles.

If your patient is scheduled for adrenal medullary autologous transplant (currently under research), follow your hospital's protocol for teaching him. The surgery involves removal of one of the adrenal glands (usually the left) and implantation of a section of the adrenal medulla into the brain tissue (usually the caudate nucleus). The patient must undergo both laparotomy and craniotomy.

Other care measures

Help the patient preserve his independence by teaching him how to adjust his daily activities to his current ability.

Enhancing mobility. Tell the patient that sitting in a chair with arms will make it easier to obtain sufficient support. Elevating the back of a favorite chair by shortening the front legs 1 to 2 inches will make it easier to get up. Suggest tying a sheet to the foot of his bed to help pull himself into a sitting position. Remind him to rise slowly to prevent orthostatic hypotension.

To help the patient maintain balance and forward momentum, instruct him to walk with a wide-based gait and to swing his arms (see *Walking with a wide-based gait,* page 181). If appropriate, show him how to use a weighted cane or a walker. Teach him how to unlock a position if he becomes temporarily fixed in it. Some common unlocking techniques include turning the head, opening the mouth, placing an arm behind the back or across the chest, tapping a leg with the hand, bending the knees slightly, or raising the toes. Tell him to use these techniques cautiously to avoid losing his balance and falling.

To prevent falls, recommend removing throw rugs and unstable furniture and moving furniture against the walls to widen traffic paths. Also tell the patient to wear sturdy shoes with good support and traction.

Combatting oily skin and increased perspiration. Explain to the patient the importance of daily bathing. Advise him to avoid oil-based soaps or lotions, and tell him to use an antiperspirant deodorant on his hands if he has sweaty palms.

Dealing with urinary urgency. Tell the patient to remain near a bathroom or to keep a urinal nearby. Suggest installing a raised toilet seat and grab bars if he has difficulty sitting and standing.

Making dressing easier. Advise the patient to wear clothing with zippers rather than buttons or to use Velcro strips. Loafer-style shoes or elastic shoelaces solve the problem of tying and untying shoes (see *Dressing aids,* page 184).

Coping with dysarthria. Instruct the patient to take his time pronouncing each word. If his voice is too soft, tell him to breathe deeply before beginning each sentence. Tell him that reading aloud (especially poetry) and singing can help his articulation, inflection, and voice projection.

Reducing stress. Teach the patient to explore a relaxation technique that will be compatible with his life-style. Avoid recommending progressive muscle relaxation, which may increase rigidity and tremor. Simple techniques, such as deep breathing and visualization, can be used spontaneously throughout the day. Teach a family member simple massage techniques to help reduce the patient's stress at the end of the day. Note that stress may result from excessive intake of sugar and caffeine and prolonged exposure to loud noise, bright lights, or extreme temperatures.

Teaching family members. Instruct the family to be alert for signs of depression in the patient, such as anorexia, insomnia, and disinterest in his surroundings. Tell them to encourage the patient's participation in family discussions, even though facial rigidity may cause him to look disinterested.

The emotional or financial crises brought on by the illness may severely strain family relationships. Throughout the patient's illness, encourage family members not to neglect themselves. Don't hesitate to suggest counseling, and encourage them to draw on community resources as well as family and friends.

Stress the importance of the patient's wearing a medical identification bracelet or necklace at all times. Refer the patient and his family to a local group or national organization for information and support.

Sources of information and support

American Parkinson Disease Association
116 John Street, Suite 417, New York, N.Y. 10038
(800) 223-2732

National Parkinson Foundation
1501 N.W. 9th Avenue/Bob Hope Road, Miami, Fla.
(800) 327-4545; Fla. residents (800) 433-7022

United Parkinson Foundation
360 West Superior Street, Chicago, Ill. 60670
(312) 664-2344

Further readings

Berry, P., and Ward-Smith, P. "Adrenal Medullary Transplant as a Treatment for Parkinson's Disease: Perioperative Considerations," *Journal of Neuroscience Nursing* 20(6):356-361, December 1988.

Delgado, J., et al. "Care of the Patient with Parkinson's Disease," *Journal of Neuroscience Nursing* 20(3):142-150, June 1988.

Lannon, M., et al. "Comprehensive Care of the Patient with Parkinson's Disease," *Journal of Neuroscience Nursing* 18(3):121-131, June 1986.

Norberg, A., et al. "The Interaction Between the Parkinsonian Patient and His Caregiver During Feeding: A Theoretical Model," *Journal of Advanced Nursing* 12(5):545-550, September 1987.

Pentland, B. "The Management of Parkinson's Disease," *Geriatric Nursing & Home Care* 8(1):12-14, January 1988.

Walking with a wide-based gait

Dear Patient:

Walking with a wide-based gait and swinging your arms will help you to maintain balance and keep moving forward. Use the following step-by-step guidelines to practice this technique. Remember to look ahead when walking and not at your feet.

1 Start by positioning your feet 8 to 10 inches (20 to 25 cm) apart. Stand as straight as you can.

2 Now lift your foot high with your toes up, taking as large a step as possible.

3 As you bring your foot down, place your heel on the ground first and roll onto the ball of your foot and then your toes. Perform the same steps with the other foot. Repeat these movements.

4 Swing your right arm forward when moving your left leg. Swing your left arm forward when moving your right leg.

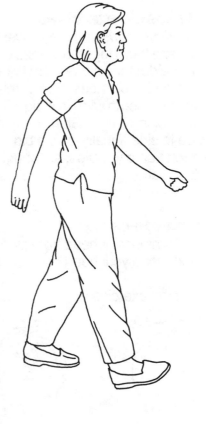

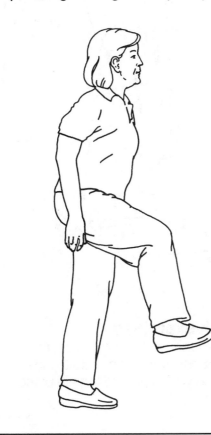

How to do stretching exercises

Dear Patient:

Your doctor has prescribed exercises to help you maintain flexibility and muscle strength. At first, do each exercise 1 to 5 times daily. Then, gradually increase to 10 to 20 times daily. If you're unable to do these exercises standing up, you can do most of them sitting down.

Facial muscle exercises
Raise your eyebrows and then lower and squeeze them together. Next, open your eyes wide; then close them tight.
　　Now, wrinkle your nose. Follow this by opening your mouth wide in a big "O" and then closing it tight. Shift your jaw from side to side. Finally, give a big smile; then purse your lips, as though trying to whistle.
　　Repeat the exercises.

Neck exercises
Begin by turning your head from side to side. Next, bend your head down and back.
　　Repeat the exercises.

Shoulder exercises
Raise your shoulders toward your ears as high as you can. Then lower them.
　　Repeat a few more times.

Arm and shoulder exercises
Raise your arms over your head. Then swing them down, extending them behind your back. Repeat.

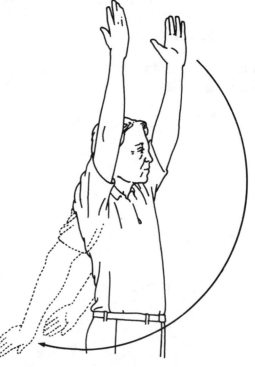

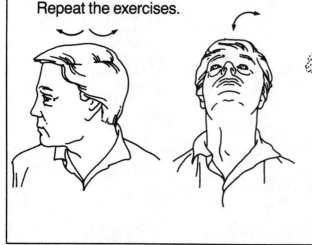

Trunk exercises
With your hands on your hips, twist your body at the waist from side to side, keeping your hips and legs in place. Repeat.

continued

How to do stretching exercises — *continued*

Hip and knee exercises

Holding on to a counter or a sturdy piece of furniture, raise your right knee toward your right shoulder. Lower it and then raise your left knee, raising it toward your left shoulder. Lower the knee and repeat these movements.

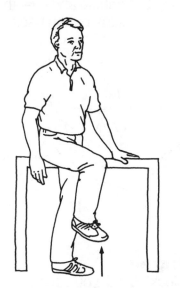

Stand facing a wall, about 8 inches (20 cm) away. Place your hands on the wall until they're above your head. Then raise your right leg up behind you, keeping your knee straight. Do the same with the left leg. Repeat.

Knee exercises

While sitting down, straighten your right knee, extending your right leg out in front of you. Then bend your right leg back under the chair as far as you can. (Keep your ankle flexed to avoid a muscle spasm.) Repeat with your left leg. Perform this exercise several times.

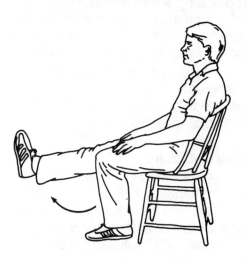

Ankle and foot exercises

While sitting down, make circles with your right foot, first in one direction and then in the other. Repeat with your left foot. Do this a few more times.

Ankle and toe exercises

While sitting down, extend your leg and point your toes toward the floor. Then point them up toward your nose. Try this several more times.

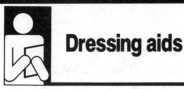

Dressing aids

Dear Patient:

Does dressing yourself seem to take a long time? If so, here are some tips to make dressing faster and easier.

First, place your clothes close by, in the order in which you'll put them on. To pull your pants on or off, lie down, sit on a bed or a chair, or lean against a sturdy piece of furniture.

Also consider using any of the dressing aids described below.

Dressing sticks

A dressing stick helps you pull garments over your shoulders. Pad one end of the stick, or tip it with a rubber thimble so that your clothes will cling to the stick. Screw a small cup hook into the other end to help you manage zippers.

To help you pull garments over your feet and up, attach cup hooks (lightly taped to protect your skin) to two dowel sticks. Slip the hooks into tape loops, which you can sew inside a garment's waistband.

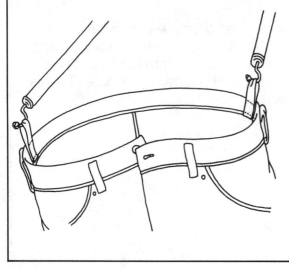

Buttonhook

If you struggle with buttons, consider getting a buttonhook. Slip this aid through the buttonhole and over the button. Then pull the button back through the hole.

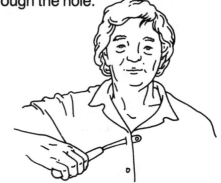

Stocking aid

With a stocking aid, you can put on stockings without bending over. If you're using an aid like the one shown, first slide the stockings over the form. Secure the stockings; then pull the form up your leg—along with the stocking.

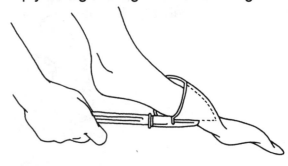

Zipper pull

A large zipper pull will make opening and closing zippers easier. Or attach an object, such as a key ring or a large paper clip, to a small zipper pull.

Alzheimer's disease

Your primary teaching goal in Alzheimer's disease consists of preparing the family to meet the spiraling demands of patient care. You'll direct most of your teaching to the primary caregivers. Offer them emotional support as you explain the inexorable course of this degenerative dementia and the measures they can take to relieve its physical, emotional, and social strains.

Expect family members to wonder why the patient's personality has changed so dramatically. Address their concerns by discussing the pathophysiology of Alzheimer's disease and its possible causes. Point out the difficulty in diagnosing the disease, explaining that diagnosis involves various examinations and tests to rule out other illnesses.

To prepare the family for the patient's progressive deterioration, discuss Alzheimer's signs, symptoms, and stages. Review diet adjustments and medications to help manage symptoms, and explain how to decrease patient stress and create a safe environment. Not to be overlooked—provide suggestions to help the caregiver avoid burnout.

Discuss the disorder

Inform the patient (if appropriate) and his family that Alzheimer's disease is a degenerative disorder of the brain. It produces progressive nerve atrophy in the frontal lobe of the cerebral cortex. Characteristic pathologic changes include neurofibrillary tangles (large, irregular fibrous strands found throughout the nerve cell) and senile or neuritic plaques (extracellular clusters of degenerating nerve terminals), which hinder cerebral cortex function. Other abnormalities include reduced oxygen metabolism, decreased blood flow in the brain, thickened capillary walls in the cerebral cortex, absence of the perivascular neural plexus, and loss of brain cells.

Explain that the cause of Alzheimer's disease isn't known, but several factors have been implicated: a deficiency in the brain's neurotransmitter substances, viruses, genetic predisposition, and environmental toxins.

Review the signs and symptoms of Alzheimer's disease. Describe its subtle, early signs, such as forgetfulness. Emphasize that the disease is more than just memory loss—it produces progressive changes in the patient's intellect, personality, sensation, motor, and overall functioning. (See *The many faces of Alzheimer's disease*, page 186.) Explain that the disease progresses in stages,

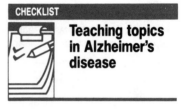

CHECKLIST

Teaching topics in Alzheimer's disease

☐ Pathophysiology and possible causes of Alzheimer's disease
☐ Signs and symptoms and stages
☐ Diagnostic workup, including a patient and family history; physical, neurologic, and psychiatric examinations; laboratory tests; and magnetic resonance imaging, electroencephalography, and other tests
☐ Need for activity and exercise to maintain mobility and help prevent complications
☐ Dietary adjustments for patients with restlessness, dysphagia, or coordination problems
☐ Medication to relieve depression and prevent seizures and experimental drugs to help increase cognitive function
☐ Home care planning—establishing a daily routine, providing a safe home environment, and avoiding overstimulation
☐ Tips for the caregiver, including the importance of adequate rest, good nutrition, and private time
☐ Source of information and support

Julie Tackenberg, RN, MA, CNRN, who wrote this chapter, is a clinical specialist at the University Medical Center, Tucson, Ariz.

The many faces of Alzheimer's disease

Although *memory loss* is commonly associated with Alzheimer's disease, families may not realize that this is only one of its many devastating signs and symptoms. Teach them that the following intellectual, personality, and stress-tolerance deficits are also signs and symptoms of the patient's disease.

Intellectual deficits
• inattention to time
• decreased attention span; increased distractibility
• difficulty making decisions
• inability to solve abstract problems
• inability to plan and complete activities
• inability to perform routine, sequential motor activities, such as dressing, bathing, or eating (motor apraxia)
• increased activity (purposeless, repetitive, and compulsive) coupled with decreased performance
• altered perception of visual and auditory cues

Personality deficits
• inappropriate affect
• lack of inhibitions (involving emotional lability, need for immediate gratification, inability to control temper, tactlessness)
• self-preoccupation and increased refusal to participate
• confabulation, perseveration, paranoia, delusions, hallucinations, and social withdrawal
• expression of hostility or helplessness when deficits are mentioned

Stress-tolerance deficits
• confusion
• nighttime awakening, pacing, and wandering
• fatigue and loss of energy
• avoidance behavior
• anxiety
• violence

---

but at an unpredictable rate. Eventually, though, the patient will suffer complete memory loss and total physical deterioration. (See *How Alzheimer's disease progresses.*)

Complications
Reinforce the need for precautions as the disease progresses to prevent the patient from injuring himself from his own violent behavior, wandering, or unsupervised activity.

Also explain that insufficient exercise and activity may lead to immobility and its complications, such as pneumonia and other infections. Stress that malnutrition and dehydration may also occur if the patient forgets or refuses to eat.

Describe the diagnostic workup
No tests directly detect Alzheimer's disease. Instead the patient will undergo several examinations and tests to rule out other diseases that cause dementia. Because several doctors may be involved in obtaining a patient and family history, performing physical and neurologic examinations, and conducting a psychiatric interview, make sure to clarify who will perform each examination and where it will be done.

The patient will also undergo laboratory and other diagnostic tests, including magnetic resonance imaging (MRI), electroencephalography (EEG), cerebral blood flow studies, and cerebrospinal fluid (CSF) analysis. Warn the family that the diagnostic workup may be lengthy, requiring several trips to the hospital. (See *Diagnosing Alzheimer's disease,* page 188, for more information.) Tell them that the process may, indeed, overwhelm the pa-

---

How Alzheimer's disease progresses

Counsel family members to expect progressive deterioration in the patient with Alzheimer's disease. To help them plan future patient care, discuss the stages of this relentless and inevitably progressive disease.

Bear in mind that family members may refuse to believe that the disease is advancing. So be sensitive to their concerns, and if necessary, review the information again when they're more receptive.

Forgetfulness
The patient becomes forgetful, especially of recent events. He frequently loses everyday objects, such as keys. Aware of this loss of function, he may compensate by relinquishing tasks that might reveal his forgetfulness. Because his behavior isn't disruptive and may be attributed to stress, fatigue, or normal aging, he usually doesn't consult a doctor at this stage.

Confusion
The patient has increasing difficulty with activities that require planning, decision-making, and judgment (such as managing personal finances, driving a car, or performing his job). However, he does retain everyday skills, such as personal grooming. Social withdrawal occurs when the patient feels overwhelmed by a changing environment and his inability to cope with multiple stimuli. Travel is difficult and tiring. As he becomes aware of his progressive loss of function, he may become severely depressed.

Safety becomes a concern when the patient forgets to turn off appliances or to recognize unsafe situations, such as boiling water. At this point, the family may need to consider day care or a supervised residential facility.

Decline in activities of daily living
The patient at this stage loses the ability to perform activities of daily living, such as eating or washing, without direct supervision. Weight loss may occur. He withdraws from the family and increasingly depends on the primary caregiver. Communication becomes difficult as his understanding of written and spoken language declines. Agitation, wandering, pacing, and nighttime awakening are linked to his inability to cope with a multistimuli environment. He may mistake his mirror image for a real person (pseudohallucination). Caregivers must be constantly vigilant, which may lead to physical and emotional exhaustion. They may also feel a sense of loss and anger.

Total deterioration
In the final stage of Alzheimer's disease, the patient no longer recognizes himself, his body parts, or other family members. He becomes bedridden, and his activity consists of small, purposeless movements. Verbal communication stops, although he may scream spontaneously. Complications of immobility may include pressure sores, urinary tract infections, pneumonia, and contractures.

---

tient, precipitating a deterioration in his behavior and intellectual performance. Reassure them, though, that you'll make every effort to minimize his stress before and between the tests.

Patient and family history
Explain that the doctor will ask the family questions about the patient's short-term memory, judgment, and decision-making and whether he shows increased fatigue or personality changes. In Alzheimer's disease, a thorough history reveals a progressive decline in cognitive function, not a stepwise decline as in other types of dementia. Mention that a medication history can rule out the possibility of drug toxicity—the most common, and most easily corrected, cause of confusion and dementia in elderly patients.

Physical examination
Inform the patient and the family that the patient will have a complete physical examination to rule out dementia caused by an underlying illness, such as congestive heart failure or pneumonia.

Diagnosing Alzheimer's disease

Inform the family that diagnosing Alzheimer's disease may be a long and painstaking process. Why? Alzheimer's disease is just one form of dementia. At least 100 other causes of demented behavior exist.

Explain that a conclusive diagnosis of Alzheimer's disease involves performing a brain biopsy and examining the neurofibrillary tangles and plaques under a microscope. However, this traumatic procedure carries a high risk of cerebral infection; therefore it's done only during autopsy.

To help standardize the diagnosis of Alzheimer's disease, the Department of Health and Human Services has established the following clinical criteria for a probable diagnosis:
• dementia confirmed by neurologic testing, with at least two cognitive-function deficits
• progressive deterioration in memory and other types of cognition
• onset of signs and symptoms between ages 40 and 90
• all other possible neurologic and systemic diseases ruled out.

The Department also named these supporting criteria to strengthen a suspected diagnosis of Alzheimer's disease:
• signs and symptoms of aphasia, apraxia, and agnosia
• depression, insomnia, incontinence, delusions, hallucinations, disinhibition, sexual disorders, weight loss, and other associated signs and symptoms
• impaired ability to perform activities of daily living
• family history of Alzheimer's disease
• normal findings on such tests as lumbar puncture, electroencephalography, and various computerized scans
• occasional plateaus in disease progression
• seizures in advanced disease stages.

Neurologic examination

Advise the patient (if appropriate) and the family that a neurologic examination (lasting about 2 hours) will assess specific deficits characteristic of Alzheimer's disease. Examples of deficits include an impaired sense of smell (usually an early symptom), impaired stereognosis (inability to recognize and understand the form and nature of objects by touching them), gait disorders, tremor, and loss of recent memory. Peculiar or inappropriate speech is also common. (In one study, 90% of Alzheimer's patients answered questions with intrusions or inappropriate repetition of answers they'd already given to earlier questions.) Explain that the patient may be asked to make calculations, solve problems, and answer questions about current events.

Tell the family that the doctor may perform a "snout reflex" test to rule out a focal problem, such as a tumor. This test involves tapping or stroking the patient's lips or the area just under his nose. Grimacing or puckering the lips is a positive sign for Alzheimer's disease. Point out that this reflex is normal in early infancy but suggests diffuse organic brain disease in adults.

Is the patient aware of his deficits? If so, warn the family that during the tests he may become frustrated and angry and refuse to answer any questions. The patient with more advanced disease may become agitated or belligerent. Tell the family that the patient with memory loss may be even more confused and restless after the tests.

Neuropsychological interview

Explain that a neuropsychological interview helps rule out severe depression, which is often mistaken for dementia or Alzheimer's disease in elderly patients. All of these conditions cause apathy, unresponsiveness, and memory loss. Explain that this is a lengthy test (4 to 6 hours) and may greatly upset the patient.

Magnetic resonance imaging

Instruct the patient (if appropriate) and the family that an MRI scan evaluates the condition of the brain and rules out intracranial lesions as the source of dementia. Mention that the test takes about 1 hour and causes no discomfort or radiation exposure. However, because it does involve exposure to a strong magnetic field, ask if the patient has any metal objects in his body, such as a pacemaker, aneurysm clips, a hip prosthesis, or bullet fragments, so the machine can be adjusted.

Describe how the patient will lie on a table that slides into a large cylinder housing the MRI magnets. Explain that he'll need to lie quietly. If the doctor thinks he will be unable to do this, he may order a mild sedative. The patient's head, chest, and arms are restrained to help him remain still so that the images won't be blurred. Warn him that he'll hear a loud knocking noise while the machine is running, and tell him that he can request earplugs or pads. Reassure him that a technician can see and hear him from another room. After the test, the patient can resume his normal activities.

Electroencephalography

Explain that an EEG records and evaluates the brain's electrical activity and helps diagnose tumors, abscesses, and other intracranial lesions that might cause the patient's symptoms. Mention that the test takes about 45 minutes.

Offer reassurance that the test is painless and that the electrodes won't cause an electric shock. Also teach about any pretest restrictions, which depend on the type of EEG (such as sleep, sleep deprivation, or photic stimulation). In addition, the patient should wash his hair 1 to 2 days before the test to remove hair spray, cream, or oil.

During the test, the patient will be positioned comfortably in a reclining chair or bed. After lightly rubbing the patient's skin to ensure good contact, the technician will apply paste and attach electrodes to the patient's head and neck. Caution the patient to lie still during the test. Then review the activities he may be asked to perform. For example, he may be asked to breathe deeply and rapidly for 3 minutes or to fall asleep, depending on the type of EEG.

After the test, the technician will remove the electrodes and remove the paste with acetone. (Warn the patient that this might sting where his skin was scraped.) He can then resume his regular activities. The patient should wash his hair to remove residual paste.

Cerebral blood flow studies

Tell the patient and the family that cerebral blood flow studies detect abnormalities in blood flow to the brain. The test takes about 30 minutes. Reassure them that the test is painless and exposes the patient to less radiation than a chest X-ray.

During the test, the patient will lie on a table, and the technician will place a frame around his head. If the inhalation technique is used, the patient will breathe through a mask or a mouthpiece (wearing noseclips) for 10 minutes as readings are taken. If the injection technique is used, he'll receive an I.V. injection and breathe through a mask or dome. Warn him to lie still during the test. Afterward, he can resume his normal activities.

CSF analysis

Teach that a CSF analysis reveals whether the patient's signs and symptoms stem from a chronic neurologic infection. This 15-minute test involves removing spinal fluid via a lumbar puncture and analyzing it. Warn the patient that he'll feel some pressure as the needle is inserted, and he may become uncomfortable from the position assumed during the test.

Describe how the patient will sit with his head bent toward his knees, or he'll lie on the edge of a bed or a table with his knees drawn up to his abdomen and his chin resting on his chest. After cleaning the lumbar area, the doctor will inject a local anesthetic. Tell the patient to report any tingling or sharp pain. Next the doctor will insert a hollow needle into the subarachnoid space surrounding the spinal cord. Tell the patient not to move to avoid dislodging the needle. Also tell him that he may be asked to breathe deeply or to straighten his legs and that the doctor may apply pressure to the jugular veins.

Explain that after the test the doctor will remove the needle and apply an adhesive bandage. The patient must then lie flat, with his head even with or below his hips, for 4 to 24 hours to prevent a headache. Tell him that he can turn from side to side but that he shouldn't raise his head. He should also drink plenty of fluids for the rest of the day to help replenish the CSF and to prevent a headache.

Teach about treatments

Alzheimer's disease has no cure, but various treatments may temporarily improve the patient's quality of life and make caring for him easier. Such treatments center on stress reduction, safety measures, drug therapy, diet modification, and physical activity.

Activity

Explain that adequate exercise and activity will help maintain the patient's mobility and prevent complications, such as pneumonia or other infections. Exercise also promotes a normal day and night routine. Encourage family members to find physical activities, such as walking or light housework, that satisfy and occupy the patient. Repetitive activity, such as folding towels, scrubbing the floor, sweeping, or indoor bicycle riding may satisfy the patient. Repetitive motions relieve the patient of making a decision about what to do next, decreasing his stress level.

Diet

Stress the importance of a well-balanced diet with adequate fiber. If the patient is hyperactive, advise the family to increase his caloric intake with between-meal supplements. But tell them to avoid stimulants, such as coffee, tea, cola, and chocolate.

Tell the family to limit the number of foods on the patient's plate, so he won't have to make decisions. If he has coordination problems, advise them to cut his food and to provide finger foods, such as fruit and sandwiches. Suggest using plates with rim guards, built-up utensils, and cups with lids and spouts.

If the patient develops dysphagia, tell the family to serve semisoft foods. Suggest freezing liquids to a slush or mixing them with other foods. If the patient can't swallow or has no interest in food, nasogastric or gastrostomy tube feedings may be necessary; instruct the family accordingly.

If the patient puts almost anything in his mouth, whether it's food or not, tell the family to keep preferred foods handy.

Medication

Explain that no medications are currently available to treat Alzheimer's disease but that several are being studied. Investigative drugs include choline chloride, lecithin, tacrine hydrochloride, and physostigmine salicylate (Antilirium). Although these substances provide little or no benefit if used alone, researchers are combining them to try to slow the disease process. For example, choline chloride and lecithin, which occur naturally in various foods and are precursors for acetylcholine synthesis, are used together to improve cognitive function by increasing acetylcholine availability. In addition, tacrine hydrochloride and physostigmine salicylate, both cholinesterase inhibitors, are being used to prolong acetylcholine action in the brain, which also increases cognitive function.

Inform the patient (if appropriate) and his family that other medications are used to manage the patient's signs and symptoms. For example, antipsychotics and antidepressants control behavioral changes, and neuroleptics control seizures. Caution the family to check with the doctor before giving the patient any unprescribed drugs, especially sedatives, because drug action may be enhanced in Alzheimer's disease.

If the patient has trouble swallowing, advise crushing tablets or opening capsules and mixing them with a semisoft food. However, caution the family always to check with the pharmacist before crushing tablets or opening capsules because specially formulated drugs shouldn't be altered. Mention that in many cases flavorful oral suspensions may be available that will ease administration problems.

Other care measures

Encourage the family to allow the patient as much independence as possible while ensuring his—and others'—safety. (See *Planning home care,* pages 193 to 195.) To combat the patient's confusion, emphasize maintaining a routine in *all* his activities. If the patient panics or becomes belligerent, advise the family to remain calm and to try distracting him.

Recommend dividing the patient's daily tasks into short, simple steps and then guiding him through them. Tell the family to use activities that stimulate or calm him appropriately. Suggest repetitive tasks, such as sanding wood and listening to music.

Also, advise the family to avoid overstimulating the patient before bedtime and to limit fluids about 3 to 4 hours before bedtime, so the patient won't need to get up to urinate. If he develops irregular sleep patterns and wanders at night, he may harm himself and others. If necessary, tell the family to lock doors and windows, barricade stairways, and use night-lights. If the patient's confused about his surroundings, tell the family to use pictures to guide him.

Teach the family about home safety measures, such as storing medication out of the patient's reach and removing throw rugs. If necessary, remind them to remove handles and buttons from appliances. (See *Promoting patient safety,* pages 196 and 197.) If the patient has coordination problems, suggest using Velcro straps instead of buttons and loafers or shoes with elastic shoelaces.

Stress that the patient can't control his behavior, although sometimes he may respond appropriately. And, even if the patient no longer recognizes his family, urge them to still include him in their activities. Last, emphasize to the family the importance of taking some time for themselves. (See *Aid for the caregiver: Avoiding burnout,* pages 198 to 200.) Refer them to a local Alzheimer's support group and to the Alzheimer's Association for more information.

Source of information and support

Alzheimer's Association
70 E. Lake Street, Suite 600, Chicago, Ill. 60601
(312) 853-3060

Further readings

Chiverton, P., and Caine, E.D. "Education to Assist Spouses in Coping with Alzheimer's Disease: A Controlled Trial," *Journal of the American Geriatric Society* 37(7): 593-98, July 1989.

Dixon, A.Y. "Environments of Care for the Patient with Alzheimer's Disease," *Journal of Advanced Medical-Surgical Nursing* 1(2):48-54, March 1989.

Fabiszewski, K.J. "Alzheimer's Disease: Overview and Progression," *Journal of Advanced Medical-Surgical Nursing* 1(2):1-17, March 1989.

Gwyther, L.P. "Overcoming Barriers: Home Care of Dementia Patients," *Caring* 8(8):12-16, August 1989.

Jaeger, M. "Alzheimer's Disease: Providing Nutritional Support," *Nursing89* 19(4):100-01, April 1989.

Johnson, L., and Keller, A.L. "Staging Alzheimer's Disease," *Geriatric Nursing* 10(4):196-97, July-August 1989.

Kaseman, D.F., and Young, S.H. "Stress: An Added Incapacitator," *Geriatric Nursing* 9(5):274-77, September-October 1988.

McGacken, A.L., et al. "The Right Environment for Alzheimer's," *Geriatric Nursing* 10(6):293-94, November-December 1989.

Niemoller, J. "Change of Pace for Alzheimer's Patients," *Geriatric Nursing* 11(2):86-87, March-April 1990.

Noyes, L.E. "Caregiving Techniques for Dementia Patients," *Caring* 8(8):18-21, August 1989.

Zook, M.L. "Living With Alzheimer's Disease: Resources for Family Caregivers," *Caring* 8(8):30-31, August 1989.

Planning home care

Dear Caregiver:

Taking care of a patient with Alzheimer's disease requires a great deal of patience and understanding. It also requires you to look at the patient's environment with new eyes. Then you have to learn how to change this environment to help him function at the highest possible level.

Keeping these points in mind, read over the following tips to help you plan your daily care.

Reduce stress

Too much stress can worsen the patient's symptoms. Try to protect him from the following potential sources of stress:
• a change in routine, caregiver, or environment
• fatigue
• excessive demands
• overwhelming, misleading, or competing stimuli
• illness and pain
• over-the-counter medications.

Establish a routine

Keep the patient's daily routine stable so he can respond automatically. Adapting to change may require more thought than the patient can handle. Even eating a different food or going to a strange grocery store may overwhelm him.

Ask yourself: What are the patient's daily activities? Then make a schedule:
• List the activities necessary for his daily care, and include ones that he especially enjoys, such as weeding in the garden. Designate a time frame for each activity.
• Establish bedtime rituals—especially important to promote relaxation and a restful night's sleep for both of you.
• Stick to your schedule as closely as possible (for example, breakfast first, then dressing) so the patient won't be surprised or need to make decisions.

> **Mitchell's daily schedule:**
>
> **7:45 - 8:30 AM Breakfast**
> • Mitchell enjoys taking his time during breakfast.
> • Serve some type of fresh fruit with breakfast.
> • If he seems interested in talking, speak slowly.
>
> **8:30 - 9:00 AM Bathing**
> • Tell Mitchell, one step at a time, how to prepare for his bath.
> • Once he has finished, gently help him out of the tub and hand him his blue terry robe.
>
> **9:00 - 9:30 AM Dressing**
> • Allow Mitchell to dress himself at his own pace. Lay out his clothes in the order he will put them on.

• Keep a copy of the patient's schedule to give to other caregivers. To help them give better care, include notes and suggestions about techniques that work for you; for instance, "Speak in a quiet voice" or "When helping Mitchell dress or take a bath, take things one step at a time, and wait for him to respond."

continued

Planning home care — *continued*

Practice reality orientation

In your conversation with the patient, orient him to the day and the activity he'll perform. For instance, say "Today is Tuesday, and we're going to have breakfast now." Do this every day.

This keeps the patient aware of his immediate environment and tells him what to expect without challenging him to remember events.

Simplify the surroundings

The patient will eventually lose the ability to interpret correctly what he sees and hears. Protect him by trying to decrease the noise level in his environment and by avoiding busy areas, such as shopping malls and restaurants.

Does the patient mistake pictures or images in the mirror for real people? If so, remove the photos and mirrors. Also avoid rooms with busy patterns on wallpaper and carpets because they can overtax his senses.

To avoid confusion and encourage the patient's independence, provide cues. For example, hang a picture of a toilet on the bathroom door.

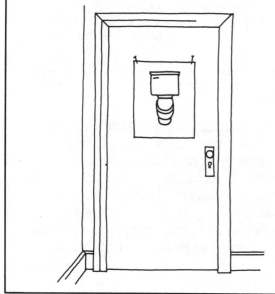

Avoid fatigue

The patient will tire easily, so plan important activities for the morning when he's functioning best. Save less demanding ones for later in the day. Remember to schedule breaks — one in the morning and one in the afternoon.

About 15 to 30 minutes of listening to music or just relaxing is sufficient in the early stages of the disease. As the disease progresses, schedule longer, more frequent breaks (perhaps 40 to 90 minutes). If the patient naps during the day, have him sleep in a reclining chair rather than in a bed to prevent him from confusing day and night.

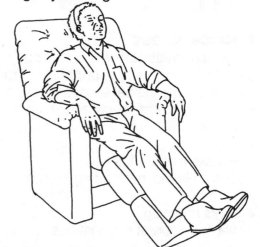

Don't expect too much

Accept the patient's limitations. Don't demand too much from him — this forces him to think about a task and causes frustration. Instead, offer help when needed, and distract him if he's trying too hard. You'll feel less stressed, too.

Prepare for illness

If the patient becomes ill, expect his behavior to deteriorate and plan accordingly. He'll have a low tolerance for pain and discomfort.

continued

Planning home care — *continued*

Never rely on the patient to take his own medicine. He may forget to take it or miscount what he has taken. Always supervise him.

Use the sense of touch
Because the patient's visual and auditory perceptions are distorted, he has an increased need for closeness and touching. Remember to approach the patient from the front. You don't want to frighten him or provoke him into becoming belligerent or aggressive.

Respect the patient's need for personal space. Limit physical contact to his hands and arms at first, then move to more central parts of his body, such as his shoulders or head.

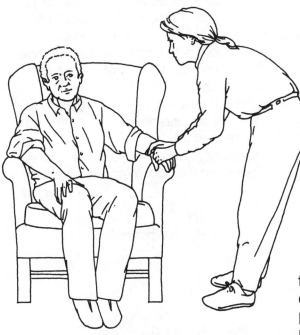

Using long or circular motions, lightly stroke the patient to help relieve muscle tension and give him a sense of his physical self. Physical contact also expresses your feelings of intimacy and caring.

Allowing the patient to touch objects in the environment can help relieve stress by providing information. Let him handle, poke, pull, or shake objects — for example, a handbag, a brush, or a comb. Make sure they're unbreakable and can't harm him.

Handle problem behavior
If the patient becomes restless or agitated, divert his attention with an appropriate activity. Good choices include walking, rocking in a rocking chair, sanding wood, folding laundry, or hoeing

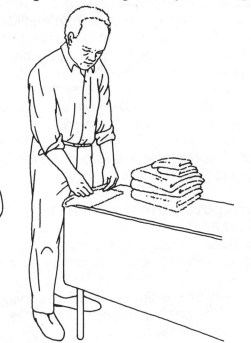

the garden. These repetitive activities don't require any particular sequence or planning. A warm bath, a drink of warm milk, or a back massage can also be calming.

Although problem behavior can be taxing for you, try to remember that the patient can't help himself. Your understanding and compassion can increase his sense of security.

Promoting patient safety

Dear Caregiver:

The patient with Alzheimer's disease requires intensive physical care as well as almost constant supervision to keep him from hurting himself. This means removing potential safety hazards from his environment and installing assistive devices where needed.

You can purchase many of these devices at large pharmacies that have geriatric departments or from medical supply stores. You can even use child-proofing devices, such as safety caps for electrical outlets, soft plastic corners for furniture, and doorknob covers. They're available from catalogs or where baby products are sold.

Use the following guidelines to help you provide a safe environment for the person in your care.

Remove potential safety hazards

- Move knives, forks, scissors, and other sharp objects beyond the patient's reach.
- Taste the patient's food before serving it so he won't burn his mouth or himself if he accidentally spills it.
- Serve the patient's food on unbreakable dishes.
- Remove the knobs from the stove and other potentially hazardous kitchen appliances, and put dangerous small appliances, such as food processors and irons, out of reach.
- Adjust your water heater to a lower temperature (no higher than 120° F. [48.8° C.]) to prevent accidental burns.

- Cover unused electrical outlets, especially those above waist level, with masking tape or safety caps.

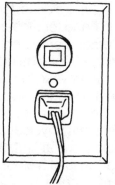

- Remove mirrors or install ones with safety glass in rooms the patient uses.
- Get rid of throw rugs and cover slippery floors with large area rugs. Place pads under the rugs, and secure them so they don't slide.
- Keep floors and stairways clear of toys, shoes, and other objects that can trip the patient.
- Camouflage doors with murals or posters so they don't look like exits, or

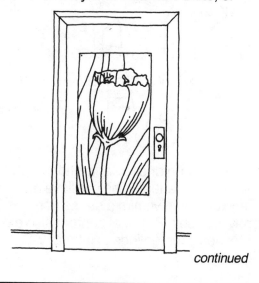

continued

Promoting patient safety — *continued*

simply lock them. Install a lock at the base of the door as an extra security measure, or install a childproofing device over the knob.
● Barricade stairways with high gates.

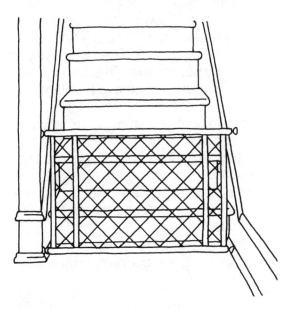

● Remove all breakable wall hangings and pictures, and attach curtains to the wall with Velcro.
● Keep traffic patterns open by moving unsafe furniture to the walls.
● Store all medications out of the patient's reach, preferably in a locked container.

Install assistive devices
● Pad sharp furniture corners with masking tape or plastic corners.
● Provide a low bed for the patient.
● Keep the house well illuminated during waking hours. Keep a night-light in the bathroom.
● If the patient uses the stairs, mark the edges with strips of yellow or orange tape to compensate for poor depth perception.

● Encourage the patient to use the bathroom by making a "path" of colored tape leading in that direction.
● Attach safety rails in the bathtub, near the toilet, and on stairways.

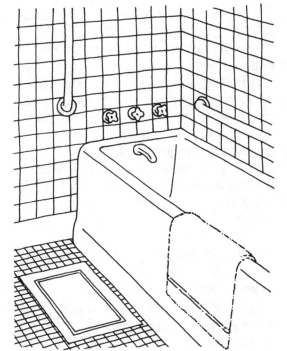

● Glue nonskid strips in the bathtub and by the toilet.
● Provide an identification bracelet for the patient, listing his name, address, phone number, and medical problems.

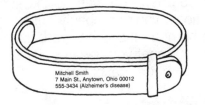

Mitchell Smith
7 Main St., Anytown, Ohio 00012
555-3434 (Alzheimer's disease)

● Give the local police a photograph and description of the patient, in case he's found wandering in the streets.

Aid for the caregiver: Avoiding burnout

Dear Caregiver:

Anyone caring for a patient who needs full-time supervision and care is a prime candidate for burnout. Seemingly endless responsibilities can leave you feeling emotionally and physically drained, with virtually no time for yourself. If you feel inadequate to handle an unexpected crisis, in the end both you and the patient suffer.

How can you cope? Start by learning the warning signs of burnout so you'll know if you're reaching your physical and emotional limits.

Ask yourself these questions:
- Do I have trouble getting organized?
- Do I cry for no reason?
- Am I short tempered?
- Do I feel numb and emotionless?
- Are everyday tasks getting harder to accomplish?
- Do I feel constantly pressed for time?
- Do I feel that I just can't do anything right?
- Do I feel that I have no time for myself?

If you answered "yes" to the above questions, you're probably suffering from burnout. If so, the tips below will help you meet your own needs so you can give better patient care.

Get enough rest
Exhaustion magnifies pressures and reduces your ability to cope. So the first step in combating burnout is getting a good night's sleep—every night, if possible. Here's how:

First, decide how much sleep you usually need—say, 7 hours—and set aside this much time. Then when you go to bed, try not to replay the day in your mind—this isn't the time to problem-solve.

To help control disturbing thoughts, try relaxation techniques, such as deep breathing, reading, or listening to soft music. Or try dimming the bathroom lights and taking a warm bath or shower to relieve muscular tension and help you wind down.

Strenuous activity can encourage sleep by tiring you out physically. It also

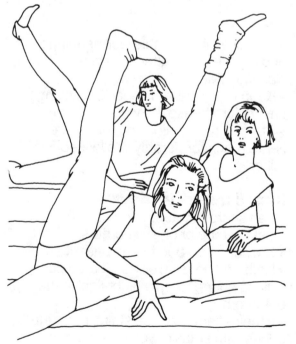

continued

Aid for the caregiver: Avoiding burnout — *continued*

increases your physical stamina, improves your self-image, brightens your outlook, and gets you out of the house.

If possible, hire a relief caretaker so you can attend aerobics classes, go for a brisk walk, or get some kind of exercise for at least 1 hour three times a week.

In addition, try to schedule three or four short breaks during the day.

Resting for 10 minutes with your feet up and your eyes closed can rejuvenate you and counteract the cycle of frantic activity that's probably keeping you up at night.

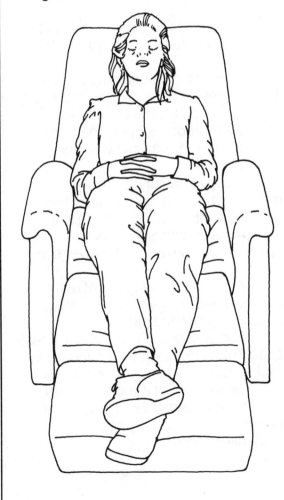

Finally, use sleeping pills and tranquilizers only as a last resort — and only temporarily. Both kinds of drugs have side effects that can cause more problems for you in the long run. Instead, to induce drowsiness, try drinking a glass of warm milk.

Eat well
Eating regular, well-balanced meals will help keep up your energy and increase your resistance to illness.

Skipping meals or eating on the run can cause vitamin and mineral deficiencies, such as anemia (a shortage of iron in the blood), that deplete your strength and make you feel exhausted.

Choose foods from the four food groups every day, avoid "empty" calories, and unless you're overweight and your doctor advises it, don't diet — you need increased calories to fuel your increased activity.

Don't try to be superhuman
After you've been giving home care for several weeks, reappraise your earlier plans. How much can you really do? How much time do you need for yourself?

Now, delegate tasks. If possible, hire extra caretakers or someone to help with housework and shopping. Send your laundry out. Remember: You don't have to do it all yourself, or do it all today, or accomplish everything on your list. Do only what's absolutely necessary, and learn to set priorities.

Just remember to save some time for pleasurable activities. If you have 15

continued

PATIENT-TEACHING AID

Aid for the caregiver: Avoiding burnout — *continued*

minutes' free time, listen to music or take a walk.

And if you want to have friends for dinner, go ahead. Just ask everyone to bring a course.

Confide in someone

A family member or close friend can help you resolve conflicts, be a sounding board for your anger and frustration, and offer emotional support. A support group can accomplish this too, as well as offer practical hints for patient care.

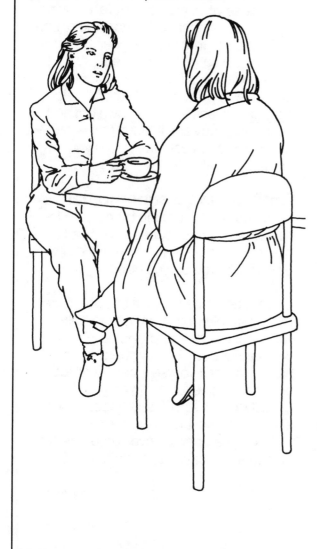

Allow yourself some quality time alone

Free time won't happen automatically — you have to schedule it. In fact, the patient also needs time for himself. So allow yourself and him some personal space and private time. If you don't, you'll become too dependent on each other.

Try to keep your life as normal as possible. Continue to do things that you enjoy, either by yourself or with your friends.

Remember: Meeting your own needs isn't selfish, even if the patient's homebound.

If you continue to feel guilty about taking some time for yourself, go for counseling.

How much time alone is necessary? The answer depends on you. At the very least, you need to take the time to attend to your important personal needs, such as bathing, washing your hair, and dressing.

At the other end of the spectrum, you might want or need to have a part-time or full-time job. If so, you'll need to arrange for a caretaker to take care of the patient while you're working away from home.

Make sure this arrangement reflects your own personality and your unique relationship with the patient.

What is your goal? To provide the best quality of life for the patient without sacrificing your own. How you accomplish this is up to you. But if you feel happy with the arrangement and the patient seems to be reasonably content, it's probably working.

Multiple sclerosis

As in other progressive degenerative disorders, multiple sclerosis (MS) requires complex teaching to help the patient adjust to the disease's physical, emotional, and psychosocial effects. A major cause of chronic disability in young and middle-aged adults, MS affects more women than men. Although most patients lead active, productive lives and enjoy prolonged remissions, a minority see the disease progress so rapidly that they have little time to adjust to their loss of abilities.

Notorious for its unpredictable and spontaneous remissions and exacerbations, MS episodes can be mild or severe. Because of this, the patient needs to know what can trigger an exacerbation, why ability levels may change unexpectedly, how to care for herself during exacerbations (and remissions), and how to cope with any residual neurologic deficits, such as sensory alterations or dysphagia. She'll need to learn what types of diet and exercise are compatible with MS and the importance of following her prescribed medication regimen. What's more, she'll need information about sexual dysfunction, and, possibly, childbearing.

Discuss the disorder

Explain that MS is thought to result from a genetic trait that causes susceptibility to autoimmune dysfunction, viral infection, or both (see *MS: Clues to its cause,* page 202). MS destroys myelin, the lipoprotein that covers axons (the impulse-conducting part of the nerve cell) in the brain and the spinal cord. This causes neurologic deficits. If the destruction involves the axon or if the myelin fails to regenerate, plaque and scar tissue form, causing permanent deficits. For more information, see *When myelin breaks down,* page 202.

Inform the patient that varied problems may come and go in no predictable pattern. These include mood swings; speech, hearing, and visual disturbances; sensory losses; bowel, bladder, and sexual dysfunction; and muscle tremors, weakness, and spasms. Confirm that a deficit may appear during an exacerbation and recede during a remission, or that the deficit may become permanent. Explain that the type of deficit—motor, sensory, cognitive, or emotional—depends on which part of the brain or spinal cord is involved.

Julie N. Tackenberg, RN, MA, CNRN, and **Janette Yanko, RN, MN, CNRN,** wrote this chapter. Ms. Tackenberg is a clinical editor at Springhouse Corporation, Springhouse, Pa. Ms. Yanko is head nurse in the Central Nervous System Unit, Allentown Hospital–Lehigh Valley Hospital Center, Allentown, Pa.

CHECKLIST

Teaching topics in multiple sclerosis

☐ Explanation of how demyelination affects neurologic function
☐ Preparation for tests, such as cerebrospinal fluid analysis, computed tomography, magnetic resonance imaging, and evoked potential studies, to diagnose and monitor multiple sclerosis
☐ Activity and dietary guidelines
☐ Energy conservation measures
☐ Using wheelchairs safely for mobility and independence
☐ Administration of drugs to relieve symptoms
☐ Preparation for plasmapheresis or stereotaxic thalamotomy, if ordered
☐ Measures for minimizing neurologic deficits
☐ Bladder and bowel retraining
☐ Methods to relieve urinary incontinence and retention, including Credé's maneuver and self-catheterization
☐ Sexual dysfunction and childbearing concerns
☐ Source of information and support

202 Multiple sclerosis

MS: Clues to its cause

When you discuss multiple sclerosis (MS) with your patient, include information about current studies. Inform her that researchers are investigating immune dysfunction and genetic factors as possible MS causes.

Probing the immune system
Studies show that patients with a progressive form of MS have about half as many of the immune system's T-4 suppressor-inducer cells as do healthy people. Theoretically, this deficiency may permit other immune system cells to lose control and attack the nervous system, leading to MS.

Searching for the genetic link
Although genetic factors have long been suspected as a cause of MS, evidence remains inconclusive. But two recent Canadian studies may change that. In the first study, identical (monozygotic) and fraternal (dizygotic) twins were selected from about 5,500 MS patients. They were studied to detect any differences in the tendency to develop the disease. Significantly, the likelihood of having MS was nearly 26% among identical twins but only 2.3% among fraternal twins. The rate for nontwin siblings was 1.9%.

A second study included 815 MS patients and 11,300 of their relatives. Researchers concluded that children of MS patients have a 30% to 50% greater risk of contracting the disease than the general population, which has a 0.1% chance of having MS. Daughters of mothers who have MS have a risk of about 5%. Rarely, when both parents have MS, the risk of their children having MS falls between 10% and 15%.

Looking ahead
Next, the specific genes influencing susceptibility to MS must be identified.

When myelin breaks down

When your patient asks what causes her symptoms, describe myelin's role in speeding electrical impulses along nerve pathways to the brain for interpretation. Then explain how multiple sclerosis (MS) short-circuits and disrupts conduction of nerve impulses in the central nervous system (CNS), sending either partial impulses or no impulses at all to the brain. Here's more detail.

Myelin, a lipoprotein complex of glial cells or oligodendrocytes, forms a sheath around the neuron's long nerve fibers (the axon).

Because of its high electrical resistance and low capacitance, myelin serves as an ideal insulator. This allows efficient conduction of nerve impulses from one node of Ranvier to the next.

However, myelin sheaths are susceptible to injury, for example, by hypoxemia, toxic chemicals, vascular insufficiency, and autoimmune responses. As a result, the myelin sheath becomes inflamed, and the membrane layers break down into smaller components that become well-circumscribed plaques (filled with microglial elements, macroglia, and lymphocytes). This process is called demyelination.

The damaged myelin sheath impairs normal conduction, causing partial loss or dispersion of the action potential and consequent neurologic dysfunction.

ABNORMAL NEURON

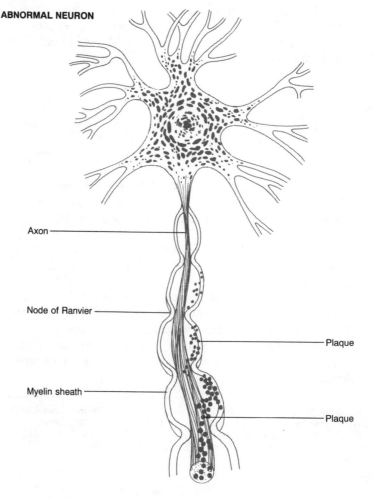

Axon

Node of Ranvier

Myelin sheath

Plaque

Plaque

Complications

Tell the patient that failure to follow the prescribed medication regimen may hasten sensory alterations or visual disturbances, leading to physical injury from falls. Also caution her that if she fails to comply with treatments for her deficits, she may develop urinary tract infections, constipation, and joint contractures. Reinforce the importance of avoiding or minimizing factors that can trigger an exacerbation.

Describe the diagnostic workup

Inform the patient that no specific test can diagnose MS. Rather, she'll undergo various tests to help distinguish MS from other neurologic disorders and to monitor its course. Discuss cerebrospinal fluid (CSF) analysis (see *Testing for MS* for tests that evaluate CSF). As appropriate, teach about computed tomography (CT), magnetic resonance imaging (MRI), positron emission tomography (PET), and evoked potential studies (visual, auditory, and somatosensory). Describe other tests to help diagnose or monitor the disease, including nerve conduction studies and possibly neuropsychological tests.

Tell the patient that she'll have blood tests to detect enzyme deficiencies and byproducts of muscle breakdown and atrophy. Mention where and when blood samples will be drawn, and advise her that she may feel transient discomfort from the needle puncture and tourniquet pressure.

CSF analysis

Explain that this test involves extracting and analyzing spinal fluid to detect abnormalities. The procedure takes about 15 minutes. Tell the patient that she'll be seated with her head bent toward her knees, or she'll lie on the edge of a bed or table, with her knees drawn up to her abdomen and her chin resting on her chest. After cleaning the spinal area, the doctor will inject a local anesthetic. The patient should report any tingling or sharp pain.

Explain that she may feel pressure as the doctor inserts a hollow needle into the subarachnoid space surrounding the spinal cord. Instruct her to stay still to avoid dislodging the needle. Also tell her that the doctor may ask her to breathe deeply or to straighten her legs and that he may apply pressure to the jugular veins.

After the doctor withdraws the spinal fluid, he'll remove the needle and apply an adhesive bandage. Instruct the patient to lie flat for 4 to 24 hours to prevent a headache. Caution her to keep her head even with or below hip level. Reassure her that though she mustn't raise her head, she can turn from side to side. Also advise her to increase fluid intake for the rest of the day to help replenish CSF and to prevent a headache.

CT scan

Inform the patient that a CT scan uses X-ray images to detect structural abnormalities, edema, or brain and spinal cord lesions that could cause MS-like symptoms. Mention that the test takes

---

Testing for MS

Inform the patient that the most recent diagnostic test for multiple sclerosis (MS) is a series of laboratory analyses of cerebrospinal fluid (CSF). Explain that in a demyelinating disease, such as MS, myelin components (lipids and proteins) are released into CSF.

Three tests evaluate the CSF for these lipids and proteins. The *CSF IgG index test* and the *oligoclonal band test* compare measured substances in the CSF with the same substances in the blood. The comparison shows whether chronic demyelination is occurring. A third test—the *myelin basic protein test*—measures myelin levels in the CSF.

between 30 and 60 minutes and causes little discomfort, although she may feel cold because the equipment requires a cool environment. Explain that she won't be allowed food or fluids for 4 hours beforehand if the test calls for contrast medium infusion.

Tell the patient that she'll lie on a movable X-ray table, with a strap restricting her movement to ensure clear X-ray images. The table will then slide into the tubelike opening of the scanner. If ordered, contrast medium infusion will take about 5 minutes. Instruct the patient to report immediately any discomfort or feelings of warmth or itching. (The technician can see and talk to her from an adjacent area.) Then describe the sounds that the scanner will make as it revolves around her.

Advise the patient that immediately after the test she can resume her usual activities and diet. Urge her to drink additional fluids for the rest of the day to eliminate the contrast medium, if used.

MRI scan

Explain that MRI helps document central nervous system changes resulting from MS. By providing clear images of the brain, the test can identify lesions. Give the patient a copy of the teaching aid *Preparing for magnetic resonance imaging,* page 211.

PET scan

Explain that a PET scan evaluates brain cell function by measuring how quickly tissues consume radioactive isotopes. Explain that the isotopes can be administered in inhalable gas or intravenously in glucose. Either way, the isotopes emit positrons. In certain cells, these positrons emit gamma rays that a computer converts into cross-sectional images of brain activity. Inform the patient that the test takes about 1 hour, is painless, and involves minimal radiation exposure.

Advise the patient that she'll lie on a movable table with her head immobilized (to prevent blurring test images) and positioned inside a ring-shaped opening in the scanner. If the doctor uses the inhalation method, tell the patient that she'll inhale a radioactive isotope tracer through a mask. Instruct her to breathe normally; she won't smell or taste anything odd. If the doctor uses the I.V. method, tell the patient that she may feel a warm sensation during the isotope's injection. Instruct her to notify the doctor or technician if she feels any discomfort. For either method, she'll have a dome-shaped hood placed over her head and face to prevent the exhaled tracer from circulating in the room.

Explain that after the PET scan, the doctor will remove the test apparatus and collect a blood sample. Then the patient can resume her usual activities.

Evoked potential studies

First explain that these tests help to determine nerve pathway integrity. They measure the nervous system's electrical response to a visual, auditory, or sensory stimulus. Tell the patient that the tests take about 1 hour and are painless. Advise her to wash her hair 1 to 2 days beforehand.

Inform the patient that she'll be positioned on a bed or table or in a reclining chair. Emphasize that for accurate results, she should stay still during the test. Then describe how a technician will clean her scalp and then apply a pastelike gel and electrodes to her head and neck. Mention that the test equipment may be noisy. With the electrodes in place, she'll be asked to perform various activities, such as gazing at a checkerboard pattern or a strobe light. She may listen through headphones to a series of clicks, or she may have electrodes placed on an arm and a leg and be asked to respond to a tapping sensation. Inform her that the technician will remove the electrodes and paste when the tests end. Then she can resume her usual activities. Tell her that shampoo will remove residual paste from her hair.

Nerve conduction studies
Inform the patient that these tests measure the speed with which electrical impulses travel along a nerve. Inform the patient that the test may make her feel uncomfortable.

Tell her that during the hour-long test she'll lie down or sit up, depending on the nerve to be tested. Then describe how the technician will clean the skin over the test area and insert shallow, needle electrodes in the area near the distal nerve ending. (These electrodes sense and record electrical impulses emitted by the nerves tested.) Then he will insert a needle electrode at various sites along the nerve route. (These electrodes deliver mild charges to stimulate each nerve and measure its response.) Caution the patient to stay still (to promote accurate test results and to avoid prolonging the test) except when asked to move. Mention that after the test she can resume her usual activities.

Neuropsychological tests
Explain that these tests evaluate simple to complex mental and verbal abilities and compile a personality inventory. Mention that the tests may take between 1 and 2 hours. Then describe some of the activities she'll be asked to perform—for example, calculations, solving problems, and answering questions about current events. Tell the patient and her family that if she has a memory loss or emotional lability, she may feel confused and agitated when the tests end.

Teach about treatments
Because symptoms and their severity vary widely among MS patients, treatment reflects the individual patient's needs. Typically, though, you'll focus on balancing rest with activity; eating a nutritious, high-fiber diet; and using prescribed medications correctly. Because bladder and bowel dysfunction embarrass the patient, be prepared to teach retraining techniques. And, as appropriate, discuss less common treatments, such as plasmapheresis or stereotaxic thalamotomy.

Activity
Fatigue, stress, and overexertion may trigger or intensify MS symptoms, so emphasize the importance of frequent rest periods,

When is a wheelchair necessary?

If your patient asks if she'll have to use a wheelchair, tell her that not everyone with multiple sclerosis needs one. And those who do may not need one all the time.

Some patients have periods of moderate disability in an otherwise normal life. Others have disability that progresses slowly. They may not need a wheelchair until 20 years or so after the disease is diagnosed.

explaining that a great deal of energy is used transmitting nerve impulses past damaged myelin. What's more, because fewer muscles are effectively innervated, the patient will tire more quickly as fewer muscles carry the added workload. Advise her to plan activity after rest periods. If she holds a job, tell her to stagger rest periods throughout working hours whenever possible.

Discuss the benefits of moderate but staggered exercise. Exercise helps decrease calcium loss from bones, prevent renal calculi, maintain muscle tone and joint mobility, and promote circulation. Advise the patient to perform slow, gentle, stretching exercises throughout the day to help diminish spasticity.

If incoordination interferes with the patient's mobility, teach her to walk with a wide-based gait or to use a weighted cane or walker, if necessary. Also suggest ways to make her home safe for daily living.

If appropriate, teach the patient how to use a wheelchair to maintain her mobility and independence (see *When is a wheelchair necessary?*). Instruct her or her caregiver how to perform safe transfers from the wheelchair to her bed or to a car. And offer her a copy of the patient-teaching aid *Learning about wheelchair transfers,* pages 212 to 214. If the patient's immobile, teach her caregiver how to perform proper turning techniques and passive range-of-motion exercises.

Diet

Discuss the nutritious, well-balanced diet the patient needs to maintain her ideal weight and to prevent constipation. Adequate fluid intake, including warm liquids, prune juice, and coffee, and high-fiber foods help prevent constipation. To help prevent renal calculi and urinary tract infections, encourage the patient to consume about 2 to 3 quarts (2 to 3 liters) of fluid daily—including some cranberry or other acidic juice.

If the patient has swallowing difficulties, suggest eating semisolid foods. She can chop or soften foods in a blender and freeze liquids to a slush or mix them with other foods to make swallowing easier. Also, suggest that she sit upright with her head tilted slightly forward while she eats. To stimulate the swallowing reflex, tell her to stroke *upward* from the base of her throat to her chin.

When swallowing is extremely difficult or aspiration may occur, show the family how to prepare and administer nasogastric or gastrostomy tube feedings.

Medication

Explain to the patient that during acute exacerbations, her doctor may prescribe corticosteroids to help alleviate symptoms. During remissions, he may prescribe antispasmodics, anticholinergics, laxatives, antipsychotics, and antidepressants, as needed.

If muscle spasms become severe, the doctor may prescribe skeletal muscle relaxants, such as baclofen (Lioresal) or dantrolene sodium (Dantrium). Explain that these drugs, which help to relax muscles and relieve spasticity and stiffness, may make her feel confused, dizzy, drowsy, or weak. If these symptoms persist, instruct her to notify her doctor and not to operate machinery or a motor vehicle. Also tell her to report constipation, headache, frequent or painful urination, and persistent nausea. Caution her not to discontinue therapy without her doctor's permission. To prevent dizziness, advise her to rise slowly from a sitting or lying position and to avoid hot baths and showers. Suggest that she take the drug with meals or milk to prevent GI distress.

Has the doctor prescribed an investigational drug for your patient? If so, discuss its potential benefits and risks (see *What's new in MS treatments?*). Also inform the patient of her rights as a participant in investigational therapy.

Procedures
Prepare the patient for plasmapheresis, if appropriate. Explain that although its success rate varies in MS, plasmapheresis may temporarily diminish the severity of symptoms. Describe how the procedure removes blood from the body, separates its components, removes antibodies suspected of causing certain MS symptoms, and then returns the clean blood to the body. Explain that the procedure involves making two puncture sites—one to remove the blood and another to replace it. After the procedure, pressure will be applied to the puncture sites for 15 to 30 minutes to stop any bleeding. Tell the patient that she'll need to rest for 3 to 4 hours afterward. Then she can resume her normal routine and medication schedule.

Surgery
If drug therapy doesn't control the intention tremors that accompany MS, tell the patient that the doctor may recommend stereotaxic thalamotomy. In this operation, the surgeon creates a surgical lesion in the thalamus on the side of the brain *opposite* the tremors. Explain that the patient's head will be shaved and cleaned and that she'll receive a local anesthetic. Inform her that the surgeon will fasten a metal frame to her head. Although the frame may feel uncomfortable, it will help to hold her head steady while the surgeon opens a small hole in her skull. Describe the drilling sound she'll hear. Tell the patient that she'll be awake during surgery so that she can respond to such commands as "Raise your arm" or "Move your hand." Explain that this helps the surgeon make the lesion precisely and safely. Inform the patient that she may have a headache after surgery.

Other care measures
Educate the patient about factors that precipitate exacerbations. Typically stress, fatigue, temperature extremes, infection, trauma, menstruation, and pregnancy can all trigger symptoms. Demonstrate stress-reduction techniques, and encourage the patient to get adequate rest. Advise her to avoid hot baths and showers, to stay indoors in unusually cold or hot weather, and to use an air conditioner when appropriate. If she lives in a warm climate, tell her to plan activities for the cooler part of the day and to avoid pro-

What's new in MS treatments?

Share encouraging news about fresh treatment approaches with your patient. For example, growing evidence of immune dysfunction in multiple sclerosis (MS) led to clinical trials of global immunosuppression with cyclophosphamide or total lymphoid irradiation in patients with progressive MS. Results show that these patients improved. Two other investigational treatments include interferon and copolymer 1 (COP 1).

Interferon
In a 2-year study, human beta interferon (IFN-B) was administered intrathecally to MS patients. The drug significantly reduced the incidence of MS flare-ups in most patients. Scientists think that IFN-B may stabilize fluctuations in the MS exacerbation-remission cycle. Or it may alter the viral trigger for exacerbations.

COP 1
Scientists synthesized a series of seven polymers that mimic myelin basic protein. The first—COP 1—suppressed MS in animals, without producing toxicity. In human trials, 25 patients with early exacerbatory-remitting MS were treated with COP 1 for 2 years. These patients had fewer relapses, and some had less cumulative disability at the end of the trial than did 23 control patients. And beneficial effects were reported in patients who had little or no disability at the study's outset.

In severe later-stage MS, studies are under way, using immunologic evaluation and magnetic resonance imaging techniques, to define how COP 1 affects the central nervous system and to compare brain lesions before and after treatment.

longed sun exposure. Recommend that she avoid crowds, seek treatment for all fevers, and report any illness to her doctor. Stress that she avoid people with known infections. Teach self-care measures for tremors and deficits involving speech, hearing, vision, short-term memory, senses, and elimination.

Tremors and spasms. If the patient has *head tremors,* suggest that she rest her head against a high-backed chair to give her some stability. Also, teach her how to apply any prescribed collars or neck braces. If she has hand tremors, teach her how and when to apply splints. Also suggest that she use weighted utensils or wrist weights weighing 1 to 2 lb (about 0.5 to 1 kg) while feeding herself. Discuss using a plate with suction cups on its base, a plate guard, and a weighted cup or a cup with a lid and lip. As appropriate, offer her a copy of the patient-teaching aid *Kitchen helpers,* pages 274 and 275.

Show the patient with *spasticity* how to use a cold pack.

Counseling about sexual dysfunction

For many patients, the neurologic and psychological disturbances that accompany multiple sclerosis (MS) produce sexual dysfunction. This compounds their apprehension and adds to their stress as the disease progresses.

As the patient's nurse, you're likely to be asked for advice. Before teaching, you'll need to establish rapport. Then review the organic and psychogenic factors that contribute to sexual function and dysfunction. Discuss the problem openly, and take a complete sexual history. Explore how MS may have changed your patient's sexual self-concept. Ask open-ended questions, such as, "How has MS changed the way you feel about yourself as a woman (man)? In what ways does MS interfere with your ability to enjoy sex? Can you describe what makes you feel less desirable to your partner?"

Encourage realistic adjustment to sexual limitations imposed by MS. Offer hope that although no cure exists for neurologically based sexual dysfunction, together the patient and partner can work toward a mutually satisfying sexual relationship, using creativity, flexibility, and sexual aids or prosthetic devices, if desired.

Counseling the female patient
Among women with MS, the most common sexual problems include inability to achieve orgasm (from decreased genital sensation), loss of libido, and spasticity.

If the patient can't achieve orgasm, encourage her and her partner to explore other erotic stimuli. Mention oral or manual stimulation as alternatives. For women with vaginal dryness, recommend using a sterile water-soluble gel, such as K-Y Jelly, for extra lubrication. For women with spasticity, suggest positional changes during intercourse, such as lying on her side or on top of her partner. Point out that prolonging foreplay with gentle stroking and massage will enhance muscle relaxation. If the doctor prescribes a muscle relaxant, tell the patient that taking it 30 to 60 minutes before intercourse may prevent muscle spasms.

Instruct the patient who loses bladder control during intercourse to drink fewer fluids beforehand. Also teach her how to perform self-catheterization to empty her bladder before intercourse.

Counseling the male patient
The most common sexual problem for men with MS is erectile dysfunction, which may stem from psychogenic or organic factors. For example, an upper motor neuron lesion in the brain stem may impair arousal, whereas a lower motor neuron lesion may impede the erection reflex. Before counseling the patient, you or his doctor will need to determine whether the problem stems from psychological or neurologic causes.

If the patient has intermittent erections, suggest that he and his partner try touching, stroking, or a using a vibrator to produce more consistent erections. Men who ejaculate prematurely may benefit from the "squeeze technique." Using this technique, the partner applies gentle finger pressure to the penis to delay ejaculation. For chronic impotence, mention that a penile prosthesis may be appropriate.

If the patient has an indwelling penile catheter because of a bladder problem, show him how to fold the catheter over his penis and hold it in place with a condom.

Also, tell her how to decrease spasticity in her legs before sexual activity. For more information, see *Counseling about sexual dysfunction.*

Speech, hearing, and visual disturbances. If the patient has *dysarthria,* a *low-pitched voice,* or *slow, scanning speech,* reinforce the need to perform phonation exercises, if prescribed. And, if appropriate, explain how to use a communication board and voice amplifiers.

Advise the patient with a *hearing deficit* to always face the speaker. Or refer her for lipreading instruction (if available), unless she also has visual disturbances. Make sure to caution her to watch for motor vehicles before crossing a street (she shouldn't rely on sound alone).

Show the patient with *diplopia* how to use an eye patch or a frosted lens over one eye, alternating the patch every 2 to 4 hours. Discuss ways to adjust to loss of depth perception if the patient has vision in only one eye. Suggest reading books with large print or listening to audiotaped publications. If the patient has corneal sensory loss, show her how to instill eye drops and use a clear eye shield.

Short-term memory deficit. If the patient has a *short-term memory deficit,* suggest that she carry a pad and pencil so that she can write down important information right away. She can refer to it later if she forgets something.

Sensory losses. If the patient has *sensory deficits,* instruct her to be cautious near extremely hot or cold objects. Tell her to use a bath thermometer to test bathwater temperature. Also tell her that she may perform activities better and more safely by observing (rather than feeling) her hand and foot movement.

Bladder and bowel dysfunction. For *urinary incontinence or retention,* advise the patient to drink about 2 to 3 quarts (2 to 3 liters) of fluid daily but to restrict fluid intake about 2 hours before bedtime. If she's *incontinent,* teach her how to reestablish a normal pattern (see *Tips for dealing with urinary incontinence*).

If *urinary retention* becomes a problem, stress methods the patient can use to completely empty her bladder (to prevent infection). As appropriate, teach her to perform intermittent catheterization and give her a copy of patient-teaching aid *For women: How to catheterize yourself,* page 215. (For a male patient, supply the teaching aid *For men: How to catheterize yourself,* page 216.) Also, recommend that the patient stimulate voiding by stroking her thighs and vulva (or, for a man, the glans penis), and by tapping the center of the abdomen below the navel about 10 to 15 times or until urination occurs. Eventually, the duration and intensity of tapping needed to produce emptying will decrease.

Credé's maneuver can also help empty the bladder. Direct the patient to tap her abdomen until she hears a dull sound indicating a full bladder. Next, tell her to use the flat part of her fingertips to knead the bladder, progressively applying more pressure. (Caution her not to grind her fingertips into her skin.) Then, to ensure complete voiding, describe the hollow sound that she'll hear when she taps her empty bladder.

Tips for dealing with urinary incontinence

Encourage your patient to deal actively with urinary incontinence. Here are some tips:
- Record fluid intake (including ice cream, gelatin, and pudding), and note excesses.
- Keep a record of urination times (both intentional urination and incontinent episodes). Review the record periodically to detect a time pattern. Then plan to urinate at the most appropriate times (for example, after meals or during the night).
- Follow a urination schedule, beginning with every 2 hours, increasing to every 3 hours, and progressing to every 4 hours. Wear a wristwatch with a time signal or set an alarm clock.
- Wear incontinence briefs during bladder retraining to prevent embarrassment and to provide a sense of security.
- Avoid plastic or rubber bed sheets. They promote skin breakdown.

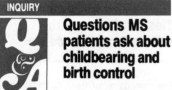

Questions MS patients ask about childbearing and birth control

Will MS keep me from having children?

Multiple sclerosis (MS) doesn't affect your reproductive capabilities, but before deciding to have children, consider carefully the physical and financial changes MS will make in your life. For example, you may find that emotional, motor, vision, and speech changes dampen your enthusiasm to parent a child. You may also discover that the health care costs accompanying MS limit your financial capacity to provide for children.

Now that I have MS, my husband and I have decided not to have children. What birth control method should I use?

The one or ones that suit your physical abilities and personal preferences. For example, if you have little uterine sensation, avoid an intrauterine device because you may not feel the pain or cramping indicating infection or perforation. If your mobility decreases, don't use oral contraceptives because these drugs may increase your risk of thrombophlebitis. If you're positive you don't want children, talk to your doctor about tubal ligation.

Before my fiancé got MS, he used a condom whenever we had sex. Now he says he won't use this method. What can I do?

You could ask your doctor about prescribing oral contraceptives, an intrauterine device, or a diaphragm for you. And you might consider using contraceptive foams or jellies. But don't overlook the possibility that your fiancé has diminished hand function and genital sensation that impairs his motivation to use a condom. If so, perhaps you could offer to help him apply the device.

For *constipation*, reinforce dietary guidelines with the patient. Explain that a nutritious, well-balanced diet and physical activity may offer relief. Also discuss a bowel retraining program—for example, using laxatives or suppositories at a prescribed time. Then suggest that she attempt to have a bowel movement about 30 minutes after a meal (usually breakfast), when the gastrocolic reflex is the strongest.

As appropriate, inform the patient that *fecal incontinence* usually results from illness, such as the flu, or from irritating substances, such as alcohol, spicy foods, or cigarettes, rather than from MS. Advise her to avoid irritating substances and hot liquids, to increase dietary fiber, and to wear incontinence briefs, if necessary.

Discuss any other question the patient may have about disease-related changes in her life—for example, childbearing concerns (see *Questions MS patients ask about childbearing and birth control*).

Source of information and support

National Multiple Sclerosis Society
205 East 42nd Street, New York, N.Y. 10017
(212) 986-3240

Further readings

Ashburn, A., et al. "An Approach to the Management of Multiple Sclerosis," *Physiotherapy Practice* 4(3):139-45, September 1989.

Henderson, J.S. "Intermittent Clean Self-catheterization in Clients with Neurogenic Bladder Resulting from Multiple Sclerosis," *Journal of Neuroscience Nursing* 21(3):160-64, June 1989.

Kassirer, M.R., and Osterberg, D.H. "Pain in Multiple Sclerosis," *American Journal of Nursing* 87(7):968-69, July 1987.

Phair, L.S. "Innovative Approaches to Multiple Sclerosis Patient Education," *Patient Education and Counseling* 8(4):419-22, December 1986.

Schmitt, D.M. "Helping Gwen to Keep Going," *Nursing89* 19(3):54-56, March 1989.

Thornton, N.G., and Dewis, M. "Multiple Sclerosis and Female Sexuality," *Canadian Nurse* 85(4):16-18, April 1989.

Zubey, R.L. "Understanding Magnetic Resonance Imaging from a Nursing Perspective," *Orthopaedic Nursing* 7(6):17-23, November-December 1989.

Preparing for magnetic resonance imaging

Dear Patient:

Your doctor wants you to have a painless test called magnetic resonance imaging—MRI for short. Unlike an X-ray, this test produces images of your body's organs and tissues without exposing you to radiation. Instead, MRI uses a powerful magnetic field and radiofrequency energy to produce computerized pictures. Here's how to prepare for it.

Before the test
You may eat, drink, and take your usual medicines. Try to use the bathroom just before the test because MRI may take up to 90 minutes.

Take off any metallic objects you may be carrying or wearing, such as a watch, rings, eyeglasses, or a hearing aid. Metals can be damaged by the strong magnetic field. Also empty your pockets of any coins or plastic card keys or charge cards with metallic strips. The scanner will erase the strips.

Let the doctor know if you have any metal objects inside your body, such as a pacemaker, aneurysm clip, joint prosthesis, metal pin, or bullet fragments, so the scanner can be adjusted.

During the test
You'll lie on a narrow, padded table throughout the test. The technician will tell you to stay still to prevent blurred images. To help you stay still, your head, chest, and arms may be secured with

straps. Remember that MRI is painless and involves no exposure to radiation.

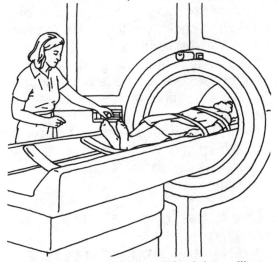

The table on which you're lying will slowly glide into the scanner's narrow tunnel. You'll notice the walls are just a few inches from your body. Inside, you'll hear fans and feel air circulating around you. And you may hear thumping noises made by the machine. The technician will probably offer you earphones, or you may request earplugs before the test.

The technician, located in an adjacent room, can see and hear you. And you'll have mirrors above your head, which will enable you to see the technician.

Afterward
Feel free to resume your usual activities. If you've been lying down for a long time, however, don't get up too quickly or you may feel slightly dizzy. Rise slowly to give your body a chance to adjust.

PATIENT-TEACHING AID

Learning about wheelchair transfers

Dear Patient:

To move from your bed to your wheelchair (and back), you'll need to master some transfer techniques.

Use a standing transfer as long as your upper body and legs will support you. Use a sitting transfer when they won't.

Now, follow these illustrated steps to move from your bed to your wheelchair. To return to your bed, reverse the steps.

How to perform a standing transfer

1 Sit at the edge of the bed with your shoes on and your feet flat on the floor. Make sure the wheelchair's positioned at a 45-degree angle to your bedside. (For example, the front of the chair's seat should be midway between facing the bedside and parallel to the bedside.)

Lock the chair's wheels, and move the footrests out of the way.

2 Position your feet slightly apart, with one foot a bit in front of the other. Then place your hands, palms down, on the bed, next to your hips. Now, lean forward slightly. Push your hands down on the bed (or the side rail, if your bed has one), and raise yourself to a standing position, as shown at the top of the next column.

If you feel your arms and legs weakening, call for assistance. If you feel all right, proceed.

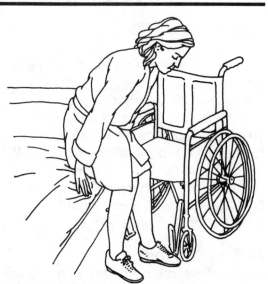

3 With your hand, grasp the wheelchair armrest that's farthest from you. (Remember, you're going to back in, so use your right hand to grab the right armrest or your left hand for the left armrest.) Your fingers will be directed outward, your thumb will be toward you.

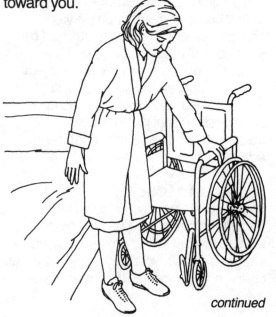

continued

PATIENT-TEACHING AID

Learning about wheelchair transfers — *continued*

4 Now, pivot, or step, to the side as you grasp the wheelchair's other armrest with your other hand. Position your back directly in front of the wheelchair's seat. The backs of your legs should be touching the edge of the seat.

Support your weight with your hands as you lower yourself into the chair. Then, replace the footrests and position yourself comfortably.

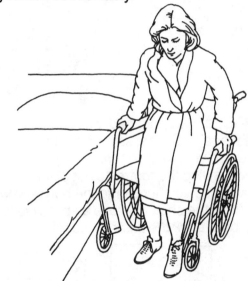

How to perform a sitting transfer

1 Sit at the edge of your bed, with your legs over the side, your shoes on, and your feet flat on the floor. Now, move the wheelchair so its right side is parallel to the left side of the bed. *Lock the wheels.*

2 To grasp the wheelchair, remove the chair's right armrest and hang it from the side of the chair. Then remove the right footrest or move it to the side. Next, place your left hand, palm down, on the wheelchair's seat. Place your right hand, also palm down, next to your right hip.

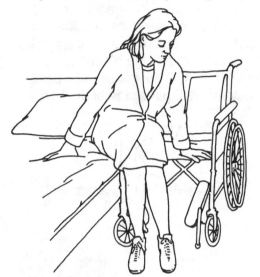

3 Push down with your right hand to lift your buttocks off the bed. Then shift your weight to your left hand as you slowly move yourself into the wheelchair's seat. Once you're in the chair, get comfortable and reattach the armrest and, if necessary, the footrest.

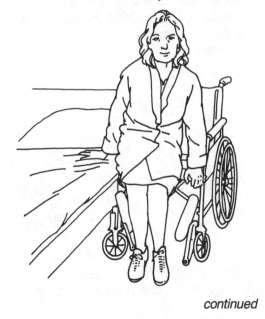

continued

Learning about wheelchair transfers — *continued*

How to perform a forward-backward sitting transfer

1 First, remove the wheelchair's footrests or swing them aside. Then, pull the front of the wheelchair as close as possible to the side of the bed. *Lock the wheels.* The seat of the wheelchair should be facing the side of the bed.

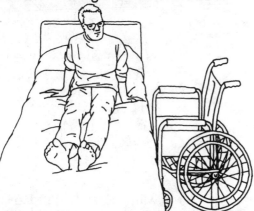

2 Make sure you're sitting in bed with your legs extended. Now, lean slightly forward. Pushing your hands down on the mattress, lift your buttocks slightly off the bed. Keeping your legs extended across the bed, inch backward to the bedside—close to the wheelchair. Stop when your back is in front of the wheelchair.

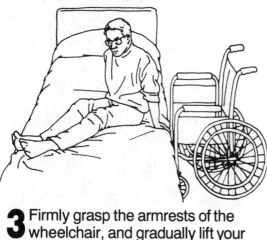

3 Firmly grasp the armrests of the wheelchair, and gradually lift your buttocks onto the seat. Unlock the wheels. Slowly push yourself away from the bed, allowing your feet to drop gently toward the floor. Replace the footrest, and get comfortable in the chair.

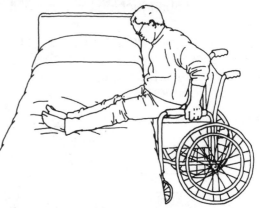

4 To get back into bed, position the wheelchair seat so it's facing the bed. Lift your legs off the footrests. Then, swing the footrests out of the way. Now, raise your legs onto the bed as you position the chair as close as possible to the bed. *Lock the chair's wheels.*

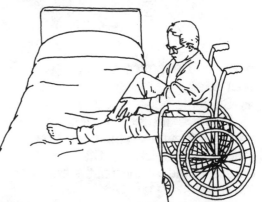

5 Next, grasp the armrests and lift your buttocks slightly off the seat. Keeping your legs extended across the bed, use a push-up motion to inch toward the middle of the bed. Once you're safely on the bed, turn yourself around and get comfortable.

PATIENT-TEACHING AID

For women: How to catheterize yourself

Dear Patient:

Follow these instructions to perform catheterization.

1 Gather the equipment: catheter, lubricant (water soluble), basin, clean washcloth, soap and water, paper towels, and plastic bag. Then wash your hands thoroughly. During the procedure, be sure to touch only the catheter equipment to avoid spreading germs.

2 Separate the folds of your vulva with one hand, and, using the washcloth, thoroughly clean the area between your legs with warm water and mild soap. Use downward strokes (front to back) to avoid contaminating the area with fecal matter. Now, pat the area dry with a towel.

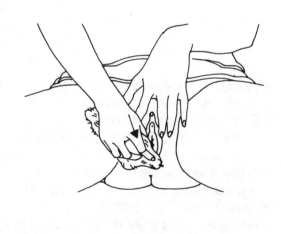

3 Open the lubricant and squeeze a generous amount onto a paper

towel. Then roll the first 3 inches of the catheter in it.

4 Spread the lips of the vulva with one hand, and, using the other hand, insert the catheter in an upward and backward direction about 3 inches into the urethra (located above the vagina). If you meet resistance, breathe deeply. As you inhale, advance the catheter, angling it upward slightly. Stop when urine begins to drain from it. Allow all urine to drain into the toilet.

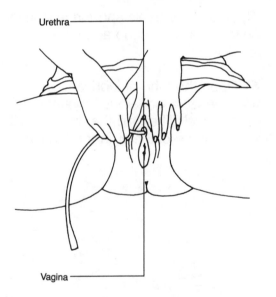

Urethra—

Vagina—

5 Pinch the catheter closed and slowly remove it. Wash it in warm, soapy water, rinse, and dry. Place it in a plastic bag until the next use. (After you've used the catheter a few times, boil it in water for 20 minutes to keep it germ-free.)

PATIENT-TEACHING AID

For men: How to catheterize yourself

Dear Patient:

Follow these instructions to perform catheterization.

1 Gather the equipment: catheter, lubricant (water soluble), basin for collecting urine, clean washcloth, soap and water, paper towels, and plastic bag. Then wash your hands thoroughly. During the procedure, touch only the catheter equipment to avoid spreading germs.

2 Wash your penis and the surrounding area with soap and water. Then pat dry.

3 Open the tube of lubricant and squeeze a generous amount onto a paper towel. Then roll the first 7 to 10 inches of the catheter in the lubricant.

right angle to your body, grasp the catheter as you would a pencil, and slowly insert it into the urethra. If you meet resistance, breathe deeply. As you inhale, continue advancing the catheter 7 to 10 inches until urine begins to flow. Allow all urine to drain into the basin or toilet.

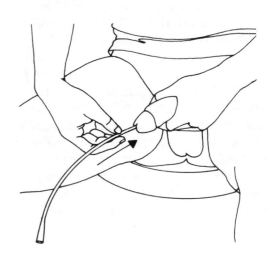

5 When the catheter stops draining, pinch it closed and slowly remove it. Empty the basin, if used; then rinse and dry it. Wash the catheter in warm, soapy water, rinse it inside and out, and dry it with a clean towel. Place it in a plastic bag until the next use. (After you've used the catheter a few times, the doctor may tell you to boil it in water for 20 minutes to keep it germ-free.)

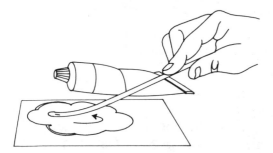

4 Put one end of the catheter in the basin or toilet. Hold your penis at a

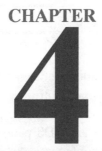

CHAPTER

4

Immune and Hematologic Conditions

Contents

Acquired immunodeficiency syndrome

No disease in recent memory has generated more misunderstanding, fear, and publicity than acquired immunodeficiency syndrome (AIDS). A serious threat to health worldwide, AIDS has killed tens of thousands of people and infected millions. Its mode of transmission and the absence of a cure make patient teaching vitally important—and highly challenging.

Teaching a patient with AIDS requires patience, perseverance, and a sound knowledge of the syndrome. Typically, the patient will feel a myriad of emotions, including shock, anger, fear, despair, and isolation. In this state of mind, he won't be receptive to learning. As a result, you'll need to plan your teaching around times when he's most responsive, and you may have to repeat much of the information. You'll also need to keep up to date on AIDS research and treatments so you can answer questions knowledgeably. What's more, you must explore your own feelings and fears about AIDS before you can establish the trusting nurse-patient relationship that's so necessary for successful teaching.

What will you teach the patient with AIDS? A comprehensive plan includes a description of how AIDS attacks the immune system, and a discussion of opportunistic infections and cancers associated with AIDS and their signs and symptoms. It also includes diagnostic tests; treatments, such as good nutrition and drug therapy; and other care measures, such as safe sexual practices and infection control in the home.

Discuss the disorder

Inform the patient that AIDS results from infection with the human immunodeficiency virus (HIV), which impairs immune function. This virus attaches to specialized white blood cells (WBCs) called T_4 or helper T cells, gradually depleting their number and hindering their response to infection. Once crippled, the immune system leaves the patient vulnerable to opportunistic infections and cancers. (See *How HIV affects immunity,* page 220, and *Signs and symptoms of AIDS-related infections,* page 221.) Explain that although no cure has been discovered for AIDS, recent scientific developments may hold promise for the future.

Tell the patient that HIV appears in body secretions, especially blood, semen, and vaginal secretions. Explain that the infection can be transmitted through unprotected vaginal or anal intercourse, needles contaminated with blood, blood transfusions, or (in infants) through transplacental contact or breast-feeding.

Lynne Kreutzer-Baraglia, RN, MS, and **Beverly A. Post, RN, CIC, MS,** wrote this chapter. Ms. Kreutzer-Baraglia is assistant professor at Concordia University-West Suburban College of Nursing, Oak Park, Ill. Ms. Post is clinical risk and infection control manager at Louis A. Weiss Memorial Hospital, Chicago.

CHECKLIST

Teaching topics in AIDS

☐ How HIV affects the immune response
☐ Opportunistic infections, cancer, and neurologic effects associated with AIDS
☐ Diagnostic criteria for AIDS
☐ Diagnostic tests, such as ELISA, Western blot, and helper T-cell count
☐ Activity modifications, including adequate rest and moderate exercise
☐ Adequate nutrition to prevent opportunistic infections
☐ Drug therapy, such as zidovudine, co-trimoxazole, and pentamidine
☐ Safe sex practices, including how to use a condom
☐ Providing home care for an AIDS patient
☐ Caring for children with AIDS
☐ Sources of information and support

How HIV affects immunity

Briefly explain normal and impaired immune function to your patient, using clear language. Include the information below in your teaching.

Normal immune function
When viruses enter a healthy body, they're identified as antigens by macrophages. Then macrophages process the antigens and present them to T cells and B cells.

The antigen-activated T cells proliferate and form several kinds of T cells. For example, helper T cells stimulate B cells, whereas suppressor T cells control the extent of T-cell help for B cells. Lymphokine-producing T cells are involved in delayed hypersensitivity and other immune reactions. Cytotoxic, or killer T, cells directly destroy antigenic agents. Memory T cells are stored to recognize and attack the same antigen on subsequent invasions.

The B cells multiply, forming memory cells and plasma cells that produce antigen-specific antibodies, which then attack and kill the invading virus.

Impaired immune function
HIV selectively infects the helper T cells, impairing their ability to recognize antigens. Now the virus is free to proliferate, causing abnormal immune system function and progressive destruction.

As immunity weakens, the patient becomes vulnerable to potentially fatal protozoal, viral, and fungal infections and to certain forms of cancer. Meanwhile, many more HIV particles are released and invade other T cells, further weakening the immune system and intensifying the problem.

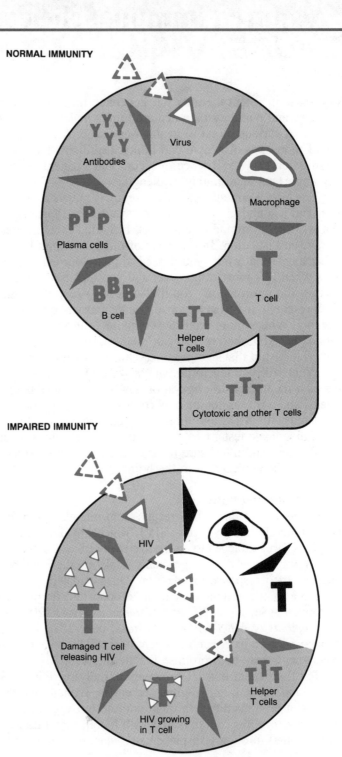

NORMAL IMMUNITY

Antibodies
Virus
Macrophage
Plasma cells
B cell
T cell
Helper T cells
Cytotoxic and other T cells

IMPAIRED IMMUNITY

HIV
Damaged T cell releasing HIV
HIV growing in T cell
Helper T cells

Signs and symptoms of AIDS-related infections

How much does your AIDS patient know about opportunistic infections? Probably not as much as he should. Explain that the more he knows about infections associated with AIDS, the better his chances are for controlling them. Teach him about the causes and symptoms of opportunistic viral, fungal, protozoal, and mycobacterial infections.

Viral infections
Cytomegalovirus (CMV) may cause pneumonia, diarrhea, colitis, encephalitis, and elevated liver enzyme levels. Eye changes include large hemorrhages and white exudates on the retina and visual changes leading to blindness. Lymphocyte tests show positive antibody titers.

Herpes simplex produces ulcers persisting longer than 1 month in the perineal, perianal, and scrotal areas in addition to the face, esophagus, and colon.

In *herpes zoster,* a disseminated weeping, pruritic rash usually appears on the buttocks, back, and legs.

Fungal infections
Candida albicans affects the mouth and esophagus, causing difficult, painful swallowing and a white coating or plaque on the oral and rectal mucosae. Skin lesions may appear on the axillae and groin.

Cryptococcus neoformans can cause acute meningitis or chronic meningoencephalitis. Its first symptoms usually are headache, vomiting, and diplopia without fever.

Protozoal infections
Pneumocystis carinii usually causes pneumonia but can initially cause diarrhea, night sweats, fever, weight loss, and unexplained lymphadenopathy. Later signs and symptoms include dyspnea, dry cough, tachypnea, cyanosis, diffuse crackles, and severe hypoxemia. Cotton-wool exudates may appear on the retina.

Toxoplasma gondii can cause brain abscess, diffuse encephalopathy, and meningoencephalitis. Asymptomatic lymphadenopathy may be accompanied by fever, malaise, sore throat, headache, and myalgias.

Infection with *Cryptosporidium* may cause GI effects ranging from soft stools to severe diarrhea.

Mycobacterial infections
Mycobacterium avium and *M. tuberculosis* produce chronic cough and hemoptysis. They also affect the liver, spleen, lymph nodes, and bone marrow. Signs and symptoms may include fatigue, weakness, weight loss, and fever.

Point out that HIV-infected patients develop AIDS at a variable rate.

Explain that some patients remain asymptomatic until they abruptly develop an opportunistic infection, such as *Pneumocystis carinii* pneumonia (PCP), or cancer, such as Kaposi's sarcoma. But more often, they have a recent history of nonspecific signs and symptoms, such as fatigue, afternoon fevers, night sweats, weight loss, diarrhea, or cough. Soon afterward, they typically develop several concurrent infections.

Complications
Emphasize the importance of recognizing symptoms, seeking medical help promptly, and following recommended treatment to limit the number of infections the patient incurs. Make sure he clearly understands that preventing further injury to his damaged immune system can help him preserve the quality of his life.

Inform the patient that the most common opportunistic infection associated with AIDS is PCP. It's caused by a one-celled protozoan that affects the pulmonary tissues of immunosuppressed people. Numerous cysts composed of clumped organisms multiply in alveolar spaces and eventually cause obstructive disease. Signs and symptoms range from a dry cough, mild fever, and dyspnea on exertion to respiratory failure. Successful management depends

Understanding HIV encephalopathy

When teaching about AIDS complications, explain that up to 90% of patients have central nervous system damage. These neurologic changes result from lymphomas; toxoplasmosis; viruses, such as papovavirus; fungal infections, such as cryptococcal meningitis; and drugs that affect the nervous system, such as hypnotics, antidepressants, and sedatives. However, the most frequent cause is HIV encephalopathy.

Signs and symptoms
Inform the patient that HIV encephalopathy results from direct HIV infection of the brain. At first, the patient has trouble concentrating; then he becomes forgetful and has trouble reading, writing, and following instructions. At this point, because he withdraws from his friends, HIV encephalopathy may be mistaken for depression.

Eventually, however, the patient's speech becomes thick and slurred, he becomes progressively more clumsy, and his spontaneous verbal and motor responses slow down. In a later stage, he becomes mute, paraparetic or paraplegic, and incontinent.

Diagnosis
Although a definitive diagnosis can't be made until autopsy, a computed tomography scan may show brain atrophy weeks or even months before the first symptoms appear. Magnetic resonance imaging may show multifocal or diffuse white matter changes in the brain and spinal cord.

Treatment
Zidovudine (Retrovir) can reverse the cognitive and motor decline caused by HIV encephalopathy.

on early detection of pulmonary involvement. Unfortunately, PCP in patients with AIDS doesn't respond well to treatment. (See *Teaching the patient with PCP.*)

Tell the patient that Kaposi's sarcoma is a common form of cancer in AIDS patients. Once seen only in elderly men of Mediterranean descent, this cancer was first linked to AIDS in 1981. In its original form, Kaposi's sarcoma affects the cutaneous tissues, usually of the legs. It can exist for a decade or longer without harming the internal organs. But in AIDS patients the cancer responds far more aggressively, affecting the endothelial tissue, compromising the blood vessels, and invading the deeper organs and tissues, especially in the GI tract. Small red or purple multicentric lesions develop over the entire body. They may be slightly raised and either isolated or linear in pattern. In advanced stages, the disease obstructs the lymphatic system, causing leg, head, and neck edema.

Teach the patient about HIV encephalopathy, a neurologic complication that occurs in 40% to 60% of AIDS patients. (See *Understanding HIV encephalopathy.*)

Describe the diagnostic workup
Inform the patient about multiple diagnostic tests to establish an initial diagnosis of HIV infection and detect associated opportunistic infections or cancer. (For more information, see *Diagnostic criteria for AIDS,* page 225.)

HIV antibody tests
Explain that two blood tests are commonly used to detect HIV antibodies: the enzyme-linked immunosorbent assay (ELISA) and the Western blot. In the ELISA, the patient's serum sample is incubated with live HIV. If HIV antibodies are present, they'll react with the test solution. If findings are positive, a Western blot assay is performed to confirm the results. This more definitive test can identify specific HIV antibodies.

Tell the patient that positive results with both tests establish HIV infection. Stress that this doesn't mean that the patient has AIDS, only that he's been infected with the virus. On the other hand, a negative result doesn't necessarily mean that he's not infected. The patient may carry HIV for several weeks to months before developing detectable antibody levels, and therefore he should be tested again at a future date.

T-cell assay
Inform the patient that an absolute helper T cell count may be performed to evaluate his immune status. When the count falls below 200, opportunistic infections occur, confirming the AIDS diagnosis. Normally, the ratio of helper T cells to suppressor T cells is 2:1; in a person with AIDS, this ratio is reversed.

Other tests
Teach the patient about other ordered tests. To diagnose PCP, a

Teaching the patient with PCP

If you care for AIDS patients, you're probably familiar with the symptoms and treatment of *Pneumocystis carinii* pneumonia (PCP) — one of the most common opportunistic infections associated with AIDS. But you may be unfamiliar with — or even confused about — the best approach to use in teaching the patient about this deadly disease.

Begin by referring to a standard teaching plan to provide direction. Then modify the plan to meet your patient's special needs. To help you do so, suppose you're caring for Lance Richards, a 32-year-old college professor who lives with his male lover.

Assess first

When you first meet Mr. Richards, you realize right away that he's not ready for patient teaching — his anxiety level is high, and he seems to be in a state of denial. Talking rapidly and gesturing with trembling hands, he says, "This can't be happening to me. I'm sure I'll feel better soon."

Mr. Richards' chart reveals that 6 months ago he started tiring easily, noticed swollen glands in his neck, and began running a fever. He also had occasional diarrhea and night sweats. Worried, he visited his doctor, who ordered an enzyme-linked immunosorbent assay. It was positive for the HIV antibody. A Western blot assay confirmed HIV infection. These results, combined with Lance's symptoms and a helper T-cell count of 200/mm³, convinced the doctor that Lance had been infected with HIV.

The doctor prescribed zidovudine (Retrovir), but Lance had such a severe adverse reaction that the drug had to be discontinued. When he developed the dry, hacking cough and fever indicative of PCP, the doctor admitted him to the hospital. On admission, Lance had a bronchoscopy, which was positive for PCP. The doctor started him on I.V. co-trimoxazole and informed him that his HIV infection had now progressed to AIDS.

During your conversation with Lance, you notice that he seems knowledgeable about AIDS transmission. He tells you, "I've never shot up drugs, and neither has my lover. But after my divorce 2 years ago, I had a few one-night stands. That's how I got it, I guess." Before you leave, you tell Lance that you'll be back when he's feeling better to teach him more about AIDS and to answer any questions.

In spite of the co-trimoxazole, Lance's condition deteriorates rapidly until he requires intubation and mechanical ventilation. He also develops a rash from the medication and is switched to I.V. pentamidine isethionate (Pentam 300). A week later, his condition improves, and the doctor extubates him and begins discussing his discharge.

In your first patient-teaching session, you find Lance slightly less anxious and considerably more aware of his situation. His bout with PCP has also left him feeling depressed and isolated, as evidenced by his statement: "I feel like a leper. No one cares about me now."

Like that of most AIDS patients, Lance's state of mind isn't conducive to learning, so you plan your teaching accordingly. You decide to keep teaching sessions brief and explanations simple, to repeat information frequently, and to leave plenty of time for questions.

Define learning needs

What should you teach Lance? Decide by comparing his knowledge of AIDS and PCP with the content of a standard teaching plan, which includes:
- an explanation of how AIDS attacks the immune system
- PCP pathophysiology
- signs and symptoms of AIDS and PCP
- tests to diagnose AIDS and PCP
- treatment for AIDS and PCP, including drug therapy, rest, and diet.

From your conversations with Lance, you determine that he's fairly knowledgeable about how AIDS is transmitted, about its signs and symptoms, and about diagnostic tests. But he knows relatively little about PCP. Therefore, your teaching plan will focus on PCP — its pathophysiology, signs and symptoms, and drug therapy. Your goal is to help Lance prevent a recurrence of PCP or at least to recognize its signs and symptoms so that he can seek treatment promptly.

Set learning outcomes

With the standard teaching plan as your guide, you help Lance set learning outcomes. Together, you decide that he should be able to:

```
-identify the causative agent of PCP
-describe how this agent affects the
respiratory system
-discuss PCP signs and symptoms
-voice his feelings about AIDS and PCP
-explain what adverse effects can occur from
his medications and why he should maintain the
treatment schedule
-discuss why he should eat a well-balanced
diet and adjust his activities to his energy
level
-explain the importance of preventing
infections.
```

continued

Teaching the patient with PCP — *continued*

Choose teaching tools and techniques

What tools and techniques will enhance your teaching? Because Lance tires easily and isn't especially receptive to learning at this time, start with *short explanations* and *brief discussions* of PCP's causes, signs, and symptoms.

Then proceed to use *booklets, posters,* and other *visual aids* that illustrate the anatomy of the lungs, the four food groups and menu planning, and other topics.

Ask the dietitian to discuss menu planning with Lance. Include a medication card to teach Lance about co-trimoxazole and its adverse effects. Remember to encourage Lance to express his feelings and fears about AIDS, and leave enough time to answer his questions.

Evaluate your teaching

What techniques will you use to measure Lance's progress and, if necessary, to redirect your teaching? *Questions and answers* can help you measure Lance's knowledge of AIDS and PCP. For example, can he list adverse effects of co-trimoxazole? Use *observation* to assess his understanding of infection prevention. For example, watch Lance wash his hands. Does he use the proper technique?

Use *discussion* to evaluate his ability to express his feelings about AIDS. For example, encourage him to talk about what's happening to him, how it makes him feel, and how he'll cope with his deteriorating health. Try *role-playing* to assess how he'll handle a typical problem, such as telling his family that he has AIDS.

bronchoscopy will be done. Brushings or washings are necessary to obtain a specimen for silver stain to identify the *P.carinii* protozoa. Chest X-rays help detect pulmonary complications such as diffuse bilateral interstitial infiltrates in PCP. Arterial blood gas studies and pulmonary function tests are routinely used to diagnose pulmonary complications and to monitor progress, especially in patients with PCP. A tissue biopsy confirms a diagnosis of Kaposi's sarcoma.

Discuss tests that confirm the diagnosis of AIDS-related disorders—for example, gallium scan, colonoscopy, bone marrow aspiration, computed tomography scan, or magnetic resonance imaging.

Teach about treatments

Although at this time there is no cure for AIDS, explain to the patient that various treatments can suppress HIV, deal with opportunistic infections, and improve his quality of life. These treatments consist of medications, diet, rest, and exercise.

Activity

Tell the patient that adequate rest is crucial to reduce the risk of infection. However, explain that moderate exercise can help him maintain muscle mass, improve circulation, and provide a feeling of well-being. Advise him to exercise regularly, to avoid overexertion, and to alternate periods of activity and rest. If he's well enough to go outdoors, recommend walking as an ideal exercise. If he spends long hours in bed, suggest lifting light hand weights. Of course, he should modify his exercise program as his condition deteriorates. Suggest that he discuss an exercise program with his doctor or a physical therapist.

Diagnostic criteria for AIDS

Inform the patient that the Centers for Disease Control (CDC) defines AIDS as an illness characterized by one or more indicator diseases (opportunistic infections or cancers) and based on laboratory evidence of human immunodeficiency virus (HIV) infection. The CDC guidelines are:

Without laboratory evidence of HIV infection
Patients with a definitive diagnosis of one or more of the following indicator diseases are diagnosed with AIDS even without laboratory evidence of HIV infection:
- bronchitis, pneumonitis, or esophagitis persisting longer than 1 month
- candidiasis of the esophagus, trachea, bronchi, or lungs
- extrapulmonary cryptococcosis
- cryptosporidiosis with diarrhea persisting more than 1 month
- cytomegalovirus (CMV) of an organ other than the liver, spleen, or lymph nodes in a patient older than 1 month
- herpes simplex virus ulcers persisting longer than 1 month
- Kaposi's sarcoma in a patient under age 60
- lymphoid interstitial pneumonia, pulmonary lymphoid hyperplasia, or both (LIP/PLH complex) in a patient under age 13
- disseminated *Mycobacterium avium* or *M. kansasii* infection at a site other than or in addition to the lungs, skin, or cervical or hilar lymph nodes
- *Pneumocystis carinii* pneumonia (PCP)
- progressive multifocal leukoencephalopathy
- toxoplasmosis of the brain in a patient younger than 1 month

With laboratory evidence of HIV infection
Patients with a definitive diagnosis of one or more of the *above* indicator diseases or one or more of the *following* indicator diseases are diagnosed with AIDS if they test positive for HIV:
- disseminated coccidioidomycosis at a site other than or in addition to the lungs or cervical or hilar lymph nodes
- HIV encephalopathy
- disseminated histoplasmosis at a site other than the lungs
- isosporiasis with diarrhea persisting longer than 1 month
- Kaposi's sarcoma
- primary lymphoma of the brain
- other non-Hodgkin's lymphoma of B-cell or unknown immunologic phenotype
- disseminated mycobacterial disease caused by other than *M. tuberculosis* at a site other than or in addition to the lungs, skin, or cervical or hilar lymph nodes
- extrapulmonary disease caused by *M. tuberculosis,* involving at least one site
- recurrent *Salmonella* (nontyphoid) septicemia
- HIV wasting syndrome (emaciation)

   Patients with a *presumptive* diagnosis of one or more of the following indicator diseases are diagnosed with AIDS if they test positive for HIV:
- candidiasis of the esophagus
- CMV retinitis with vision loss
- Kaposi's sarcoma
- LIP/PLH complex in a patient under age 13
- disseminated mycobacterial disease (acid-fast bacilli with species not identified by culture) involving at least one site other than or in addition to the lungs, skin, or cervical or hilar lymph nodes
- PCP
- toxoplasmosis of the brain in a patient older than 1 month

Diet
Teach the patient the importance of maintaining adequate nutrition to prevent infection and weight loss. Encourage eating small, frequent, high-calorie, high-protein meals, and emphasize the importance of drinking plenty of fluids. Discuss ways to stimulate his appetite, facilitate food preparation, and make mealtimes more pleasant. (See *Tips for sound nutrition,* page 231.) If he continues to lose weight, show him how to keep a calorie count, and teach him about commercial dietary supplements.

Medication
Educate the patient about drugs used to modify HIV infection (zidovudine), related infections (co-trimoxazole and pentamidine), and cancer (chemotherapeutic drugs). Also teach him about drugs currently under testing. Advise him to check with the doctor about the availability of investigative drugs.

    Zidovudine. Tell the patient that no drug has been discovered to restore immune function, but that zidovudine (Retrovir) can limit the replication of HIV. This drug slows the progression of AIDS, relieving many of its incapacitating symptoms and decreasing the number of opportunistic infections. It's also used prophylactically in patients who test HIV positive but don't yet have AIDS.

    Review how and when the patient should take zidovudine, emphasizing that the drug doesn't cure AIDS. Point out the drug's possible adverse effects. Immediately reportable reactions include chills, fever, pallor, sore throat, unusual bleeding or bruising, and unusual tiredness or weakness. Other adverse effects include altered taste perception, diarrhea, headache, insomnia, anorexia, nausea and vomiting, restlessness, transient agitation, and rash. Reassure the patient that most reactions will subside in 2 to 3 weeks and that the doctor may prescribe an antiemetic (Compazine) or a benzodiazepine (Xanax) if symptoms persist. Ibuprofen (Motrin) may also help relieve minor discomforts.

    Inform the patient that long-term use of zidovudine can cause anemia and granulocytopenia. Explain that in severe anemia, the doctor may discontinue the drug for 7 to 10 days and order a transfusion of 2 to 3 units of blood. Once the patient's hemoglobin level returns to baseline, drug therapy can resume. Patients with macrocytic, megaloblastic anemia, which is usually mild, can continue taking zidovudine at full dosage, but they may require blood transfusions if their hemoglobin levels drop below 8 g/dl.

    In a patient with advanced AIDS who has granulocytopenia, the zidovudine dosage is usually decreased when the granulocyte count falls below $750/mm^3$ and is discontinued when the count drops below $500/mm^3$. Reassure the patient that his dosage will be increased as his count rises.

    In a patient with less-advanced AIDS, the dosage is decreased only when the granulocyte count falls to 50% of baseline. Again, reassure the patient that if his count rises, the dosage will be increased.

Co-trimoxazole. Teach the patient that co-trimoxazole (sulfamethoxazole and trimethoprim [Bactrim, Septra]) is the drug of choice for PCP. Discuss how and when to take the drug and its possible adverse effects. Tell the patient to report aching joints or muscles; fever; itching; pallor; skin blistering, peeling, rash, or redness; sore throat; unusual bleeding, bruising, fatigue, or weakness; vomiting; and yellowing of the eyes or skin. Mention that he may also experience anorexia, diarrhea, dizziness, headache, nausea, and photosensitivity.

Instruct the patient to complete the prescribed course of therapy and to take each dose as ordered. Warn him to avoid direct sunlight to prevent a photosensitivity reaction and not to drive a car or perform other activities requiring full alertness until his reaction to the drug is known.

Pentamidine. If the patient is allergic to sulfa drugs or if co-trimoxazole isn't effective in treating PCP, the doctor may order pentamidine isethionate (Lomidine, Pentam 300). Given by injection, this drug can cause severe hypotension. Instruct the patient to lie down while receiving it. Tell him that the nurse will take his blood pressure when she administers the drug and several times afterward until it stabilizes.

Warn the patient that pentamidine may lower his WBC count, increasing his chance of infection. It may also lower his platelet count, increasing the risk of bleeding. Advise him to avoid people with colds or other infections and to check with the doctor immediately if he thinks he's getting a cold or other infection. He should also contact the doctor if he notices any unusual bleeding or bruising. Tell him to brush and floss his teeth carefully, to check with the dentist for other ways to clean his teeth and gums, and to contact the doctor before having any dental work done. Instruct him to use an electric shaver (instead of a safety razor) and to use fingernail and toenail clippers cautiously.

Advise the patient to report adverse effects of pentamidine, which can occur up to several months after drug discontinuation. Such effects include drowsiness, flushed, dry skin, fruity breath odor, increased urination and thirst, and hunger or loss of appetite. He should also report anxiety, chills, cold sweats, cool, pale skin, rash, nausea, rapid or irregular pulse, shakiness, and unusual tiredness or weakness. What's more, he should report blurred vision, confusion, headache, dizziness, fainting or lightheadedness, fever, hallucinations, and sore throat.

Other possible effects include hardness, pain, or a sore at the injection site; redness or flushing of the face, especially following I.V. injection; an unpleasant metallic taste in the mouth; and vomiting.

Chemotherapy. Inform the patient that vincristine and vinblastine form the cornerstone of Kaposi's sarcoma treatment, although etoposide, doxorubicin, and alpha-interferon may also be used. Give the patient a copy of the teaching aid *How to control the side effects of chemotherapy and radiation therapy*, pages 306 to 309.

Procedures

Although medication, diet, and rest constitute the main treatments for opportunistic infections in AIDS, two procedures are sometimes used to treat Kaposi's sarcoma. If the sarcoma affects only the skin, the lesions may be treated with electron beam therapy. If the sarcoma invades deeper tissues, radiation therapy or chemotherapy may be used. If the doctor orders radiation, explain the procedure to the patient.

Other care measures

Take the time to educate the patient and his caregivers about other measures that will help them cope with AIDS.

Infection control. Make sure you emphasize the importance of prevention or early detection and treatment of infections. Give the patient a copy of the teaching aid *Preventing infection—and recognizing its symptoms,* page 236.

AIDS transmission. Besides stressing the importance of prompt treatment, teach the patient how to prevent transmitting AIDS to others. Tell him not to donate blood, blood products, organs, tissue, or sperm. Warn him to inform potential sex partners and health care workers that he's HIV positive. If he uses I.V. drugs, caution him not to share needles and to warn any persons with whom he shared needles in the past that he's infected.

Inform the patient that high-risk sexual practices for AIDS transmission are those that exchange body fluids—for example, receptive or insertional anal intercourse without a condom, vaginal intercourse without a condom, fellatio without a condom, cunnilingus, insertion of a fist or foreign object into the rectum followed by anal intercourse without a condom, and oral-anal stimulation.

Discuss safe sexual practices with your patient. Tell him that these include hugging, petting, massaging, mutual masturbation, social kissing, using sex toys (but not sharing them), and having protected sexual intercourse. Give him a copy of the patient-teaching aid *How to use a condom,* pages 232 and 233.

Teach the patient about precautions in activities of daily living so that friends, roommates, and family members don't contract AIDS. Reinforce your instruction by providing a copy of the patient-teaching aid *Caring for an AIDS patient at home,* pages 234 and 235.

AIDS in children. If your patient is a child, teach his caregivers about the special concerns and precautions involved. (See *Caring for the HIV-infected child.*) Tell them about programs that help the child cope with a terminal illness.

AIDS in pregnancy. Warn the pregnant patient that her infant may become infected before birth, during delivery, or during breast-feeding—so caution her not to breast-feed. Advise the female patient of childbearing age to postpone getting pregnant until more is known about the AIDS virus and pregnancy.

Alternate therapy and support services. Because conventional treatments often fail to achieve the desired results, be prepared to tell the patient about alternative therapies if he asks. These treat-

Caring for the HIV-infected child

Infants of mothers who are at high risk for HIV infection should be tested for HIV after age 4 months. (Before this time, B cells may be too immature for an immune response.)

Because maternal antibodies may cause false-positive test results, the infant should be tested again at age 6 months.

If your patient is a child, tell the parents and other caregivers to use the same precautions as they would for an adult HIV-infected patient. In addition, inform them of the following special precautions and concerns.

Vaccines

HIV-infected children should receive only killed vaccines. They shouldn't be given tubercular vaccines containing Calmette-Guérin bacillus or vaccines for measles, mumps, or rubella. Such inactivated vaccines as *Haemophilus influenzae* Type B and pertussis as well as diphtheria and tetanus toxoids can be administered on schedule.

An inactivated polio vaccine rather than the activated oral form should be given. Polio vaccines should be administered along with pertussis vaccine and diphtheria and tetanus toxoids at 2, 4, 6, and 18 months, and at ages 4 to 6.

Older children at high risk for HIV infection should undergo testing before receiving live-virus vaccines. If a parent won't allow testing, the child shouldn't be inoculated.

Fevers

Children with HIV infections can run fevers of 101° to 105° F. (38.3° to 40.6° C.) for weeks. If tests don't reveal a bacterial infection, HIV is assumed to be the cause.

To treat fevers, keep the child warm and comfortable, change the bed linens often, and use extra blankets. Give sponge baths and fluids to control the fever.

Clean the thermometer after every temperature reading. Wash it with soap and water, soak it in 70% to 90% ethyl alcohol for 30 minutes, then rinse under running water. If the child has chronic diarrhea, take his temperature under his arm, rather than rectally.

Nutrition

Feed the child a high-protein, high-calorie diet supplying 100% to 150% of the recommended daily allowance for his weight. Try to make the food as appealing as possible.

Blood products

Blood or blood products to be given to children with HIV infection or AIDS require irradiation to prevent graft-versus-host disease.

Umbilical stumps

To prevent infection, clean the umbilical stumps of infants of mothers at high risk daily until they fall off or are removed.

Circumcision

Infants of mothers at high risk for HIV infection shouldn't be circumcised because of the risk of infection.

Protective clothing

Wear gloves when changing diapers, a mask and glasses if you may be splashed with body secretions or excretions, and a gown when handling an infant.

Use an artificial airway when performing cardiopulmonary resuscitation—don't use mouth-to-mouth resuscitation.

Wear gloves when handling newborns until after their first baths and when handling the placenta.

Other considerations

The child's home environment and relationship with family members will greatly influence how he copes with his illness. Allow the child to lead as normal a life as possible. He should attend school unless he presents an infection risk to classmates, or unless they pose a risk to him. Seek occupational therapy for older children who fall behind in motor development because of illness, or work with them at home.

---

ments include acupuncture, Chinese herbals, megavitamins, coenzyme Q, and diets (such as macrobiotic, immune power, or yeast-control). Suggest that he contact a local or national AIDS organization for information and referrals before starting an alternative therapy. Also encourage him to continue with his prescribed regimen even if he uses an alternative therapy and to let the doctor know what other therapies he's trying.

Last, provide information about local and national AIDS organizations and support groups for patients, their partners, and family members. Tell the patient about various services, ranging from one-on-one volunteer counseling to assistance with medical insurance. Urge him to seek support from these organizations, and if necessary, help him contact them.

Sources of information and support

AIDS Health Project
Box 0884, San Francisco, Calif. 94143-0884
(415) 476-6430

AIDS Health Services Program and AIDS Resource Program
1326 Third Avenue, San Francisco, Calif. 94143-0936
(415) 476-6430

Gay Men's Health Crisis
P.O. Box 274, 132 West 24th Street, New York, N.Y. 10011
(212) 807-7035

Gay Rights National Lobby/AIDS Project
P.O. Box 1892, Washington, D.C. 20012
(202) 546-1801

Health Education Resource Organization (HERO)
101 West Reed Street, Suite 825, Baltimore, Md. 21201
(301) 685-1180

Mothers of AIDS Patients (MAP)
P.O. Box 3132, San Diego, Calif. 92013
(619) 234-3432

National AIDS Hotline
Centers for Disease Control (CDC)
1-800-342-AIDS

National AIDS Network
2033 M Street, NW, Suite 800, Washington, D.C. 20036
(202) 293-2437

National Association of People with AIDS (NAPA)
2025 I Street, NW, Suite 415, Washington, D.C. 20006
(202) 429-2856

National Gay Health Coalition
206 N. 35th Street, Philadelphia, Pa. 19143
(215) 386-5327

Further readings

Bernstein, L.J., et al. "AIDS in Children and Adolescents," *Patient Care* 23(18):80-83, 86, November 15, 1989.
Caring for the Person with AIDS at Home. Midland, Mich.: Mid-Michigan Health Care Systems, 1988.
Clement, M., et al. "Managing the HIV-Positive Patient," *Patient Care* 23(17):51-54, 56, 58+, October 30, 1989.
Flaskerud, J. *AIDS/HIV Infection: A Reference Guide for Nursing Professionals.* Philadelphia: W.B. Saunders Co., 1988.
Scherer, P. "How AIDS Attacks the Brain," *American Journal of Nursing* 90(1):44-53, January 1990.

Tips for sound nutrition

Dear Patient:

Eating right can keep your body functioning at its maximum and help you ward off infections. In fact, you may need up to 5,000 calories a day because AIDS causes your body to burn calories rapidly. By following the nutrition tips below, you'll help prevent weight loss and conserve your strength.

If you don't feel hungry
Most patients with AIDS lose their appetites. To combat this, make breakfast your biggest meal, and eat small, frequent meals throughout the day, resting beforehand.

Don't fill up on fluids during meals, but drink at least six glasses of water a day. Drink nutritional supplements (such as Ensure) for between-meal snacks.

Don't take recreational drugs, such as cocaine, because they'll further suppress your appetite and your immune system.

If food tastes unsavory
AIDS can alter your sense of taste, so try eating well-cooked poultry and fish instead of red meat, and serve high-protein foods at room temperature or colder to make them more palatable.

If you have mouth sores
If eating is painful because of mouth sores, ask your doctor to prescribe a topical anesthetic to apply to your mouth before eating. Eat soft foods or puree foods in a blender, and avoid acidic, spicy, or salty foods.

If you're too tired to cook
If you're tired at mealtimes, pick a time when you're less tired, and make soups, stews, or other foods in large quantities to freeze for later use. Consider using a microwave oven to heat leftovers or commercial frozen dinners. Ask a friend to help with cooking and food shopping.

If you have nausea, vomiting, or diarrhea
If GI symptoms are a problem, don't cook strong-smelling foods, such as onions, and avoid high-fiber foods, such as bran cereals, and high-fat foods, such as french fries. Buy lactose-reduced milk. Ask your doctor about antiemetics, antidiarrheals, and electrolyte supplements.

If you're depressed
Eating alone can be depressing, so share mealtimes with others. Try to provide a pleasant setting and engage in pleasant conversation.

Other tips
Check the expiration dates on food packages to ensure freshness. Cook meats and eggs thoroughly to prevent salmonella infection. Wash vegetables and fruits well, and peel them before eating. Never drink unpasteurized milk or use cracked eggs. Don't use wooden cutting boards, which can harbor germs.

How to use a condom

Dear Patient:

Sexual abstinence is the only sure way to prevent sexual transmission of AIDS. But if you use a new condom every time you have sex—and use it correctly—this will help protect your partner from infection. The suggestions below will help you choose, store, and use condoms.

Buying condoms

Buy only American-made, latex condoms. They give better protection. Avoid those made of lambskin.

Be sure the condom has a reservoir tip (or receptacle end). Notice that the package has a manufacturer's date—and an expiration date if the product contains a spermicide.

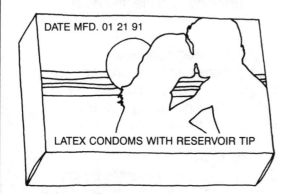

DATE MFD. 01 21 91

LATEX CONDOMS WITH RESERVOIR TIP

Storing condoms

Store unused condoms in a cool, dry place. Don't keep them in a warm place, such as your hip pocket or the glove compartment of your car. Heat can damage the latex.

Using condoms

Follow these steps to apply and remove a condom.

1 Open the wrapper carefully because a jagged fingernail can tear the condom. Hold the rolled condom by the reservoir tip to squeeze out the air and make room for the semen when you ejaculate.

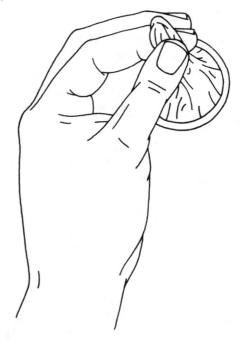

2 If the condom isn't lubricated inside, apply a water-based lubricant or plain water to your penis to increase sensation.

Once you have an erection, pull back the foreskin if you're uncircumcised.

continued

How to use a condom — *continued*

Next, place the rolled condom on the end of your penis.

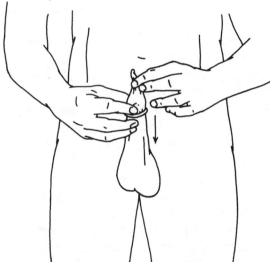

3 Hold the reservoir tip with one hand, and unroll the condom onto your erect penis with the other hand. Unroll it until it touches your pubic hair. If the condom doesn't have a reservoir tip, keep ½ inch free at the end to collect semen.

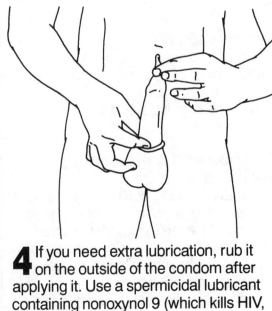

4 If you need extra lubrication, rub it on the outside of the condom after applying it. Use a spermicidal lubricant containing nonoxynol 9 (which kills HIV, the AIDS virus) for vaginal intercourse and a water-based lubricant for anal intercourse. Don't use petroleum jelly or oil — they can weaken the latex.

If the condom breaks or tears during intercourse, have your partner insert contraceptive foam, cream, or jelly containing nonoxynol 9 into her vagina or his rectum immediately.

5 After you ejaculate, hold the condom firmly while withdrawing your penis. To reduce the risk of spilling semen, withdraw your penis while it's still erect.

6 To remove the condom, pinch the tip with one hand to keep the semen from spilling, and roll the condom off your penis with the other hand.

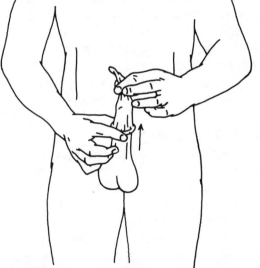

7 Flush the condom down the toilet immediately, or discard it in a closed, rigid plastic or metal container, such as a coffee can. Never use a condom twice.

8 Wash your penis and hands with soap and water.

Caring for an AIDS patient at home

Dear Caregiver:

You can care for a patient with AIDS at home without exposing yourself or other family members to the virus and without giving the patient a new infection. How? By ensuring that no one comes into contact with the patient's blood, semen, or vaginal secretions. Although the virus that causes AIDS may be detected in saliva, urine, feces, mucus, perspiration, or other body secretions, no one has developed AIDS from contact with these body fluids.

The precautions below take time and planning, but they'll soon become second nature. Remember, though, precautions shouldn't be so exaggerated that the patient feels isolated.

To prevent AIDS transmission at home, follow these guidelines:

Hand washing
Use soap and water to wash your hands, arms, and any other body surfaces that touch the patient before and after all patient contact and before preparing food or eating.

Don't touch your own body or your mouth during patient care. Also remind the patient to wash his hands frequently, especially before eating and after using the bathroom.

Gloves, gowns, and masks
Protective clothing isn't needed for general care or during casual contact, such as when bathing intact skin or feeding the patient. However, it should be worn in the following instances.

Use *gloves* when touching body secretions or excretions—for example, in blood contact during mouth, wound, or nose care, or when caring for a woman who's menstruating or who's just given birth.

Also wear gloves when handling soiled diapers, sheets, or clothing, when the patient has vomited or been incontinent, or when caring for a patient with rectal or genital lesions (sores or blisters). Remember to wash your hands after removing gloves.

Wear a *gown* if you may be splattered with body fluids. Wear a *mask* if the patient has *Mycobacterium tuberculosis* and is coughing. Wear a *mask* and *protective eyewear* to prevent vomit or saliva from splashing into your eyes, nose, or mouth.

Eating utensils
Wash dishes used by patients with AIDS in hot, soapy water, and dry them after washing. But you needn't keep the patient's dishes isolated from other dishes.

Kitchen and bathroom facilities
Patients with AIDS don't need separate kitchen and bathroom facilities. The patient may use the same toilet as other family members without special precautions unless he has diarrhea, herpes lesions, or incontinence.

If he does, disinfect the toilet with a

continued

Caring for an AIDS patient at home — *continued*

1:10 solution of bleach and water after each use. Wait 10 minutes, then rinse with clear water.

Cleanups

If blood, urine, or other body fluids spill, clean them up promptly with hot, soapy water. Then disinfect the washed surface with a 1:10 bleach solution, and rinse with clear water after 10 minutes.

Soak sponges or mops used to clean up body fluids in a 1:10 bleach solution for 5 minutes. Don't rinse them in sinks where food is prepared, and don't use them to clean food-preparation areas.

Pour mop water down the toilet. If the patient uses a bedpan or an emesis basin, pour the body fluids and excretions down the toilet.

Clean up the kitchen and bathroom as you normally do. To prevent growth of fungi and bacteria, wash surfaces regularly with soap and water and scouring powder. Clean the refrigerator regularly, and mop the floors at least once a week.

Disinfect the bathroom and shower floor with a commercial disinfectant or a 1:10 solution of bleach and water. Pour a small amount of full-strength bleach

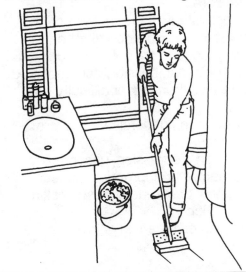

down the toilet. Clean up spills as soon as they occur, and don't use the same sponge to clean the bathroom and kitchen food-preparation areas.

Laundry

Wear gloves when handling soiled items. Always launder towels and washcloths after the patient uses them. Seal laundry soiled with body fluids in heavy-duty, double plastic bags until you can wash them. Soak items soiled with body fluids in cold water and an enzymatic detergent, then wash in hot water, detergent, and one cup of bleach. Machine dry on hot. Do all of the patient's laundry separately.

Disposable items

Place disposable, soiled gloves, diapers, underpads, tissues, and other items in sealed, heavy-duty, double plastic bags before discarding. Regular trash pickup is usually adequate, but follow your community's regulations for disposal.

Injection needles

Dispose of a used needle immediately in a sealed, rigid, puncture-proof plastic or metal can. Never recap or break a needle. Follow your community's regulations for disposal.

Personal items

Never share the patient's toothbrush, razor, or other personal items that might be contaminated with blood.

Glass thermometers can be shared as long as they're cleaned thoroughly first. Wash them with soap and cold water, soak them in 70% to 90% ethyl alcohol for 30 minutes, then rinse under running water.

PATIENT-TEACHING AID

Preventing infection – and recognizing its symptoms

Dear Patient:

Because AIDS damages your immune system and impairs your body's ability to fight infections, preventing infections is extremely important.

However, if you do come down with an infection, remember that early recognition and treatment are equally important.

Appropriate and timely treatment may prevent your condition from getting worse.

Preventing infection

To help prevent infection, review these guidelines and follow them whenever possible:
• Avoid crowds and people with known infections, such as herpes, influenza, mononucleosis, and cytomegalovirus. Even stay away from people who have minor colds.
• Get adequate sleep at night, and rest often during the day.
• Eat small, frequent meals, even if you've lost your appetite and have to force yourself to eat.
• Practice good hygiene, especially good oral hygiene. Don't use commercial mouthwashes because their high alcohol and sugar content may irritate your mouth and provide a medium for bacterial growth.
• Don't used any unprescribed intravenous drugs — or at least don't share needles with anyone else.
• Avoid traveling to foreign countries. If you must travel, however, consider drinking only bottled or boiled water and avoiding raw vegetables and fruits to prevent a possible intestinal infection.
• Wear a mask and gloves to clean bird cages, fish tanks, or cat litter boxes.
• Keep rooms clean and well ventilated, and keep air conditioners and humidifiers cleaned and repaired so they don't harbor infectious organisms.

Recognizing symptoms of infection

Contact your doctor immediately if you notice any of these symptoms:
• persistent fever or nighttime sweating not related to a cold or the flu
• swollen lymph nodes in your neck, armpits, or groin that last more than 2 months and aren't related to any other illness
• profound, persistent fatigue unrelieved by rest and not related to increased physical activity, longer work schedules, drug use, or a psychological disorder
• loss of appetite and weight loss
• open sores
• dry, persistent, unproductive cough
• persistent, unexplained diarrhea
• a white coating or spots on your tongue or throat, possibly accompanied by soreness, burning, or difficulty swallowing
• blurred vision or persistent, severe headaches
• confusion, depression, uncontrolled excitement, or inappropriate speech
• persistent or spreading rash or skin discoloration
• unexplained bleeding or bruising.

Hemophilia

A rare, inherited bleeding disorder, hemophilia affects about 1 in 4,000 males. Fortunately, early recognition and treatment of bleeding episodes can prevent the many complications that were common before clotting factor concentrates and home I.V. infusion programs were developed. Most likely, you'll emphasize this point as you explain the patient's condition and discuss measures he can take to manage bleeding episodes.

Discuss the disorder

Begin by explaining how the body normally responds to bleeding. First, the injured blood vessels constrict to impede blood flow. Then, platelets rush to the injury site to plug leaking capillaries. Next, clotting factors (special plasma proteins) activate to form a firm fibrin clot. This clot continually breaks down and re-forms until the injury heals.

In a person with hemophilia, an injured vessel will constrict and platelets will plug the capillaries as usual. But because one of the blood's 10 clotting factors is missing or abnormal, the clotting process goes awry. Compare the hemophilic clotting process to the domino effect. Imagine the 10 clotting factors as the dominoes. Explain that the removal or misalignment of one falling domino in the chain breaks the chain reaction. Interrupted in this way, the clotting process produces a mushy, ineffective clot.

Make it clear to the patient with hemophilia that he doesn't bleed faster than anyone else. However, because of the missing or defective clotting factor, he may have prolonged or delayed oozing. Explain that bleeding typically occurs with injuries to the kidneys, joints, muscles, and subcutaneous tissue, where the missing factor plays the most important role in coagulation. Identify which of his clotting factors is defective or missing.

Explain that hemophilia is inherited and that the disorder almost always affects males because the causative genetic abnormality occurs on the X chromosome. Women have two X chromosomes, so they have two chances to inherit an X chromosome with the normal gene. Men have an X and a Y chromosome, so they have only one chance to inherit the normal gene. (The Y chromosome doesn't affect production of Factors VIII and IX.) If a woman has an X chromosome with a hemophilia gene on it, she's considered a carrier. Clarify the inheritance pattern

Regina B. Butler, RN, Maribel J. Clements, RN, MA, and **Brenda Shelton, RN, MS, CCRN, OCN,** contributed to this chapter. Ms. Butler is a hemophilia coordinator and hematology nurse specialist at Children's Hospital of Philadelphia. Ms. Clements is a clinical associate at Puget Sound Blood Center in Seattle. Ms. Shelton is a critical care instructor at Johns Hopkins Oncology Center in Baltimore.

 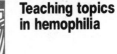

CHECKLIST

Teaching topics in hemophilia

☐ Explanation of normal and abnormal clotting processes
☐ Hemophilic inheritance patterns
☐ Type and severity of hemophilia
☐ Importance of recognizing bleeding episodes and seeking treatment promptly
☐ Initiation of early treatment to prevent complications
☐ Diagnostic tests, such as blood studies
☐ Activity restrictions to avoid injury
☐ Clotting factor replacement therapy and other medications
☐ Administration of I.V. clotting factors
☐ Prevention of hepatitis and AIDS
☐ Importance of avoiding aspirin and other drugs that affect platelets
☐ First-aid measures
☐ Preventive dental care
☐ Sources of information and support

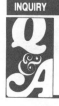

INQUIRY

Questions parents ask about transmitting hemophilia

No one in either of our families ever had hemophilia. How did our son get hemophilia?

In 20% to 25% of families with a hemophiliac, there's no family history of the disorder. Evidently, there's a high mutation (change) rate in the genes responsible for producing clotting factors VIII and IX. The mutation may occur in the child, in either parent, or elsewhere in the family tree.

What are our chances of having another child with hemophilia?

Each son of a carrier has a 50-50 chance of being a hemophiliac, and each daughter, a 50-50 chance of being a carrier. Your hemophilia treatment center can tell you more about testing and probability.

Because our son has hemophilia, will his children also have it?

If your son marries a carrier, your grandsons may have hemophilia. If your son marries someone who isn't a carrier, your grandsons won't have hemophilia, and they won't pass on the gene. All of their sisters will be carriers, though, and your great-grandsons may have hemophilia. The diagram below shows how a sex-linked recessive disorder occurs only in males and is transmitted only by a female carrier. The diagram's second row (the second generation) shows that each son of a carrier has a 50-50 chance of having hemophilia, and each daughter has a 50-50 chance of being a carrier. The last two rows represent the third generation if the second generation offspring mate with normal partners.

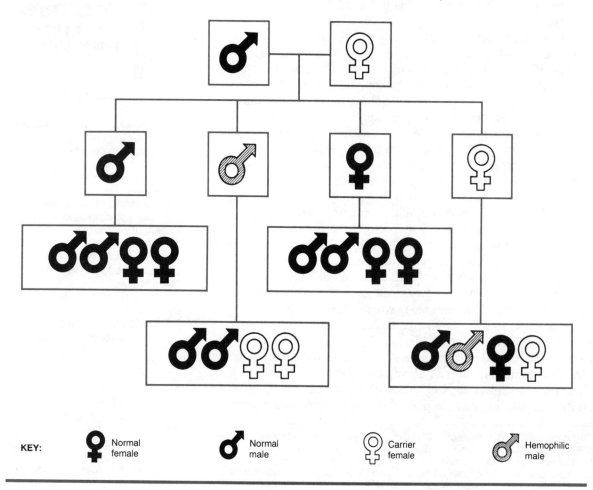

KEY: Normal female — Normal male — Carrier female — Hemophilic male

that results in hemophilia. (See *Questions parents ask about transmitting hemophilia.*)

Review the patient's type of hemophilia and classify it as mild, moderate, or severe (see *Explaining the difference between hemophilia A and hemophilia B*). Tell him that the severity depends on the degree of his clotting factor deficiency. Explain that the normal range for all 10 clotting factors is 50% to 150% of a baseline figure.

Tell the patient that abnormal bleeding usually doesn't occur unless clotting factor levels fall below 35%. If the patient has a clotting factor value between 5% and 25%, he has *mild hemophilia.* This hemophilia may be so mild as to go undiagnosed until adulthood. That's because a mild case doesn't cause spontaneous bleeding or bleeding after minor trauma. Rather, the patient has prolonged bleeding after major trauma, surgery, or tooth extractions. Postoperative bleeding continues as a slow ooze or ceases and starts again, up to 8 days after surgery.

If the patient's clotting factor values range from 1% to 5%, tell him that he has *moderate hemophilia.* He may bleed abnormally after relatively mild trauma, such as a hard bump or a sprain. What's more, bleeding episodes may occur as often as once a month or no more than once every several years. Moderate hemophilia causes symptoms similar to severe hemophilia, but the patient experiences spontaneous bleeding only occasionally.

With *severe hemophilia,* clotting factor levels fall below 1% of the normal value and spontaneous bleeding may result. Typically, the patient's first sign is excessive bleeding after circumcision. Later, spontaneous bleeding or severe bleeding after minor trauma may produce large subcutaneous and deep intramuscular hematomas. Bleeding into joints and muscles causes pain, swelling, extreme tenderness, and, possibly, permanent deformity.

Even in nonhemophiliacs, small blood vessels in the synovial membranes rupture from time to time. Normally, though, the bleeding stops almost immediately. In a patient with severe hemophilia, however, the vessel will continue oozing until the pressure in the joint becomes great enough to stop the bleeding. This usually takes several days. The only other way to stop the bleeding is to give the patient an infusion of the missing clotting factor. Patients with severe hemophilia may have bleeding episodes as often as once a week.

Complications

Urge the patient and his family to comply with treatment measures. Point out that most hemophiliacs can expect a normal life span, although damage from abnormal bleeding still poses a serious threat. Explain that bleeding near peripheral nerves may cause peripheral neuropathy, pain, paresthesia, and muscle atrophy. If bleeding impairs blood flow through a major vessel, ischemia and gangrene may result. Of greater concern are pharyngeal, lingual, intracardial, intracerebral, and intracranial bleeding, which can cause shock and death. To prevent significant blood loss and

Explaining the difference between hemophilia A and hemophilia B

Tell your patient and his family that when blood studies confirm the hemophilia diagnosis, he'll learn which type of hemophilia he has. Typically he'll have type A or type B, which reflect the most common clotting factor deficiencies.

Hemophilia A, or classical hemophilia, occurs with deficient Factor VIII, and hemophilia B, or Christmas disease (named for a patient), results from deficient Factor IX.

Explain that both hemophilia types cause the same symptoms, but treatment for each type differs. Knowing which type of hemophilia the patient has helps the doctor prescribe the most effective treatment. As appropriate, clarify test findings in hemophilia A and hemophilia B.

Hemophilia A
Tell the patient with hemophilia A that his Factor VIII assay value may be 0% to 30% of normal and that test findings will reflect a prolonged activated partial thromboplastin time (PTT). However, he will have a normal platelet count and function and normal bleeding and prothrombin times.

Hemophilia B
Inform the patient with hemophilia B that his test findings will show that his blood lacks Factor IX. What's more, he'll have baseline coagulation values similar to those for hemophilia A but normal amounts of Factor VIII.

Recognizing and managing bleeding

Bleeding in hemophilia may occur spontaneously or stem from an injury. Inform your patient and his family about possible types of bleeding and their associated signs and symptoms. Accordingly, advise them when to call for medical help.

BLEEDING SITE	SIGNS AND SYMPTOMS	NURSING INTERVENTION
Intracranial	Change in personality or wakefulness (level of consciousness), headache, nausea	Instruct the patient or his family to notify the doctor immediately and treat symptoms as an emergency.
Joints (hemarthroses) Most often affects the knees, followed by elbows, ankles, shoulders, hips, and wrists	Joint pain and swelling, joint tingling and warmth (at onset of hemorrhage)	Tell the patient to begin antihemophilic factor (AHF) infusions and then to notify the doctor.
Muscles	Pain and reduced function of affected muscle; tingling, numbness, or pain in a large area away from the affected site (referred pain)	Urge the patient to notify the doctor and start an AHF infusion if the patient's reasonably certain that bleeding results from recent injury (otherwise, call the doctor for instructions).
Subcutaneous tissue or skin	Pain, bruising, and swelling at the site (delayed oozing also may occur after an injury)	Show the patient how to apply appropriate topical agents, such as ice packs or absorbable gelatin sponges (Gelfoam), to stop bleeding.
Kidney	Pain in the lower back near the waist, decreased urine output	Notify the doctor and start AHF infusion if bleeding results from a known recent injury.
Heart (cardiac tamponade)	Chest tightness, shortness of breath, swelling (usually occurs in hemophiliacs who are very young or who have severe disease)	Instruct the patient to contact the doctor or go to the nearest emergency department at once.

chronic joint disease, the patient must recognize the signs and symptoms of internal bleeding and respond promptly to them (for more information, see *Recognizing and managing bleeding*).

Describe the diagnostic workup

Explain that a family history or a history of prolonged bleeding after trauma or surgery (including tooth extractions) or of spontaneous bleeding into muscles or joints usually indicates a defect in the hemostatic mechanism. However, the patient will need specific coagulation factor assays to confirm and identify the type and severity of hemophilia.

Inform the patient that blood studies are the key diagnostic tool for assessing hemophilia. Point out that additional tests may be ordered periodically to evaluate complications caused by bleeding. For example, computed tomography (CT) would be used for suspected intracranial bleeding, arthroscopy or arthrography for certain joint problems, and endoscopy for GI bleeding.

Blood studies

Inform the patient that the usual blood tests for any suspected bleeding disorder include a bleeding time, a platelet count, coagulation screenings, and clotting factor assays. Tell him that most of these tests require collection of a blood sample. Once test findings confirm the diagnosis, regularly required tests include specific clotting factor assays and an occasional inhibitor screen, all of which can be done with one venous blood sample.

Describe the *bleeding time* test. Explain that this test requires a slight incision, so it may or may not be done. If the patient has the test, tell him that the study measures the time it takes for a clot to form and for bleeding to stop. Usually the test takes 10 to 20 minutes. Explain that first his forearm will be cleaned with an antiseptic solution and a blood pressure cuff applied to his upper arm. Inform him that two small cuts will be made on his forearm. Then the nurse or technician will use filter paper to blot drops of blood until a platelet plug forms and oozing stops.

Teach about treatments
Inform the patient that he may go for years without requiring treatment. Emphasize, however, that he must always act cautiously to prevent injury and that, when necessary, he must receive intravenous clotting factors promptly.

Activity
Discuss the benefits of regular, moderate exercise. Advise the patient that strong muscles protect the joints. This, in turn, decreases the incidence of hemarthroses (bleeding into the joints). Add that isometric exercises that strengthen surrounding muscles—for example, quadriceps exercises after hemarthrosis in the knee—can help prevent muscle weakness and recurrent joint bleeding.

Urge the patient, though, to avoid such sports as football, lacrosse, and boxing. These obviously increase his risk for serious bleeding. Stress that all hemophiliacs (including those with mild hemophilia) must avoid rough contact sports or activities that increase the risk for intracranial bleeding. Tell patients with chronic joint disease to avoid such sports as soccer, basketball, skiing, aerobic exercises, or ice hockey because these activities stress the joints and carry a high risk for joint injury.

Besides avoiding certain sports, caution the patient to steer clear of activities that increase his risk for injury and prolonged bleeding. These include heavy lifting and carrying and using potentially harmful equipment, such as power tools.

Alternatively, encourage the patient and his family to take up swimming, hiking, or biking. If the patient's a child, review appropriate safety precautions with his parents. The child with severe hemophilia may require supervision and protective apparel, such as a helmet, elbow and knee pads, and leg guards, to prevent injury. Be sure to offer the parents a copy of the patient-teaching aid *Caring for a child with hemophilia,* pages 249 and 250.

Medication
Inform your patient (or his family) that I.V. infusion of the missing clotting factor is the primary treatment for hemophilia. Which

Teaching about adverse reactions to blood products

Teach any hemophilic patient—especially the one who infuses replacement factors at home—to recognize and promptly treat adverse reactions to blood products. The most common reactions and treatments include:
• *flushing, headache, or tingling.* These reactions occur most often with freeze-dried concentrate. They usually aren't serious. Slowing the infusion rate may cause symptoms to abate.
• *fever and chills.* Indicating an allergy to white blood cell antigens, this reaction occurs most often with plasma infusions. Reassure the patient that this reaction usually isn't serious and that acetaminophen (Tylenol) may relieve discomfort.
• *hives.* The most common reaction to cryoprecipitate or plasma, this hypersensitivity sign results from an allergy to a plasma protein. Hives usually subside with diphenhydramine or another antihistamine. Ideally, patients who develop hives frequently should receive an antihistamine about 45 minutes before a clotting factor infusion.
• *anaphylaxis.* The same plasma proteins that cause hives may occasionally cause anaphylaxis. Review the signs and symptoms of anaphylaxis: rapid or difficult breathing, wheezing, hoarseness, stridor, and chest tightness. Teach the patient to administer epinephrine and then to contact the doctor at once.

Clotting factor replacement products

Even though your patient may lack only one clotting factor, the medications used to replace that factor vary. Inform him that each factor replacement product has distinct specificity, composition, and storage and administration requirements. To ensure optimum treatment effectiveness, teach your patient about the replacement factor prescribed for him.

Cryoprecipitate
• Contents: Factor VIII (70 to 100 units/bag); no Factor IX
• Storage: can freeze for up to 12 months; must use within 6 hours of thawing
• Administration: given through a blood filter; compatible only with normal saline solution.

Lyophilized Factor VIII
• Contents: derived from monoclonal antibodies
• Storage: may be freeze-dried and labeled with exact units of Factor VIII contained in vial (vials range from 200 to 1,500 units of Factor VIII or IX each and contain 20 to 40 ml after reconstitution with diluent); can store for 2 years at temperatures ranging from 36° to 46° F. (2° to 8° C.) or for 6 months at room temperature not exceeding 88° F. (31° C.)
• Administration: no blood filter needed; usually given by slow I.V. push through a butterfly infusion set.

Fresh-frozen plasma
• Contents: Factor VIII (approximately 75 units/ml) and Factor IX (approximately 1 unit/ml); impractical for most hemophiliacs because a large volume is needed to raise factors to hemostatic levels
• Storage: can freeze for up to 12 months; must use within 2 hours of thawing
• Administration: given through a blood filter; compatible only with normal saline solution.

Anti-inhibitor coagulant complex
• Contents: derived from human plasma and used in patients having Factor VIII inhibitor; may be heat- or vapor-treated and labeled with the units of Factor VIII correctional activity contained in each vial
• Storage: can refrigerate 35° to 46° F. (2° to 8° C.) before reconstitution with diluent; must not refrigerate after reconstitution
• Administration: varies according to product—give within 1 hour (for Autoplex T), within 3 hours (for Feiba VH Immuno) after reconstitution.

replacement factor or other preparation he receives depends on the type and severity of his hemophilia. If he's receiving a clotting factor replacement, mention that the short half-life of clotting factors may necessitate repeated infusions (see *Clotting factor replacement products*).

Other treatment includes medication, such as desmopressin (DDAVP or Stimate) to prevent bleeding from surgery or tooth extraction, or fresh-frozen plasma to control bleeding from a traumatic injury. Emphasize that in most cases prompt treatment can prevent complications, although some adverse reactions may occur (see *Teaching about adverse reactions to blood products*). Teach the patient (and his parents) how to recognize his need for therapy, and discuss the preparation that he'll use (see *Teaching about drugs for hemophilia,* pages 244 and 245).

Factor VIII cryoprecipitate. Tell the patient that with *severe or moderate hemophilia A,* he'll typically receive an infusion of Factor VIII. Also called the antihemophilic factor (AHF), Factor VIII comes in two forms: single-donor, frozen concentrate (cryoprecipitate) that's administered by I.V. drip and a commercially prepared, freeze-dried concentrate extracted from plasma contributed by a pool of donors. Reconstituted in a small amount of sterile water, this form is usually given by I.V. push.

Desmopressin. Inform the patient with *mild hemophilia A* that he may receive desmopressin rather than a clotting factor concentrate. Explain that desmopressin stimulates the release of stored Factor VIII and temporarily doubles or triples the patient's Factor VIII level. Tell him that he'll take this intravenously every day or every other day for three or four doses.

Prothrombin complex concentrate. Advise the patient that this preparation treats or prevents bleeding in patients with *severe or moderate hemophilia B.* This freeze-dried preparation, which contains Factor IX, comes in a powder reconstituted with 20 to 30 ml of sterile water. It's given by I.V. push.

Fresh-frozen plasma. State that bleeding episodes in patients with *mild hemophilia B* may be treated with fresh-frozen plasma to reduce the risk of exposure to hepatitis and other viruses. Mention that each unit infusion takes at least 30 minutes; adult patients characteristically receive 4 or 5 units per infusion.

Procedures

You'll need to teach the patient or his parents how to give an infusion, how to care for veins, how to mix the infusion and calculate the dosage, and how to keep accurate records. You'll also need to outline possible complications, such as blood-borne infection and factor inhibitor development related to replacement factor procedures.

Home infusion (or self-infusion). Most parents learn to administer clotting factor to their child by the time he enters school. To qualify for home infusion, the child must have reasonably accessible veins and must be able to remain still. Hemophilic children usually learn to perform self-infusion between ages 8 and 12. After you teach the patient and his parents the technique, offer them the teaching aid *Learning self-infusion,* pages 251 and 252.

Protecting veins. Impress the patient with the importance of preserving his veins for lifelong therapy. Instruct him not to apply pressure to the puncture site until after he removes the needle. Warn him that putting pressure on the needle as he withdraws it will damage the vein. Then show how to apply firm pressure with one finger for 3 to 5 minutes. Instruct him to keep his arm straight, not bent.

Also instruct him to remind medical caregivers to use stainless steel butterfly needles whenever possible and to remove them after each infusion. The reason for this: plastic inside-the-needle catheters may inflame and scar the vein, especially if they're left

Teaching about drugs for hemophilia

DRUG	ADVERSE REACTIONS	TEACHING POINTS
Blood derivatives		
antihemophilic factor (AHF) (Hemofil, Koate-HT)	• Watch for breathing difficulty, chills, fever, flushing, hives, itching, and wheezing.	• Demonstrate sterile infusion techniques if the patient will self-infuse this product. • Explain how to calculate an accurate dose: multiply the patient's weight in kilograms by the percent desired. Then multiply this figure by 0.4 to find the number of AHF units needed. *Note:* The doctor will specify the percent desired (higher for a major bleeding episode, so the dose will be larger). • Urge the patient to keep and submit accurate self-treatment records. • Emphasize precautions to prevent transmission of blood-borne disease – especially proper disposal of I.V. equipment. • Advise the patient to call the treatment center if problems arise. • Instruct him to keep concentrates in the refrigerator.
anti-inhibitor coagulant complex (Autoplex T, Feiba VH Immuno)	• Watch for anaphylaxis, disseminated intravascular coagulation (DIC), and hypersensitivity (changes in blood pressure and pulse rate, chills, fever, and rash). • Other reactions include flushing and headache.	• Explain that rapid infusion may cause changes in pulse rate and blood pressure, headache, and flushing. If these symptoms develop, instruct the patient to discontinue the infusion until the symptoms subside and then to resume the infusion at a slower rate. • Tell the patient to store the medication in the refrigerator 35° to 46° F. (2° to 8° C.) but not to freeze it. Instruct him, however, not to refrigerate the medication after he reconstitutes it. • Advise him to administer Autoplex T within 1 hour of reconstitution and to administer Feiba VH Immuno within 3 hours.
prothrombin complex concentrates (Factors II, VII, IX, and X) (Konyne, Proplex)	• Watch for chest pain, chills, coughing, fever, flushing, hives, and respiratory distress. • Other reactions include headache.	• Explain that this product treats bleeding when clotting factors II, VII, IX, and X are missing or deficient. • Teach the patient sterile I.V. infusion technique. Emphasize the importance of slow infusion (no more than 3 ml/minute) to reduce the risk of thrombosis. • Tell him to stop the infusion immediately if chest pain or breathing difficulties occur. • Teach the patient how to calculate dosage by multiplying his weight in kilograms by the percent desired. Then multiply this figure by 0.6 to get the needed dose. *Note:* The doctor will specify the percent desired (higher for a major bleeding episode, so the dose will be larger). • Urge the patient to keep and submit accurate treatment records. • Also emphasize the importance of preventing blood-borne disease by properly disposing of I.V. equipment. • Remind the patient to call the treatment center if problems arise. • Tell him to use only concentrates labeled "heat-treated." • Instruct him to refrigerate concentrate.

continued

Teaching about drugs for hemophilia—*continued*

DRUG	ADVERSE REACTIONS	TEACHING POINTS
Hemostatics		
aminocaproic acid (Amicar)	• Watch for anuria, chest pain, diarrhea, dysuria, leg pain, nausea, severe muscle pain or weakness, thrombosis, and unusually slow or irregular heart rate. • Other reactions include dizziness, headache, nasal congestion, red eyes, rhinitis, and skin rash.	• Inform the patient that this drug treats excessive bleeding. • Warn against taking the drug within 6 to 12 hours of infusing prothrombin complex concentrates. Instruct the patient to check first with the treatment center. • Emphasize the importance of taking medication for the prescribed length of time, even after bleeding has stopped. • Encourage parents to review dosage with the treatment center as their child grows.
desmopressin (DDAVP, Stimate)	• Watch for coma, confusion, drowsiness, and seizures. • Other reactions include flushing, headaches, mild abdominal cramps, nausea, rhinitis, vulval pain, and weight gain.	• Inform the patient that this drug will stop spontaneous bleeding and bleeding from injury. • Explain that this drug, which isn't derived from blood, alleviates the hazard of possible contamination.

in place for several days. Besides, a new venipuncture should be performed for each infusion. (The exceptions are situations requiring continuous I.V. fluids or antibiotics or with patients—for example, young children—on whom venipuncture is especially difficult.)

Administering clotting factor. Teach the patient with severe or moderate hemophilia—or his parents—how to mix and administer clotting factor concentrates. This will prevent treatment delays and, in instances of minor bleeding, may save the patient a trip to the doctor's office or the hospital.

Explain how to calculate the amount of clotting factor concentrate needed to control the bleeding episode. Then stress the importance of contacting the doctor or treatment center if major bleeding occurs—for example, GI bleeding, head injury, and prolonged joint bleeding. Emphasize that home care (or self-infusion) isn't intended to replace medical care.

Keeping infusion records. Show the patient and his family how to keep accurate treatment records. Recommend that they write down the problem that required infusion treatment, the nature of the treatment, and the treatment's outcome. Advise patients to send or take this information to their treatment center at least once a month. For minor bleeding episodes, explain that most patients learn to first infuse clotting factor concentrate and then to record the treatment. For major bleeding episodes, tell the patient to first infuse the clotting factor concentrate, call the doctor or treatment center for further instructions, and then record the facts about the bleeding episode.

Reviewing possible complications. Inform the patient and his parents that self-infusion may be complicated by infection. Hepatitis, for example, may be transmitted through blood products.

Urge the patient to be immunized against hepatitis B. (Point out that no vaccines exist for hepatitis C or hepatitis D.)

Instruct the patient to prevent spreading blood-borne communicable diseases (such as hepatitis) to family members and others by disposing of all needles, syringes, and blood-contaminated waste in a hard plastic or cardboard container and returning the container to the hospital or hemophilia treatment center for disposal. Advise placing larger wastes contaminated with blood in an impermeable plastic bag and returning this package as well.

You'll also need to answer questions about other potential infections. For example, the patient may express concern about contracting acquired immunodeficiency syndrome (AIDS) through blood products. Explain that all donated blood and plasma is screened for antibodies to the human immunodeficiency virus (HIV) that causes AIDS. Also, all freeze-dried products are routinely heat-treated to kill HIV. These precautions make contracting AIDS through blood products highly unlikely.

Of course, a hemophiliac who received clotting factor concentrate before these products were heat-treated may already be exposed to HIV. This is also true of a patient who received cryoprecipitate and plasma before blood donors were screened carefully. This patient needs your reassurance. Point out that AIDS has developed in less than 1% of all hemophiliacs exposed to HIV through a blood product. If appropriate, though, refer an anxious patient to a hemophilia treatment center for follow-up information and counseling.

Between 10% and 20% of patients with severe hemophilia will develop inhibitors. This means that their body produces such an abnormal Factor VIII or IX that it recognizes the normal (infused) factors as foreign proteins. In response, the body produces antibodies, called inhibitors, against normal Factors VIII and IX. The antibodies destroy the clotting factor as quickly as it's infused. Because of this risk, tell patients to call their doctor if their home infusions don't seem to be controlling bleeding episodes.

Tell the patient that factor inhibitor levels can be measured to diagnose this condition. If confirmed, the condition may be treated with anti-inhibitor coagulant complex (Autoplex T, Feiba VH Immuno). Additional occasional treatment with desmopressin or aminocaproic acid (Amicar) may help. Explain that this condition's severity commonly depends on the hemophilia's severity.

Other care measures
Although clotting factor infusions are the major treatment for hemophilia, don't overlook emotional support, general preventive care, and first-aid measures. If your patient's a child, remember that emotional problems can be as disabling as physical ones (for more information, see *Helping parents cope with their child's hemophilia*). You may need to tactfully remind parents that overprotectiveness, permissiveness, and even withdrawal are typical parental responses to hemophilia and that these responses may cause serious social or emotional problems. If appropriate, offer to refer the family for counseling.

Helping parents cope with their child's hemophilia

Hemophilia can dramatically influence the way parents respond to their child who has it. Help them act constructively by teaching them to identify ways that they react to their child's illness.

Curbing overprotectiveness
When parents learn that their child has a bleeding disorder, it's only natural for them to want to protect him from getting hurt. Overprotectiveness, however, may interfere with their child's normal development—especially his exploratory behaviors and physical activities. The child, depending on his personality, may respond to protectiveness by exhibiting dependence, passivity, and fearfulness, *or* by acting rebellious, angry, or dangerously daring.

Telling parents that their carefulness usually can't keep the child from having bleeding episodes typically falls on deaf ears. Rather, ask them to tell you how they treat their hemophilic child differently from their other children. In the telling, they may realize their excessive protectiveness. If they don't have other children, ask them to compare their protective practices with their friends' and neighbors' practices. Also suggest that they keep track of how often they warn, "Watch out" or "Be careful."

Avoiding permissiveness or indulgence
Parents may also adopt a permissive or indulgent attitude toward their hemophilic child. Perhaps they feel sorry for him (or guilty themselves) because he has hemophilia or because they've restricted so many of his activities. If so, they may try to make it up to him by giving in on other matters or by showering him with toys, treats, and special privileges. They may relax rules that they would enforce for their other children. Or they may require the child to be less responsible in learning self-discipline and contributing to family operations—for instance, by doing chores regularly.

Unfortunately, this doesn't help the child—especially if permissiveness leads to a disregard for social rules and self-control. An overindulged child may throw temper tantrums and adopt manipulative behavior to empower himself. Or he may exhibit qualities of laziness or passivity. What's more, he may be easily bored and expect his parents or society to entertain and provide for him.

Conversing about how well-meaning permissiveness or indulgence can cause more harm than good may help parents overcome these perfectly normal responses to a child with a disability. The child needs attention and encouragement, of course, but giving in to unreasonable demands and excusing him from responsibilities won't help him to function successfully in school or in life at large.

Discouraging hypochondriasis or self-absorption
Another common parental reaction may lead to hypochondriasis in the child when the parents become alarmed about the risk of abnormal bleeding episodes. If the child gets too much attention whenever he has a bleeding episode or if he's encouraged to stay home from school, he may think of himself as ill or defective. He may even use his hemophilia to excuse himself from school or other responsibilities that he perceives as unpleasant or unrewarding. Urge parents to encourage regular school attendance. Bleeding episodes should be treated matter-of-factly and not as a reason to withdraw from daily activities or general commitments.

Protecting against withdrawal and rejection
The most devastating parental reactions are withdrawal and rejection. If parents reject their child because he has hemophilia, the child may develop feelings of inferiority, a poor self-image, and a fear of failure.

Fortunately, complete withdrawal or rejection is rare among parents of hemophilic children. Parents usually express shock and grief when they hear their child's diagnosis, but most eventually adjust. Meeting with professionals from a hemophilia treatment center and with other parents of hemophilic children may ease their adjustment.

Prevent a bleeding episode. Advise hemophilic patients to avoid taking aspirin, combination medications containing aspirin, and over-the-counter anti-inflammatory agents, such as ibuprofen compounds (Advil, Motrin). These medications decrease platelet function—aspirin significantly and ibuprofen to a lesser extent. However, both medicines could amplify the frequency and severity of bleeding episodes. Tell the patient to ask his pharmacist for a list of medications containing these compounds and then to avoid them. Instruct him to take acetaminophen (Tylenol) for mild pain or fever, but to consult his doctor for any sign of inflammation.

Give first aid. Mention that application of pressure is usually the only treatment needed for surface cuts and nosebleeds. Deeper cuts may stop temporarily with pressure. (With cuts deep enough to require suturing, the patient will need clotting factor infusions to prevent further bleeding.)

Suggest applying ice packs and elastic bandages to alleviate pain from hemarthrosis. Emphasize, however, that these measures are not a substitute for clotting factor infusions.

Observe general precautions. Urge the patient to wear medical identification, such as a Medic Alert necklace or bracelet. This will help to ensure that the patient receives clotting factor infusions as soon as possible after major accidents or a loss of consciousness.

Preventive dental care is important for everyone, of course, but especially for the patient with hemophilia. Make sure he understands that dental caries can be filled and teeth extracted, but emphasize that he'll need clotting factor infusions before some of these procedures. Emphasize that poor dental hygiene can lead to bleeding from inflamed gums.

The patient obviously has much to learn, all of which you can't possibly teach him in a few sessions while he's hospitalized. That's why you should refer him to the nearest comprehensive hemophilia center for evaluation and follow-up teaching. Refer interested family members, too. Explain that these centers typically offer carrier testing, prenatal diagnosis, and other genetic counseling services.

Sources of information and support

American Society of Pediatric Hematology-Oncology (ASPHO)
c/o Carl Pochedly, M.D., Wyler Children's Hospital
5841 South Maryland Avenue, Chicago, Ill. 60637
(312) 702-6808

Children's Blood Foundation (CBF)
424 East 62nd Street, Room 1045, New York, N.Y. 10021
(212) 644-5790

National Hemophilia Foundation (NHF)
110 Green Street, Room 406, New York, N.Y. 10012
(212) 219-8180

Further readings

Fletcher, M. "Haemophilia Research," *Nursing 1990* 4(6):38, March 8-21, 1990.

Smith, A.A., et al. "The Burned Hemophiliac," *Journal of Burn Care and Rehabilitation* 9(4):389-90, July-August 1988.

Turner, T. "A Helping Hand for Haemophiliacs. . . Paediatric Haemophiliac Service," *Nursing Times* 84(49):26-29, December 7-13, 1988.

Weinstein, B.D., and DeNeffe, L.S. "Hemophilia, AIDS, and Occupational Therapy," *American Journal of Occupational Therapy* 44(3):228-32, March 1990.

Wilson, P.A., et al. "Psychosocial Responses to the Threat of HIV Exposure Among People with Bleeding Disorders," *Health Social Work* 14(3):176-83, August 1989.

Caring for a child with hemophilia

Dear Parents:

Your child has hemophilia, a lifelong bleeding disorder. With proper care, he can lead a nearly normal life, attending school regularly and taking part in most activities. Follow these guidelines to promote his health and well-being.

Prevent injury
Protect your child from injury, but avoid unnecessary restrictions that impair his normal development. For example, if your son's a preschooler, add padded patches to the knees and elbows of clothing to protect these joints when he falls.

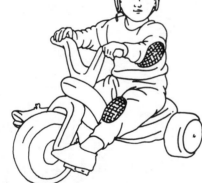

You must forbid an older child to participate in contact sports, such as football, but you can encourage him to swim or to play golf.

Administer first aid
If your child is injured, administer first aid as you would for anyone else. Remember, he won't bleed any faster than normal. He'll just bleed longer. If he's not treated promptly, he may have prolonged or delayed oozing that can cause pain and disability. Injuries to the head, neck, or eye are serious.

If your child says he has pain, starts limping, or stops using an arm or leg, suspect that he's bleeding into a joint or muscle. Arrange for prompt treatment.

Watch for bleeding
Be alert for signs of bleeding, especially in the head area and especially if your child suffered a blow or bump on his head in the last 4 or 5 days. Called "intracranial bleeding," this problem causes upset stomach, vomiting, headache, irritability, and drowsiness.

If he vomits blood or material that looks like coffee grounds, or if he passes stools that are black and sticky (tarry), suspect bleeding in the stomach or intestinal area.

Blood in the urine points to kidney bleeding and should be treated by giving fluids and clotting factor.

Whenever your child's injured or appears to be bleeding abnormally, call your doctor or hemophilia treatment center immediately.

Learn to infuse clotting factors
When your child reaches age 6 or 7, you may want to learn how to give him clotting factor infusions at home. This provides him with treatment as quickly as possible after you (or he) notice signs and symptoms of abnormal bleeding. This also may eliminate the need for a hospital stay.

Your son's nurse or doctor or special-

continued

Caring for a child with hemophilia — *continued*

ists at the hemophila treatment center can teach you. Once you know how to give an infusion, remember to keep the blood factor concentrate and infusion equipment handy at all times — even (or especially) during family vacations.

Be alert for illness

Naturally, because your child will be receiving blood products, he'll be exposed to hepatitis. Watch for early signals of this disease, which may appear from 3 weeks to 6 months after treatment with blood components. Signs and symptoms include headache, fever, decreased appetite, nausea, vomiting, abdominal tenderness and pain in the same area.

Be sure your child receives the hepatitis B vaccine along with his regularly scheduled immunizations.

Take important precautions

● Make sure your child wears a Medic Alert bracelet or necklace at all times.
● Never give him aspirin. It may increase the frequency or severity of his bleeding episodes. Examine all medicine labels for these words — "aspirin," "acetylsalicylic acid," or "ASA." They are all names for the same medicine: aspirin.
● Teach your child to care for his teeth regularly with careful toothbrushing. This may prevent the need for future dental procedures, such as scaling, restoration, or surgery. Have him use a soft toothbrush to avoid gum injury.

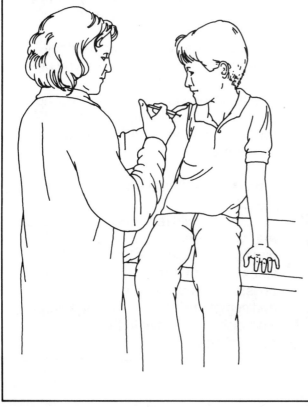

● Keep routine follow-up examinations with the doctor or at the local hemophilia center.
● To answer your son's (or your) questions about the vulnerability of his (or your) future offspring, ask for information from a genetic counselor or contact the National Hemophilia Foundation.
● Your daughters may want to consider genetic screening, too. This can detect whether they carry the hemophilia gene.

Learning self-infusion

Dear Patient:

These instructions will help you give yourself clotting factors at home.

Remember, if you're infusing clotting factors for a minor bleeding episode, keep a record of it. Write down when you did the infusion, why you needed it, and how much clotting factor you used. Be sure to take this information with you the next time you go to the doctor.

If you give yourself clotting factors for major bleeding, call your doctor afterward to tell him about it.

Now use these directions to help you do what your nurse or doctor taught you. And to avoid infection, be sure to use only new needles and syringes every time you give yourself an infusion.

1 Gather your equipment. Make sure you have your clotting factor concentrate and sterile water, syringe, a butterfly needle set, a tourniquet, alcohol wipes, gauze pads, and tape.

2 Thoroughly wash and rinse your hands with soap and water.

3 Remove the flip-top lids on the clotting factor concentrate bottle and the sterile water bottle. Use the alcohol wipes to clean the stoppers. Add sterile water from the water bottle to the powder in the concentrate bottle to make a liquid.

4 If you're using *nonvacuum bottles,* inject air into the sterile water bottle and withdraw the water. Inject water into the concentrate bottle. Direct the water against the bottle's side so you don't make any bubbles or foam.

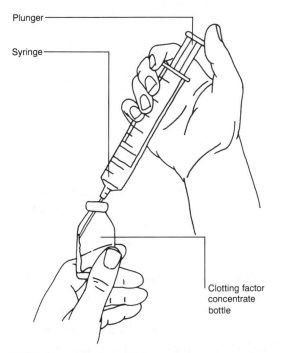

Plunger

Syringe

Clotting factor concentrate bottle

Withdraw air to relieve pressure, and then withdraw the needle. Put a cap on the needle.

If you're using *vacuum bottles,* the idea's the same. Insert the double-ended needle into the water bottle. Then turn the needle and bottle upside down and insert the other end of the needle into the bottle that contains the concentrate.

continued

Learning self-infusion — *continued*

Direct the stream of water against the side of the bottle so you don't make bubbles or foam.

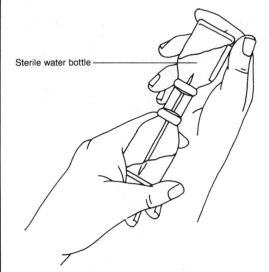

Sterile water bottle

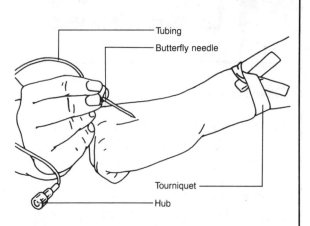

Tubing

Butterfly needle

Tourniquet

Hub

Lift the water bottle off the needle (to release the vacuum). Pull the needle from the concentrate, and rotate or roll the bottle gently in your hands until the powder dissolves completely. Clean the stopper of the concentrate bottle with a new alcohol wipe.

Next, transfer the dissolved concentrate into your syringe that has a needle and a filter. To do this, use the syringe to inject air into the concentrate bottle. Then pull back on the plunger to draw the reconstituted concentrate into the syringe.

5 Wrap the tourniquet around your lower arm about 3 inches above the place where you'll insert the needle into your vein. Clean the area with an alcohol wipe and let it dry.

Then loosen the hub at the end of the butterfly needle tubing to break the vacuum. Now, uncap the needle and insert it at a 30- to 45-degree angle through your skin into the center of the

vein. When you see blood return, lower the needle to make it level with your skin. Slide the needle slightly forward so that it won't slip from the vein.

6 Take off the tourniquet and tape the butterfly needle to your skin. Now, remove the filter section of your syringe. Attach the syringe part holding the liquid concentrate to the hub of the butterfly needle's tubing. Pull back gently on the plunger of the syringe to fill the tubing with blood. Then infuse the concentrate slowly as directed by your nurse or doctor.

7 When the infusion's finished, place a gauze pad over the site and remove the needle. *Don't apply pressure to the site as you remove the needle. It can damage the vein.*

8 When you've removed the needle, apply firm pressure to the venipuncture site for 3 to 5 minutes.

9 To prevent the spread of infection, put used needles and syringes into a special box or plastic container. Return them to the hospital or clinic. Wrap other equipment in plastic and return it as well.

Sickle cell syndrome

Comprising several disorders, sickle cell syndrome includes sickle cell anemia (SCA) and sickle cell trait, among other disorders. SCA is an inherited disease, which occurs mostly in blacks and sometimes in persons from Mediterranean cultures. Chronic and incurable and shrouded by myth and misinformation, this painful disease calls for sensitive teaching. Because patients and families typically experience fear and anxiety, your teaching will focus on relieving apprehension and discomfort, preventing sickle cell crises, avoiding complications, and understanding hereditary transmission.

Because the patient with sickle cell anemia usually has periodic crises, he may be discouraged and depressed, which can delay learning. You may need to help him express his feelings before implementing your teaching plan. Also, because sickle cell anemia is a chronic disease, you'll need to determine how much the patient already knows before you start teaching. If he's been hospitalized before, point out that there's always more to learn about his condition. And the more he learns, the better prepared he'll be to guard against complications. (For more information, see *Teaching the patient with sickle cell anemia,* page 254.)

Discuss the disorder

Explain that SCA results from an inherited mutation in hemoglobin, the blood component that carries oxygen to body tissues. Red blood cells (RBCs) containing this substance (hemoglobin S) have normal oxygen capacity but become abnormally rigid, rough, and elongated (sickle-shaped) when they lose oxygen. Normal RBCs, which carry normal hemoglobin A, remain disklike and pliable.

Inform the patient that sickling typically occurs with activities or conditions that increase the body's need for oxygen, such as running at high altitudes. Inform him, too, that as sickle cells increase—during strenuous exercise, for example—they tend to clump together, obstructing circulation and depriving tissues of oxygen (see *The sickle cell cycle: A closer look,* page 255). Warn the patient that without intervention, tiny obstructions can become large infarctions. Explain further that heavy concentrations of sickled cells can thicken the blood and slow circulation. Mention that dehydration—from vomiting, diarrhea, excessive sweating, or diuretic use—causes the blood to thicken and makes the condition worse.

Contributors to this chapter include **Regina Butler, RN,** coordinator and hematology nurse specialist at Children's Hospital of Philadelphia; **Maribel J. Clements, RN, MA,** clinical associate at Puget Sound Blood Center in Seattle; **Joan E. Mason, RN, EdM,** clinical editor and consultant at Springhouse Corporation, Springhouse, Pa.; and **Dolores Shrimpton, RN, MA,** assistant professor at Kingsborough College, Brooklyn, N.Y.

CHECKLIST

Teaching topics in sickle cell syndrome

☐ Explanation of sickle cell anemia (SCA), sickle cell trait, and inheritance patterns
☐ Complications of SCA—especially those requiring immediate medical attention, such as vaso-occlusive crisis
☐ Precipitating factors for vaso-occlusive crisis
☐ Explanation of blood tests and other diagnostic procedures
☐ Principles of good nutrition, especially adequate intake of fluids and foods containing folic acid
☐ Infection prevention measures, including immunizations and prophylaxis
☐ Home care for vaso-occlusive crisis
☐ Special care measures, including genetic counseling and precautions related to surgery and pregnancy
☐ Sources of information and support

Teaching the patient with sickle cell anemia

Because sickle cell anemia (SCA) is usually diagnosed in childhood, an ideal teaching plan will be flexible enough to meet the needs of parents and patients at different developmental levels. For example, a grade schooler might learn about self-care by playing a board game about nutrition and exercise. A teenager might learn more from videos. You'll need to use a standard teaching plan as your springboard. Then customize the plan so that it instructs the caregiver while providing age-appropriate information for the patient. Here's one example.

Assess first
You're the primary nurse assigned to 8-year-old Chevron Brown. Admitted to the hospital with vaso-occlusive crisis, he seems ill and has flulike symptoms: a cough, runny nose, and slightly red throat. He has a fever of 100° F (37.8° C), a pulse rate of 100 beats/minute, and a respiratory rate of 22 breaths/minute. His chest is clear to percussion and auscultation, except for occasional crackles. Tearfully holding his abdomen, Chevron whimpers, "My belly hurts." His chart tells you that this is his third admission. Talking with his mother, you learn that Chevron's in second grade, and he loves bike riding, basketball, and Cub Scouts. Mrs. Brown suspects that Chevron got sick at school, where the flu is rampant. She concedes that she waited too long to call the doctor. "I know I should have brought Chevron in sooner, but he's so afraid of shots. I hoped he'd get over it himself."

What are the Browns' learning needs?
To determine what to teach the Browns, compare what they know about SCA and vaso-occlusive crisis with the contents of a standard teaching plan. Then decide which points to include or modify. A standard teaching plan includes:
• an explanation of SCA and inheritance patterns
• complications of SCA
• symptoms that require prompt medical attention
• tests to diagnose SCA
• infection-prevention measures, such as proper nutrition, regular immunizations, and prescribed drugs.
• home treatment for vaso-occlusive crisis.

From your conversation with Mrs. Brown, you realize she understands basic facts about SCA—but she could use some reinforcement on vaso-occlusive crisis and its prevention. So your teaching plan will focus on home treatment of vaso-occlusive crisis, when to seek medical care, and ways to prevent recurrence. You'll include Chevron in your teaching sessions. The youngster seems eager to learn.

What learning outcomes will you set?
With the standard teaching plan as your guide, you work with the Browns to set learning outcomes. They decide that they should be able to:

-describe what happens in vaso-occlusive crisis
-list measures to prevent infection and dehydration
-select foods and beverages that will meet folic acid and fluid needs
-explain how to increase fluid intake during illness and ways to limit physical and emotional stress
-explain the benefit of complying with immunizations and prescribed medication
-demonstrate home care measures for vaso-occlusive crisis, such as applying warm compresses
-name symptoms that require prompt care.

What teaching methods and tools will you use?
You and Mrs. Brown *discuss* what happens in vaso-occlusive crisis and how to prevent it. Then you *reinforce* key facts, such as the importance of increasing fluid intake at the first sign of a cold or other illness.

With Chevron, you schedule your teaching for a time when he's free of pain and in the mood to learn. Because school-age children learn best by *demonstration,* you show him what happens in vaso-occlusive crisis by placing marbles in a tube. He watches how easily the marbles pass through. Then you give him some paper clips to put in the tube. These bunch up and tangle, passing through with difficulty. This exercise allows Chevron to participate actively in learning, enabling him to see how sickled cells clog blood vessels.

Next, you use *flash cards* or a *game* to help Chevron remember self-care strategies, such as which foods contain rich amounts of folic acid. Teaching tools for Mrs. Brown include *pamphlets* on SCA, good nutrition, and childhood immunizations. Before giving her the pamphlets, you review them to make sure the advice is consistent with Chevron's therapy.

Throughout your teaching, you treat Chevron as a basically well person who happens to be sick. You emphasize to Mrs. Brown the importance of helping Chevron to develop a positive self-image, cautioning her to avoid casting her son in a "sick role."

How will you evaluate your teaching?
To assess the Browns' progress, ask them to *simulate* what they would do to prevent another vaso-occlusive crisis. For example, can they specify what they would do at the first sign of a cold? What symptoms would prompt them to call the doctor? Also use *discussion* and *direct observation* to evaluate their progress and identify additional learning needs.

Reassure the patient that reoxygenation usually returns most sickled cells to a normal, round shape, but some cells may remain permanently deformed. That's when chronic anemia occurs because deformed RBCs survive for only 15 to 20 days. Normally formed RBCs survive and function for about 120 days.

Make sure to include an explanation of inheritance patterns and the sickle cell trait as you discuss SCA and the risk of passing on the disorder to offspring. Explain that persons with sickle cell trait have one hemoglobin S gene and one hemoglobin A gene. This means that they can pass on the gene that causes SCA but that they don't have the disease itself (see *Reviewing sickle cell inheritance patterns,* page 256).

Complications

Urge the patient to comply with prescribed therapy. Emphasize that with SCA he's susceptible to serious infection, especially meningitis, pneumonia, and sepsis. One reason for this is the spleen's inability to function properly, which naturally limits the body's defenses. Serious infection can start suddenly and quickly worsen. Although young children are at greater risk, SCA patients of any age can incur serious infection. Besides risking infection, the patient also risks vaso-occlusive crisis. The most common complication of SCA, this painful condition can result from infection, dehydration, and excessive fatigue.

Describe the diagnostic workup

Tell the patient and his family that blood tests—notably hemoglobin electrophoresis—can confirm the SCA diagnosis. If SCA is confirmed, encourage all family members to be tested.

Prepare the patient for other tests as needed, such as routine blood counts, blood chemistry profiles, and urinalysis to detect early organ damage. Complications of SCA may require additional blood tests and possibly X-rays.

Mention that the doctor may order a lateral chest X-ray to detect the "Lincoln-log deformity." This spinal abnormality develops in many adults and some adolescents with SCA, leaving the vertebrae resembling logs that form the corner of a cabin.

Explain that another simple diagnostic tool includes an ophthalmoscopic examination to detect corkscrew- or comma-shaped vessels in the conjunctivae, another possible sign of SCA.

Teach about treatments

Although SCA can't be cured, stress that treatments can alleviate symptoms and prevent painful crises. Urge the patient to modify his activities and to adopt eating habits that ensure adequate dietary folic acid. Discuss such infection prevention measures as routine immunizations. Make sure to highlight signs and symptoms of vaso-occlusive crisis and home care measures.

Activity

Inform the patient that he can participate in physical activities promoting health and fitness, such as gym classes, as long as he

The sickle cell cycle: A closer look

Use a picture to show the difference between normal and sickled red blood cells (RBCs) and to illustrate how sickle cell anemia (SCA) threatens health.

Normal RBCs
Point out that normal RBCs look like disks with an indented center. Their round shape and pliability ease their circulation through the blood vessels.

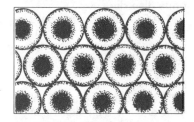

Sickle-shaped RBCs
On the other hand, RBCs that contain hemoglobin S, the genetic defect responsible for SCA, can become sickle- or crescent-shaped when they deliver oxygen. As these cells circulate, their shape causes them to tangle, trapping one another and jamming the blood vessels.

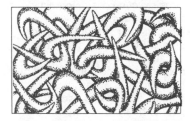

Consequently, oxygen isn't delivered to body tissues and ischemia results. This sets up a risky situation: Clogged vessels lead to capillary blood backups. Then hypoxia increases, and more RBCs are needed to meet increased oxygen needs. As more RBCs lose oxygen, more sickling occurs, and a dangerous cycle begins. Without interruption, the "sickle cycle" can be life-threatening.

Reviewing sickle cell inheritance patterns

Besides concern about his own health, the patient with sickle cell anemia (SCA) may be quite concerned about the health of his descendants. To help him assess the risks of passing on this genetic disease, review basic inheritance patterns and differentiate SCA from sickle cell trait or other less common disorders in sickle cell syndrome.

Homozygous vs. heterozygous disorders

Define SCA as a *homozygous* disorder, meaning that at conception the potential offspring with SCA receives two sickle cell genes—one from each parent.

If he receives one sickle cell gene and one normal gene, at birth he will have the *heterozygous* disorder called sickle cell trait. This makes him a "carrier." A carrier can pass the sickle cell gene to his offspring.

Tell the carrier with sickle cell trait that he'll never have SCA. However, caution him to avoid activities that induce hypoxia, such as mountain climbing or scuba diving. Explain that strenuous oxygen-consuming activities may provoke a sickling crisis (similar to that which occurs in SCA patients). That's because 20% to 40% of this person's total hemoglobin will be hemoglobin S. Reassure him, though, that he can usually expect to be symptom-free and have a normal life span.

Genetic possibilities

For the patient with SCA or the family member with sickle cell trait, review the various inheritance patterns at right. State that the chances of having a child with SCA or sickle cell trait are the same with each pregnancy.

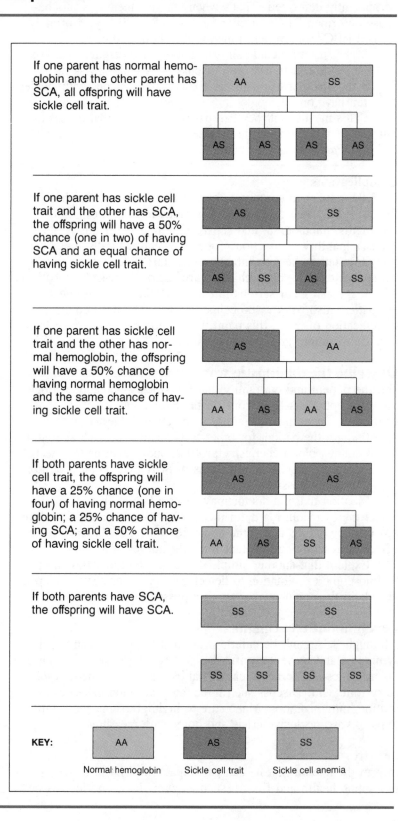

If one parent has normal hemoglobin and the other parent has SCA, all offspring will have sickle cell trait.

If one parent has sickle cell trait and the other has SCA, the offspring will have a 50% chance (one in two) of having SCA and an equal chance of having sickle cell trait.

If one parent has sickle cell trait and the other has normal hemoglobin, the offspring will have a 50% chance of having normal hemoglobin and the same chance of having sickle cell trait.

If both parents have sickle cell trait, the offspring will have a 25% chance (one in four) of having normal hemoglobin; a 25% chance of having SCA; and a 50% chance of having sickle cell trait.

If both parents have SCA, the offspring will have SCA.

KEY:
AA — Normal hemoglobin
AS — Sickle cell trait
SS — Sickle cell anemia

rests frequently, increases his fluid intake, and doesn't overdo it. Warn him that fatigue can contribute to vaso-occlusive crisis. One further caution: The patient with splenomegaly should be told to avoid contact sports to minimize the risk of a ruptured spleen.

Diet
Adequate nutrition is essential for SCA. Because folic acid deficiency will exacerbate anemia and may lead to bone marrow depression from increased demands to replace RBCs, urge the patient to add folic acid-rich foods (leafy, green vegetables) to his diet. Also, remind him to avoid consuming alcohol and smoking cigarettes.

Discuss ways to maintain adequate hydration to minimize RBC sickling. Suggest that parents offer a child more fluids, such as eggnog, ice pops, and milk shakes.

Medication
Although drugs can't cure SCA, certain vaccines, anti-infectives, and chelating agents can minimize complications resulting from SCA or from possible transfusion therapy. Other medications, such as analgesics, may help to relieve the pain of vaso-occlusive crisis. Emphasize infection prevention measures—especially for a child with SCA. Tell parents that immunization against childhood diseases is a must, as is strict adherence to a prescribed medication regimen when an infection develops.

Vaccines. Discuss the advantages of polyvalent pneumococcal vaccine, which the child may receive at age 6 months and again at age 2 years. Add that he'll need booster vaccines every 4 years. Mention the *Haemophilus influenzae* B vaccine as another immunization to consider. Explain that the child usually receives this vaccine at age 15 months.

Anti-infective drugs. Review prophylactic anti-infective therapy. Low-dose oral penicillin administered twice daily until the child reaches age 6 may reduce his risk for pneumococcal infections. After age 6 this preventive measure may not be needed.

Although parents must understand the importance of complying with these measures, they should also realize that prophylaxis isn't foolproof. They'll still have to watch for early signs and symptoms of infection. Typically, appropriate antibiotic therapy will be prescribed to treat infections. Forewarn parents that the child may need to be hospitalized for antibiotic therapy.

Chelating agent. If a patient with SCA receives regular transfusions, he may require deferoxamine (Desferal), a chelating agent. This medication helps to remove dangerous iron deposits caused by repeated transfusions. The patient can take the drug at home, but first he or his parents will need detailed instructions on how to mix and administer it (subcutaneously or intravenously). Before giving these instructions, consult your institution's procedures manual and consult a hematology nurse.

Instruct the patient or his parents to contact the doctor as soon as possible if the following adverse reactions occur: dyspnea, hearing or visual impairment, pain at the injection site, or skin rash. Explain that the drug may color urine orange-red.

Uncommon crises in sickle cell anemia

Besides infection and vaso-occlusive crisis, other conditions pose a menace to the patient with sickle cell anemia (SCA). Help him or his caregiver to recognize the warning signs that require urgent medical attention.

Aplastic (megaloblastic) crisis
This condition results from bone marrow depression related to SCA. It's characterized by pallor, lethargy, sleepiness, dyspnea, and possibly coma. Clinical findings include markedly decreased bone marrow activity and red blood cell (RBC) hemolysis.

Acute sequestration crisis
Although rare, this can affect infants between the ages of 8 and 24 months. Without treatment, this sudden, massive entrapment of RBCs in the spleen and liver can lead to hypovolemic shock and death. Signs and symptoms include lethargy, increasing pallor, rapid pulse rate, shallow breathing, and abdominal pain.

Hemolytic crisis
This rare condition may affect patients who have SCA and glucose-6-phosphate dehydrogenase deficiency. Liver congestion and enlargement may result from degenerative changes. Signs and symptoms include jaundice and abdominal swelling and tenderness.

Analgesics. The patient with SCA may need medication to relieve pain, especially that related to vaso-occlusive crisis. Recommend acetaminophen. Or, if the doctor prescribes a narcotic analgesic, tell the patient to follow his instructions and to report persistent pain.

Other care measures
Because sickle cell disorders affect not only the patient but also those closest to him, make sure to offer guidelines for giving crisis care, maintaining emotional and physical support, and obtaining genetic and psychological counseling as needed.

Guide crisis care. Review the signs and symptoms of vaso-occlusive crisis so that the patient or his parents will recognize and treat it early. As appropriate, explain how to care for this condition at home, and provide a copy of the teaching aid *Managing vaso-occlusive crisis,* page 260.

Inform parents that an infant's first vaso-occlusive crisis may be called the "hand-foot crisis" because the infant's hands or feet, or both, swell and become painful. Advise them to begin home treatment measures but to call the doctor if symptoms persist or worsen.

If the patient must be hospitalized for a vaso-occlusive crisis, explain that I.V. fluids and parenteral analgesics may be given. Sometimes, the patient also may receive oxygen and blood transfusions.

Again, review symptoms that need immediate medical attention. For example, instruct parents of young children (ages 8 to 24 months) to report signs of acute sequestration crisis (see *Uncommon crises in sickle cell anemia*). Stress that this crisis, though rare, constitutes a medical emergency.

Other symptoms requiring urgent care include fever over 101° F. (38.3° C.), stiff neck, difficulty speaking or walking, numbness, weakness, or in infants, priapism.

Offer emotional support. Because delayed growth and late puberty are common among SCA patients, reassure adolescent patients that they will grow and mature. Tell them they should catch up with their friends by age 17 or 18.

Promote general health. Forewarn parents that urinary frequency may prevail. What's more, bedwetting may begin around age 6. Explain that this results not from disobedience or behavior problems, but from the SCA patient's inability to concentrate urine.

Encourage parents to schedule their child for a yearly eye examination to detect and treat retinal damage resulting from SCA.

Stress meticulous leg and foot care because leg ulcers commonly develop during the late teens.

Promote normal intellectual and social development by cautioning parents against overprotectiveness. Although the SCA patient must avoid strenuous exercise, he can safely enjoy most everyday activities.

Suggest counseling. Refer parents of children with SCA for genetic counseling to answer their questions about SCA in future offspring. Recommend screening for other family members to determine whether they're SCA carriers. Besides genetic counseling, parents may benefit from psychological counseling to help them cope with possible guilt feelings. Accordingly, suggest they join an appropriate support group.

Explain special situations. Discuss how special conditions, such as surgery or pregnancy (or both) may affect SCA patients.

Urge the patient to make sure all health care providers know that he has SCA before he undergoes any treatment—especially major surgery. That's because during any procedure that requires general anesthesia, the patient with SCA will need adequate ventilation to prevent hypoxic crisis. Urge the patient to wear medical identification stating that he has SCA.

Inform women that SCA makes pregnancy hazardous. Also hazardous to their health are oral contraceptives. If appropriate, refer female patients to a gynecologist for counseling. However, if the patient *does* become pregnant, offer guidelines for maintaining a balanced diet. Also suggest she ask her doctor about taking a folic acid supplement.

Acknowledge that in men with SCA, sudden, painful bouts of priapism may develop. Reassure the patient that these common episodes have no permanent harmful effects.

Finally, because SCA affects all body systems and many aspects of a patient's life-style, it requires multidisciplinary care involving hematologists, nurses, social workers, and other therapists. Encourage the patient to take full advantage of available resources.

Sources of information and support

National Association for Sickle Cell Disease
4221 Wilshire Boulevard, Suite 360, Los Angeles, Calif. 90010
(213) 936-7205

Sickle Cell Disease Foundation of Greater New York
One West 125th Street, Room 206, New York, N.Y. 10027
(212) 427-7762

Further readings

Burghardt-Fitzgerald, D.C. "Pain-Behavior Contracts: Effective Management of the Adolescent in Sickle-Cell Crisis," *Journal of Pediatric Nursing* 4(5):320-24, October 1989.

Davies, S. "Obstetric Implications of Sickle Cell Disease," *Midwife Health Visitor and Community Nurse* 24(9):361-63, September 1988.

Gibson, S. "Pediatric Management Problems: Hand Foot Syndrome of Sickle Cell Disease," *Pediatric Nursing* 13(6):418-19, November-December 1987.

Kirk, S.A. "Sickle Cell Disease and Health Education," *Midwife Health Visitor and Community Nurse* 23(5):200, 204, 206, May 1987.

Platt, A.F. Jr., and Eckman, J.R. "The Multidisciplinary Management of Pain in Patients with Sickle Cell Syndrome," *Journal of the American Academy of Physician Assistants* 2(2):104-13, March-April 1989.

Schechter, N., et al. "The Use of Patient-Controlled Analgesia in Adolescents with Sickle Pain Crisis: A Preliminary Report," *Journal of Pain Symptom Management* 3(2):109-13, Spring 1988.

Vichinsky, E., et al. "Newborn Screening for Sickle Cell Disease: Effect on Mortality," *Pediatrics* 81(6):749-55, June 1988.

Managing vaso-occlusive crisis

Dear Caregiver:

Because the person that you're caring for has sickle cell anemia, he's at risk for a serious complication called vaso-occlusive crisis. If this crisis occurs, the tips below can help you treat it and maybe prevent it from recurring.

What goes wrong?

In sickle cell anemia, some (*not all*) red blood cells change from a normally round shape to a sickle shape. When this happens, the sickled cells clog small blood vessels and keep blood from reaching vital organs. This condition, called vaso-occlusive crisis, causes pain and, possibly, cell damage.

Some things that cause a crisis are:
- infection, such as a cold or the flu
- dehydration — from not drinking enough fluid or from sweating, vomiting, or diarrhea
- low oxygen levels — for example, from a visit to the mountains
- temperature extremes.

Recognizing a crisis

Suspect a crisis if the person has:
- pain, especially in the stomach area, chest, muscles, or bones
- paleness, usually around the lips, tongue, and fingernails
- unusual sleepiness or irritability
- a low-grade fever that lasts 2 days
- dark urine.

Responding to a crisis

First, call the doctor and describe the person's symptoms. For a mild crisis, the doctor may suggest home care.

Here's how to help the person at home:
- Apply warm, moist compresses to painful areas. Cover the person with a blanket to prevent a chill. *Never* use ice packs or cold compresses. These could be harmful.
- Ease pain with acetaminophen (Panadol, Tylenol).
- Tell the person to stay in bed. Let him sit up if that's more comfortable.
- Make sure the person drinks lots of fluids so he doesn't get dehydrated.
- Call the doctor if symptoms persist or get worse.

Preventing a crisis

Although these precautions aren't fool-proof, they may help to prevent another crisis. Discuss these do's and don'ts with the person in your care.

Do's

- Stay up-to-date with immunizations.
- Prevent infections: Take meticulous care of wounds, eat well-balanced meals, have regular dental checkups, and learn proper tooth and gum care.
- Seek treatment for any infection.
- Drink fluids at the first sign of a cold or other infection.

Don'ts

- Avoid tight clothing that could block circulation.
- Never exercise strenuously or excessively. This could trigger a crisis.
- Avoid drinking lots of ice water or exposing yourself to sizzling hot or freezing cold temperatures.
- Steer clear of mountain climbing, unpressurized aircraft, and high altitudes.

Rheumatoid arthritis

Afflicted with an insidious, chronic, and painful disorder, the patient with rheumatoid arthritis (RA) can easily become discouraged. However, you can help him overcome this feeling by pointing out that effective treatments for inflammation and joint pain do indeed exist. Discovering what best meets his individual needs may take time, though. As a result, you'll need to motivate the patient to experiment with self-care measures and assistive devices.

Your teaching should include an explanation of how the disease occurs. You'll also want to teach him about blood and synovial fluid tests and X-rays. What's more, you'll need to point out the significance of medication, diet, and a balanced program of exercise and rest. In severe RA, you may need to discuss surgery.

Discuss the disorder

Early on, the patient may experience pain, tenderness, swelling, or stiffness in the synovial joints—the shoulder, elbow, wrist, hand, hip, knee, and foot. Explain that he has a chronic, systemic inflammatory disorder. Difficult to predict, it may progress slowly or rapidly. The patient can expect exacerbations and remissions.

What causes RA? No one knows for sure. Researchers suspect that it involves an autoimmune response to the patient's own immunoglobulin G (IgG). Apparently, synovial lymphocytes (B cells) produce IgG that acts as an antigen. The immune system fails to recognize the IgG antibodies as self, stimulating an immune response within the joint. The production of anti-IgG antibodies (rheumatoid factors) stimulates formation of immune complexes in the synovium. These complexes initiate and sustain an inflammatory response (see *Understanding rheumatoid arthritis,* page 262).

Subsequently, pannus—formation and thickening of the synovial membranes—develops. Inflammation may spread to cartilage, tendons, ligaments, and, eventually, bone. The patient may suffer joint deformities, subluxations, contractures, pain, and loss of function.

Complications

Warn the patient that improperly treated RA can lead to excruciating joint pain. If he fails to follow his drug regimen, irreversible joint damage and severe deformities may occur. If he fails to follow his prescribed exercise program, muscle strength and joint

Lynne Kreutzer-Baraglia, RN, MS, and **Beverly A. Post, RN, MS, CIC,** contributed to this chapter. Ms. Kreutzer-Baraglia is an assistant professor at West Suburban College of Nursing, Oak Park, Ill. Ms. Post is a risk manager and infection control manager at Louis A. Weiss Memorial Hospital, Chicago.

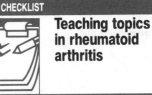

CHECKLIST

Teaching topics in rheumatoid arthritis

☐ Description of rheumatoid arthritis
☐ Explanation of its suspected cause
☐ Importance of complying with treatment to prevent complications
☐ Preparation for blood tests and, if ordered, synovial fluid analysis
☐ Administration of salicylates or other medication, such as nonsteroidal anti-inflammatory drugs
☐ A balanced program of rest and activity, with tips for improving quality of sleep
☐ Exercise program
☐ Dietary considerations, including devices to ease meal preparation
☐ Surgical options, when appropriate
☐ Use of good body mechanics and assistive devices
☐ Application of heat or cold
☐ Discussion of sexual activity and alternative treatments
☐ Sources of information and support.

Understanding rheumatoid arthritis

What causes the pain and swelling of rheumatoid arthritis?

Begin your explanation by describing to the patient the structure of a normal joint. Illustrate for him the location of the synovium. This is the inner layer of an articular capsule that surrounds a freely movable joint and that secretes the thick fluid which normally lubricates the joint.

Next, explain how rheumatoid arthritis is characterized by an autoimmune response. Synovial lymphocytes (B cells) produce IgG, which acts as an antigen. This stimulates an immune response within the joint, with the production of anti-IgG antibodies (rheumatoid factors) leading to the formation of immune complexes.

The immune complexes activate the classic and alternative complement system. This activation initiates the inflammatory response, which results in progressive enlargement and thickening of the synovium and damage to cartilage and bone.

JOINT STRUCTURE

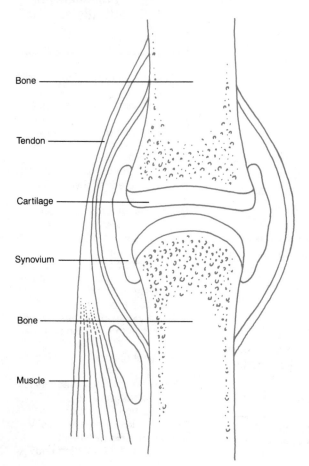

Bone

Tendon

Cartilage

Synovium

Bone

Muscle

DEVELOPMENT OF RHEUMATOID ARTHRITIS

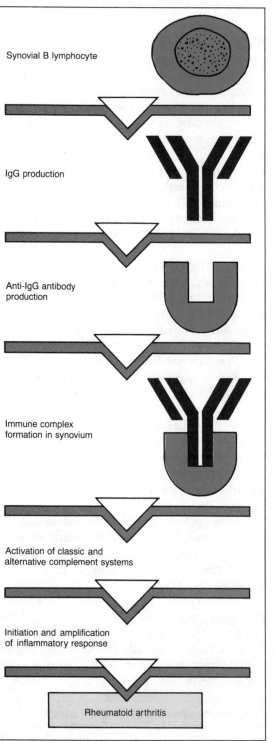

Synovial B lymphocyte

IgG production

Anti-IgG antibody production

Immune complex formation in synovium

Activation of classic and alternative complement systems

Initiation and amplification of inflammatory response

Rheumatoid arthritis

mobility may be reduced. Weakness in hip flexor and quadriceps muscles can also lead to gait problems, demanding extra energy and placing further stress on other joints.

Describe the diagnostic workup

Teach the patient about three blood tests: rheumatoid factor (RF), erythrocyte sedimentation rate (ESR), and complete blood count (CBC). Each requires a small blood sample. The RF test, which detects anti-IgG antibodies, is positive in about 80% of RA patients. The ESR may detect inflammation, whereas the CBC can detect anemia, a frequent finding in RA. No single blood test provides a conclusive diagnosis.

Also teach the patient about synovial fluid analysis, which helps determine the cause of joint inflammation and swelling. Describe the aspiration process: A needle is inserted, usually in the knee joint, to obtain a fluid sample. Aspiration may decrease pain and prevent joint destruction. Warn the patient that although he will be given a local anesthetic, he may feel temporary discomfort when the needle penetrates the joint. He should report any increased pain or fever (indications of joint infection) experienced afterward.

Because X-rays of affected joints help to assess damage, tell the patient that he may undergo repeat X-rays at varying intervals to monitor bone erosion and joint deformity.

Teach about treatments

Your goal is to impart the knowledge and skills needed to effectively manage a chronic illness. Emphasize that the patient's well-being depends on his willingness to comply with the treatment regimen and thereby prevent worsening pain and deformity.

Activity

Highlight the importance of balancing activity with rest. Recommend sleeping 8 to 10 hours a night and lying down for ½ hour twice each day. If the patient experiences a flare-up, advise him to simplify his schedule. Tell him that it's appropriate to ask for help with daily tasks.

Counsel the patient who can't sleep well because of pain (see *Tips for getting a good night's sleep*). Tell him to maintain correct body position during rest, with joints extended rather than flexed. Advise using a firm mattress supported by a bed board and a small, flat pillow. If splints are prescribed, tell the patient to wear them in bed and whenever possible during the day. Caution against placing a pillow under his knees, which fosters joint deformity. Impress on the patient the importance of using good body mechanics at all times (see *A joint effort,* page 271).

Encourage the patient to pace himself and to set realistic goals for activities. How can he know when it's time to slow down? He may experience increased pain or fatigue and progressive loss of dexterity in involved joints. If pain lasts for 2 hours or

---

Tips for getting a good night's sleep

The patient with rheumatoid arthritis needs adequate sleep in addition to resting between activities. Tell him that if he can get a good night's sleep, his arthritic pain may be reduced during the day.

Provide these tips:
- Go to bed each night at the same time and awake each day at the same time.
- Participate in regular exercise.
- Avoid eating large meals before going to bed.
- Avoid caffeine and alcohol before going to bed.
- Try not to use over-the-counter medications to go to sleep.
- Learn deep-breathing and relaxation exercises.
- Focus on a mental image of a pleasant place or event before falling asleep.
- If sleep problems persist, consult the doctor.

Energy-saving tips

The patient with rheumatoid arthritis needs to conserve his energy. Suggest that he:
• use dressing aids, including a long-handled shoehorn, a reacher, elastic shoelaces, a zipper pull, and a buttonhook.
• wear mittens, if he has trouble putting his fingers into gloves.
• use helpful household items, such as a hand-held shower nozzle, hand rails, grab bars, and easy-to-open drawers.
• keep needed materials, utensils, and tools organized and handy.
• when possible, sit down while performing activities that may tire him, such as dressing or cooking, to prevent stress on weight-bearing joints.

more after completing a task, the patient should do a little less the next time or find ways to simplify his effort (see *Energy-saving tips*).

Exercise. What can exercise do for the patient? First of all, it can make flexing and extending joints easier, reduce pain and stiffness, and help prevent loss of joint function. It may even help him regain joint function.

Recommend that an exercise program become part of the patient's daily routine. Remind him to consult with his doctor or therapist before beginning. Underscore the importance of staying within reasonable limits; an exercise program shouldn't be too difficult in light of his condition. Warn against strenuous exercise during acute inflammatory episodes. If the patient experiences muscle cramping or pain while exercising, advise him to stop exercising and gently massage the cramped muscle. When symptoms diminish, he can resume activity. Encourage him to take advantage of moments when he has the least pain and stiffness and the most energy and when his medication achieves its peak effect (see *Restoring strength and relieving pain,* pages 272 and 273).

Discuss the significance of therapeutic and recreational exercise. Therapeutic exercises are prescribed by a doctor or physical or occupational therapist to meet the patient's individual needs with maximum efficiency. A therapeutic program may include range-of-motion exercises to facilitate joint mobility and flexibility and strengthening exercises.

Eating better means living better

For the patient with rheumatoid arthritis, a healthful diet takes on a special significance.

If the patient is overweight, diplomatically inform him that he's placing extra stress on his joints, which can lead to further pain and damage. Help motivate him to lose weight until he reaches his ideal weight. Instruct him to eat slowly, take smaller portions, and avoid seconds.

Discuss how the patient prepares food. Instruct him to broil or bake using water or meat or vegetable juices rather than butter or oil. To lessen excess fat, he should trim fat from meats and remove skin from poultry.

Instruct the patient to limit the following foods:

• butter, cream, lard, shortening, hard cheeses like cheddar, and margarine
• salt and sugar
• caffeine
• alcohol
• high-fat baked goods
• fried foods.
   Tell the patient he can eat these foods freely:
• fresh fruits
• vegetables, especially raw ones
• fish and poultry (low in fat and high in protein)
• lean red meat (high in iron)
• whole-grain breads and cereals (iron-enriched, the extra fiber will help satisfy the patient)
• low-fat milk, cheese, and yogurt.

Recreational exercises, such as group exercises, sports, games, crafts, and hobbies, can help maintain or improve strength, joint mobility, and endurance. However, they cannot substitute for a therapeutic exercise program. A local Arthritis Foundation chapter may be able to recommend a group exercise program adapted for people with arthritis.

Diet

Communicate the importance of a balanced diet. Foods high in vitamins, proteins, and iron promote tissue building and repair. Make sure the patient knows how to select among the four basic food groups to meet daily requirements. Advise frequent, small meals if his appetite is poor (see *Eating better means living better*).

Teach techniques for making meal preparation easier. Tell the patient to plan breaks between cooking chores. When symptoms become severe, convenience foods may offer the best bet. Promote the use of assistive devices and appliances (see *Kitchen helpers*, pages 274 and 275).

Medication

The patient should understand that drug therapy aims to control inflammation and pain and arrest RA's progress. Achieving this may require several types of drugs:

• *Anti-inflammatory drugs* reduce inflammation, thereby diminishing pain. Nonsteroidal anti-inflammatory drugs work by blocking prostaglandin synthesis. (Prostaglandins precipitate the inflammatory response, which includes edema, pain, warmth, and redness at the site of tissue injury.) Corticosteroids inhibit the immune response by suppressing or preventing cell-mediated immune reactions.

• *Disease-modifying agents,* such as gold compounds and antimalarials, slow the disease process.

• *Immunosuppressants,* such as azathioprine, methotrexate, and cyclophosphamide, inhibit the autoimmune response seen in RA. Because immunosuppressant therapy heightens the risk of severe infection, teach the patient infection control measures.

For more information, see *Teaching patients about rheumatoid arthritis drugs,* pages 266 and 267.

To help the patient remember his medication schedule, devise a medication calendar. Urge him to notify the doctor if symptoms worsen during therapy. If he has weak or deformed hands or if moving them hurts, suggest that he ask his pharmacist not to use childproof caps. If appropriate, provide a copy of the patient-teaching aid *Learning about naproxen,* page 276.

Surgery

Joint surgery may relieve pain, increase mobility, and improve appearance. Explain to the patient relevant surgical procedures, which may include:

• synovectomy—removal of the synovium to reduce pain and swelling.

continued on page 268

INQUIRY

Questions patients ask about arthritis treatments

Should I be taking "arthritis-strength" aspirin?
Over-the-counter drugs advertised as "arthritis-strength" are really just more expensive versions of the regular-strength drug sold under the same product name. These products contain larger doses of the drug, but that doesn't make them more effective in relieving pain. However, because you need to take fewer tablets per dose, this convenience may be worth the extra cost.

Will I benefit from using ointments and liniments?
Ointments and liniments depend on skin irritants, such as oil of wintergreen, for their effects. When applied, these external analgesics increase blood flow to the upper layers of your skin, resulting in redness, a warm sensation, and increased skin temperature. They provide brief relief. Be aware that substances contained in these products are absorbed through the skin, and can cause problems if used too often.

How effective are the diets advertised to cure arthritis?
There's no scientific evidence that any diet, food, or vitamin can cure rheumatoid arthritis. If you're overweight and your hips, knees, ankles, or feet are affected by arthritis, then losing weight can help you. You'll feel less pain and reduce stress on weight-bearing joints.

Teaching patients about rheumatoid arthritis drugs

DRUG	ADVERSE REACTIONS	PATIENT-TEACHING POINTS
Anti-inflammatory agents		
Aspirin and salicylates **aspirin** (Bayer) **aspirin combinations** (Anacin, Excedrin) **buffered aspirin** (Bufferin) **enteric-coated aspirin** (Ecotrin)	• Watch for gastric distress, hearing loss, hyperventilation, nausea and vomiting, and tinnitus. • Other reactions include confusion, diaphoresis, and thirst.	• Warn the patient not to substitute acetaminophen for a salicylate. He shouldn't take additional aspirin or over-the-counter products that contain salicylates while on this medication. • Warn against taking antacids, nonsteroidal anti-inflammatory drugs, or alcohol. • If the drug causes GI distress, advise him to take each dose with food or a full glass of water. • Warn him against crushing or chewing enteric-coated aspirin. • Tell him to report symptoms of GI bleeding to his doctor.
Nonsteroidal anti-inflammatory drugs		
diclofenac (Voltaren) **ibuprofen** (Motrin) **naproxen** (Naprosyn) **piroxicam** (Feldene)	• Watch for blurred vision, diarrhea, dizziness, drowsiness, fluid retention, heartburn, hematuria, indigestion, nausea, sore throat, tinnitus, vertigo, vomiting, and wheezing. • Other reactions include cystitis and decreased visual acuity.	• Warn the patient not to take this medication with aspirin, alcohol or over-the-counter products that contain aspirin. • If he experiences GI distress, tell him to take his medication with meals. He may use antacids with a doctor's approval. • Advise him to limit salt intake. These drugs can cause fluid retention. • Explain that he may not notice improvement for at least a month after beginning treatment.
Corticosteroids		
prednisone (Deltasone, Orasone)	• Watch for abdominal pain, acne, hypertension, marked weight gain, melena, menstrual irregularity, mental status changes, unusual tiredness and vomiting. • Other reactions include back or rib pain, diaphoresis, easy bruising, fever, increased facial and body hair, mild mood swings, mild nausea, and sore throat.	• Explain to the patient that corticosteroids can cause widespread adverse reactions. Emphasize, however, that reactions are unlikely with short-term administration, even at high doses. • Advise him to avoid products containing aspirin or other salicylates, over-the-counter drugs containing sodium, and alcohol. • Tell him to take the drug with food or milk to decrease risk of GI irritation. Low-sodium antacids, such as Maalox, may help prevent GI distress. • Advise the patient on long-term therapy to wear a medical identification tag or carry a wallet card. • Urge him to notify other health care providers, such as his dentist, of his therapy. • Tell the patient taking a single daily dose to take it early in the morning. He should take a missed dose upon remembering it, but not the next day. Warn him not to double dose. • If the patient taking a divided daily dose misses one portion, tell him to take the next dose on schedule. • Tell the patient taking an alternate-day dose not to take a missed dose if he remembers that same day. Instead, he should take the missed dose the next morning, skip a day, then resume alternate-day therapy.
Disease-modifying agents		
Gold salts **auranofin** (Ridaura) **aurothioglucose** (Solganal) **gold sodium thiomalate** (Myochrysine)	• Watch for bleeding and infection, dermatitis, diffuse glossitis, GI disturbances (with auranofin), edema, gingivitis, intestinal pneumatosis, metallic taste (preceding diffuse glossitis or gingivitis), pulmonary fibrosis, rash, stomatitis, upper respiratory tract inflammation, vaginitis, and weight gain. • Other reactions include conjunctivitis and skin pigmentation.	• Explain that his medication may take several months to work. • Tell him to prevent possible renal damage by avoiding over-the-counter nonsteroidal anti-inflammatory drugs, such as ibuprofen. • To prevent inducing or aggravating gold-induced dermatitis, advise him to avoid exposure to sunlight. • To treat mild mouth ulcers, suggest a mouth rinse of 1 teaspoon of salt in 8 oz of water. Advocate good oral hygiene. • Explain that he must undergo frequent blood tests to monitor drug toxicity.

continued

Teaching patients about rheumatoid arthritis drugs — *continued*

DRUG	ADVERSE REACTIONS	PATIENT-TEACHING POINTS
Disease-modifying agents — *continued*		
Antimalarials **chloroquine** (Aralen) **hydroxychloroquine** (Plaquenil)	• Watch for diarrhea, heartburn, indigestion, nausea and vomiting, tinnitus, and visual disturbances. • Other reactions include anxiety, dizziness, and weakness.	• Warn the patient to avoid alcohol. • Stress the importance of regular eye exams during therapy. • Advise taking his medication with food to lessen GI distress. • Remind him to report any unusual disturbances, such as tinnitus.
penicillamine (Cuprimine, Depen)	• Watch for bleeding, bruising, GI disturbances, generalized pruritus and rashes, infection, kidney dysfunction (proteinuria, hematuria), tinnitus, visual disturbances, and weight gain. • Other reactions include asthma, alopecia, hot flashes, pulmonary fibrosis, and thrombophlebitis.	• Tell the patient not to take iron or iron preparations within 2 hours of penicillamine. Doing so may impair the drug's effectiveness. • Advise him to take the drug on an empty stomach — 1 hour before or 3 hours after meals. • Tell him that complete blood and platelet counts will be done twice a month for the first three months of therapy and then once every month.
Immunosuppressants		
azathioprine (Imuran)	• Watch for bleeding gums, blood in stools, easy bruising, fever, hemorrhaging, lowered resistance to infection, nausea and vomiting (in the first few months of therapy) and sore throat. • Other reactions include alopecia, diarrhea, and rash.	• If the patient experiences GI upset, advise him to take azathioprine with food and in divided doses. • Stress the need for scrupulous oral and personal hygiene. • Tell him to avoid crowds and people who have infections. • Urge him to postpone immunizations until after therapy. • Warn female patients of childbearing age to avoid becoming pregnant during and up to 4 months after therapy. • Emphasize that prescribed laboratory tests and periodic monitoring by the doctor are essential. • Stress the importance of notifying the doctor of any untoward reactions.
cyclophosphamide (Cytoxan)	• Watch for agitation, amenorrhea, chills, confusion, cough, dizziness, edema, fever; lower back, side, or stomach pain; shortness of breath; tachycardia; tiredness; unusual bleeding or bruising; and weakness. • Other reactions include black, tarry stools; frequent urination; sores in mouth and on lips; unusual thirst; and yellow eyes or skin.	• Tell the patient to drink at least 2½ quarts of fluid a day and to urinate as often as possible. • Suggest that he avoid coffee and tea, which have a diuretic effect. • Advise him to take his medication early in the day and to urinate before going to bed. • Stress the need for scrupulous oral and personal hygiene. • Tell him to avoid crowds and people who have infections. • Urge him to postpone immunizations until after therapy. • Warn female patients of childbearing age to avoid becoming pregnant during and up to 4 months after therapy. • Emphasize that prescribed laboratory tests and periodic monitoring by the doctor are essential. • Stress the importance of notifying the doctor of any untoward reactions.
methotrexate (Folex, Mexate)	• Watch for acute pneumonitis with fever, cough, and shortness of breath; alopecia; clay-colored stools; dark urine; diarrhea; nausea and vomiting; photosensitivity; stomach pain; stomatitis; unusual bleeding or bruising; and yellow eyes or skin. • Other reactions include back pain, blurred vision, dizziness, drowsiness, headache, seizures, and unusual tiredness or weakness.	• Teach the patient the symptoms of liver dysfunction and explain the importance of avoiding alcoholic beverages. • Tell him that he may have to undergo frequent blood tests and liver function studies before and during therapy. • Encourage fluid intake to prevent renal damage. • Advise him to wear sunglasses and use sun block when appropriate. • Stress the importance of reporting cough, fever, and shortness of breath to the doctor. • Stress the need for scrupulous oral and personal hygiene. • Tell him to avoid crowds and people who have infections. • Urge him to postpone immunizations until after therapy. • Warn female patients of childbearing age to avoid becoming pregnant during and up to 4 months after therapy. • Stress the importance of notifying the doctor of any untoward reactions.

Sex matters

Feeling himself less attractive and less agile, the rheumatoid arthritis patient may believe he has lost his ability to have an enjoyable sex life. Create an opportunity to discuss family and social life. Talking openly about his sexual concerns can prove a great help.

First, make it clear that he's not alone in his fears and that information is available: guidelines for adapting sexual positions to arthritic needs do indeed exist.

But what should you say to the patient who wants to know more—now? Start by encouraging him to plan for pleasure. He should schedule sexual activity for when he feels best. Pacing his daily activities will help him to avoid fatigue.

To relax joints before sex, tell the patient to perform range-of-motion exercises and take a warm bath or shower. Taking analgesics beforehand will help to relieve joint pain.

When making love, the patient will need to try out different positions so he can find those that put less strain on painful joints. Suppose, for instance, a patient has hip or knee involvement. He can try making love while lying on his back, using pillows for support. His partner can lie on top of him, supporting her weight with her elbows and knees. Another example: A woman with severe contractures may try lying on her back with her knees flexed during intercourse.

Of course, you'll tailor this teaching to the patient's learning needs and his sensitivities. However, your message will remain the same: if the patient's willing to make adaptations, rheumatoid arthritis needn't prevent him from having and enjoying sex.

• osteotomy—cutting and resetting a bone to correct a deformity.
• resection—removal of a bone or part of a bone, frequently performed on the feet to increase comfort when walking.
• arthrodesis—bone fusion to diminish pain.
• arthroplasty—repairing or replacing joints to reduce pain and increase flexibility and mobility (see *Teaching about joint replacement*).

Urge the patient to comply with his prescribed postsurgical regimen—his recovery may well depend on it. Physical therapy constitutes a key part of this regimen. Tell him that he'll experience pain early on during therapy; however, it will be muscle, not joint, pain. Assure him that it will lessen with time. Depending on the type of surgery, he may have to prepare for several months of therapy.

Other care measures

Coping with RA can be made easier by learning about proper clothing and heat and cold therapy.

Clothing. Because cold drafts can cause muscle tension, tell the patient to wear warm clothing. If arthritis affects the patient's feet, he may relieve pain by inserting special pads or metatarsal bars in his shoes. A severe foot deformity may call for custom-made shoes.

Heat and cold therapy. Applying heat and cold locally may relieve pain and inflammation. Applying heat before exercising will also relieve stiffness.

Encourage the patient to experiment to determine what works best for him. Discourage him from purchasing costly devices for applying heat or cold; home methods usually prove effective.

For moist heat, suggest standing in a warm shower, soaking in a tub, or applying wet towels to stiff or painful joints. Tell the patient that mild heat will produce results; it should feel soothing, not hot.

For dry heat, recommend wrapping a heating pad in a towel before placing it against the skin. If the patient has diminished sensation, tell him never to set the heating pad on the highest setting, and to check often for burns. Advise using heat for about 20 minutes to achieve full benefit.

For cold application, suggest using moist towels or ice packs for 10 to 15 minutes. To make an ice pack, the patient can fill a plastic bag with crushed ice.

The patient may benefit from using a combination of heat and cold. Instruct the patient to first soak his hands or feet in warm water (110° F. [43° C.]) for about 3 minutes and then soak them in cold water (65° F. [18° C.]) for about a minute. He should repeat this process three times, ending with warm water.

Addressing patient concerns. Because arthritis changes the way he looks and moves, the patient may need reassurance that he can still enjoy a satisfying sexual relationship (see *Sex matters*). Advise the woman of childbearing age with RA to let her doctor

Teaching about joint replacement

Your patient may receive total or partial replacement of a joint with a synthetic prosthesis to restore stability and relieve pain. Joint replacement may also provide an increased sense of independence and self-worth. The illustrations below depict common joint replacement sites.

Preparing the patient for recovery
Get the patient ready for the lengthy postoperative recovery and rehabilitation period. He'll probably remain in bed for up to 6 days after surgery. Explain that even while he's confined to bed, he'll begin an exercise program to maintain joint mobility. As appropriate, show him range-of-motion exercises or demonstrate the continuous passive motion device that he'll use during recovery.

Point out that he may not experience pain relief after surgery and that in fact pain may actually worsen for several weeks. Reassure him that pain will diminish dramatically once edema subsides. Emphasize that analgesics will be available as needed.

Preparing the patient for home care
Reinforce the exercise regimen prescribed by the doctor and physical therapists. Remind the patient to adhere closely to his schedule and not to rush rehabilitation, no matter how good he feels.

Review prescribed limitations on activity. Depending on the location and extent of surgery, the doctor may order the patient to avoid bending or lifting, extensive stair climbing, and sitting for prolonged periods (including long car trips or plane flights). He'll also caution against overusing the joint, especially if it's a weight-bearing one.

Caution the patient to promptly report signs of possible infection, such as persistent fever and increased pain, tenderness, and stiffness in the joint and surrounding area. Remind him that infection may develop several months after joint replacement.

Tell the patient to report a sudden increase of pain, which may indicate dislodgment of the prosthesis.

ELBOW REPLACEMENT

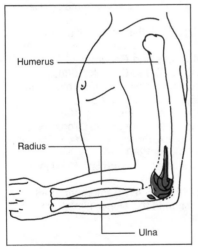

FINGER JOINT REPLACEMENTS

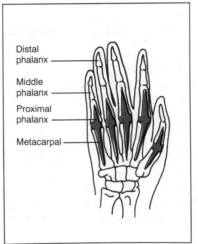

TOTAL HIP REPLACEMENT

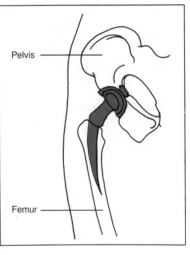

SHOULDER REPLACEMENT

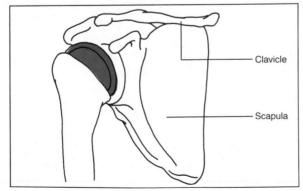

KNEE REPLACEMENT

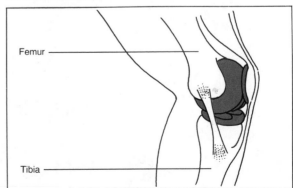

Straight talk about alternative treatments

Like it or not, most arthritis patients will try one or more unproven remedies. Any unproven remedy, no matter how seemingly benign, can cause harm if it provides an excuse to neglect prescribed therapy.

Impress on the patient that repeated scientific studies have failed to prove the efficacy of these remedies. Many in fact are known to be unsafe. Warn him never to substitute an unproven remedy for his therapeutic regimen.

Some remedies for arthritis are considered harmless. These include:
● acupuncture
● copper bracelets
● mineral springs
● topical creams
● vibrators
● vinegar and honey.

Other remedies, however, have proved to be harmful. These include:
● dimethyl sulfoxide (DMSO)
● large doses of vitamins
● snake venom.

Still other remedies haven't had their safety established. These include:
● bee venom
● biofeedback
● dietary changes
● fish oil
● laser treatments
● vaccines
● yucca.

know if she plans to become pregnant. He may adjust her medication dosage.

Discussing alternative cures. Make it clear that RA has no miracle cures despite claims to the contrary. Encourage the patient to notify you, his doctor, or the local chapter of the Arthritis Foundation *before* trying any alternative treatment (see *Straight talk about alternative treatments*).

Sources of information and support

American Rheumatism Association
17 Executive Drive, NE, Suite 480, Atlanta, Ga. 30329
(404) 633-3777

Arthritis Foundation
1314 Spring Street, SW, Atlanta, Ga. 30309
(404) 872-7100

Association for People with Arthritis
Six Commercial Street, P.O. Box 954, Hicksville, N.Y. 11802
(800) 323-2243

Further readings

Agnew, P.J. "Joint Protection in Arthritis: Fact or Fiction?" *British Journal of Occupational Therapy* 50(7):227-30, July 1987.
"Arthritis & Self Care: The Patient's Role in Disease Management," *Caring:* 18-25, January 1989.
Arthritis Foundation. *Exercise & Your Arthritis.* Atlanta: Arthritis Foundation, 1987.
Crosby, L.J. "Stress Factors, Emotional Stress and Rheumatoid Arthritis Activity," *Journal of Advanced Nursing* 13(4):452-61, July 1988.
Docken, W.P., et al. "Rheumatologic Causes of Pain: Rheumatoid Arthritis," *Hospital Practice* 23(1):57-61, 65, January 15, 1988.
"Empty Promises," *Arthritis Today:* 12-19, January-February 1989.
Fairleigh, A., et al. "Post-operative Metacarpophalangeal Arthroplasty: Dynamic Splint for Patients with Rheumatoid Arthritis," *Canadian Journal of Occupational Therapy* 55(3):141-46, June 1988.
Mate, C., et al. "Cervical Myopathy in Rheumatoid Arthritis," *Nursing Times* 83(40):71-72, October 7-13, 1987.
"Rheumatoid Arthritis," *Medical Times* 116(9):45-47, September 1988.
Wadsworth, T.G., et al. "Joint Reconstruction in the Upper Limb," *Physiotherapy* 73(12):679-84, December 1987.

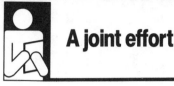

A joint effort

Dear Patient:

You can help to protect your joints from injury by following these guidelines.

Using your strengths
Use your largest and strongest joints. When stirring a pot, for example, use your elbow and whole arm instead of just relying on your wrist and hand to do the work. Support weak or painful joints as much as possible.

When using stairs, lead with your stronger leg going up and your weaker leg going down.

If you carry a purse, place its strap over your shoulder rather than carry it in your hand. This will help protect a painful elbow or wrist or painful fingers.

Sitting and standing
Sit in a straight-backed chair that is high enough for your feet to remain flat on the floor. This will help relieve joint stress. Consider buying a raised seat for your toilet so you can get up more easily.

Avoid bending, stooping, or holding the same position for a long time.

Pushing
Push open a heavy door with the side of your arm, not with your hand and outstretched arm.

Grasping and lifting
When grasping an object, put your hands near the center of your body. This will let you draw strength from your whole body, not just from your hands and arms.

When lifting an object that's low or on the ground, bend your knees and lift with your back straight. This spreads the

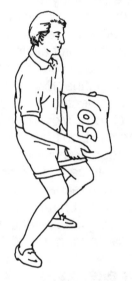

weight of the object over many joints, instead of just relying on your hands, wrists, and elbows. Whenever possible, slide objects instead of lifting them.

Carry heavy loads in your arms instead of gripping them with your fingers or hands. Use both palms to lift and hold cups, plates, pots, and pans, rather than gripping them with your fingers or only one hand.

Straightening
Keep your fingers stretched out, instead of bent in, as much as possible. This will help prevent exaggerating deformities. Bend your knuckles as briefly as possible to hold objects.

Spread your hand flat over a sponge or rag instead of squeezing it with your fingers.

Restoring strength and relieving pain

Dear Patient:

Don't underestimate the benefits of exercise. Done regularly, it can help you overcome the pain and stiffness of rheumatoid arthritis, restore and maintain strength, and limber up your joints. It can also improve your circulation.

Develop a routine. Perform 5 to 10 repetitions of selected exercises once or twice each day. Move in a slow, steady manner. Don't bounce. If a joint is inflamed, gently move it as much as you comfortably can. Have someone help you, if necessary.

Don't hold your breath during exercise. Instead, slowly breathe in and out. You may count out loud.

Shoulder exercises
Try these two exercises for your shoulders.

1 Lie on your back. Raise one arm over your head, keeping your elbow straight and your arm close to your ear. Then return your arm slowly to your side. Repeat with your other arm.

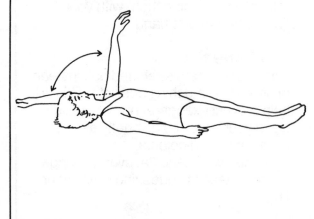

2 While standing, place your hands behind your head. Move your elbows back as far as you can. As you move your elbows back, tilt your head back. Return to the starting position and repeat.

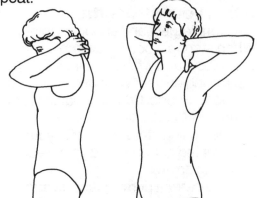

Knee and hip exercises
Try these five exercises for your knees and hips.

1 Lie on your back with one knee bent. Keep the other leg as straight as possible. Now bend the knee of the straight leg and bring it toward your chest. Push the leg into the air and then lower it to the floor. Repeat, using the other leg.

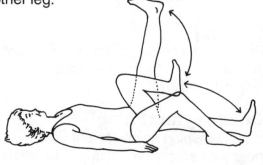

continued

PATIENT-TEACHING AID

Restoring strength and relieving pain — *continued*

2 Lie on your back with your legs as straight as possible, about 6 inches apart. Keep your toes pointed up. Roll one hip and knee from side to side, keeping your knees straight. Repeat with your other hip and knee.

3 To strengthen your knees even more, try this. While lying on your back with both legs out straight, try to push the back of your knee against the floor. Then tighten the muscle on the front of your thigh. Hold it tight and slowly count to 5. Relax. Repeat with the other knee.

4 Lie on your back with your legs straight and about 6 inches apart. Point your toes up. Slide one leg out to the side and return. Try to keep your toes pointing up. Repeat with your other leg.

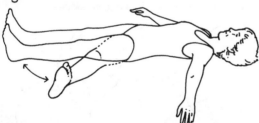

5 Sit in a chair that is high enough for you to swing your leg. Keep your thigh on the chair and straighten your knee. Hold a few seconds. Then, bend your knee back as far as possible. Repeat with the other knee.

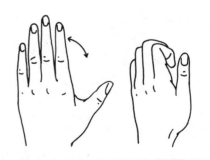

Ankle exercise
While sitting, keep your heels on the floor and lift your toes as high as possible. Then lower your toes to the floor and lift your heels as high as possible. Lower your heels and repeat.

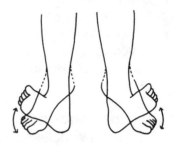

Thumb exercise
Open your hand and straighten your fingers. Reach your thumb across your palm until it touches the base of your little finger. Stretch your thumb out and repeat. Repeat with the other thumb.

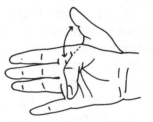

Finger exercise
Open your hand, with fingers straight. Bending all the finger joints except the knuckles, touch the top of your palm with your fingertips. Open your hand and repeat.

Kitchen helpers

Dear Patient:

Adjusting to arthritis needn't mean giving up the satisfaction of accomplishing daily tasks, such as preparing meals. To help you around the kitchen, select from this menu of assistive devices and appliances:

Counter-top appliances

Appliances such as slow cookers and toaster ovens can eliminate the bending required when cooking with an oven. Another energy-conserving tip: Obtain a wheeled dolly or plant stand for moving heavy items across counters.

Cutting board

Simple modifications to a cutting board can make chopping and slicing easier. The example here comes with suction cups underneath to hold it firmly to the counter or table. You can drive a few rustproof nails into the board to prevent food from sliding off (corks can be placed over the nails when not in use). Consider attaching a raised lip along one edge of the board to secure bread for buttering.

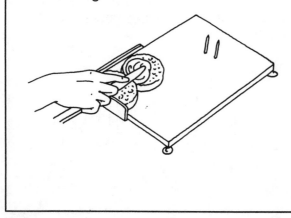

Cookware

Use lightweight plastic dishes and aluminum pots and pans. Double-handled pots and pans will enable you to lift with both hands.

Knives

If you have a good grasp, you may want to try the rocker knife. As you rock its handle up and down, the sharp, curved blade slices through the food.

If your grasp is weak, consider the quad knife. This knife also cuts with a rocking motion, but you don't have to grasp its handle firmly.

If you have use of only one hand, try the rolling knife, which is similar to a pizza cutter.

QUAD KNIFE   ROLLING KNIFE

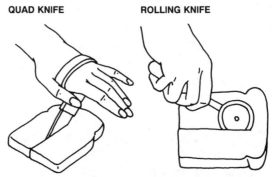

Utility brush

A brush with suction cups on its base may help to clean vegetables or fruit or to scour silverware. Wet the suction cups and then secure the brush to the sink. To remove it, slide it up the side of the sink.

You can also use utility brushes to clean dentures or scrub your nails.

continued

Kitchen helpers — *continued*

Peelers

For peeling vegetables or fruit, a floating blade peeler is safer than a knife. To make it easier to grasp, you can build up the handle. You can also fasten the peeler to a metal clamp, as shown here. Or use a large-loop peeler if your fingers are stiff or weak.

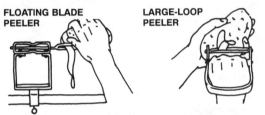

FLOATING BLADE PEELER

LARGE-LOOP PEELER

Bowl holder and nonskid mats

A metal or wooden bowl holder can help you keep a bowl level and steady for mixing, or on its side for scraping and pouring, as shown here.

Placing a nonskid rubber or plastic mat under a bowl will keep it steady. You can also place a mat under a jar to make its lid easier to twist off.

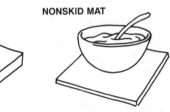

BOWL HOLDER

NONSKID MAT

Graters

A grater with a wooden support can be fixed to the wall, allowing you to use the grater with one hand. Or you can use a grater that fits on a support and nails driven into a cutting board.

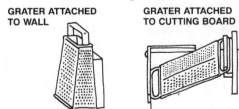

GRATER ATTACHED TO WALL

GRATER ATTACHED TO CUTTING BOARD

Draining aids

Several aids can help you safely pour hot liquid from cooking pots. A lock-on lid that clamps onto the pot will enable you to drain liquid using one hand.

You can also use a bulb baster to transfer small quantities of hot liquid to and from a pan.

Can and bottle openers

Do you have trouble opening jars or bottles? Using a wedge-type opener attached to a wall or under a shelf offers one solution. This opener has metal teeth that grip a jar's lid while you twist the jar with one or both hands.

You can also use a rubber gripper or vise-grip opener for jars or a hand-held electric can opener that can be manipulated with one hand.

To open a ring-top can, press down and then pry up the top with a table knife.

To open a can of liquid with one hand and without spilling, wedge the can firmly in the corner of a drawer. Tuck a folded towel underneath it to bring the top of the can to the right height and open with a can opener.

USING WEDGE-TYPE OPENER   OPENING RING-TOP CAN

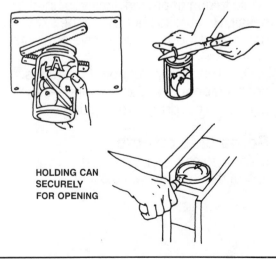

HOLDING CAN SECURELY FOR OPENING

Learning about naproxen

Dear Patient:

Your doctor has prescribed naproxen (the label may also read Naprosyn) to reduce the joint pain, swelling, and stiffness you're experiencing because of arthritis.

Be sure to take your naproxen exactly as the label directs. Take it with a full glass of water and remain upright for about 30 minutes afterward.

If naproxen gives you heartburn, check with your doctor. He may tell you to take the drug with your meal instead. Or, he might tell you to take it with an antacid.

If you miss a dose, take it as soon as your remember. However, if it's almost time for the next dose, skip the missed one—you should never take two doses at once. To help you remember, take it at the same time every day—when you first get up, for example, or just before bed.

A few precautions
While taking naproxen, limit your intake of salt. Be sure to check the labels on processed foods for excessive amounts of salt.

Don't drink any alcoholic beverages, not even beer or a glass of wine. And don't take the drug with aspirin.

Some side effects
Be sure to call your doctor right away if any of these side effects occur:

- you find yourself urinating less often than usual
- there's blood in your urine
- you have diarrhea or black stools
- you get a sore throat or start wheezing
- you feel light-headed, dizzy, or very drowsy
- you hear ringing in your ears
- your ankles are swollen
- you get a rash
- your vision is changing.

A few reminders
Keep taking your naproxen even if you don't notice a decrease in joint pain or stiffness right away. It may take a month for naproxen to achieve its effect.

Ask your pharmacist to put your medication in a non-childproof bottle for easier opening (unless a child lives in your house).

Don't let anyone else take your naproxen—and don't be tempted to take a friend's or relative's naproxen. The dosage could be different because your doctor wrote your prescription with your special needs in mind.

Don't postpone taking a dose to make the drug last longer than the doctor intended.

Check the expiration date on your naproxen periodically. Throw it away and get a new bottle if the expiration date has passed.

If the drug makes you feel drowsy, don't drive or operate machinery.

Systemic lupus erythematosus

A chronic inflammatory disorder, systemic lupus erythematosus (SLE) poses difficult but not insurmountable teaching problems. The disorder's chronicity, its periodic flareups, and its unpredictable remissions can interfere with learning and hinder compliance. When the patient experiences a long remission, for instance, she may lose her motivation to comply with therapy. Alternatively, she may meticulously comply with it but become discouraged when flareups persist. Before your teaching can succeed, you'll have to help her accept the reality of lifelong treatment and periodic flareups.

During SLE's early stages, you'll need to prepare the patient for a lengthy diagnostic workup. After diagnosis, your focus turns to providing her with an understanding of the disorder and communicating the importance of adhering to prescribed treatment. You'll need to encourage her to perform gentle exercises, maintain proper diet, and take other steps to preserve health. You'll have to reinforce the need to minimize exposure to sunlight and possibly prepare her for apheresis. What's more, you may need to advise her about pregnancy and family planning.

Discuss the disorder

Explain that SLE is a chronic disorder that leads to structural changes in the connective tissue, the fibers that support many other body tissues. Its unpredictable course includes exacerbations interspersed with long periods of complete or near-complete remission. SLE may produce only mild effects. However, its effects on the heart, blood vessels, kidneys, lungs, and central nervous system may be life-threatening. It strikes women 8 times as often as men and has a higher incidence among nonwhites—especially among blacks. Most patients are between the ages of 20 and 50.

Tell the patient that SLE causes varied signs and symptoms. The most common include a butterfly-shaped rash on the face (facial erythema), hair loss, stiff and aching joints, musculoskeletal deformity, and photosensitivity. The patient may also experience fatigue, weight loss, chills, fever, sensitivity to heat and cold, and musculoskeletal pain.

Explain the pathophysiology of SLE. The disorder's cause remains uncertain, but researchers believe antibodies develop against the body's own tissues—mostly deoxyribonucleic acid (DNA), but sometimes ribonucleic acid (RNA), clotting factors,

Geri Budesheim Neuberger, RN, MN, EdD, Lynne Kreutzer-Baraglia, RN, MS, and **Beverly Post, RN, MS, CIC,** contributed to this chapter. Ms. Neuberger is an associate professor at University of Kansas School of Nursing, Kansas City, Kan. Ms. Kreutzer-Baraglia is an assistant professor at West Suburban College of Nursing, Oak Park, Ill. Ms. Post is a risk manager and infection control coordinator at the Louis A. Weiss Memorial Hospital in Chicago.

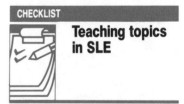

CHECKLIST

Teaching topics in SLE

☐ Explanation of the disorder, emphasizing its unpredictable exacerbations and remissions
☐ Complications of systemic lupus erythematosus (SLE)
☐ Preparation for repeated diagnostic tests
☐ Importance of gentle exercise and ample rest
☐ Drug therapy
☐ Apheresis to treat acute flareups or life-threatening complications
☐ Preventing infection and skin breakdown
☐ Minimizing exposure to sunlight
☐ Coping with Raynaud's phenomenon
☐ Pregnancy and family planning, if needed
☐ Sources of information and support

and blood cells. This autoimmune response generates immune complexes, which damage connective tissue and cause inflammation. (See *Immunity gone awry*.) Explain that because immune complexes may reside anywhere in the body, different symptoms appear at different times, with varying severity.

Point out that heredity may predispose some patients to SLE; the disorder has been found in certain families for several generations. Explain that certain factors may trigger the onset of symptoms; these include physiological or emotional stress, streptococcal or viral infection, inadequate rest, or exposure to direct or indirect sunlight, ultraviolet light, vaccines, or X-rays. Throughout the course of illness, these same factors may trigger periodic flareups. Certain drugs, including sulfonamides, hydralazine, procainamide, penicillin and other antibiotics, and some oral contraceptives, also may cause acute exacerbations.

Complications

Explain that failure to comply with treatment will heighten the risk of exacerbations, but that even full compliance can't guarantee protection against a flareup. Communicating this reality early in treatment may help the patient avoid needless self-recrimination later on.

Because SLE is a systemic disease, complications depend largely on the organs affected. The patient may develop vasculitis, possibly leading to infarctive ulcers, necrotic leg ulcers or digital gangrene; Raynaud's phenomenon; cardiopulmonary abnormalities such as myocarditis, endocarditis, tachycardia, parenchymal infiltrates and pneumonitis; renal abnormalities such as hematuria, urinary tract infections, and kidney failure; and central nervous system complications such as emotional instability, organic brain syndrome, and headache.

Describe the diagnostic workup

Advise the patient that definitive diagnosis of SLE may require months of observation, many laboratory tests and, possibly, measurement of her response to different medications. Ask her to provide a precise history of her symptoms to aid diagnosis.

Inform the patient that blood tests will help to evaluate her immune system and to detect certain antibodies. The antinuclear antibody test yields positive results in about 95% of SLE patients. A positive lupus erythematosus factor test strongly suggests SLE, especially in the presence of clinical symptoms. However, the anti-DNA antibody test remains the most specific test for SLE ; it rarely gives positive results in other disorders. Notify her that tests may be repeated periodically to monitor the effectiveness of therapy.

Explain to the patient that she may undergo a complete blood count, an erythrocyte sedimentation rate, a urinalysis, a chest X-ray, an electrocardiogram, and renal function tests to evaluate SLE's effects.

Immunity gone awry

Inform the patient with systemic lupus erythematosus (SLE) that she has an *autoimmune disease,* in which her immune system malfunctions. Normally, her antibodies fight off harmful bacteria. In SLE, though, they attack her body's own healthy tissues. Why does this occur? So far, no one can say for sure. Use the illustrations below to help explain how SLE may occur.

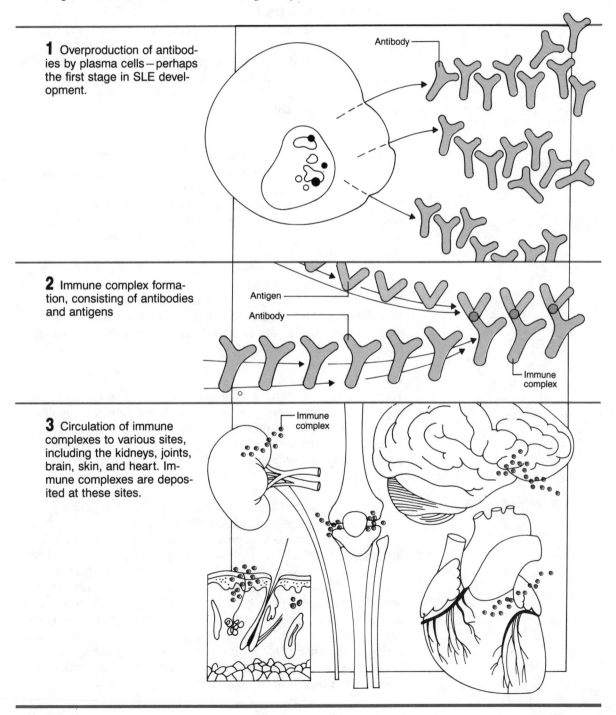

1 Overproduction of antibodies by plasma cells—perhaps the first stage in SLE development.

Antibody

2 Immune complex formation, consisting of antibodies and antigens

Antigen

Antibody

Immune complex

3 Circulation of immune complexes to various sites, including the kidneys, joints, brain, skin, and heart. Immune complexes are deposited at these sites.

Immune complex

Tell the patient scheduled for a renal biopsy to fast for 6 hours beforehand. Explain that the biopsy involves inserting a needle through the back and obtaining a small tissue sample from her kidney. Inform the patient that she'll receive a mild sedative and a local anesthetic. Tell her she'll have to lie on her stomach with a sandbag under her abdomen; to hold her breath during needle insertion; and to remain in bed up to 24 hours after the test.

Teach about treatments

Explain that treatment for SLE combines drug therapy and measures to prevent complications. These measures may include gentle exercise, ample rest, dietary changes, precautions against infection and photosensitivity reactions, coping with Raynaud's phenomenon, preparing for apheresis, and family planning for women in their childbearing years.

Activity

If the patient suffers from joint stiffness and inflammation, inform her about the benefits of moderate exercise, including range-of-motion exercises. Such activity will promote optimal health and help maintain joint mobility. Recommend using moist or dry heat before exercising to decrease discomfort. Warn her not to exercise to the point of fatigue, to stop during a flareup, and to resume exercise slowly thereafter.

Because fatigue commonly occurs in SLE, recommend 10 to 12 hours of sleep each night and periodic rests during the day. Make sure the patient understands the need to curtail activities before she tires. Also encourage her to maintain a calm, stable environment, if possible, and to practice relaxation exercises and other stress-reduction techniques.

Diet

While no diet will cure or even improve SLE, recommend foods high in protein, vitamins, and iron to help the patient maintain optimum nutrition and prevent anemia. If she has lost weight, suggest increasing caloric intake with between-meal snacks or commercially available high-protein, high-calorie supplements.

Medication

Explain to the patient that the doctor will tailor drug therapy according to her symptoms and severity of illness.

If your patient takes aspirin or other nonsteroidal anti-inflammatory drugs (NSAIDs), explain that these drugs not only relieve pain and fever but also fight inflammation. Warn her that common side effects include gastric upset and ulcers. Advise her to report unintended weight gain and GI symptoms, including loss of appetite, nausea, vomiting, diarrhea, or abdominal cramps. Urge her to call her doctor immediately if she has black, tarry stools or if her vomit contains blood or resembles coffee grounds.

For severe SLE or acute exacerbations, systemic corticosteroids are the treatment of choice. Initial high doses often bring noticeable improvement within 48 hours. When symptoms come under control, dosage is tapered slowly. Although corticosteroids may provide dramatic symptomatic relief, their long-term use can cause severe adverse reactions. Consequently, advise the patient to report mood disturbances, GI upset, acne, fever, easy bruising, weight gain, menstrual irregularities, and unusual tiredness. Caution her never to stop the drug or alter the dosage without consulting her doctor. Before undergoing any dental work or surgery, she must inform the dentist or doctor of corticosteroid therapy.

Topical corticosteroids, such as flurandrenolide, may also be used to treat skin or mucosal lesions. Demonstrate proper application of cream to the patient and warn her not to use nonprescription preparations without her doctor's approval. Mention that local adverse effects may include burning, itching, irritation, dryness, acne, hypopigmentation, hypertrichosis, allergic contact dermatitis, secondary infection, and atrophy.

If the patient takes antimalarial drugs, such as chloroquine and hydroxychloroquine, explain that these drugs treat skin and mucosal lesions. Tell her to report mild nausea, vomiting, diarrhea, ringing in her ears or loss of hearing, mood changes, sore throat, fever, and unusual bleeding or bruising. Because antimalarials can cause retinopathy, recommend that an ophthalmologist examine her eyes every 3 to 4 months to detect early signs of retinal damage. If she notices any changes in her vision, such as blurring or blind spots, tell her to contact her doctor immediately. Inform her that she must take the drug regularly and that she may not achieve full benefits for up to 6 months.

If the patient fails to respond to NSAIDs, corticosteroids, or antimalarials, the doctor may prescribe an immunosuppressive drug, such as cyclophosphamide, chlorambucil, methotrexate, or azathioprine. Explain that these drugs hinder the inflammatory responses that lead to SLE symptoms but can cause serious adverse reactions. Tell her to watch for and immediately report unusual bleeding or bruising, chills, fever, and sore throat. Also, encourage her to comply with regular blood tests, which can determine if the drug interferes with blood cell production. Warn her that she may experience some hair loss; hair will grow back when she stops taking the drug.

Procedures
If the patient has life-threatening complications or an acute flare-up that resists corticosteroids, she may undergo therapeutic apheresis. Explain that a needle will be inserted in each arm and that her blood will be pumped through a machine to remove the circulating immune complexes that exacerbate her disorder. Tell her that her pulse and blood pressure will be monitored and that she should report any tingling sensations around her mouth or in her hands or feet.

Other care measures
Underscore the importance of minimizing exposure to infection, especially if the patient takes corticosteroids, which suppress the

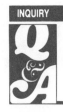

Questions SLE patients ask about pregnancy

Does becoming pregnant make lupus worse?
In about 25% of women, systemic lupus erythematosus (SLE) gets worse during pregnancy. For the rest, it stays the same or even improves. After the birth of your baby, there's a small chance that your disease will flare up. Unfortunately, doctors can't predict how pregnancy and childbirth will affect your symptoms. Before pregnancy, you and your spouse need to discuss the possibility that your condition may worsen.

Before I get pregnant, is there anything special I should do?
Ideally, you should try to get pregnant when your disease is in remission or under good medical control. Let your doctor know about your plans well before you try to become pregnant. He will need to discontinue any drugs you're taking that could possibly harm a fetus. Birth defects caused by drugs may oc-

cur in the first few weeks of pregnancy, long before you're aware you're pregnant.

Will I need special care during pregnancy?
You'll probably need to see your obstetrician more often than you would without the condition. Certain problems of pregnancy, such as toxemia, occur more commonly in SLE. To minimize complications, make sure you keep all medical appointments, and follow through with recommended blood, urine, and other diagnostic tests.

What are my chances of having a healthy baby?
It's very unlikely that your baby will be born with SLE. Unfortunately, women with lupus face a greater risk of miscarriages and stillbirths. Following your doctor's advice throughout your pregnancy will greatly improve your chances of having a healthy baby.

---

immune response. Advise her to avoid crowds and people with known infections and to consult her doctor about influenza and pneumococcal vaccines. Caution against excessive bathing because it can dry or break down the skin, leaving it vulnerable to infection. However, each day she should clean and pat dry areas where two skin surfaces touch, such as the underarm or genital areas. Tell her to regularly inspect these areas for signs of infection or skin breakdown.

Emphasize meticulous mouth care for preventing and treating oral lesions. Advise the patient to use a soft toothbrush and to avoid commercial mouthwashes because of their high sugar content and the irritating and drying effect of the alcohol base. Instruct her to have regular dental checkups and to call her doctor upon noticing white plaques in her mouth—possible signs of fungal infection. Suggest soft, bland foods if she has open sores.

Sunlight exposure may cause severe urticaria and bullous lesions. Even brief exposure (20 minutes or less) may produce a rash. Caution the patient to avoid sunlight, even when reflected from sand or snow. Provide a copy of the patient-teaching aid *Protecting your skin,* page 284.

If the patient has Raynaud's phenomenon (a common occurrence in SLE), tell her to protect her hands and feet from cold temperatures to prevent vasospasm. Instruct her to avoid cold water and to wear gloves when handling cold items, such as frozen foods.

Because many female SLE patients are in their childbearing years, provide counseling about pregnancy and family planning, as needed. (See *Questions SLE patients ask about pregnancy.*) Explain that the patient may experience menstrual irregularities during flareups but her normal cycle will resume during remissions. If she wishes to become pregnant, tell her that keeping her disorder under control and obtaining good prenatal care increase her chances of having a healthy baby. Advise choosing an obstetrician who specializes in high-risk pregnancies, ideally one with experience in caring for pregnant SLE patients.

If the patient wishes to avoid pregnancy, discuss birth control options. Explain that oral contraceptives may aggravate the disorder and that many doctors recommend a diaphragm. If your patient is unfamiliar with the diaphragm, explain how to obtain and use one. Warn her against becoming pregnant and possibly exposing a fetus to potentially teratogenic medications.

Finally, tell the patient to call the doctor if fever, cough, or skin rash occurs or if chest, abdominal, muscle, or joint pain worsens.

Sources of information and support

American Lupus Society
23751 Madison Street, Torrance, Calif. 90505
(213) 373-1335

Arthritis Foundation
1314 Spring Street, NW, Atlanta, Ga. 30309
(404) 872-7100

Lupus Foundation of America
1717 Massachusetts Avenue, NW, Suite 203, Washington, D.C. 20036
(202) 328-4500

Further readings

Bergman, H.D. "The Treatment of Systemic Lupus Erythematosus,"*Journal of Practical Nursing* 39(1):50-57, March 1989.

Hooker, R.S. "Systemic Lupus Erythematosus," *Physician Assistant* 12(1):71-72, 74-75, 79-80, January 1988.

Lockshin, M.D., and Rothfield, N.F. "A Better Prognosis in Lupus," *Patient Care* 22(4):75-79, 82, 85-86, February 29, 1988.

Regan-Gavin, R. "The War Within: A Personal Account of Coping with Systemic Lupus Erythematosus," *Health and Social Work* 13(1):11-19, Winter, 1988.

Rothfield, N.F. "The Diagnostic Features of SLE," *Hospital Practice* 24(1A):37-46, January 30, 1989.

Whitney, R. "Unlock the Mystery of Lupus," *Today's OR Nurse* 11(3):10-12, 30-32, March 1989.

Protecting your skin

Dear Patient:

Exposure to the sun, or even to fluorescent lights, may make your condition worse. Excessive exposure, in fact, may cause rashes, fever, arthritis, and even damage to the organs inside your body.

You needn't spend your waking hours in the dark to be safe though. Just follow the precautions below.

Prepare for going outdoors

Wear a wide-brimmed hat or visor to shield yourself from the sun's rays. Protect your eyes by wearing sunglasses. Put on a long-sleeved shirt and trousers to filter out harmful rays. In hot weather, choose clothing made of lightweight loosely woven fabrics, such as cotton.

Buy a sunscreen containing PABA (para-aminobenzoic acid) with a skin protection factor of 8 to 15. If you're allergic to PABA, choose a PABA-free product offering equivalent sun protection.

Before you go outside, rub the sunscreen onto unprotected parts of your body, such as your face and hands. Read the label to determine how often to reapply it. Usually, you'll use more after swimming or perspiring.

Avoid strong sunlight

Try to stay indoors during the most intense hours of sunlight, from 10 a.m. to 2 p.m. The ideal time to garden, take a walk, play golf, or do any other outdoor activity is just after sunrise or just before sunset.

Remove fluorescent light

At home, replace any fluorescent fixtures or bulbs with incandescent ones. At work, though, avoiding fluorescent light may be difficult. Consider asking your supervisor about moving to a work area closer to a window, so you can use natural light. If you have a fluorescent light above your desk, turn it off and request a lamp that uses incandescent bulbs.

Be careful with soaps and drugs

Certain toiletries, including deodorant soaps, may increase your skin's sensitivity to light.

Try switching to nondeodorant or hypoallergenic soaps. Certain drugs, including tetracyclines and phenothiazines, also make you more sensitive to light.

Always check with your doctor or pharmacist before taking any new medication.

Recognize and report rashes

Be alert for the key sign of a photosensitivity reaction: a red rash on your face or other exposed area. If you discover a suspicious rash or other reaction to light, call your doctor. Remember, prompt treatment can prevent damage to the tissues beneath your skin.

Iron deficiency anemia

For patients with this prevalent nutritional disorder, you'll need to focus on promoting compliance with therapy. Affecting 10% to 30% of adults in North America, iron deficiency anemia occurs most commonly in premenopausal women, premature and low-birth-weight infants, children, and adolescent girls. Unfortunately, because the disorder is so common, many patients consider it trivial and fail to comply with treatment. As a result, you'll need to convince patients that iron deficiency can lead to severe problems.

Begin by explaining the disorder and its characteristic signs and symptoms. Point out the complications if anemia goes untreated, and explain laboratory tests to diagnose the disorder. Finally, discuss the treatment regimen, including an iron-rich diet, iron supplements, and adequate rest and follow-up care.

Discuss the disorder

Inform the patient that the body's iron reserves can be rapidly depleted when its demand for iron isn't met. Discuss the role of red blood cells (RBCs). (See *How red blood cells work,* page 286.) Explain how body tissues become starved for oxygen (a condition called hypoxia) when iron deficiency impairs the body's oxygen-transporting capacity.

The resultant signs and symptoms of iron deficiency anemia usually don't materialize until the problem is severe, so the typical patient may postpone seeking medical attention. Classic advanced signs and symptoms include dyspnea with exertion, fatigue, listlessness, pallor, inability to concentrate, irritability, headache, frequent infections, and tachycardia. A cardinal sign is pica—the desire to eat nonfood substances, such as dirt or ice. Other key signs of long-standing iron deficiency include brittle, spoon-shaped nails, cracks in the corners of the mouth, smooth tongue, dysphagia, vasomotor disturbances, numbness and tingling of the hands and feet, and neuralgic pain.

Tailor your teaching about iron deficiency anemia to the patient's age. If your patient's an infant, tell the parents that natural iron stores are depleted by age 4 to 6 months, so an infant given prolonged, unsupplemented breast-feedings or bottle feedings (especially of cow's milk) typically has iron deficiency anemia. Tell the teenager and her parents that a rapid growth period, such as adolescence, increases the body's need for iron. If the body must

Jo Ann Kelly Gottlieb, RN, MS, Lynne Kreutzer-Baraglia, RN, MS, and **Beverly A. Post, RN, MS, CIC,** contributed to this chapter. Ms. Gottlieb is an assistant professor of nursing at Barry University School of Nursing, Miami Shores, Fla. Ms. Kreutzer-Baraglia is an assistant professor at West Suburban College of Nursing, Oak Park, Ill. Ms. Post is a risk and infection control manager at Louis A. Weiss Memorial Hospital, Chicago.

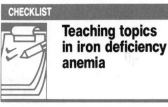

CHECKLIST

Teaching topics in iron deficiency anemia

☐ Explanation of iron deficiency anemia, including the role of red blood cells and iron
☐ Signs and symptoms of iron deficiency anemia
☐ Causes and age-related risk factors
☐ Diagnostic blood studies
☐ The role of diet in treatment, including ways to stimulate the appetite and how to choose iron-rich foods
☐ Iron supplements: how to take them, special precautions, and possible adverse effects
☐ Importance of continuing care, obtaining adequate rest, and treating infections promptly
☐ Source of information and support

How red blood cells work

If your patient thinks of iron deficiency anemia as just a minor malady, she may neglect to comply with treatment. So encourage her to grasp the disorder's seriousness by explaining the oxygen-carrying role of red blood cells (RBCs) and describing how they develop. Highlight the crucial role played by iron.

Where do RBCs come from?

Explain that RBCs begin in stem cells in the bone marrow. During this process called erythropoiesis, a nucleated RBC precursor (hemocytoblast) matures into a nucleus-free RBC (reticulocyte). From the early basophil stage, during which hemoglobin synthesis begins, to the later normoblast stage, in which the cell nucleus wanes to allow greater mobility, the cell produces hemoglobin. This substance accounts for the blood cell's reddish color and allows it to carry oxygen. Hemoglobin also contains about two-thirds of the body's iron.

Where do RBCs go?

When the RBC's hemoglobin concentration reaches about 34%, the cell loses its nucleus and leaves the bone marrow to circulate in the bloodstream as a reticulocyte. Within about 24 hours, the young reticulocyte matures into an erythrocyte. The entire process

(from hemocytoblast to erythrocyte) takes about 4 days and occurs continuously in the body.

What happens to old RBCs?

Explain that an RBC lives for about 120 days. When it completes its cycle, it attracts a macrophage. This scavenger cell—found in the spleen, liver, bone marrow, and other tissues—devours the worn-out RBC and breaks down the hemoglobin molecules into reusable elements. One of these elements—heme—gives the hemoglobin molecule its oxygen-carrying capacity. And iron released from the heme molecules mixes with a serum globulin called transferrin. This mixture then becomes new hemoglobin and also goes to the liver, spleen, and other cells for storage.

What difference does iron make?

Tell the patient that with adequate intake, iron will circulate continuously through her body. On the other hand, inadequate intake will gradually deplete the body's iron reserves. As a result, erythrocytes, hemoglobin levels, and RBC volume will diminish. This will impair the blood's oxygen-carrying capacity and lead to tissue hypoxia and eventually, symptoms of iron deficiency anemia.

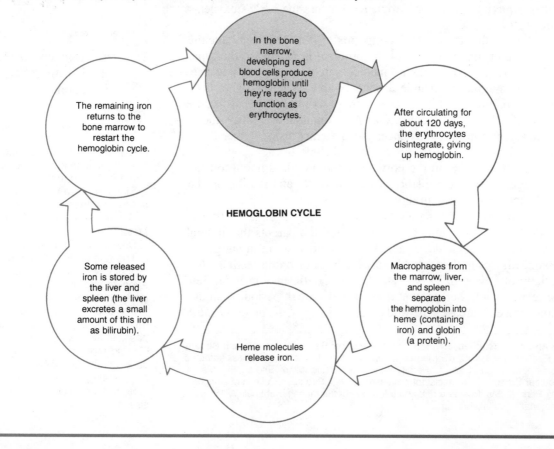

In the bone marrow, developing red blood cells produce hemoglobin until they're ready to function as erythrocytes.

After circulating for about 120 days, the erythrocytes disintegrate, giving up hemoglobin.

Macrophages from the marrow, liver, and spleen separate the hemoglobin into heme (containing iron) and globin (a protein).

Heme molecules release iron.

Some released iron is stored by the liver and spleen (the liver excretes a small amount of this iron as bilirubin).

The remaining iron returns to the bone marrow to restart the hemoglobin cycle.

HEMOGLOBIN CYCLE

draw on unreplenished iron stores, anemia will result. If your patient's a woman, explain that she may have iron deficiency from blood loss during menstruation, especially if her iron stores are already low. Tell a pregnant patient that much of her body's iron supply is being diverted to the fetus for erythropoiesis.

Mention that iron deficiency anemia also may result from chronic diarrhea; gastrectomy; celiac disease and other iron malabsorption disorders; blood loss from traumatic injury, GI bleeding, cancer, or varices; and erythrocyte trauma caused by heart valve replacement.

Complications
Stress that failure to comply with therapy can lead to a chronic lack of oxygen, possibly producing persistent fatigue and dyspnea, an increased susceptibility to infection, and other advanced symptoms of iron deficiency. The body tries to compensate for oxygen deprivation by increasing both heart rate and cardiac output, resulting in tachycardia.

Describe the diagnostic workup
Explain that the doctor will order blood tests to diagnose iron deficiency anemia and to determine its severity. Routine tests to measure iron levels include serum iron, total iron-binding capacity, and ferritin analyses. A complete blood count may be ordered to evaluate hemoglobin levels and detect morphologic changes in RBCs. Add that blood tests may be repeated to monitor the patient's progress through treatment.

Teach about treatments
Inform the patient that iron deficiency anemia typically improves with iron supplementation and an iron-rich diet. Instruct her also to get adequate rest, to treat infections promptly, and to keep all follow-up medical appointments. If the patient's disorder is particularly severe, prepare her for possible blood transfusions.

Diet
Inform the patient that diet alone can't cure iron deficiency anemia but that it does play a leading role in therapy. Discuss which foods contain the most iron, and encourage her to include them in her daily diet. Explore her eating habits. Does she have a poor appetite? This may contribute to the disorder. Then offer her the patient-teaching aid *Choosing iron-rich foods,* page 289. Also refer to *Tips for improving the appetite.*

Medication
Explain that the doctor may prescribe iron supplements to replenish the patient's iron supply. These supplements are usually taken orally—the safest, most effective, and least expensive treatment. However, they may be given parenterally if the patient doesn't take oral supplements as prescribed or if they trigger an adverse reaction, such as nausea or constipation.

Inform the patient that she'll need a prescription for some supplements, whereas she can obtain others over the counter.

Tips for improving the appetite

If your patient has a poor appetite (common in iron deficiency anemia), offer these suggestions for improving it:
- Plan your day to include frequent rest periods so you'll have more energy for eating.
- Eat five or six small meals a day instead of three large ones.
- Wear comfortable, loose clothing during meals. Try pants with elastic waistbands or drawstring waists.
- Refresh yourself before meals by brushing your teeth and washing your face and hands.
- Set the table with brightly colored napkins and plates. Or decorate with a centerpiece of fresh flowers. Yellow, orange, and red stimulate the appetite; blue, green, and dark colors depress it.
- Eat with friends or family members and hold a pleasant conversation—one of the best stimulants.
- Sit in a comfortable chair, relax, and eat slowly. Adjust the room temperature and lighting to a comfortable level. Listen to soothing music.
- Avoid foods that cause abdominal fullness and gas, such as broccoli, beans, or cabbage.
- Include foods from the four food groups at each meal.
- Add zest and interest to food with herbs and spices.
- Introduce variety by serving different colored foods at the same meal.
- Drink liquids after eating, not right before or during a meal. Liquids make you feel full.

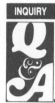

Questions anemic patients ask about iron

How long will I have to take iron supplements?

Probably no longer than 6 months. The iron levels in your body will begin to rise shortly after you start taking supplements. However, the replenishing process takes time because the rate of iron absorption decreases as your iron level rises. Your doctor will probably continue therapy for 2 to 4 months after levels return to normal.

The first iron pill I took irritated my stomach, so now I'm on enteric-coated supplements. What does this mean?

Enteric tablets or capsules have a special coating that doesn't dissolve until the pill reaches the small intestine. This prevents the iron from being released in the stomach, where it can cause irritation, nausea, and constipation.

Unfortunately, iron isn't absorbed as well in the small intestine, making enteric-coated tablets less effective. Sometimes stomach irritation can be avoided by reducing the number of iron tablets you take to one a day. Then you can try gradually adding additional tablets as tolerance increases. Or trying a different type or brand of iron may help. Ask your doctor about these alternatives.

Is it true that cooking in cast-iron pots will help me get more iron?

Yes, but only when you cook certain types of food and cook them for a long time. Acidic foods like tomato sauce will absorb iron from pots.

The age of your cookware and how well you care for it also affects the amount of iron absorbed by food. Old, rusty pans actually provide more iron than new ones.

Then teach her how to take the iron supplement her doctor prescribes, and point out possible adverse effects. (For more information, see *Questions anemic patients ask about iron*.) Common iron supplements include ferrous fumarate (Feostat, Ircon), ferrous gluconate (Fergon, Ferralet), ferrous sulfate (Feosol, Slow Fe), and iron dextran (Imferon, K-FeRON). Reinforce your instructions with a copy of the teaching aid *Getting the most from oral iron supplements*, page 290.

Other care measures

Encourage the patient to keep follow-up appointments with the doctor and to continue the prescribed therapy even after her condition improves. Explain that once hemoglobin levels return to normal, she'll probably need to continue therapy for at least 2 more months to replenish the body's depleted iron reserves. Caution her also that iron deficiency may recur.

Advise the patient to pace her activities to include frequent rest periods. If shortness of breath, weakness, light-headedness, or palpitations develop during the day, suggest changing positions or moving about slowly to minimize dizziness and other symptoms.

If the patient's a child, promote health maintenance through immunizations and prompt treatment of infections.

Explain to the patient with severe iron deficiency anemia that she may need transfusions of packed RBCs. Mention that this treatment will increase circulating hemoglobin levels and improve tissue oxygenation. Supplied by I.V. infusion, a packed RBC transfusion may take up to 2 hours to complete.

Source of information and support

Children's Blood Foundation
424 East 62nd Street, Room 1045, New York, N.Y. 10021
(212) 644-5790

Further readings

"Anemia from Lithium?" *Nurses Drug Alert* 11(1):2, January 1987.
"CDC Criteria for Anemia in Children and Childbearing-Aged Women," *Morbidity and Mortality Weekly Report* 38(22):400-04, June 9, 1989.
Farley, P.C., and Foland, J. "Iron Deficiency Anemia. How to Diagnose and Correct," *Postgraduate Medicine* 87(2):89-93, 96, 101, February 1, 1990.
Froberg, J.H. "The Anemias: Causes and Courses of Action," *RN* 52(1):24-30, January 1989.
"Iron Deficiency in Adolescent Athletes," *Emergency Medicine* 21(17):51, 55, 58, October 15, 1989.
Waterworth, S. "Management of Anemia," *Nursing* (London) 3(40): 12-15, August 1989.
Wheby, M.S. "Sizing Up the Seriousness of Anemia," *Emergency Medicine* 21(14):179-81 +, August 15, 1989.
Wolfe, D.W. "Hematologic Complications of Malignancy," *Topics in Emergency Medicine* 8(2):13-24, July 1986.

Choosing iron-rich foods

Dear Patient:

Although many everyday foods contain large amounts of iron, your body typically absorbs only a small portion of it. So you'll need to choose foods that contain lots of iron. But which ones should you choose? First of all, pick foods from all of the four major groups: milk and dairy, meat, bread and cereal, and fruit and vegetable. Then modify the amount from each group by considering your other dietary needs. For instance, if you need to cut back on cholesterol, don't pick liver.

Select wisely
Keep in mind that the iron in grains and vegetables isn't absorbed as readily as the iron in meat, fish, and poultry. On the other hand, eating meat, fish, or poultry *along with* grains and vegetables increases iron absorption. So does eating a food that contains vitamin C—an orange, tomato, or potato, for example. In fact, eating a tomato with a hamburger quadruples iron absorption. (On the other hand, drinking tea with the same meal lowers iron absorption.)

Know how much iron you need
Recommended amounts are 18 milligrams a day (mg/day) for women age 50 and under and 10 mg/day for men and women over age 50. Your doctor will tell you exactly how much iron you should consume. Consult the list at right to find the foods highest in iron.

Food	Quantity	Iron (mg)
Oysters	3 ounces	13.2
Beef liver	3 ounces	7.5
Prune juice	½ cup	5.2
Clams	2 ounces	4.2
Walnuts	½ cup	3.75
Ground beef	3 ounces	3.0
Chick-peas	½ cup	3.0
Bran flakes	½ cup	2.8
Pork roast	3 ounces	2.7
Cashew nuts	½ cup	2.65
Shrimp	3 ounces	2.6
Raisins	½ cup	2.55
Navy beans	½ cup	2.55
Sardines	3 ounces	2.5
Spinach	½ cup	2.4
Lima beans	½ cup	2.3
Kidney beans	½ cup	2.2
Turkey, dark meat	3 ounces	2.0
Prunes	½ cup	1.9
Roast beef	3 ounces	1.8
Green peas	½ cup	1.5
Peanuts	½ cup	1.5
Potato	1	1.1
Sweet potato	½ cup	1.0
Green beans	½ cup	1.0
Egg	1	1.0
Turkey, light meat	3 ounces	1.0

PATIENT-TEACHING AID

Getting the most from oral iron supplements

Dear Patient:

Your doctor has prescribed an oral iron supplement to correct your iron deficiency. Although most people get enough iron from their diets, some must take additional iron to boost the iron supplies in their bodies.

Before you start

Tell the doctor if you've ever had an allergic reaction to iron. Also tell him which other drugs you take regularly (including nonprescription drugs). They might interfere with iron absorption. Tell him also if you're breast-feeding, pregnant, or have any medical problem.

How to take iron supplements

• For best absorption, take iron supplements on an empty stomach with a full glass of water, tomato juice, or citrus juice. If your stomach feels upset, take iron with food — but call the doctor if this problem persists.

• Avoid consuming calcium supplements, antacids, eggs, dairy products, whole-grain breads and cereals, coffee, tea, and alcohol for 1 hour before or 2 hours after taking your iron supplement. All interfere with iron absorption.

• Don't crush pills. If you have trouble swallowing them, ask the doctor about taking liquid iron.

• To keep liquid iron supplements from staining your teeth, mix each dose with 8 ounces of water or fruit juice, and drink from a straw placed away from your

teeth. If iron does stain your teeth, remove the stains by brushing with baking soda or 3% hydrogen peroxide.

• If you miss a dose, skip it and go back to your regular schedule. Double-dosing can cause iron poisoning.

Special instructions

• Unabsorbed iron will color your stools dark green or black — a harmless reaction. In fact, if your stools don't turn dark, call your doctor. The iron tablets may be breaking down improperly, and you may not be getting enough iron.

• If taking iron causes constipation, eat fibrous foods, such as bran and raw fruit and vegetables. Taking a powdered psyllium product may help too.

• Rarely, iron supplements cause toxic reactions. Call your doctor or poison control center immediately if you have any of the following: severe diarrhea with cramping; vomiting; unusual weakness; tarry stools or stools with red streaks; pale, clammy skin; or an unusually fast or irregular heartbeat.

• Take iron supplements only as long as your doctor orders — usually from 2 to 4 months after your deficiency is cured.

• Don't switch to over-the-counter supplements afterward, and don't take oral supplements along with iron injections — this can cause poisoning.

• Remember to add the iron in foods when calculating your iron intake.

• Keep iron supplements out of children's reach. Even small doses of adult iron can be fatal to children.

CHAPTER
5
Cancer

Contents

Lung cancer

Teaching your patient and his family about lung cancer may be among the greatest challenges you'll face as a nurse. A frightening diagnosis for most patients, lung cancer is the leading cause of cancer death. Among women, it has surpassed breast cancer as the leading cancer killer. Among all lung cancer patients, only 13% live 5 or more years after diagnosis.

Despite these grim statistics, you can help your patient adjust to the diagnosis by educating him about the disease and his treatment options so that informed decisions can be made. Your support and instruction will be needed throughout treatment so that the patient can derive the greatest benefit from therapy and learn to manage side effects.

You'll also help your patient and his family form realistic expectations about treatment outcomes without providing false hope. Despite lung cancer's overall poor prognosis, you'll emphasize that treatment possibilities include cure, control, or symptomatic relief as you review the options of chemotherapy, radiation therapy, and surgery.

Discuss the disorder

Begin your discussion by describing lung anatomy. Use a drawing to show the patient that he has two lungs—a right and a left. The right lung has three lobes, the upper, middle, and lower; the left lung has two lobes, the upper and lower. Explain that air reaches the lungs through the trachea, a tube that forks into two parts to form the left and the right mainstem bronchi. This bronchial tree then subdivides into smaller branches called bronchioles. At the end of the bronchioles are the alveoli, where the exchange of oxygen and carbon dioxide occurs.

Explain that epithelial cells line the tracheobronchial tree to protect the lungs from irritants. However, repeated exposure to airborne carcinogens, such as cigarette smoke or asbestos, causes these cells to lose their protective properties. This may precipitate lung cancer.

Inform the patient and his family that lung cancer is 10 times more common in smokers than in nonsmokers; indeed, at least 85% of lung cancer patients are smokers. Air pollution and industrial carcinogens also are risk factors, especially when combined with cigarette smoking. For more information, see *Lung cancer*

Valerie A. Woebkenberg, RN,C, MSN, OCN, a nurse practitioner at Temple University Hospital, Philadelphia, wrote this chapter.

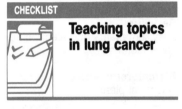

Teaching topics in lung cancer

☐ Explanation of lung anatomy and disease progression
☐ Discussion of major types of lung cancer
☐ Complications from metastasis
☐ Preparation for diagnostic tests, such as pulmonary function tests, bronchoscopy, and computed tomography
☐ Treatments: chemotherapy, radiation therapy, and surgery
☐ Ways to manage or minimize treatment side effects
☐ Pain management techniques, such as relaxation and stimulation
☐ Promoting health and avoiding lung cancer risk factors, including smoking and industrial carcinogens
☐ Sources of information and support

Lung cancer and the workplace

Almost everyone knows that cigarette smoking is a risk factor for lung cancer. But not everyone knows that other airborne pollutants are villains, too. In particular, exposure to industrial carcinogens can cause lung cancer, especially among smokers.

Refer to the list below to help patients identify and avoid (or at least protect themselves from exposure to) these known workplace carcinogens.

Acrylonitrile
Fiber mills (blankets, carpets, clothing, draperies, synthetic furs, and wigs)

Arsenic
Copper smelting and metallurgical industries, mines, insecticide and pesticide plants (and products), tanning factories

Asbestos
Asbestos factories (and asbestos removal work sites); insulation, rubber, and textile plants; mines and shipyards

Beryllium
Beryllium plants and electronic-parts and missile-parts factories

Bis(chlorethyl)ether
Chemical plants

Cadmium
Cadmium factories; battery, chemical, jewelry, paint and pigment plants; electroplating and metallurgical industries

Coal tar pitch volatiles
Aluminum potrooms, foundries, steel mills

Coke oven emissions
Coke plants, steel mills

Dimethylsulphate
Chemical, drug, and dye plants

Epichlorohydrin
Chemical plants

Hematite
Hematite mines

Mineral oils, soot, and tars
Construction sites, roofing plants (and roofs), chimney sweep businesses, heavy industry

Nickel
Nickel refineries

Vinylchloride
Plastics and vinylchloride polymer plants

and the workplace, and *Questions patients ask about lung cancer.*

As appropriate, discuss the most common lung cancer types—for example, adenocarcinoma, small cell (oat cell) carcinoma, or epidermoid (squamous cell) carcinoma. Inform the patient that a pathologist determines the type after reviewing the tissue samples obtained during the diagnostic workup and that the type of treatment he receives depends on the cancer's type and the tumor's stage.

Complications
Explain that by following the treatment plan the patient boosts his chances for cure or control and for avoiding complications from cancer's spread or from treatment's side effects. Nevertheless, despite the patient's compliance, the primary tumor may grow and invade neighboring tissues. Or, cancer cells may be carried to other parts of the body by the circulatory or the lymphatic systems. Lung cancer most commonly spreads to the brain, bones, liver, and adrenal glands.

Because early lung cancer is difficult to detect, disease complications may constitute the presenting symptoms. For example, as the tumor grows, the patient may cough, wheeze, have difficulty breathing or swallowing, or cough up blood. The tumor may press against a nerve and cause arm and shoulder pain, or it may compress and partially occlude the superior vena cava, causing swelling of the head and neck.

Describe the diagnostic workup

Because so many lung cancer patients remain symptom-free while the disease advances, metastasis has occurred in about 70% of patients by the time of diagnosis. Tell the patient that he may undergo diagnostic tests to detect a tumor and to determine its location, type and size, extent of metastasis, and appropriate therapy. (For more information, see *Staging lung cancer,* page 296.)

The patient may also have blood tests to monitor the disease and treatment. These tests include a complete blood count, blood chemistries, arterial blood gas (ABG) studies, and liver function studies. When the doctor orders a blood test, tell the patient who will perform the venipuncture and where, and inform him of any pretest restrictions. Also, if ordered, show him how to collect a sputum sample for analysis.

When teaching the patient about the following diagnostic tests, explain that he may undergo them one time only or periodically for evaluation.

Chest X-ray

Inform the patient that a chest X-ray may detect lung tumors. Tell him the test takes only a few minutes, but that the technician may need more time to check film quality.

Before the test, instruct him to remove all clothing except his pants, socks, and shoes and to put on a gown without snaps. Remind him to remove all jewelry and other metallic objects from his neck and chest. If he's having the X-ray in the radiology department, he'll stand or sit in front of a machine. If the X-ray's done at bedside, someone will help him sit up before sliding a hard film plate behind his back. He'll be asked to take a deep breath and to hold it for a few seconds while the technician snaps the X-ray picture. Urge him to remain still for those few seconds. Reassure him that he'll receive minimum radiation exposure.

Lung tomography

Explain that lung tomography helps diagnose and monitor lung lesions. Just before the test, tell the patient to remove all jewelry. Then describe how he'll lie on his back on a hard X-ray table while the X-ray tube swings above him and takes numerous films from different angles. Instruct him to stay still, relax, and breathe normally during the test. Explain that movement may invalidate test results and necessitate repeated testing.

Pulmonary function tests

Teach the patient that pulmonary function tests estimate the degree of lung dysfunction resulting from lung cancer. Instruct him not to smoke for 4 hours before the test and to avoid eating a

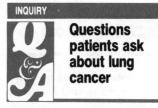

Questions patients ask about lung cancer

How long can I live with lung cancer?
No one can predict how long you'll live. But in general, the earlier your cancer was diagnosed, the better the outlook. The outlook is best for patients with stage I cancer, in which the tumor hasn't spread to the lymph nodes or other sites. Up to 65% of these patients are alive after 5 years. In more advanced cancers, the survival rate drops. However, statistics don't tell the whole story. Your response to treatment is what matters most.

If I stop smoking, will my lung cancer go away?
Giving up smoking won't cure your lung cancer or make the tumor disappear. However, it will improve your lung capacity and ease your breathing. You'll tolerate your treatments better and be less likely to develop a lung infection.

Do you think X-rays caused my lung cancer?
Although X-rays have been implicated as a risk factor in some cancers, they haven't been shown to contribute to lung cancer.

Staging lung cancer

Tell the patient that his treatment plan and prognosis depend on his type of lung cancer and its stage. Explain that a cancer's stage is determined by the size and characteristics of the primary tumor, the extent of lymph node involvement, and metastasis to distant sites.

The American Joint Committee on Cancer assigns the following labels and descriptions to lung cancer.

Tumor classifications
T0: No evidence of primary tumor
TX: Tumor proved by malignant cells in bronchopulmonary secretions but undetected by X-ray or bronchoscopy
TIS: Carcinoma in situ
T1: Tumor 3 cm thick or less, surrounded by normal lung or visceral pleura
T2: Tumor more than 3 cm thick or of any size that invades the visceral pleura or extends to the hilar region; tumor lies within a lobar bronchus or at least 2 cm from the carina; any related atelectasis or obstructive pneumonitis involves less than entire lung
T3: Tumor of any size that extends into neighboring structures, such as the chest wall, diaphragm, mediastinal pleura, or pericardium without involving the heart, great vessels, trachea, esophagus, or vertebral body; or a tumor within the main bronchus within 2 cm of the carina without involving it
T4: Tumor of any size that invades the mediastinum and involves the heart, great vessels, trachea, esophagus, vertebral body, or carina; or malignant pleural effusion

Nodal involvement
N0: No detectable metastasis to lymph nodes
N1: Metastasis to the peribronchial or the ipsilateral hilar lymph nodes
N2: Metastasis to the ipsilateral mediastinal and the subcarinal lymph nodes
N3: Metastasis to the contralateral mediastinal or the hilar lymph node, the ipsilateral or the contralateral scalene, or the supraclavicular lymph nodes

Metastasis
M0: No known metastasis
M1: Distant metastasis at specific site or sites

Occult carcinoma
TX, N0, M0: Malignant cells in bronchopulmonary secretions but no other evidence of tumor or metastasis

Stage 0
TIS, N0, M0: Carcinoma in situ

Stage I
T1, N0, M0 or T2, N0, M0: Tumor can be T1 or T2 without nodal involvement or metastasis

Stage II
T1, N1, M0 or T2, N1, M0: Tumor can be T1 or T2 with metastasis extending only to the peribronchial or the ipsilateral hilar lymph nodes

Stage IIIa
T3, N0, M0 or T3, N1, M0 or T1 to T3, N2, M0: Tumor is more extensive than T2 but doesn't invade a vital structure; or any tumor up to T3 with metastasis to the ipsilateral mediastinal or the subcarinal lymph nodes

Stage IIIb
Any T, N3, M0 or T4, any N, M0: Tumor that invades vital mediastinal structures or metastasizes to inoperable nodes but not beyond the thorax

Stage IV
Any T, any N, M1: Tumor that metastasizes beyond the thorax and the regional lymph nodes—for example, the scalene or supraclavicular lymph nodes

large meal or drinking a lot of fluid before the test. Suggest he wear loose, comfortable clothing. If he wears dentures, tell him to keep them in to help form a tight seal around the breathing tube's (spirometer) mouthpiece. Just before the test, advise him to void.

Explain that during the test he'll wear a noseclip and sit upright. Or he may sit in a small, airtight box called a body plethysmograph (then he won't need a noseclip, but he might experience claustrophobia). Assure him that he can communicate with the technician through the window in the box. He'll breathe through a mouth tube for each test and be instructed to breathe in several ways; for example, to inhale deeply and exhale completely or to inhale quickly. Mention that arterial blood may be drawn during the test to analyze ABG levels. Tell him to report any swelling or bleeding at the puncture site or any numbness, tingling, or pain in the punctured arm or leg.

Emphasize that the test will proceed quickly if he follows directions and keeps a tight seal around the mouthpiece or tube. These measures also will promote accurate results. Forewarn him that he may experience shortness of breath and fatigue during the test, but that he'll be allowed to rest periodically. Instruct him to inform the technician, however, if he experiences dizziness, chest pain, palpitations, nausea, severe dyspnea, or wheezing.

Bronchoscopy

Explain that this test allows direct visualization of the patient's airway to confirm the diagnosis. Discuss the procedure in detail; then give the patient a copy of the teaching aid *Preparing for bronchoscopy,* page 305, for review.

Needle biopsy

Explain that a percutaneous needle biopsy is used to diagnose and stage the disease. Mention that this test can take 30 to 60 minutes. Then inform the patient that he'll receive a local anesthetic before the doctor makes a small incision and introduces a biopsy needle through the incision, chest wall, and pleura into the lung tumor. After obtaining a tissue sample for analysis, the doctor will withdraw the needle and apply pressure and a small bandage to the incision site.

Thoracentesis

Tell the patient that thoracentesis provides tissue or fluid samples from areas surrounding the lungs, which helps the doctor determine the extent of lung disease. Explain that the patient will wear a hospital gown during the test. His vital signs will be taken and the area around the needle insertion site will be cleansed and shaved.

Then he'll be positioned with his arms on pillows or over a bed table or he'll lie partially on his side in bed. The doctor will cleanse the needle insertion site with a cold antiseptic solution, then inject a local anesthetic. Warn the patient that he may feel a burning sensation as the doctor injects the anesthetic, and that he'll feel pressure during needle insertion and withdrawal. Instruct him to remain still during the test to avoid risking lung injury.

Encourage him to relax and breathe normally during the test, and warn him not to cough, breathe deeply, or move. Instruct him to notify the doctor if he has breathing difficulties or feels weak and sick. These responses may indicate respiratory distress. Tell him also that after the needle's withdrawn he'll feel the doctor apply pressure and a bandage to the puncture site.

Reassure him that after the test the nurse will monitor his blood pressure, heart rate, and breathing for several hours. Tell him to report any fluid or blood leakage from the needle insertion site and to report respiratory distress signs as well; for example, shortness of breath, palpitations, wheezing, dizziness, weakness, or profuse sweating. Explain that he'll have a chest X-ray to document how well he's recovering and to detect any complications.

Mediastinoscopy

Inform the patient that this test, which is performed in the operating room, allows the doctor to visualize the mediastinal area and to obtain tissue samples for analysis. This helps determine appropriate treatment. Caution the patient not to eat or drink for 8 hours before the test. Inform him that he'll receive an I.V. sedative before the test and then a general anesthetic.

Explain that while the patient's anesthetized, the doctor will insert an endotracheal tube to ensure an open airway during the surgical procedure. Then he'll make a small incision in the patient's chest and insert a mediastinoscope to obtain tissue specimens for analysis.

Advise the patient that when he awakens in the recovery room, the endotrachael tube may remain in place for several hours or overnight. He can expect a nurse to monitor his vital signs frequently for the first 4 hours after the test.

Warn him that he may have pain or tenderness at the incision site, a sore throat, and hoarseness. He may also experience nausea, vomiting, and a sense of unreality from the anesthetic. Reassure him that these effects are temporary and that he may request analgesics for pain.

Computed tomography scan

Inform the patient that a computed tomography (CT) scan uses computer technology to help diagnose and monitor pulmonary lesions. To enhance the images obtained by CT scan, the doctor may use a contrast medium. If he does, advise the patient not to eat or drink anything for 4 hours before the test. Explain that after he removes all jewelry and other metal objects from his head and neck area, he'll lie on his back on a narrow table that will glide slowly into the center of a large, noisy, tunnel-shaped machine.

If the patient is having a contrast study, the doctor will inject a dyelike substance called a contrast medium into an arm vein. Inform the patient that he may experience nausea, flushing, warmth, and a salty taste but that these symptoms will subside. Advise him to alert the technician immediately if he feels burning in his arm.

Inform him that he'll be asked not to move during the test. Instruct him to relax and breathe normally. Tell him that movement may invalidate test results and necessitate repeated testing.

Bone scan

Explain that a bone scan permits skeletal imaging with a scanning camera after the patient receives an I.V. radioactive tracer compound. Tell the patient that this test can detect tumors and show where the cancer has spread.

After the patient receives an I.V. injection of the tracer and imaging agent, encourage him to increase his fluid intake for the next 1 to 3 hours to boost renal clearance of the circulating free tracer that isn't taken up by the bone. Instruct him to void immediately before the procedure. Then describe how he'll lie on the X-ray table while the scanner moves back and forth over his body. He may be repositioned several times to obtain adequate views. Assure him that the scan itself, which takes about 60 minutes, is painless and that the isotope emits less radiation than a standard X-ray machine.

Gallium scan

Explain that this scan helps detect primary and metastatic tumors. Inform the patient that he needn't restrict food or fluids for this test, which takes 30 to 60 minutes. The doctor usually schedules the test for 24 to 48 hours after the I.V. injection of radioactive gallium citrate (^{67}Ga). Warn the patient that he may experience transient discomfort from the needle puncture during the injection. Reassure him, however, that the substance is only slightly radioactive and is not harmful.

If the radiologist uses a gamma scintillation camera, assure the patient that the uptake probe and detector head may touch his skin but won't cause discomfort. If he uses a rectilinear scanner, describe the soft, irregular clicking noise it makes as it registers radiation emissions. Inform the patient that he may be positioned erect or prone or in an appropriate combination of these positions, depending on his physical condition and which views (or angles) the doctor chooses. Tell him that he won't need any special care after the test.

Liver-spleen scans

Inform the patient that these scans can show metastasis to the liver and spleen through pictures taken with a special scanner or camera. Reassure him that the test is painless and that it takes about 60 minutes.

Explain that he will receive an injection of a radioactive isotope ^{99m}Tc—technetium Tc 99m sulfur colloid—through an I.V. line in his hand or arm. Tell him to report flushing, feverishness, light-headedness, or difficulty breathing. Assure him that the injection contains only trace amounts of radioactivity and rarely produces side effects. If the test equipment includes a rectilinear scanner, he'll hear a soft, irregular clicking noise as it moves across his abdomen. If the test equipment includes a gamma scintillation camera, he'll feel the camera lightly touch his abdomen. Instruct him to lie still, relax, and breathe normally. He may be asked to hold his breath briefly to ensure clear, high-quality pictures. Tell him that he'll need no special after-test care.

Teach about treatments

Inform the patient that treatment depends on the disease's type and stage. Surgery, radiation therapy, and chemotherapy are all options. Teach him about the benefits and risks of each so that he knows what to expect.

Medication

Discuss analgesic medications to relieve pain and anticancer drugs to treat lung cancer.

Analgesics. If the patient's taking a narcotic drug, such as morphine (Duramorph) or hydromorphone (Dilaudid), advise him to avoid driving and other activities that require alertness. Instruct him not to drink alcohol or use other central nervous system depressants while taking his medication. Tell him to take the drug exactly as prescribed, even when his pain subsides. To prevent constipation, suggest that he use a stool softener.

Chemotherapy. If the patient's undergoing chemotherapy, explain that this form of drug therapy kills cancer cells by interfering with their reproduction. He'll receive these drugs by mouth or by injection into his veins, muscles, or spinal fluid. Typically, they're given in specific cycles and sequences, so that his body can recover during the drug-free period.

Identify the type and sequence of drugs that he'll receive. For example, the doctor may order combinations of cyclophosphamide (Cytoxan), doxorubicin (Adriamycin), and etoposide (Vepesid); or methotrexate (Mexate) and vincristine (Oncovin).

If appropriate, provide instructions for administering chemotherapy at home, including advice for taking liquids, tablets, pills, or capsules. If he'll receive chemotherapy through an implanted infusion port (such as Infus-A-Port or Port-A-Cath), explain that he'll need no dressing or special care after the incision heals. Inform the patient of any harmful drug interactions.

Explain that side effects occur during chemotherapy because the drugs can affect *any* rapidly growing cells in the body—normal cells as well as cancer cells. The normal cells most likely to be affected are in the bone marrow, digestive tract, reproductive organs, and hair follicles.

Teach him prophylactic measures to decrease the side effects of chemotherapy. For example, inform him that proper mouth care from the start of chemotherapy can help prevent mouth ulcers. Suggest that he rinse his mouth hourly with normal saline. Give him a copy of the patient-teaching aid *How to control the side effects of chemotherapy and radiation therapy,* pages 306 to 309.

Stress that every person responds differently to chemotherapy. Some have few or no side effects; others have a more difficult time. Reassure the patient that if a drug causes severe side effects, the doctor can adjust the dosage or prescribe medications to relieve those side effects. Explain that most side effects subside before or shortly after treatment ends.

During chemotherapy, encourage the patient to balance activity with rest. Tell him that compliance with these measures will help him to tolerate his treatments. Explain that the side effects of chemotherapy may leave him anemic and more tired than usual. Mention, too, that the fatigue some patients experience during chemotherapy may linger after treatment ends.

At the same time that you advise the patient to get lots of rest, warn him not to become too inactive. This may lead to deconditioning and even more fatigue. Help him plan his daily routine to make the most of his limited energy.

With the dietitian, teach the patient how to balance his diet and eat foods high in calories and protein to promote healing. For example, you might suggest adding milk or cream to soups and casseroles. Also provide tips to stimulate his appetite if his desire for food lags during chemotherapy. And for easier digestion, suggest eating five or six small meals a day instead of three big ones. Tell him that drinking plenty of fluids will help flush the toxic byproducts produced by chemotherapy or tumor breakdown from his body.

Procedures

Explain to the patient that radiation therapy destroys the cancer cells' ability to grow and multiply and that it also affects normal cells. However, normal cells usually recover quickly. Make sure the patient understands when and where he'll receive radiation therapy and who will administer it. Reinforce his doctor's explanations, and answer any questions. Tell him to notify the doctor if side effects persist or become especially troublesome or if he has a fever, cough, or unusual pain. For activity and diet teaching points during radiation therapy, refer to the guidelines for controlling the side effects of chemotherapy and radiation therapy mentioned earlier.

Surgery

If the patient's scheduled for surgery, supplement and reinforce the doctor's explanation of the disease and the surgery. Using the illustrations in *Teaching about lung surgery,* page 302, point out which part of his lung will be removed.

Inform the patient that the surgeon will perform a thoracotomy—an incision of the chest wall—to remove the cancerous lung tissue. Show him the area where he can expect to feel the incision after surgery (for example, posterolateral, anterolateral, or mediastinal).

Next, discuss possible complications—most notably, atelectasis and acute respiratory failure. Explain how lung cancer limits cardiopulmonary reserve and increases the risk for complications. Reassure the patient that the health care team will monitor his condition after surgery to minimize atelectasis and to reverse it promptly. Note that significant atelectasis could prolong his need for intubation and mechanical ventilation as well as lead to pneumonia, sepsis, and acute respiratory failure. Then, as appropriate, tell him what he'll need to know about postoperative care measures.

Endotracheal intubation. Inform the patient that he'll remain intubated for 4 to 6 hours after surgery, or perhaps overnight, to support his breathing and to clear mucus from his lungs. Explain that the endotracheal tube may be uncomfortable and that he

---

Teaching about lung surgery

If your patient has operable lung cancer and is scheduled for surgery, discuss the type of operation he'll have. Explain that the surgeon may perform one of four procedures.

Lobectomy
In lobectomy, the surgeon removes a cancerous lobe from the lung.

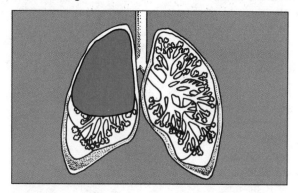

Segmentectomy
By removing one or more lung segments, the surgeon attempts to preserve as much functional, healthy tissue as possible.

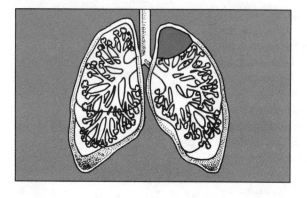

Wedge resection
The surgeon removes lung tissue without regard to segmental planes. This operation's reserved for small cancers in patients with poor pulmonary reserve.

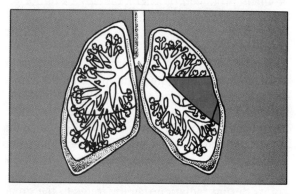

Pneumonectomy
The surgeon removes an entire cancerous lung.

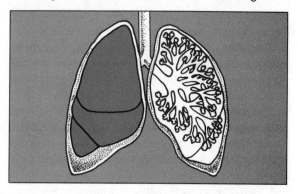

---

won't be able to talk while it's in place. Warn him that trying to remove the tube may cause larnygeal injury.

Explain that the nurse will suction accumulated mucus through the tube, possibly causing him brief dyspnea and coughing. Assure him that after suctioning, he'll receive extra breathing help with a hand-held resuscitator (Ambu bag) or a respirator.

Chest tube placement. Unless the patient's scheduled for a pneumonectomy, inform him that he'll have a chest tube in place after surgery to drain blood and fluid and to help expand his lung. Add that the drainage system will be attached to suction, which makes a bubbling noise. Warn him that the chest tube will cause discomfort.

Positioning. Prepare the patient for frequent position changes after surgery. Forewarn him that he'll be repositioned at least once an hour immediately after surgery and then every 2 hours for the first day after surgery.

Bronchial hygiene. Emphasize that coughing and deep-breathing exercises after surgery will promote free breathing passages. Give him the teaching aid *How to use a flow incentive spirometer,* page 310.

Also teach him segmental breathing exercises, which use biofeedback. Have him place his hand over the incision and apply moderate pressure. Then, tell him to relax and concentrate on getting air to the lung segment underneath his hand. Have him do pursed-lip breathing until he can expand this segment with minimal effort.

Pain control. Tell the patient that he'll receive analgesics postoperatively, but that the dosage won't be strong enough to relieve pain fully. Explain that analgesics depress respiration and interfere with bronchial hygiene.

Mobility measures. Tell the patient that as soon as his vital signs stabilize, he'll begin taking steps to regain his mobility. First he'll sit and dangle his legs over the bedside; next he'll sit in a chair; and then he'll begin walking with assistance. While he's in bed, show him how to do ankle circles and leg- and arm-raising exercises to promote muscle tone and circulation.

Other care measures
Because both chemotherapy and radiation therapy typically increase the patient's susceptibility to infection, warn him to stay out of crowds and to avoid individuals with known infections. Suggest that he avoid his friends if they have colds or other infections. Also show him proper hand-washing techniques to prevent infection.

Pain-management skills are another teaching priority for the lung cancer patient. Explain pain reduction methods, such as relaxation or stimulation techniques, to help him manage anxiety, nausea, vomiting, and discomfort.

If appropriate, inform the patient and his family about hospital and community sources of support. Refer them to a social worker, psychologist, or religious or spiritual counselor, and arrange an appointment if they wish you to do so. Take the time to respond to the patient's questions about his illness, without burdening him with more information than he needs or wants to know. If the patient has terminal cancer, offer advice on local counseling services and hospice or home care.

Educate high-risk patients in ways to reduce lung cancer risks. Refer smokers to local branches of the American Cancer

Society or groups that offer stop-smoking programs. Alert patients and their families to occupational health hazards, and urge them to limit their exposure to these hazards by adopting safety measures, such as protective clothing and ventilator masks. Encourage them to join or form groups to support or initiate effective ventilation and air-filtration programs.

Sources of information and support

American Cancer Society
90 Park Avenue, New York, N.Y. 10016
(212) 599-8200

American Lung Association
1740 Broadway, New York, N.Y. 10019
(212) 315-8700

National Institute for Occupational Safety and Health
U.S. Department of Health and Human Services, Parklawn Building, 5600 Fishers Lane, Rockville, Md. 20857
(301) 443-2140

Occupational Safety and Health Administration (OSHA)
U.S. Department of Labor, 200 Constitution Avenue, Washington, D.C. 20210
(202) 523-6138

Office of Cancer Communications
National Cancer Institute, Bethesda, Md. 20014
(800) 638-6694

Further readings

Friedman, P.J. "Lung Cancer: Update on Staging Classification," *American Journal of Roentgenology* 150(2):261-64, February 1988.
Groenwald, S.L., ed. *Cancer Nursing Principles and Practice.* Boston: Jones and Bartlett, 1987.
Irmonato, L., et al. "Estimates of the Proportion of Lung Cancer Attributable to Occupational Exposure," *Carcinogenesis* 9(7):1159-65, July 1988.
Kottke, T.E., et al. "Smoking Cessation Strategies and Evaluation," *Journal of the American College of Cardiologists* 12(4):1105-10, October 1988.
Naruke, T., et al. "Prognosis and Survival in Resected Lung Carcinoma Based On the New International Staging System," *Journal of Thoracic and Cardiovascular Surgery* 96(3):440-47, September 1988.
Risser, N.L. "The Key to Prevention of Lung Cancer: Stop Smoking," *Seminars in Oncology Nursing* 3(3):228-36, August 1987.
Strohl, R.A. "The Nursing Role in Radiation Oncology: Symptom Management of Acute and Chronic Reactions," *Oncology Nursing Forum* 15(4): 429-34, July-August 1988.
Ziegfeld, C.R., ed. *Core Curriculum for Oncology Nursing.* Philadelphia: W.B. Saunders Co., 1987.

Preparing for bronchoscopy

Dear Patient:

Here are some facts you'll want to know about the bronchoscopy the doctor has scheduled for you.

This test permits the doctor to examine your airway (your windpipe and lungs) with a thin, flexible instrument called a bronchoscope.

By looking through the instrument's eyepiece, the doctor can see abnormalities and obstructions. With another part of the instrument, he can obtain tiny tissue samples to help diagnose your illness. And he can remove foreign bodies or excess mucus.

Before the test

Don't eat for 8 hours before the test and don't drink any alcoholic beverages for 24 hours beforehand either. Food and alcohol can cause test complications and create problems with any sedatives you're given.

Do continue to take any prescribed drugs, unless the doctor says not to.

Just before the test, you'll receive a local anesthetic to numb the back of your throat and to stop you from gagging. This helps the bronchoscope slide easily inside your trachea.

You'll receive a sedative to help you relax.

During the test

The test takes 30 to 60 minutes. You'll lie on your back or sit upright, depending on your comfort and the doctor's preference. Once the doctor suppresses your gag reflex with an anesthetic, he'll insert the end of the bronchoscope through your nose or your mouth.

As he advances the instrument, he'll flush small amounts of liquid anesthetic through it to decrease any coughing and wheezing you may have. The instrument will slide through your major airways. Now you may experience some discomfort with breathing. Remember to stay calm. If necessary, the doctor will give you extra oxygen.

When the examination's over, the doctor will remove the bronchoscope.

After the test

About every 15 minutes, the nurse will monitor your blood pressure, heart rate, breathing, and temperature to make sure you're recovering well. You'll lie comfortably with your head raised. Until the anesthetic wears off and your gag reflex returns, you won't be allowed to eat, drink, or take oral medications. You may be hoarse or have a sore throat, but this is only temporary. You may gargle or suck on throat lozenges once your gag reflex returns.

Soon after the test, you'll have a chest X-ray — also to make sure you're doing well.

Your sedative may not have worn off by the time you're ready to go home. So for safety's sake, arrange for someone to take you home from the hospital or clinic.

Call the doctor or nurse immediately if you have any of these symptoms: bloody mucus, difficulty breathing, wheezing, or chest pain.

How to control the side effects of chemotherapy and radiation therapy

Dear Patient:

Your doctor has ordered chemotherapy or radiation therapy (or perhaps both) to treat your cancer. Besides treating cancer, these therapies often cause unpleasant side effects. Fortunately, you can sometimes prevent them. Other times you can do things to make yourself more comfortable. Just follow the advice below.

Mouth sores
• If you're going to have radiation therapy, see your dentist beforehand.
• Keep your mouth and teeth clean by brushing after every meal with a soft toothbrush.

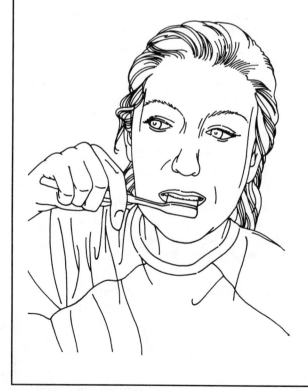

• Don't use commercial mouthwashes that contain alcohol, which tends to irritate your mouth during radiation therapy. Instead, rinse with water, water mixed with baking soda, or a mouthwash containing equal parts of Kaopectate and Benadryl Elixir. Floss daily, and apply fluoride if your dentist recommends it. If you have dentures, remove them often for cleaning.
• Until your mouth sores heal, avoid foods that are difficult to chew (such as apples) or irritating to your mouth (such as acidic citrus juices). Also avoid drinking alcohol, smoking, and eating extremely hot or spicy foods.
• Eat soft, bland foods, such as eggs and oatmeal, and soothing foods, such as ice pops. Your doctor might also prescribe medication for mouth sores.

Dry mouth
• Frequently sip cool liquids and suck on ice chips or sugarless candy.
• Ask your doctor about artificial saliva. Moisten your food with water, juices, sauces, and dressings to soften the food and make it easier to swallow. Don't smoke or drink alcohol, which can further dry your mouth.

Nausea and vomiting
• Before a radiation treatment, try eating a light, bland snack, such as toast or crackers. Or don't eat anything—some patients find that fasting controls nausea better.
• Keep unpleasant odors out of your

continued

How to control the side effects of chemotherapy and radiation therapy — *continued*

dining area. Avoid strong-smelling foods. Also brush your teeth before eating to refresh your mouth.
- Eat small, frequent meals and avoid lying down for 2 hours after you eat. Try small amounts of clear, unsweetened liquids, such as apple juice, and then progress to crackers or dry toast. Stay away from sweets and fried or other high-fat foods. It's best to stay with bland foods.
- Take antiemetic drugs, as your doctor orders. Be sure to notify him if vomiting is severe or lasts longer than 24 hours, or if you are urinating less, feel weak, or have a dry mouth.

Diarrhea
- Stick with low-fiber foods, such as bananas, rice, applesauce, toast, or mashed potatoes. Stay away from high-fiber foods, such as raw vegetables and fruits and whole-grain breads. Also avoid milk products and fruit juices. Cabbage, coffee, beans, and sweets can increase stomach cramps.
- Because potassium may be lost when you have diarrhea, eat high-potassium foods, such as bananas and potatoes. Check with your doctor to see if you need a potassium supplement.
- After a bowel movement, clean your anal area gently and apply petroleum jelly to prevent soreness.
- Ask your doctor about antidiarrheal medications. Notify him if your diarrhea doesn't stop or if you urinate less, have a dry mouth, or feel weak.

Constipation
- Eat high-fiber foods unless your doctor tells you otherwise. They include raw fruits and vegetables (with skins on),

whole-grain breads and cereals, and beans. If you're not used to eating high-fiber foods, start gradually to let your body get accustomed to the change — or else you could develop diarrhea.
- Drink plenty of liquids — unless your doctor tells you not to.
- If changing your diet doesn't help, ask your doctor about stool softeners or laxatives. Check with your doctor before using enemas.

Heartburn
- Avoid spicy foods, alcohol, and smoking. Eat small, frequent meals.
- After eating, don't lie down right away. Avoid bending or stooping.
- Take oral medications with a glass of milk or a snack.
- Use antacids, as your doctor orders.

Muscle aches or pain, weakness, numbness or tingling
- Take acetaminophen (Tylenol). Or ask your doctor for acetaminophen with codeine.
- Apply heat where it hurts or feels numb.

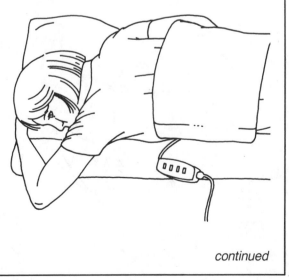

continued

PATIENT-TEACHING AID

How to control the side effects of chemotherapy and radiation therapy — *continued*

• Be sure to rest. Also, avoid activities that aggravate your symptoms.
• If symptoms don't go away and pain focuses on one area, notify your doctor.

Hair loss

• Wash your hair gently. Use a mild shampoo and avoid frequent brushing or combing.
• Get a short hair cut to make thinning hair less noticeable.
• Consider wearing a wig or toupee during therapy. Buy one before radiation begins. Or use a hat, a scarf, or a turban to cover your head during therapy.

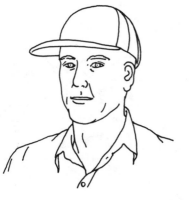

Skin problems

• For sensitive or dry skin, ask your doctor or nurse to recommend a lotion. Don't use petroleum jelly or nonprescription creams and powders. They could leave a coating that will interfere with your radiation treatments.

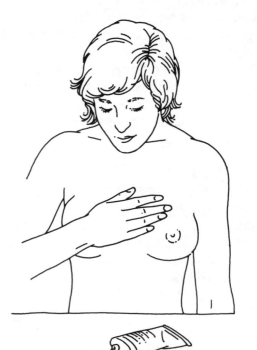

• Use cornstarch to absorb moisture, and avoid tight clothing over the treatment area. Be sure to report any blisters or cracked skin to the doctor.
• Stay out of the sun during the course of therapy. You may even have to avoid the sun for several months afterward, so check with your doctor, especially if you're planning a vacation to a sunny area. When you *can* go out in the sun

continued

How to control the side effects of chemotherapy and radiation therapy — *continued*

again, wear light clothes over the treated area, and wear a hat, too. Cover all exposed skin with a good sun block lotion (SPF 15 or above).

Tiredness
- Limit activities, especially sports.
- Get more sleep.
- Try to reduce your work hours until the end of treatments. Discuss your therapy schedule with your employer.
- If at all possible, schedule radiation treatments at your convenience.
- Ask for help from family and friends, whether it's pitching in with daily chores or driving you to the hospital.

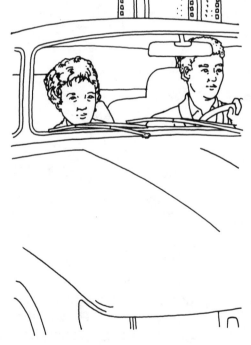

Most people are glad to help out — they just need to be asked.
- If you lose interest in sex during

treatments, either because you're too tired or because of hormonal changes, bear in mind that sexual desire usually returns after treatments end. One special note: Avoid sex if you're receiving radiation treatments to your abdomen — intercourse may be painful. This should also improve after treatment ends.

Risk of infection
You're more likely to get an infection during therapy, so follow these tips:
- Avoid crowds and people with colds and infections.
- Use an electric shaver instead of a razor.

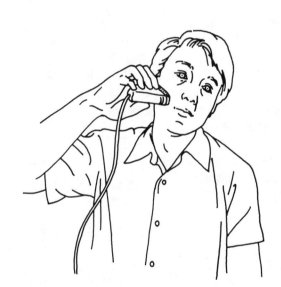

- Use a soft toothbrush. It will help you avoid injuring your gums — a frequent site of infection.
- Tell your doctor if you have a fever, chills, a tendency to bruise easily, or any unusual bleeding.

How to use a flow incentive spirometer

Dear Patient:

Your doctor wants you to use a breathing aid called an incentive spirometer. This device encourages you to breathe deeply and provides instant feedback to show how well you're doing.

    Several types of incentive spirometers are available. The type shown here has one ball. You use them all in the same way. Just follow these steps:

1 Sit up as straight as you can to help your lungs expand fully. Hold the spirometer's mouthpiece with one hand and the meter with your other hand. Position your hands so the instrument is nearly level with your mouth.

2 Exhale normally. Now place your lips tightly around the spirometer's mouthpiece.

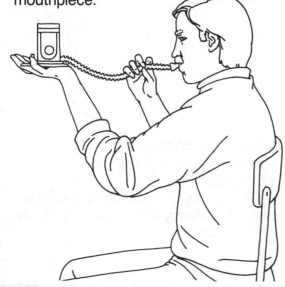

3 With the spirometer at its lowest setting, slowly inhale through the mouthpiece as much as you can. Watch the ball in the spirometer to see how deeply you've inhaled. Usually, a rising ball marks your progress.

    The more fully you expand your lungs, the higher the ball will rise. Now hold your breath and count to 3 (even though the ball drops).

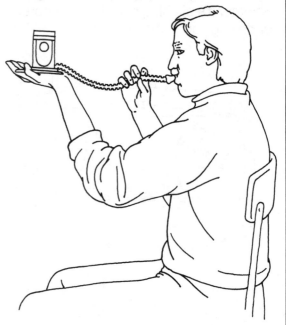

4 Finally, remove the mouthpiece from your mouth, and exhale normally. Rest for a moment. Repeat the exercise about 10 times, resting after each time.

    As you increase your lung capacity, you'll see the ball rise higher. And as you master one level on the spirometer, aim for the next level of difficulty.

Colorectal cancer

Diagnosis of colorectal cancer is certain to spark myriad emotions in a patient—and pose a twofold challenge for you. First, you'll need to support him as he confronts his fears about death, cancer, and treatment. What's more, you'll need to ensure that he and his family have accurate and adequate information for making decisions about treatment, participate in care throughout treatment and recovery, and maintain a positive attitude. (See *Teaching the patient with newly diagnosed colorectal cancer*, page 312.)

Initially, you'll prepare the patient for diagnostic tests. Then you may need to clarify their results: explaining how the tumor type and location, its stage, and the patient's overall health help determine the most effective therapy. You'll discuss treatments, which may include surgery, radiation, and chemotherapy, and you may teach about stoma care.

Point out that 5-year survival rates for patients with colorectal cancer (without metastasis) are relatively high: about 80% for those with rectal cancer and over 85% for those with colon cancer. Helping the patient to appraise his condition realistically may help him come to terms with his prospects for recovery.

Discuss the disorder

Tell the patient that colorectal cancer is one of the most common cancers affecting men and women. Point out that about 95% of tumors are adenocarcinomas. Outline the risk factors for this disease (see *Identifying colorectal cancer risk factors*, page 313).

Inform the patient that most colorectal cancers grow slowly and cause few, if any, symptoms until the disease is well advanced. Review the symptoms of colorectal disease with the patient and his family:
• rectal bleeding
• a change in bowel habits (diarrhea or constipation)
• thin, pencil-like stools
• persistent fatigue
• abdominal cramps or bloating
• fecal urgency
• a sensation of incomplete defecation (tenesmus)
• weight loss
• pain (a late symptom in the relatively insensitive colorectal area).

Explain that tumors can spread by direct invasion, or they can infiltrate the blood or lymphatic system. Mention that the tumor size doesn't necessarily correlate with the extent of metastasis.

Louise P. Joffrion, RN, MSN, CNS, who wrote this chapter, is coordinator, nursing of adults, at the Baton Rouge General School of Nursing, Baton Rouge, La.

CHECKLIST

Teaching topics in colorectal cancer

☐ An explanation of colorectal cancer
☐ Risk factors, such as age and high-fat, low-fiber diet
☐ Symptoms, including rectal bleeding and a change in bowel habits
☐ Complications, such as intestinal obstruction and anemia
☐ Preparation for diagnostic workup, including fecal occult blood test, barium enema, colonoscopy, and sigmoidoscopy
☐ Dukes staging system
☐ Chemotherapy
☐ Radiation therapy
☐ Explanation of surgery, such as low anterior resection, Hartmann's procedure, and loop colostomy
☐ Postoperative care
☐ Colostomy care and life-style alterations
☐ Sources of information and support

Teaching the patient with newly diagnosed colorectal cancer

When a patient first learns that he has colorectal cancer, he's likely to be overwhelmed by feelings of denial, anger, and fear. However, you may be able to help mitigate these feelings by giving clear information about cancer and its treatment.

But what will you teach the patient about colorectal cancer? And what options and techniques should he learn about? Start by reading the following account of John Martin's experience to learn how to modify a standardized teaching plan to suit the patient's needs.

Reviewing the patient's condition
Mr. Martin, a 54-year-old mechanic, has just been diagnosed with colorectal cancer. He tells you that his father and uncle had colorectal cancer years ago, so his diagnosis isn't a complete surprise.

Mr. Martin was first suspected of having colorectal cancer after a fecal occult blood screening turned out to be positive. He knew then that "something was wrong." He had been constipated for 2 or 3 months and had narrowed stools, but attributed these symptoms to "not enough exercise."

The doctor ordered a flexible sigmoidoscopy with biopsy, which revealed malignant polyps in the sigmoid colon. Fortunately, other tests were negative for metastasis. Although encouraged by the news that his cancer hasn't spread, Mr. Martin is apprehensive about his impending surgery.

What are Mr. Martin's learning needs?
Using a standard teaching plan as a guide, you decide what information to include or adapt in your teaching about colorectal cancer. A standard plan for colorectal cancer addresses:
• GI function, including anatomy
• risk factors, signs and symptoms, stages, and complications
• preoperative diagnostic studies
• radiation and chemotherapy
• surgical options
• care of a colostomy
• life-style alterations, including activity, diet, and medications.

After reviewing the standard plan, you conclude that Mr. Martin knows little about colorectal cancer. Furthermore, his current state of distress impairs his ability to learn. He recalls how much pain his father and uncle experienced with cancer. Also his limited education prevents lengthy teaching sessions with complex material. You decide to give him a simple explanation of his disease and focus on teaching about his surgery. You also reassure him about today's better postoperative pain control measures.

You explain the type of surgery he'll most likely undergo, and you briefly outline the purpose and function of a colostomy. Later, you'll teach about activity restrictions, stoma and skin care, colostomy appliances, dietary modifications, and drugs.

Setting learning outcomes
Based on Mr. Martin's current discharge needs, you develop his learning outcomes together. For example, Mr. Martin will be able to:
- describe GI function and dysfunction
- relate personal symptoms of colorectal cancer
- explain reasons for diagnostic tests
- state the purpose of colostomy surgery
- report postoperative complications that require prompt medical attention
- demonstrate colostomy self-care, including pouch changes and irrigation
- describe dietary and skin care considerations for colostomy patients
- relate characteristics of a healthy stoma
- discuss the type and size of the colostomy pouch and supplies he'll require
- identify sources for colostomy supplies and assistance.

Selecting teaching techniques and tools
After assessing Mr. Martin and talking with him preoperatively, you choose brief *one-to-one discussions* about GI function, cancer risks, surgery, colostomy care, and dietary and skin considerations. Because on discharge he must be able to perform ostomy care, including skin barrier and pouch changes and colostomy irrigation, you *demonstrate* these skills.

Mr. Martin is worried and easily overwhelmed, so you provide only a few *simple teaching booklets,* with lots of pictures. You'll want to review your discussions and the booklets with him frequently. You also supply real *examples of pouches and other supplies* he'll use. Other appropriate materials may include *diagrams* and *videotapes.*

Evaluating your teaching
Will Mr. Martin be able to care for his ostomy? Is he aware of dietary and preventive skin care measures he'll need to follow? To find out, you'll need to evaluate your teaching. Do this by *question and answer discussions.* For example, ask him to describe the equipment he'll need to irrigate his colostomy.

Return demonstration is another way of evaluating teaching. Because ostomy care requires so many hands-on skills, ask Mr. Martin to show you how he'll change his skin barrier and ostomy pouch and irrigate his colostomy. Evaluating Mr. Martin's new skills and knowledge will help you determine his progress in meeting learning outcomes. Then you can revise your teaching plan accordingly.

Complications
Untreated colorectal cancer is invariably fatal. Explain that as the tumor grows and encroaches on abdominal organs, abdominal distention and intestinal obstruction occur. Untreated rectal bleeding can lead to anemia.

Describe the diagnostic workup
Prepare the patient for serial tests to diagnose and stage colorectal cancer or to monitor its recurrence or progress. Besides a digital rectal examination and fecal occult blood test, he may have a barium enema or a double contrast barium enema, sigmoidoscopy or colonoscopy, excretory urography, or computed tomography (CT) scan, and several specific blood tests. Inform him that preoperative test results help to determine which surgical procedure he'll undergo.

If appropriate, briefly explain the Dukes classification system, which the pathologist uses to stage colorectal cancer (see *Staging colorectal cancer,* page 314).

Digital rectal examination
Inform the patient that a digital rectal examination can detect suspicious rectal and perianal lesions. Explain that this test is an essential part of every GI workup. Performed in the doctor's office, the hospital, or the clinic, it takes only a few minutes.

Tell the patient that the doctor will apply a lubricant to a gloved finger to minimize the patient's discomfort and possible bleeding. Then he'll insert the finger into the rectum and palpate for masses and enlarged lymph nodes.

Fecal occult blood test
Inform the patient that this simple test is used to detect occult blood in the stool. Explain that rectal bleeding, a warning sign of colorectal cancer, isn't always visible in the stool. Mention that the American Cancer Society recommends this test yearly for everyone over age 50. Depending on the doctor's orders, tell the patient how to use a home test kit to analyze a stool sample or how to collect the sample and deliver it to the doctor's office (or the laboratory) for analysis. Reinforce your instructions with a copy of the patient-teaching aid *Testing for blood in your stool,* page 323.

Barium enema studies
Explain that these radiologic studies use barium, and sometimes air, to examine the large intestine. If the study uses barium and air, tell the patient it's called a double-contrast barium enema test. The test is useful for detecting abnormalities in an obstructed colon region that can't be observed by endoscopy.

Explain that food or fluid in the GI tract prevents a clear outline of the lower GI tract. That's why pretest procedures focus on completely cleansing the intestine. Advise the patient to follow a low-residue diet for 1 to 3 days and then a clear liquid diet for 24 hours before the test. To further cleanse the intestine, the patient will receive a laxative the afternoon before the test and

Identifying colorectal cancer risk factors

Although you can't tell your patient exactly what causes colorectal cancer, you can discuss the following risk factors linked to its development:
• high-fat, low-fiber diet. Explain that fats produce bile acids, which are converted to chemical carcinogens by colon bacteria. Then if too little dietary fiber slows bowel motility, these carcinogens have prolonged contact with the bowel mucosa, increasing the opportunity for cancer development.
• age (increased incidence over age 40)
• adenomatous intestinal polyps
• familial polyposis, Gardner's syndrome, or family cancer history
• personal cancer history
• inflammatory bowel disease (ulcerative colitis or Crohn's disease)
• colon injury or surgery
• sedentary life-style
• occupational exposure to carcinogens, such as organic dyes, solvents, or abrasives.

314 Colorectal cancer

Staging colorectal cancer

Named for pathologist Cuthbert Dukes, the Dukes cancer classification assigns tumors to four stages. These stages (with substages) reflect the extent of bowel mucosa and bowel wall infiltration, lymph node involvement, and metastasis. Use this summary to clarify your patient's cancer stage and prognosis.

Stage A
Malignant cells are confined to the bowel mucosa, and the lymph nodes contain no cancer cells. Treated promptly, about 80% of patients remain disease-free 5 years later.

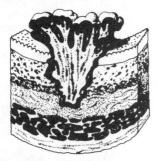

Stage B
Malignant cells extend through the bowel mucosa but remain within the bowel wall. The lymph nodes are normal. In substage B_2, all bowel wall layers and immediately adjacent structures contain malignant cells, but the lymph nodes remain normal. About 50% of patients with substage B_2 survive for 5 years or more.

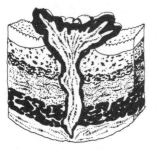

Stage C
Malignant cells extend into the bowel wall and the lymph nodes. In substage C_2, malignant cells extend through the entire thickness of the bowel wall. The lymph nodes also contain malignant cells. The 5-year survival rate for patients with stage C disease reaches about 25%.

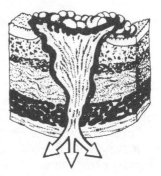

Stage D
Metastasized to distant organs via the lymph nodes and mesenteric vessels, malignant cells typically lodge in the lungs and liver. Only 5% of patients with stage D cancer survive 5 years or more.

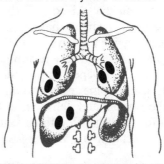

cleansing enemas the evening before or morning of the test. Or the doctor may order a saline lavage.

Inform the patient that during the test he may be secured to a tiltable table, and the doctor will take an X-ray to make sure the large intestine's empty. Then the patient will lie on his left side while the doctor inserts a small lubricated tube into the patient's rectum. Once the tube's inserted, the barium can be instilled slowly to fill the bowel while X-rays are taken.

Instruct the patient to keep his anal sphincter tightly contracted against the tube to hold it in position and prevent barium leakage. Stress the importance of retaining the barium because accurate test results depend on adequately coating the large intestine. (Assure him that the barium is easy to retain because it's cool.)

If the doctor also will instill air through the tube, tell the patient that the table may be tilted and that he'll be assisted into various positions to aid filling. Inform him that he should breathe slowly and deeply through his mouth to ease the discomfort if he feels cramps or the urge to move his bowels as the barium or air fills the large intestine.

Inform the patient that after the test he can expel the barium into a bedpan or toilet. Because barium hardens, causing intestinal obstruction or impaction, he'll receive another laxative and an enema to flush any remaining barium from the intestine. Remember to describe the light color that barium gives the stool for up to 3 days after the test. Inform the patient that he may resume eating and taking medications, as ordered. Encourage fluid intake to prevent dehydration from the bowel preparations and the test. Also, encourage rest because the test is tiring.

Sigmoidoscopy and colonoscopy
Explain that these tests allow the doctor to see inside the lower GI tract with an endoscope (a flexible fiber-optic tube) inserted into the rectum. If the patient's over age 50, point out that he should have a sigmoidoscopic examination every 3 to 5 years (after having two yearly examinations with normal findings). For more information, see *Preparing for a sigmoidoscopy or a colonoscopy,* pages 324 and 325.

Excretory urography
Inform the patient that this test visualizes the urinary tract after the injection of an I.V. contrast medium. Test results can demonstrate a colorectal tumor pressing against the ureters or kidneys or show whether the cancer has spread to the bladder. Tell the patient that a radiologist performs this 45-minute test.

Before the test, ask if the patient's allergic to iodine or I.V. contrast media. If he's had a reaction to these substances in the past, tell him that he may receive diphenhydramine (Benadryl) and prednisone (Deltasone) before and after the test to prevent a reaction. Instruct him not to eat or drink anything after midnight before the test. Explain that moderate dehydration ensures better concentration of the contrast medium, improving visualization. Inform him that he'll receive a laxative or an enema on the test morning. Mention that an X-ray will be taken before the test to verify that his bowel is clear.

Describe how the patient will lie on an X-ray table during the test. Inform him that he may experience some temporary discomfort from the needle puncture. Other transient sensations may include facial flushing, a feeling of warmth, and a salty taste when the contrast medium's injected.

Explain that X-rays will be taken at specific times (usually at 1, 5, 10, 15, 20, and 30 minutes) after injection of the contrast medium. Tomograms also may be taken to identify a mass.

Tell the patient that after the test he'll be assisted to the bathroom to void. Then another X-ray will be taken to determine whether his bladder's completely empty. Explain that he may then resume his previous diet. Encourage him to drink plenty of fluids to reverse the mild dehydration resulting from the test preparations.

CT scan
Inform the patient that a CT scan produces three-dimensional X-ray images of abdominal organs. The test usually follows a barium enema test that yields inconclusive results. It's also ordered if the doctor suspects that cancer's spread to the pelvic lymph nodes. Painless, the test takes about 30 minutes.

Instruct the patient to fast for 4 hours before the test to ensure that food in the stomach or small intestine won't obscure details of the structures being studied. Tell him that he'll also receive laxatives or enemas before the scan to ensure that nothing remains in his bowel. If the CT scan occurs on the same day as other tests, such as excretory urography, he won't need additional laxatives or enemas. If an I.V. contrast medium will be used in the test, be sure to ask the patient if he has known allergies to such agents.

Explain that during the test the patient will lie on his back on an X-ray table. Instruct him to lie still and remain quiet because movement will blur the X-ray image. Reassure him that he can communicate with the test staff, especially if he feels claustrophobic in the tunnel-like scanner. If the doctor injects an I.V. contrast medium, inform the patient that he may experience discomfort from the needle puncture and sensations of warmth, flushing, or a salty taste on injection. Describe the noises the scanner will make as it takes pictures of his abdomen, from the xiphoid process to the pelvic area. Tell him that he'll be able to resume his normal diet after the test.

Blood tests
Describe blood tests that may be ordered to spot anemia, evaluate liver function, and monitor recurrence or metastasis.

Complete blood count. Inform the patient that this test can determine whether he's anemic. Add that anemia commonly accompanies tumors of the right, or ascending, colon.

Liver function studies. Tell the patient that these studies are used to monitor liver function and disease progression. (Colorectal cancer commonly metastasizes to the liver.) Explain that elevated liver enzyme levels may prompt the doctor to order a liver scan and biopsy.

Carcinoembryonic antigen test. Inform the patient that blood levels of carcinoembryonic antigen (CEA), a biological tumor marker, rise in colorectal cancer before treatment. Mention, however, that the test isn't useful for mass screening and detection because elevated CEA levels aren't specific to colorectal cancer. Explain further that CEA levels usually decline after the tumor's removed. A postoperative increase in CEA levels may suggest disease recurrence or metastasis.

Teach about treatments

Because surgical resection of the tumor forms the mainstay of treatment for colorectal cancer, your teaching will focus on preparing the patient to undergo and recover from surgery and, as appropriate, continue treatment through chemotherapy or radiation therapy or both. As needed, offer the patient the teaching aid *How to control the side effects of chemotherapy and radiation therapy,* pages 306 to 309.

Medication

Explain that sometimes when surgery isn't possible—or successful—chemotherapy with fluorouracil (5-fluorouracil) may offer remission or improvement. (Other cytotoxic drugs may be tried as well, but studies suggest that combination therapy may be no more effective than fluorouracil alone.)

Describe the common side effects of fluorouracil I.V. administration: nausea and vomiting soon after treatment, and diarrhea, mouth soreness, and swallowing difficulties between 5 and 8 days later. Instruct the patient to watch for and report stomatitis and ecchymoses, petechiae, and easy bruising. Other side effects include hair loss, hyperpigmentation of the face and hands, hypotension or weakness, itchy eyes, leukopenia, and a rash.

Discuss measures for reducing discomfort. For example, advise the patient that he may receive an antiemetic before he receives fluorouracil. This will minimize nausea. Also explain that he'll have frequent blood tests to ensure that he can take the drug safely.

Procedures

Inform the patient that radiation therapy may be recommended before surgery to shrink a tumor or after surgery (perhaps combined with chemotherapy) to halt any remaining cancer cell growth and to prevent recurrence. Explain that bombarding cancer cells with high-level radiation destroys their ability to grow and multiply. Point out that radiation also affects normal cells, but they usually recover quickly.

Tell the patient that the duration of preoperative radiation therapy depends on the dose. For instance, if he receives low-dose radiation (500 rads), he may have a single treatment. If he receives moderate-dose radiation (2,000 to 2,500 rads), treatment may occur over 2 weeks, with surgery following 2 weeks later. If he has high-dose radiation (4,500 to 5,000 rads), therapy may last over 4 to 6 weeks, with surgery following in 6 weeks. Postoperative radiation therapy usually begins about 1 month after surgery.

Surgery

Inform the patient that surgery—the treatment of choice for colorectal cancer—aims to remove the tumor and surrounding tissue, including regional lymph nodes (to aid staging). Explain that the type of surgery will depend on the tumor's location. Point out that an end-to-end anastomosis is created whenever possible; if not, a colostomy may be necessary.

If appropriate, discuss colostomies, answering the patient's

318 Colorectal cancer

Teaching about surgery and colostomies

A patient facing surgery for colorectal cancer is bound to have questions. To help you answer them, refer to an illustration or a model of the colon when you explain the tumor's location, the type of surgery and, if appropriate, the type of colostomy. As appropriate, point out the bowel sections that will be removed (shown here by dotted lines). Your discussion may help him begin to cope with surgery and a potentially altered self-image.

Inform the patient that the type of surgery depends on the tumor's extent and location. If an anastomosis isn't feasible, the surgeon may construct a colostomy—an outside opening (or stoma) formed from a section of the colon. A colostomy may be permanent if the patient requires removal of portions of the large intestine, including the rectum and anus. Or it may be temporary if the patient has a diseased, inflamed, or injured bowel that requires rest.

Discuss surgery for rectal cancer
If the patient has a tumor in the upper third of the rectum, the surgeon may perform a *low anterior resection.* This involves excising the diseased tissue and then reattaching the rectal structures (an end-to-end anastomosis).

If the tumor lies in the lower part of the rectum, the surgeon may do an *abdominoperineal resection.* In this procedure, he excises the tumor, the rectum, and the anus through an incision in the perineum. Then he creates a *permanent* colostomy through the abdomen. (If the patient's having this surgery, prepare him for one of three postoperative results: His incision will be closed immediately after surgery, closed partially with a drain, or left open and packed. Mention that the wound heals slowly with this procedure.)

Discuss surgery for rectosigmoid colon cancer
If the patient's tumor lies in the rectosigmoid colon, the surgeon may perform *Hartmann's procedure,* creating a colostomy that may be temporary or permanent. This operation leaves the rectum in place, sealing it off as a blind pouch or bringing it through the abdominal wall to create a mucus stoma. Then the proximal end of the colon becomes a functional stoma. Hartmann's procedure allows the bowel to be reconnected later when the wound heals and diagnostic studies confirm no disease.

Describe three types of colostomy
If the patient will have a colostomy, tell him that the most common is the *single-barrel (or end) colostomy,* which is constructed by folding the colon back on itself (like a trouser cuff).

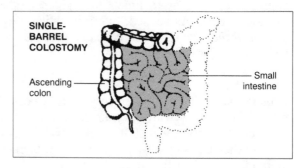

If the surgeon uses both ends of the colon to create a colostomy, tell the patient that he'll have a *double-barrel colostomy.* Explain further that one stoma (fashioned from the proximal colon) acts functionally, whereas the other one (constructed from the distal colon) secretes only mucus. If the surgeon places the two stomas beside each other, the patient can use the same ostomy pouch for both openings. Otherwise, he can wear a small dressing over the mucus-secreting stoma.

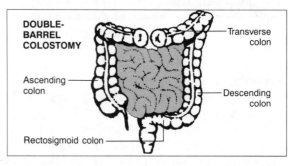

For a *loop colostomy,* the surgeon brings an intact bowel loop through the abdominal wall, then secures the loop with a stabilizing device or a fascial bridge. This keeps the loop in place until it adheres to the abdominal surface in 7 to 10 days. Explain that this temporary procedure diverts fecal matter from the anastomosis site, promoting healing. (Or the procedure may be palliative, performed to overcome an obstruction in a patient with terminal cancer.)

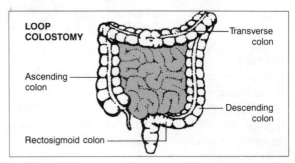

questions about types, permanence, placement, and care (for more information see *Teaching about surgery and colostomies*).

Preoperative considerations. Tell the patient that he'll need to follow a low-residue diet for 3 to 5 days before surgery. Then he'll consume only clear liquids for 1 to 3 days. Explain that the doctor may prescribe an antibiotic to decrease the bacterial count in the colon. Inform him that he'll probably receive enemas or saline lavage for 4 or 5 days before surgery to ensure thorough cleansing of the GI tract.

Inform the patient that after surgery he'll probably have a nasogastric tube in place. Explain that he'll have the tube for several days to remove air and stomach fluids and aid healing.

Postoperative instruction. Because postoperative complications may not develop until after the patient's discharge, caution him to contact the doctor should he suspect or have anastomotic leaks, hemorrhage, irregular bowel function, phantom rectum, ruptured pelvic peritoneum, stricture, urinary dysfunction, or wound infection.

Then describe ways the patient can cope with common postoperative discomforts and speed his recovery. Then, if he has a colostomy, you'll focus on *stoma care*. Initially, discuss the stoma's function and appearance (large, protruding, and swollen after surgery). Explain that swelling will subside over 6 to 9 weeks. Then tell the patient that the stoma won't hurt when touched because it has no nerve endings capable of detecting sharp pain. Add that the stoma should appear red, moist, and soft. If it looks dusky or gray, instruct him to contact the doctor. Explain further that he won't be able to control the stoma at will because it has no muscles. However, he can learn to control his bowel movements by irrigating his colostomy. Make sure to offer him the patient-teaching aid *How to irrigate your colostomy*, pages 326 to 328. For additional teaching tools on colostomy care, use the patient-teaching aids *Removing an ostomy pouch*, page 434; *Applying an ostomy pouch*, page 435; and *Draining an ostomy pouch*, page 436.

Reassure the colostomy patient that his pouch shouldn't show under most garments. Caution him to avoid tight belts or underwear because they can irritate the stoma and block stool drainage.

Discuss ways for *adapting the patient's life-style* during recovery. Tell the patient to limit activity and to avoid heavy lifting or strenuous exercise until he's fully recovered (about 6 weeks). Point out that he'll need the doctor's permission to return to work. If he has a colostomy, reassure him that it shouldn't prevent him from enjoying an active life-style, with the exception of contact sports or weight lifting. (See *Questions colostomy patients ask about life-style changes*, page 320.)

Emphasize that having a colostomy usually doesn't change the patient's desire or capacity for a fulfilling sex life. Suggest that the patient empty the pouch before sexual intercourse or that he use a stoma plug. Mention that some men experience temporary impotence after a colostomy. If the patient encounters such a problem, suggest that he talk with the doctor, enterostomal therapist, or a professional counselor.

Questions colostomy patients ask about life-style changes

How can I take a bath or shower?
You can bathe or shower with or without your pouch. Soap and water won't hurt the stoma and water can't flow into the opening. Be sure to rinse well, though, because soap residue will interfere with pouch adhesion. If you shower, don't let the water hit your stoma directly.

If you decide to keep your pouch on, apply extra tape around the edge of the skin barrier to prevent it from loosening.

Will I be able to exercise?
Having a colostomy shouldn't prevent you from exercising regularly. Check with the doctor first, though. He'll probably tell you to avoid weight lifting and rough contact sports like football.

If you swim, you'll need to ask the doctor or enterostomal therapist about using a stoma plug. This soft foam plug fits into your stoma to block drainage for up to 24 hours. It can't be seen under a bathing suit, and it filters gas without noise or odor.

If you are very active and perspire heavily, you may need to change your pouch more frequently and increase your fluid intake.

Can I go on business trips?
With a little advance preparation, you can travel for business and pleasure. Take along enough colostomy supplies for the entire trip, or call ahead to order replacements if necessary. Always pack your supplies and any prescription medicines (especially for diarrhea or constipation) in your carry-on luggage, so that you can care for yourself if your luggage gets lost.

And remember, use only safe drinking water to irrigate your colostomy.

However, after an abdominoperineal resection that results in a colostomy, nearly all men and many women experience sexual dysfunction. In men, partial or complete dysfunction depends on whether the nerve fibers controlling erection remain intact. In women, dysfunction may result from scarring or contracture at the surgical site.

Give the patient tips for *eating sensibly*. Inform him that he'll probably follow a low-residue diet for 1 to 2 weeks after surgery. He'll be able to resume a normal diet after his bowel heals. To promote regularity, advise him to eat three meals of about the same size daily and to avoid between-meal or late-night snacks. Suggest that he schedule meals at the same time every day.

If the patient has a colostomy, add that he needn't observe any special dietary restrictions. Point out, however, that foods that caused gas or diarrhea before surgery will probably still do so. Suggest that he omit or eat small amounts of these foods.

Give the patient guidelines for *controlling flatulence*. Advise him to eat slowly and chew his food well to prevent swallowing air and subsequent bloating. To identify foods that cause gas, recommend that he keep a daily record of the foods he eats and his reactions to them. Gas-producing foods include apple juice, beer, broccoli, cabbage, carbonated beverages, dairy products, dried beans, and onions. Point out that he may want to eat such foods only at home.

Or suggest odor-proof pouches, pouch deodorants, or a vented stoma plug to control odor. If gas builds up in the pouch, instruct the patient to "burp" the pouch rather than pierce it. Also tell him that simethicone (Mylicon, Phazyme) may relieve belching or bloating. Advise him to take this medication after meals and at bedtime. If he's taking tablets, tell him to chew them thoroughly.

Recommend *relieving constipation* by increasing activity or by increasing fluid intake to at least eight full (8-oz) glasses daily. Eliminating certain constipating medicines, such as iron preparations or narcotic-containing pain relievers, may help too.

Encourage the patient to increase his fiber intake. Point out that eating more fresh fruits and vegetables, whole-grain cereals, nuts, and prunes usually prevents constipation.

If the patient must take an occasional laxative, advise him to ask the doctor to recommend a mild one, such as docusate salts (Colace, Surfak). If he's taking a bulk-forming laxative such as psyllium (Metamucil) or methylcellulose (Cologel), instruct him to avoid bowel impaction by drinking at least eight full glasses of fluid daily. Caution him further to take laxatives (and diuretics) only as recommended by the doctor. In this way he can avoid upsetting his fluid and electrolyte balance. If he becomes mildly dehydrated, such liquids as bouillon, tea, or Gatorade may promote rehydration.

Discuss strategies for *managing diarrhea*. Suggest eating applesauce, bananas, or rice to relieve occasional diarrhea. Inform the patient that some medications, such as antibiotics, can cause diarrhea. Advise him to consult the doctor for an alternative medication if a prescription drug causes diarrhea. If the doctor recommends an antidiarrheal preparation, however, caution the patient to take only this medication. Occasional diarrhea usually responds to a nonprescription product, such as kaolin and pectin (Kaopectate), bismuth subsalicylate (Pepto-Bismol), or loperamide (Imodium). Or the doctor may prescribe diphenoxylate (Lomotil) or paregoric. Warn the patient that paregoric usually relieves severe diarrhea but is habit-forming. Caution him to take it only as directed.

Discuss diarrhea as related to the location of the patient's stoma. If the patient has an ascending or right transverse colostomy, tell him to expect semiliquid to soft stools. Point out that he'll need to routinely empty his pouch several times each day. If he must empty his pouch more often, he may have diarrhea. Instruct him to consult the doctor if he experiences diarrhea for more than a day.

If the patient has a descending or sigmoid colostomy, tell him that he'll have semiformed to formed stools. Point out that he'll probably have one or two bowel movements at predictable times each day. Tell him to consult the doctor about more frequent bowel movements that persist for more than 2 days.

Other care measures

Stress the importance of regular physical examinations. For patients over age 40, emphasize the need for colorectal cancer screening, including annual sigmoidoscopy and rectal examinations.

Discourage smoking, which contributes to altered bowel motility. Help the patient establish a regular bowel routine. Finally, make sure to encourage the patient recovering from colorectal cancer to use support services offered by such groups as the United Ostomy Association and other community organizations.

Sources of information and support

American Cancer Society
1599 Clifton Road, NE, Atlanta, Ga. 30329
(404) 320-3333

International Association for Enterostomal Therapy
2081 Business Circle Drive, Suite 290, Irvine, Calif. 92715
(714) 476-0268

Make Today Count
101½ Union Street, Alexandria, Va. 22314
(703) 548-9674

National Cancer Institute Office of Cancer Communications
Building 31, Room 10A24, Bethesda, Md. 20892
(800) 422-6237

National Hospice Organization
1901 North Moore Street, Suite 901, Arlington, Va. 22209
(703) 243-5900

United Cancer Council
1803 North Meridian Street, Indianapolis, Ind. 46202
(317) 879-9900

United Ostomy Association
36 Executive Park, Suite 120, Irvine, Calif. 92714
(714) 660-8624

Further readings

Alterescu, K.B. "Colostomy," *Nursing Clinics of North America* 22(2):281-89, June 1987.
Fleischer, D., et al. "Detection and Surveillance of Colorectal Cancer," *Journal of the American Medical Association* 261(4):580-85, January 27, 1989.
Guthrie, J.F., et al. "On the Alert for Colorectal Cancer," *Patient Care* 23(8):19-26, 33, April 30, 1989.
Otte, D.M. "Nursing Management of the Patient with Colon and Rectal Cancer," *Seminars in Oncology Nursing* 4(4):285-92, November 1988.
Weinrich, S.P., et al. "Timely Detection of Colorectal Cancer in the Elderly: Implications of the Aging Process," *Cancer Nursing* 12(3):170-76, June 1989.
Wicks, L.J. "Treatment Modalities for Colorectal Cancer," *Seminars in Oncology Nursing* 2(4):242-48, November 1986.
Witt, M.E. "Questions on Colon and Rectum Radiation Therapy," *Oncology Nursing Forum* 14(3)79-82, May-June 1987.

Testing for blood in your stool

Dear Patient:

A home fecal occult blood test is an easy, inexpensive way to detect blood in your stool. For accurate results, follow the directions given by the nurse or doctor, read the instructions included with the test kit, and review these steps.

How to get ready

Don't eat red meat or raw fruits and vegetables for 3 days before you take the test or during the test period. Also avoid diet supplements containing iron or vitamin C and painkillers containing aspirin or ibuprofen (for example, Advil or Nuprin) for 3 days before the test or during the test period. All of these substances can affect test results.

Increase your intake of high-fiber foods, such as whole-grain breads and cereals. Your doctor may also ask you to eat popcorn or nuts.

How to perform the test

1 Make sure all your supplies are in one place. They may include your test cards (or slides), a chemical developer, a wooden applicator, and a watch with a second hand.

2 Obtain a stool sample from the toilet bowl. Use the applicator to smear a thin film of the sample onto the slot marked "A" on the front of the test card. Smear a thin film of a second sample from *a different area of the same stool* onto the slot marked "B" on the same side of the card.

3 *If the doctor or a laboratory* will be analyzing the test samples, close slots A and B. Put your name and the date on the test kit, and return the card (or slide) to the doctor or lab as soon as possible.

If you're doing the test yourself, turn the card over and open the back window. Apply 2 drops of the chemical developer to the paper covering each sample. Wait 1 minute, then read the results.

If either slot has a bluish tint, the test results are positive for blood in the stool. *If neither slot looks blue,* the test results are normal. Write down the results.

4 Repeat the test on your next two bowel movements. Report the results of all of the tests to the doctor. Even if only one of the six test results is positive, the doctor may recommend other tests.

Discard any unused supplies when you've completed all tests.

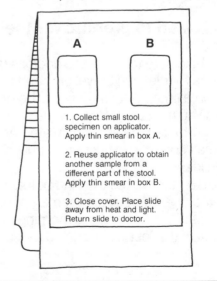

A   B

1. Collect small stool specimen on applicator. Apply thin smear in box A.

2. Reuse applicator to obtain another sample from a different part of the stool. Apply thin smear in box B.

3. Close cover. Place slide away from heat and light. Return slide to doctor.

Preparing for a sigmoidoscopy or a colonoscopy

Dear Patient:

The doctor wants you to undergo a flexible sigmoidoscopy. (If you're scheduled for a colonoscopy, read on because the two tests are similar except for a few differences. These are listed at the end of this patient-teaching aid.)

A sigmoidoscopy allows the doctor to see inside the *lower* part of the large bowel, which includes the sigmoid colon, rectum, and anus. To do this, he'll gently insert a flexible fiber-optic tube called an endoscope into the rectum.

Why is this test necessary?

Sigmoidoscopy allows careful examination of the lower bowel and rectum for bowel disease. (These areas are difficult to visualize by X-rays.) If needed, this test will also enable the doctor to take a biopsy specimen for further testing or to remove polyps.

Will I need to prepare for the test?

Yes. Make sure to follow the doctor's directions for diet and bowel preparation. Stay on a liquid diet for 48 hours beforehand. You may drink clear juices without pulp, broth, tea, gelatin, and water. And you may continue to take prescription medicine.

Take a laxative the evening before the test and give yourself an enema (for example, a Fleet enema) the morning of the test. If the test is scheduled for early morning, don't consume anything past midnight.

Just before the test, you'll take off your clothes and put on a hospital gown. Leave your socks on for warmth. Also empty your bladder.

What can I expect during the test?

The test is done by the doctor and an assistant in an office or a special procedures room. It will last about 15 to 30 minutes. Before the test begins, the assistant will help you lie on your left side with your knees flexed. Next, he'll drape you with a sheet.

Once you're in position, the doctor will gently insert a well-lubricated, gloved finger into the anus to examine the area and dilate the rectal sphincter.

Next, the doctor will gently insert the endoscope through the anus into the rectum. As it passes through the rectal sphincters, you may feel some lower abdominal discomfort and the urge to move your bowels. Bear down gently as the endoscope is first inserted. Also breathe slowly and deeply through your mouth to help you relax. This will help to ease the passage of the endoscope through the sphincters. The doctor will gradually advance the endoscope through the rectum into the lower bowel.

Sometimes air is blown through the endoscope into your bowel to distend it and permit better viewing. If you feel the urge to expel some air, try not to control it and don't be embarrassed. The passing of air is expected and necessary.

continued

PATIENT-TEACHING AID

Preparing for a sigmoidoscopy or a colonoscopy — *continued*

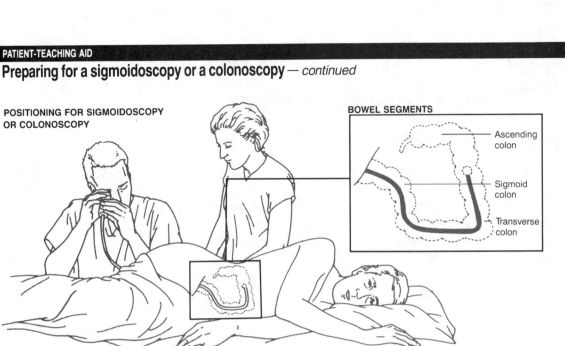

POSITIONING FOR SIGMOIDOSCOPY
OR COLONOSCOPY

BOWEL SEGMENTS

Ascending colon

Sigmoid colon

Transverse colon

You may hear and feel a suction machine removing any liquid that obscures the doctor's view during the test. This machine is noisy but painless.

The doctor will advance the endoscope slowly about 24 inches into the lower bowel. Continue to breathe slowly and deeply through your mouth to help the test go smoothly.

The doctor may remove biopsy specimens or polyps from the lining of the bowel at any time during the test. These procedures also are painless because the bowel lining doesn't sense pain.

Toward the end of the test, the doctor may insert a rigid anoscope into the lower rectum. This instrument will provide a clearer view of the anal wall, revealing any abnormalities that the flexible endoscope might miss.

What can I expect afterward?

The assistant will monitor your vital signs for about an hour afterward. Because air was introduced into your bowel, you'll begin to pass large amounts of gas. Also you may expect to have slight rectal bleeding if the doctor

removed tissue specimens. Notify the doctor immediately if you experience heavy, bright red bleeding; fever; abdominal swelling; or tenderness after the test.

How does a colonoscopy differ from a sigmoidoscopy?

The two tests are similar except a colonoscopy allows the doctor to visualize *all* of your large bowel.

To prepare for this test, follow the doctor's directions for a clear liquid diet and bowel preparation. The bowel preparation is one of two kinds: You may be instructed to drink a large amount of an electrolyte solution (GoLYTELY or Co-Lyte). This solution will clear your bowel in about 4 hours. So plan to stay at home after drinking it. Or you may be asked to take a laxative for two nights before the test and give yourself enemas the morning of the test.

Just before a colonoscopy you'll receive a sedative to help you relax and ease any discomfort you may experience as the doctor advances the endoscope past the curves of the bowel.

How to irrigate your colostomy

Dear Patient:

Irrigating your colostomy at about the same time each day can help you establish a regular bowel pattern and avoid the inconvenience of unexpected bowel movements.

   Choose a time (about 1 hour) when you won't be rushed or interrupted, preferably after a meal. Follow the instructions given by the nurse or doctor. Also read the instructions that come with the irrigation kit, and review the illustrated procedure below.

1 First lay out your supplies in one handy place. You'll need gauze pads, a water-soluble lubricant, a drainage bag, and an irrigator bag, stoma cone, tubing, clamp, gasket,

and belt (if the drainage bag isn't self-adhering). Also make sure you have an irrigation solution and a clean colostomy pouch to replace your used one.

2 Now, sit on the toilet or on a chair next to the toilet. Remove your colostomy pouch.

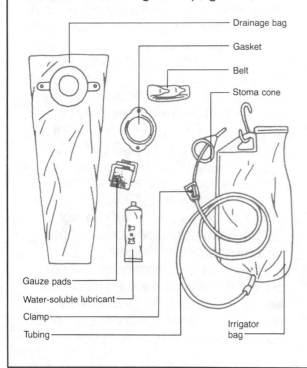

Drainage bag
Gasket
Belt
Stoma cone
Gauze pads
Water-soluble lubricant
Clamp
Tubing
Irrigator bag

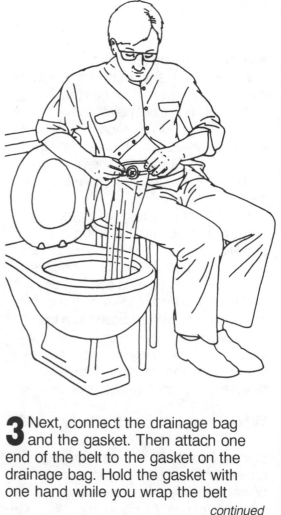

3 Next, connect the drainage bag and the gasket. Then attach one end of the belt to the gasket on the drainage bag. Hold the gasket with one hand while you wrap the belt

continued

How to irrigate your colostomy — *continued*

around your waist with your other hand. Then, attach the other end of the belt to the gasket.

4 Carefully encircle the stoma with the gasket, adjust the belt to fit, and dangle the bottom end of the drainage bag into the toilet.

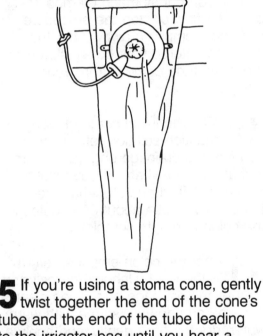

5 If you're using a stoma cone, gently twist together the end of the cone's tube and the end of the tube leading to the irrigator bag until you hear a snap.

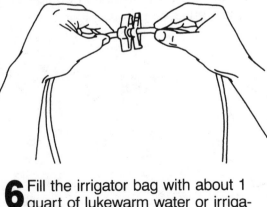

6 Fill the irrigator bag with about 1 quart of lukewarm water or irrigation solution, as the doctor orders. Hang the filled bag on a towel rack or

a hook placed next to the toilet. During irrigation, the bag should be above your stoma at your shoulder level.

7 Hold the end of the irrigator tube over the toilet. Open the control clamp and allow a small amount of water or irrigation solution to flow through the tubing. This will force any trapped air out of the tubing. Then close the control clamp.

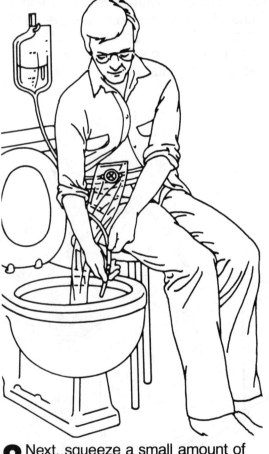

8 Next, squeeze a small amount of water-soluble lubricant onto a gauze pad and roll the first 3 inches of the tube in the lubricant.

Now, slowly slide the tube through the open top of the drainage bag and

continued

How to irrigate your colostomy — *continued*

into your stoma. If you meet resistance, don't force the tube.

Instead try to relax, and pull the tube out slightly. Unclamp the flow control and allow a small amount of water or irrigation solution to flow into the colon. Wait about 5 minutes and then try again to insert the tube. If you have repeated trouble inserting the tube, notify the doctor.

If the doctor wants you to irrigate your colostomy with a *stoma cone* instead of a tube, first lubricate the tip of the cone. Then insert the lubricated tip through the open end of the drainage bag and into your stoma (as shown).

To prevent backflow, always hold the cone in place against the stoma during irrigation.

9 Open the flow clamp of the irrigator bag, and let the water or irrigation solution run slowly into your colon. This should take about 10 to 15 minutes. If you get stomach cramps, reduce the flow or stop the procedure until the cramps go away. After the fluid has entered your colon, slowly remove the tube or cone from your stoma.

10 After the initial surge of water or irrigation solution returns, you can fold the drainage bag back, clamp it shut, and do whatever you want to until all the fluid and stool have returned. It will take about 30 minutes for the colon to empty completely.

11 After the colon empties, return to the toilet. Unhook the belt and remove the drainage bag. Then clean the area around your stoma with warm water, dry the area gently, and apply a clean colostomy pouch. Finally, wash, rinse, and store the irrigation equipment for reuse.

Laryngeal cancer

Few challenges are greater than helping a cancer patient learn to cope with his diagnosis, treatment, and aftercare. Understandably, the patient's fears about cancer and its effects are usually uppermost in his mind. And this can distract him from learning. However, when the patient has laryngeal cancer, your challenge grows because the primary treatment—laryngectomy—will dramatically affect his life-style and self-image.

If surgery involves removal of all or part of the larynx, the patient will be temporarily or permanently unable to speak after surgery. If it involves removal of the upper trachea, he'll have to breathe through a tracheostomy. If it also involves removal of the epiglottis, he'll have difficulty swallowing. As a result, the patient may be especially concerned about how he'll sound, look, and, in some cases, eat after surgery. His concerns may increase if he requires a radical neck dissection—a procedure that may disfigure his face and neck and interfere with muscle function.

Besides emotionally preparing the patient for laryngectomy and its aftermath, you'll need to prepare his family. For example, they'll need to know how to perform such daily procedures as tracheal suctioning and stoma care. And they may need to learn how to respond positively to the patient, helping him to adapt successfully.

Discuss the disorder

Distinguish the patient's type of laryngeal cancer: glottic carcinoma, which involves the structures around the glottis, or supraglottic carcinoma, which involves structures above the glottis, such as the epiglottis and false vocal cords. Using an illustration or a diagram, show the patient the laryngeal structures affected by his cancer. (See *Identifying laryngeal structures,* page 330.)

If your patient has *glottic carcinoma,* tell him that hoarseness (an early cancer sign) stems from one or more tumors impinging on the true vocal cords, which prevents the cords from coming close together during speech. Explain that these tumors occur in the earliest stage of this type of laryngeal cancer. Typically, they remain localized. However, if they spread, the cancer usually involves only the local structures higher in the neck or the regional lymph nodes.

Lynn Adams, RN, MS, OCN, and **Judith Schilling McCann, RN, BSN,** wrote this chapter. Ms. Adams is a nurse clinician specializing in outpatient chemotherapy at Memorial Sloan Kettering Cancer Center, New York City. Ms. McCann is a nursing consultant and clinical editor with Springhouse Corporation, Springhouse, Pa.

CHECKLIST

Teaching topics in laryngeal cancer

☐ Explanation of the type of laryngeal cancer: glottic or supraglottic carcinoma
☐ Description of affected laryngeal structures
☐ Diagnostic tests, including indirect or direct laryngoscopy
☐ Preparation for chemotherapy or radiation therapy
☐ Preparation for partial or total laryngectomy or radical neck dissection
☐ Self-care measures, such as tracheal suctioning, stoma care, and exercises after surgery
☐ New ways to speak and to swallow
☐ Emergency measures, such as mouth-to-stoma resuscitation
☐ Sources of information and support

Identifying laryngeal structures

How can you help your patient understand his type of laryngeal cancer? Begin by taking a few minutes to explain how normal laryngeal structures look and work.

Tell the patient that the larynx, a boxy, tubelike structure, lies in the neck between the base of the tongue and the trachea. The epiglottis seals off the trachea from the esophagus so that food and fluids can't enter the lungs.

Lining the larynx are two sets of folds: the vocal cords. One set, the true vocal cords, vibrate to make speech as air moves through a passageway called the glottis. The second set, the false vocal cords, are located directly above. They're also involved in sound production.

After teaching the patient about the location and function of laryngeal structures, discuss the areas affected by his type of cancer.

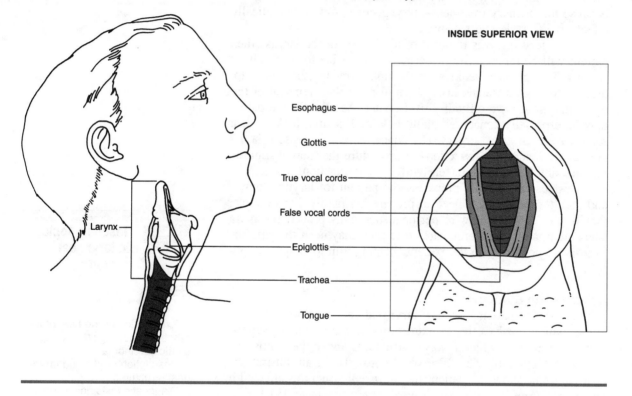

INSIDE SUPERIOR VIEW

Esophagus
Glottis
True vocal cords
False vocal cords
Epiglottis
Trachea
Tongue

Larynx

Inform the patient with *supraglottic carcinoma* that this type of cancer originated in some laryngeal structure other than the true vocal cords. Discuss its sometimes vague symptoms, which include coughing, difficulty swallowing, the sensation of "a lump in the throat," changes in voice pitch, a long-lasting sore throat (more than 6 weeks), pain in the laryngeal prominence, and a burning sensation after drinking hot liquids. Hoarseness is a late sign. If appropriate, tell him that this type of laryngeal cancer grows more aggressively than glottic carcinoma and metastasizes more rapidly to associated structures and to lymph nodes in the neck—a reason not to delay treatment.

Complications
Emphasize that the cancer will spread and cause death if it remains untreated. Explain that with glottic carcinoma, the patient

will experience difficulty swallowing and pain as the tumor grows. And with untreated supraglottic carcinoma, swallowing will become increasingly difficult, too. Hoarseness and severe pain will accompany the tumor's spread to the true vocal cords.

Describe the diagnostic workup

Prepare the patient for tests to confirm laryngeal cancer and determine its extent. Explain that diagnosis may begin with indirect laryngoscopy, usually an office procedure. If this examination reveals a suspicious lesion, the doctor will order direct laryngoscopy and perform a biopsy for a definitive diagnosis.

Indirect laryngoscopy

Tell the patient that the doctor will use a mirror to see possible laryngeal lesions. Mention that the inspection takes between 15 and 30 minutes.

Advise the patient that he'll sit comfortably in a chair, placing his buttocks well back on the seat so that his posture helps the doctor get the best view of the larynx. He'll see a mirror in front of his mouth and a light shining from behind. Then, with a piece of gauze, the doctor will grasp the tip of the patient's tongue and hold it in position with a tongue depressor. Tell the patient who gags easily that the wall of his throat, his soft palate, and the back of his tongue may be anesthetized first to relieve discomfort and prevent gagging. Next, the doctor will direct a small, warmed, long-handled mirror to the back of the patient's mouth and observe the larynx at rest and during phonation.

Explain that if the doctor requires a more detailed look, he may use a *rod lens telescope,* which magnifies the laryngeal structures, giving clear, large views. Again (with the patient still seated and his throat still numb) the doctor will grasp the patient's tongue as he advances the right-angled telescope into the patient's mouth and down his throat. As he does so, he'll ask the patient to say "e-e-e-e-e." This sound helps depress the tongue and elevate the larynx, thereby easing the instrument's passage.

If the doctor chooses to use a *flexible fiberscope,* tell the patient that this instrument can photograph his vocal cords. Describe the instrument as a thin, flexible tube with an eyepiece at one end and a camera at the other end. Explain that after the doctor sprays the patient's nostrils with an anesthetic, he'll pass the instrument through the patient's nose and into the larynx. Reassure him that the procedure is painless and doesn't cause gagging. Next, describe how he'll sit erect with his head supported by a headrest. The doctor will tell the patient to breathe through his nose to ease tube insertion. When the tube's in place, the doctor will instruct him to talk, cough, or sing as the doctor observes and photographs the vocal cords.

Direct laryngoscopy

Inform the patient that this procedure permits direct laryngeal examination and procurement of tissue samples for histologic analysis. During the examination, the doctor can also remove small,

332 Laryngeal cancer

Staging laryngeal cancer

After the patient learns his cancer stage, use the following classification, developed by the American Joint Committee on Cancer, to clarify its implications. For example, if the doctor classifies a primary tumor (T) as T1S, you can tell the patient that the tumor hasn't spread.

Glottic tumor stages
T1S—Carcinoma in situ
T1—Tumor confined to the vocal cords, which retain normal motion
T2—Tumor extends to supraglottic or subglottic area or both; vocal cord motion normal or impaired
T3—Tumor confined to larynx; vocal cord loses motion
T4—Massive tumor extending beyond the larynx or destroying thyroid cartilage or both.

Supraglottic tumor stages
T1S—Carcinoma in situ
T1—Tumor confined to its source; vocal cords retain normal motion
T2—Tumor extends to neighboring areas or glottis; vocal cords retain motion
T3—Tumor confined to larynx, but vocal cords lose motion; or tumor extends to the postcricoid area, the pyriform sinus, or the preepiglottic space and vocal cords lose motion; or both
T4—Massive tumor extending to the oropharynx, neck, or thyroid cartilage.

localized lesions. Designed to pass through the patient's mouth to the larynx, the laryngoscope is a thin, hollow tube containing a light and a special lens.

Before the test, provide instructions. Tell the patient that the test takes place in an operating room. Instruct him to refrain from eating, drinking, and taking nonprescription drugs for 8 hours before the test. Just before the procedure, tell him to remove any contact lenses, dentures, and jewelry. He should also remember to use the bathroom. Inform him that he'll receive medication to help him relax and to reduce his oral secretions.

If the patient will have a local anesthetic, explain that he may feel uncomfortable, but he shouldn't feel pain. Prepare him for the unpleasant taste and coldness of the anesthetic spray that suppresses the gag reflex. Explain that his head will be positioned and held in place while the doctor passes the laryngoscope through his mouth and throat and on to the larynx. Reassure the patient that he'll be able to breathe.

If appropriate, mention that besides obtaining a tissue sample the doctor may perform minor surgery. For example, he may do endoscopic laser surgery to remove a small, localized glottic tumor.

Inform the patient that after the test his blood pressure, heart rate, and breathing will be monitored for about 15 minutes. Instruct him to lie on his side or sit with his head elevated at least 30 degrees until his gag reflex returns—usually in about 2 hours. In the meantime, he should avoid food, fluids, and oral drugs. Tell him that he'll have a sore throat and hoarseness temporarily. Suggest that he use throat lozenges or a soothing gargle when his gag reflex returns.

Advise the patient to spit out saliva rather than swallow it for up to 8 hours after the test. During this time, he should avoid clearing his throat and coughing because these actions may dislodge blood clots at the biopsy site and possibly cause hemorrhage. Show him how to wear an ice collar to prevent or minimize swelling.

Subsequent tests
If biopsy confirms laryngeal cancer, the doctor may order tests to gauge the cancer's extent (see *Staging laryngeal cancer* for more information). These may include various scans, neck radiography, tomography, and contrast studies. Be sure to explain each test's purpose, preparation, procedure, and aftercare to the patient.

Teach about treatments
Explain that treatment has two goals: to eliminate the cancer and to preserve as much normal speech as possible. The most common treatment is partial or total laryngectomy. Other treatments may include chemotherapy, radiation therapy, or a combination of these. Offer patients undergoing these therapies a copy of the teaching aid *How to control the side effects of chemotherapy and radiation therapy,* pages 306 to 309.

Medication

If the patient will receive chemotherapy, explain how the drugs affect the cancer, how he'll receive the drugs, how often he must take them, and what side effects he can expect.

Procedures

If the patient has a localized cancer in an early stage, tell him that the doctor may recommend radiation therapy as the primary treatment instead of surgery. Radiation therapy may also be used before surgery to shrink large laryngeal tumors or after surgery to prevent metastasis or to treat recurrent cancer.

Discuss why the patient needs radiation therapy and how it will affect the disease. Then describe the procedure. Also discuss the side effects, and tell the patient how to manage them. For instance, warn him that most patients experience taste changes, decreased salivation, and skin changes.

Surgery

Inform the patient that laryngoscopic surgery may eliminate early localized glottic tumors. Tell him that his speech won't be affected and that he can return to his usual activities shortly afterward. To remove more extensive tumors, the surgeon may perform partial laryngectomy (laryngofissure, vertical hemilaryngectomy, horizontal supraglottic laryngectomy) or total laryngectomy. For advanced disease, he'll perform a total radical neck dissection. Make sure the patient and his family understand the extent of the planned surgery. Then reinforce the surgeon's explanation and clear up any misconceptions (see *Teaching about laryngeal cancer surgery,* page 334).

Tell the patient about standard preoperative procedures, including fasting before surgery, skin preparation, and I.V. therapy. Inform him that he'll receive a general anesthetic.

Next, carefully explain postoperative measures, including suctioning, nasogastric feeding, and tracheostomy tube care. If appropriate, prepare the patient for monitoring in the intensive care unit or the recovery room in the first 24 to 48 hours after surgery.

Explain communication. Encourage the patient to express his concerns if surgery will cut off vocal communication. Help him choose an alternate means of communication, such as writing, sign language, or a communication board. Reassure him that the hospital staff will know that he can't speak and that his call light will be answered immediately. Offer to arrange a meeting with another laryngectomee to discuss the patient's concerns.

If the patient's having a partial laryngectomy, explain that he can speak when his doctor determines that he can use his voice, usually 2 or 3 days after surgery. Then, caution him to whisper until his throat heals. If he's having a total laryngectomy, reassure him that speech rehabilitation can help him talk again. Offer to have a speech pathologist discuss this with him (see *Reviewing alternative speech methods,* page 335).

Teaching about laryngeal cancer surgery

For most laryngeal cancer patients, treatment means surgery. Use the information below to help the patient and his family understand the purpose, extent, and effects of the planned surgery.

Endoscopy with laser surgery
Explain that this procedure, performed during laryngoscopy, uses a laser beam to remove a glottic tumor that's confined to a small area—usually a single true vocal cord. Tell the patient that the laser beam will effectively eliminate the cancerous growth, that he'll retain his voice, and that he can resume his usual activities shortly after the procedure, as his doctor permits.

Laryngofissure
Inform the patient that this procedure removes larger glottic tumors confined to a single vocal cord. The surgeon makes an incision in the thyroid cartilage and removes the diseased vocal cord.

Tell the patient that after surgery he'll have a temporary tracheostomy and his voice may be hoarse but that hoarseness will abate as scar tissue replaces the vocal cord.

Vertical hemilaryngectomy
Explain that this procedure removes a widespread tumor. It involves excision of about half the thyroid cartilage and the subglottic cartilage, one false cord, and one true cord. Then the surgeon rebuilds the area with strap muscles.

Tell the patient that he won't have a laryngectomy stoma but that he will have a temporary tracheostomy. Reassure him that postoperative hoarseness will subside as scar tissue replaces the vocal cord.

Horizontal supraglottic laryngectomy
Explain that this operation removes a large supraglottic tumor. The surgeon removes the top of the larynx (the epiglottis, the hyoid bone, and the false vocal cords), leaving the true vocal cords intact.

Tell the patient that although he won't have a laryngectomy stoma, he will have a temporary tracheostomy to ensure a patent airway until swelling subsides. Also explain that he won't lose his voice, but that he may have swallowing difficulties without the epiglottis.

Total laryngectomy
Inform the patient that this procedure removes the true vocal cords, false vocal cords, epiglottis, hyoid bone, cricoid cartilage, and two or three tracheal rings. Neighboring areas may also be removed, depending on the tumor's extent.

The operation's also performed to remove a large glottic or supraglottic tumor attached to the vocal cord.

Because the surgeon must create a permanent tracheostomy and a laryngeal stoma, the patient will lose his speech.

Radical neck dissection
Explain that when cancer spreads to surrounding tissues and glands, the surgeon extends the supraglottic or total laryngectomy to remove the cervical chain of lymph nodes, the sternomastoid muscle, the fascia, and the internal jugular vein.

Because this operation leaves the patient with little muscle control and support for the head and neck, teach him exercises to strengthen accessory support muscles.

And because radical neck dissection disfigures the face and neck, you'll need to provide strong emotional support along with your teaching before surgery and throughout the recovery period.

Discuss suctioning. Inform the patient that when he awakens from surgery he'll have a tracheostomy tube in place. Advise him that secretions accumulating in the tube will be removed by suctioning. Decide on a signal that he can use to tell you that he needs suctioning. Assure him that his breathing will be monitored frequently. If the patient has a laryngectomy tube after surgery (shorter and thicker than a tracheostomy tube but requiring the same care), tell him that it's usually removed within 10 days.

Review feeding. Explain that the patient will have a nasogastric tube in place and that he'll receive food through this tube until the surgical site heals.

If the patient must continue nasogastric tube feedings at home, teach him and his family the procedure.

Reviewing alternative speech methods

Let your patient know that the speech pathologist can teach him new ways to speak. Then review the possibilities discussed below.

Esophageal speech
The patient talks by drawing air in through his mouth, trapping it in the upper esophagus, and releasing it slowly while forming words with his mouth. With training and practice, a highly motivated patient can master esophageal speech in about a month. Inform the patient that his speech will be choppy at first but will become smoother and more easily understood as he gains skill.

Because esophageal speech requires strength, an elderly patient or one with asthma or emphysema may find it too physically demanding to learn. And because it also requires frequent sessions with a speech pathologist, a chronically ill patient may find esophageal speech overwhelming.

Artificial larynges
The throat vibrator and the Cooper-Rand device are the two basic artificial larynges. Both types vibrate to produce speech that's easy to understand despite sounding monotonous and mechanical.

Tell the patient to operate a throat vibrator by holding it in place against his neck. A pulsating disc in the device vibrates the throat tissue as the patient forms words with his mouth. The throat vibrator device may be difficult to use immediately after surgery,

when the patient's neck wounds still feel sore.

The Cooper-Rand device vibrates sounds piped into the patient's mouth through a thin tube, which the patient positions in the corner of his mouth. Easy to use, this device may be preferred soon after surgery.

Surgically implanted prostheses
Most surgical implants generate speech by vibrating when the patient manually closes the tracheostomy, forcing air upward. One such device is the Blom-Singer voice prosthesis. Only hours after it's inserted through an incision in the stoma, the patient can speak in a normal voice. The surgeon may implant the device when radiation therapy ends or within a few days (or even years) after laryngectomy.

To speak, the patient covers his stoma while exhaling. Exhaled air travels through the trachea, then passes through an airflow port on the bottom of the prosthesis, and exits through a slit at the esophageal end of the prosthesis, creating the vibrations needed to produce sound.

Not all patients are eligible for tracheoesophageal puncture, the procedure needed to insert the prosthesis. Considerations include the extent of the laryngectomy; pharyngoesophageal muscle status; stomal size and location; and the patient's mental and emotional status, visual and auditory acuity, hand-eye coordination, bimanual dexterity, and self-care skills.

If the patient's scheduled for a total laryngectomy, mention that he'll start eating again (thick, easy-to-swallow foods, such as gelatin or ice cream) about a week after his surgery, when he can swallow normally.

Discuss swallowing. If the patient's undergoing a supraglottic laryngectomy, begin teaching him the new swallowing technique that he'll use after the operation. Give him the patient-teaching aid *Learning a new way to swallow,* page 338, and encourage him to practice before surgery. Keep in mind that this swallowing technique requires a lot of energy and patience. What's more, it can leave the patient feeling frustrated and frightened for a while. After surgery, continue to encourage him, and plan to have someone stay with him during meals until he feels comfortable using the new technique.

Although the patient won't experience much discomfort at the incision site, tell him that he may feel pain when he first attempts to swallow. Encourage him to request pain medication early—before the pain becomes unbearable. Reassure him that the pain will diminish with time.

Discharge instructions. If the patient will be going home with a tracheostomy tube, teach him and his family how to suction and

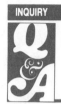

Questions patients ask about stoma care

How should I clean my stoma?
First wash your hands thoroughly. Then wash the skin around your stoma several times a day. Make sure you use a clean, moist cloth—not a cotton-tipped swab or cotton ball, which might stick. Remove dry, crusted secretions gently with sterile tweezers. Then apply a water-soluble gel, such as K-Y Jelly, to moisten the surrounding skin.

How can I keep water and dust from getting into my stoma?
Consider taking a bath instead of a shower—and don't go swimming. You can also wear a stoma shower shield or direct the shower head away from your throat. Hand-held shower heads are convenient for this.

To filter out dust or other foreign objects, wear a biblike covering for your stoma. Wear a foam one in the winter—to warm the air you breathe—and a crocheted one when the weather's milder.

How will I know if my stoma is closing?
You may find it harder to breathe through the stoma. Or you may notice new tissue growing around the stoma, decreasing its size. If either occurs, call your doctor at once. To prevent your stoma from closing, be sure to keep your tracheostomy or laryngectomy tube in place.

care for the trach tube. Give them copies of the teaching aids *How to care for your trach tube,* pages 339 to 341, and *How to suction a tracheostomy,* pages 342 and 343.

After a radical neck dissection, stress the importance of exercising to support the patient's shoulders and to strengthen his back muscles. Give him a copy of the teaching aid *Strengthening exercises after radical neck surgery,* page 344. If the patient will wear a prosthesis, teach him how to apply and remove it and how to check the surgical site for signs of infection, such as redness or tenderness. Tell him to notify the doctor if he experiences wheezing, stridor, fever, or milky drainage from the stoma (especially after meals).

If the patient's had a total laryngectomy or radical neck dissection, he'll need to cope with the effects surgery will have on his life-style and functioning. Coordinate visits by a social worker, who will direct the patient and his family to available community resources and help them obtain or rent equipment and supplies.

Other care measures
As you assist the patient to adapt to a new life-style, be prepared to answer questions on a wide range of issues, especially about stoma care (see *Questions patients ask about stoma care*). Also cover preventing infection, humidifying the air, and other precautions. Finally, discuss how to deal with emergencies.

Preventing infection. Caution the patient that bacteria can now reach his lungs more easily, making him more susceptible to colds and other respiratory infections. Advise him to check with his doctor before taking over-the-counter cold medicines containing ingredients that could dry mucous membranes.

Stress the importance of maintaining good oral hygiene to prevent infection. Advise him to rinse his mouth several times a day with mouthwash or a solution of 3% hydrogen peroxide and water.

Humidifying the air. Also advise him to keep his home and workplace (if possible) well humidified. Suggest using pans of water (changed daily so that germs don't accumulate and grow in the water) and houseplants to add moisture to the air. He can also increase the humidity to his airway by sitting in a steam-filled bathroom for 20 minutes two or three times a day or by wearing a damp, thin piece of gauze over his stoma. If the patient uses a humidifier, caution him to follow the manufacturer's care and cleaning instructions carefully to prevent an accumulation of infection-causing bacteria.

Tell him to cover his stoma with a scarf made of cotton or other porous material if he must be out in the cold. Breathing cold, dry air can be especially irritating to the patient's lungs.

Taking other precautions. Mention that heavy lifting and strenuous activity will be difficult after surgery because the patient won't be able to hold his breath to increase the pressure in his chest when straining. Discuss any specific restrictions ordered by his doctor.

Also explain to the patient that he won't be able to hold his breath and bear down to have a bowel movement. Advise him to eat foods with high-fiber content to prevent constipation. Or suggest that he ask his doctor about using a stool softener.

Emergencies. Teach the patient who's had a total laryngectomy to notify his doctor immediately if he has pain, difficulty swallowing, or bloody or purulent sputum. Urge him to carry a hemostat with him at all times to remove foreign bodies from his trachea. Suggest that he obtain a Medic Alert tag and carry an identification card with these instructions: "In case of emergency, open my collar. I breathe through my neck."

Show the patient's family how to perform mouth-to-stoma resuscitation. If the patient lives alone, suggest that he and a friend or a neighbor arrange a "buddy" system so that he has daily contact with another person who can summon help if needed. Discuss possible referrals to community health and service agencies—for example, the local visiting nurse's association.

Emphasize that despite a tracheostomy, the patient can lead a full and healthful life. Refer him and his family to the local chapter of the American Cancer Society for more information. Also inform him about services and support provided by the International Association of Laryngectomees.

Sources of information and support

American Cancer Society
90 Park Avenue, New York, N.Y. 10016
(212) 599-8200

International Association of Laryngectomees
3340 Peachtree Road, N.E., Atlanta, Ga. 30029
(404) 320-3333

Medic Alert Foundation International
P.O. Box 1009, Turlock, Calif. 95381-1009
(800) 344-3326

Further readings

Biggs, C. "The Cancer That Can Cost a Patient His Voice," *RN* 50(4):44-51, April 1987.
Chasin, W.D., et al. "What a Problem Voice Tells You," *Patient Care* 21(3):60-62, 67-69, 73-74, February 15, 1987.
Chisholm, S., and Jaros, T. "Duck-Bill Prosthesis: Words of Hope for the Laryngectomy Patient," *Nursing86* 16(3):29, 31, March 1986.
Feinstein, D. "What to Teach the Patient Who's Had a Total Laryngectomy," *RN* 50(4):53-54, 56-57, April 1987.
Hancher, K. "Social Adjustments of Laryngectomy Patients," *Journal: Society of Otorhinolaryngology Head-Neck Nurses* 6(2):4-8, Spring 1988.
Harris, L.L., and Kraege, J. "After T-E Puncture: Relearning to Speak... Tracheo-esophageal Puncture... The Blom-Singer Voice Prosthesis," *American Journal of Nursing* 86(1):55-58, January 1986.

Learning a new way to swallow

Dear Patient:

After surgery, you'll need to learn a new way to swallow to prevent food and fluids from flowing the wrong way and entering your trachea (windpipe) and lungs. The nurse will show you how before surgery, so you can start practicing. Then she'll review the steps with you after surgery, when you're ready for your first meal.

Practice steps

1 To begin, place a small amount of food at the back of your throat.

2 Take a deep breath and hold it. This pulls your vocal cords together and closes the entrance to your trachea.

3 Now use a gulping motion to swallow. Then cough. Repeat this step once or twice to prevent any food left in your throat from entering your trachea.

After surgery

You'll have your first meal several days after surgery. It will consist of soft, easy-to-swallow foods, such as mashed potatoes. As you get better at swallowing, you'll progress to foods that are harder to swallow, until you're able to swallow liquids.

Swallowing tips

Here are some tips to help you swallow comfortably:
● Eat slowly. It's the best way to avoid choking.
● Lean forward slightly as you eat. This position helps prevent food from entering your trachea.
● Stay calm. If some food does enter your trachea, the nurse will remove it immediately by suctioning it through your tracheostomy tube.

How to care for your trach tube

Dear Patient:

As part of your laryngectomy, the doctor created a permanent tracheostomy—a small opening, or stoma, in your throat.

Inserting a tube into the tracheostomy makes breathing easier because the tube keeps your windpipe open. A tracheostomy tube—for short, a "trach" (rhymes with cake) tube—features three parts:
- an inner cannula
- an outer cannula
- an obturator.

The inner cannula fits inside the outer cannula, which you insert with the obturator.

How to clean the inner cannula

To prevent infection, remove and clean the inner cannula regularly, as your doctor orders.

1 Gather this equipment near a sink: a small basin, a small brush, mild liquid dish detergent, a gauze pad, a pair of scissors, and clean trach ties (twill tape).

Or, open a prepackaged kit that contains the equipment you need. Now wash your hands. Position a mirror so that you can see your face and throat clearly.

2 Unlock the inner cannula and remove it by pulling steadily outward and downward.

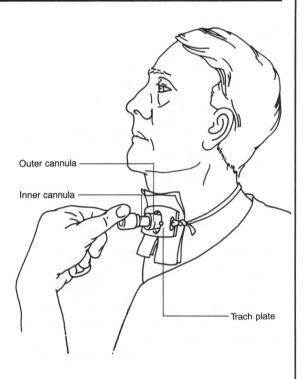

Outer cannula

Inner cannula

Trach plate

Prepare to clean the soiled cannula immediately for reinsertion. (Or put this soiled cannula aside and slip a clean inner cannula inside the outer cannula.)

If you start to cough, cover your stoma with a tissue, bend forward, and relax until the coughing stops.

3 Next, clean the soiled cannula. Here's how: soak the cannula in mild liquid dish detergent and water. Then clean it with a small brush. If your cannula is heavily soiled, try soaking it in a basin of hydrogen peroxide solution. You'll see foaming as the solution reacts with the secretions coating the cannula.

continued

PATIENT-TEACHING AID

How to care for your trach tube — *continued*

When the foaming stops, clean the cannula with the brush.

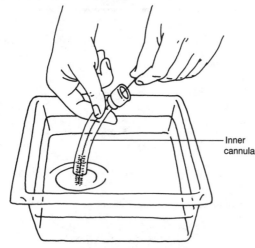

Inner cannula

You can obtain a special trach tube brush at a medical supply company or pharmacy. However, the small brushes used to clean coffee pots work just as well. They're inexpensive and available at hardware stores. Just make sure to use the brush only for your trach tube.

4 Rinse the inner cannula under running water. Make sure you've removed all of the cleaning solution. Shake off the excess water and reinsert the clean, moist cannula immediately. Don't dry it; the water drops remaining help lubricate the cannula, making reinsertion easier.

5 After you lock the clean inner cannula in place, replace the soiled trach ties that secure the trach plate. Use scissors to carefully clip and remove one trach tie at a time. Knot the end of each clean trach tie to prevent fraying, then cut a ½-inch slit in each tie. Thread the end that isn't knotted through the opening on the trach plate.

Then, feed the end through the slit, as shown below, and gently pull the tie taut. Do the same for the other tie.

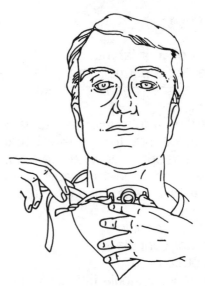

6 Secure the ties at the side of your neck with a square knot. Leave enough room so you can breathe comfortably.

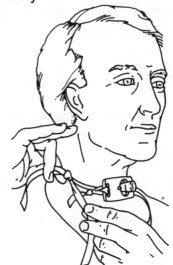

You should be able to slip two fingers between the side of your neck and the knot.

continued

How to care for your trach tube — *continued*

7 Finally, place a 4-inch by 4-inch gauze bib behind the tube to protect your neck. To make the bib, cut a slit down the middle of the gauze pad until you reach the center. Next, cut a hole in the center just big enough to go around the trach tube. Carefully insert the

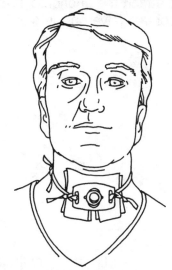

gauze bib under the trach plate. If you have heavy discharge draining from the stoma, you can insert the gauze bib from below.

How to reinsert your trach tube

Suppose you accidentally cough out your trach tube. *Don't panic.* Follow these simple steps to reinsert it.

1 Remove the inner cannula from the dislodged trach tube. If you're using a cuffed tube, be sure you deflate the cuff first.

2 Insert the obturator into the outer cannula. Then, use the obturator to reinsert the trach tube into your stoma.

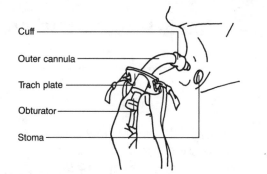

Cuff

Outer cannula

Trach plate

Obturator

Stoma

3 Hold the trach plate in place and immediately remove the obturator.

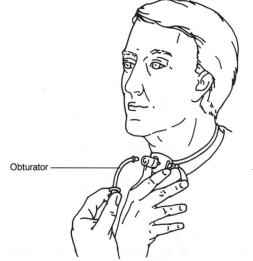

Obturator

Then insert the inner cannula into the trach tube. Next, turn the inner cannula clockwise until it locks in place. Chances are you'll cough or gag while you're doing this, so be sure to hold onto the trach plate securely.

4 Now, insert the tip of a syringe into the tube's pillow port. Inflate the cuff, as your doctor orders. The inflated cuff will help prevent the tube from accidentally being dislodged again.

5 After inflating the cuff, secure the trach ties and tuck a gauze pad under the trach plate.

How to suction a tracheostomy

Dear Patient:

The nurse will show you how to suction your tracheostomy to remove secretions that accumulate there. Then use these directions to help you remember the steps.

1 Gather the equipment:
• the suction machine
• the connecting tubing
• basin
• water
• suction catheter.

You can sterilize normal tap water by boiling it for 5 minutes. As the water cools, put a lid on the pot so the water stays germ-free. Keep a supply of sterile water in a glass jar that has been sterilized by boiling. You can also buy sterile water.

Also keep a bulb syringe nearby, in case the suction machine malfunctions or there's a power failure.

Wash your hands thoroughly. Then fill the basin with sterile water and set it aside.

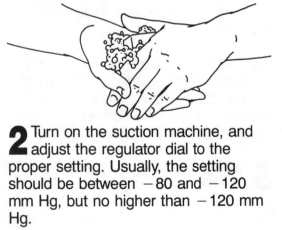

2 Turn on the suction machine, and adjust the regulator dial to the proper setting. Usually, the setting should be between -80 and -120 mm Hg, but no higher than -120 mm Hg.

3 Remove the suction catheter from its wrapper or airtight container.

4 Now, attach the suction catheter to the control valve on the suction tubing.

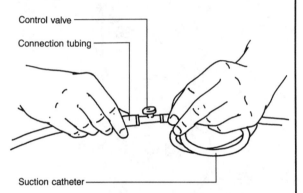

Control valve
Connection tubing
Suction catheter

5 Dip the loose tip of the catheter into the sterile water. This will help the catheter glide more easily.

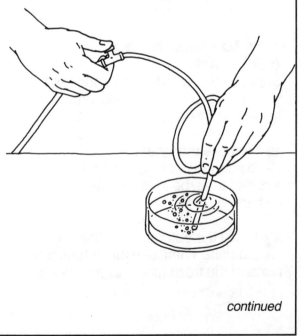

continued

How to suction a tracheostomy — *continued*

6 Take a few deep breaths and gently insert the moist catheter between 5 and 8 inches into the trachea through your tracheostomy tube or stoma until you feel resistance.

Caution: Take care not to injure yourself. Be careful not to cover the catheter's suction port during insertion. The suction pressure that results will damage the tissues that line your trachea.

ter from the trachea, rolling it between your thumb and finger as you go. This should take no more than 10 seconds. (Longer than that steals oxygen from your lungs.)

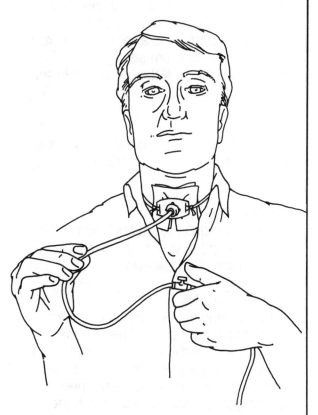

7 With your thumb, alternately cover and uncover the catheter's suction port to start and stop the suction. As you do this, slowly withdraw the cathe-

8 Put the catheter tip in the sterile water to clean the suction catheter and the connection tube. Then turn off the suction machine and disconnect the catheter from the connection tubing. Discard the disposable catheter in a plastic-lined wastebasket.

If you're using a reusable catheter, sterilize it according to the manufacturer's instructions.

PATIENT-TEACHING AID

Strengthening exercises after radical neck surgery

Dear Patient:

Here are some exercises to help you strengthen the muscles in your neck, shoulders, and arms after surgery. You can do most of them sitting down. Try to do them twice a day, or as often as your doctor directs.

Head turns
Turn your head as far to the right as you can. Then turn it as far to the left as you can.

Head tilts
Tilt your head to the left and then to the right. Straighten your head. Next, tilt it forward and then backward.

Head circles
Tilt your head forward and try to touch your chin to your chest. Then slowly rotate your head in a circle, passing your left ear over your left shoulder, tilting your head over your back, and then passing your right ear over your right shoulder, until your chin touches your chest again. Repeat in the opposite direction.

Shoulder rolls
First, sit straight in a chair. Now roll your shoulders forward and then backward.

Shoulder lifts
Still sitting in the chair, grasp each elbow with the opposite hand. Use your hand to lift your shoulder toward your ear. Repeat with the opposite shoulder.

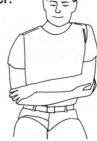

Arm swings and circles
Place the hand of your unaffected arm on a table or chair back for support. Let the arm on your affected side hang loosely. Now swing your affected arm forward and backward from your shoulder.

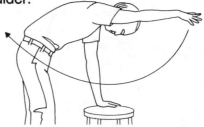

Then swing it in a circle. Be sure the motion comes from your shoulder joint and not from your elbow.

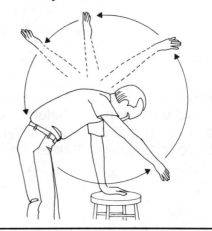

Leukemia

When you teach about leukemia, a cancer of the blood-forming tissues, you'll be dealing with patients who are understandably frightened and depressed about their condition. As you teach, try to establish a trusting relationship with the patient, helping to calm his fears and encourage communication. Because many leukemia patients are children, be especially sensitive to their emotional needs and those of their families.

Once you've established rapport with your patient, teach him about leukemia's different types. Help him to understand his particular type and its treatment. Inform him about diagnostic tests, including blood studies and bone marrow aspiration or tissue biopsy. Discuss the need for chemotherapy, possible radiation therapy, dietary changes, activity restrictions, and, if appropriate, bone marrow transplantation.

Above all, encourage the patient to comply with therapy. Emphasize that therapy aims to achieve and maintain remission and to minimize complications.

Discuss the disorder

Tell the patient that leukemia refers to a group of disorders in which certain blood cells grow and multiply uncontrollably. Explain that leukemia usually involves white blood cells (WBCs), called leukocytes. Rarely, it involves red blood cells (RBCs), or erythrocytes. Leukemia can originate in the bone marrow or the lymph nodes. In either case, the disorder leads to the growth of functionally impaired, immature cells called blasts. As these cells multiply, they accumulate in the bone marrow, where they inhibit the normal growth of WBCs, RBCs, and platelets. As a result, the production of normal blood cells diminishes, leading to anemia, leukopenia, and thrombocytopenia—a condition collectively known as pancytopenia.

Explain that leukemic cells also spill into the bloodstream, where they travel throughout the body. They may infiltrate and cause complications in the spleen, lymph nodes, central nervous system (CNS), kidneys, testes, skin, tonsils, and gums.

Although the precise cause of leukemia remains unknown, tell the patient that exposure to certain chemicals (such as benzene) or large doses of radiation may play a role. Other possible factors include viral infections, immunologic defects, and genetic abnormalities.

Arlene L. Androkites, RN, BSN, CRNP, and **Rosemary Drigan, RN, MEd, CRNP,** who contributed to this chapter, are nurse practitioners in oncology. Both practice at the Dana Farber Cancer Institute in Boston.

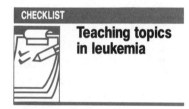

CHECKLIST

Teaching topics in leukemia

☐ How leukemia develops
☐ Major types of leukemia
☐ Preparation for diagnostic tests, such as bone marrow aspiration or biopsy
☐ Activity restrictions and need for adequate rest
☐ Foods to eat and avoid
☐ Chemotherapy
☐ Ancillary treatments, such as radiation therapy
☐ Preparation for bone marrow donation
☐ Preparation for bone marrow transplantation, if necessary
☐ Risk of graft-versus-host disease
☐ Tips to prevent bleeding and infection
☐ Sources of information and support

How leukemia develops

Tell your patient how bone marrow cells may give rise to four major leukemia types. Explain that all white blood cells (WBCs) derive from pluripotent stem cells. As the pluripotent cells mature, they differentiate into lymphoid stem cells and myeloid stem cells.

These stem cells normally develop into mature WBCs: lymphoid stem cells become lymphocytes, and myeloid stem cells become granular leukocytes. In leukemia, one or the other type of stem cell begins to grow uncontrollably. The disorder may be acute or chronic.

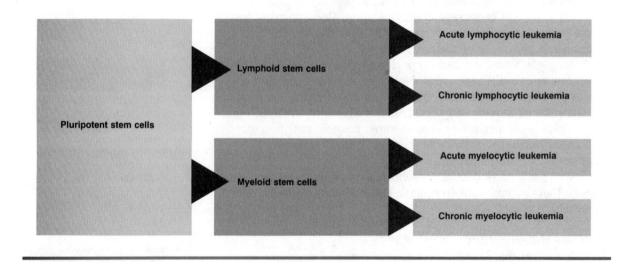

Leukemia types

Teach the patient about his specific type of leukemia (see *How leukemia develops*). In acute leukemia, symptoms occur suddenly and progress rapidly. In chronic leukemia, symptoms appear gradually. Both acute and chronic leukemia are further divided into subclasses, depending on which type of WBC has become cancerous.

Acute leukemia. The two main types are acute myelocytic leukemia (AML), in which granulocytes or monocytes proliferate, and acute lymphocytic leukemia (ALL), in which lymphocytes grow unchecked. Acute leukemia produces immature, undifferentiated WBCs.

Acute leukemia occurs most commonly in young children. The incidence declines after adolescence but then rises again in later adulthood. Acute leukemia has a higher incidence among people with certain genetic conditions, such as Down's syndrome.

Chronic leukemia. The two types are chronic myelocytic leukemia (CML) and chronic lymphocytic leukemia (CLL). Chronic leukemia produces relatively more mature and competent cells than acute leukemia does.

Explain that chronic leukemia most commonly strikes people over age 20. Incidence increases with age, peaking among those age 60 to 70. CLL seldom affects people under age 45.

If your patient has CML, inform him that this disorder may

be characterized by an abnormal chromosome called the Philadelphia chromosome. This genetic abnormality may result from exposure to radiation or carcinogenic chemicals.

Complications
Point out that acute leukemia, if untreated, typically causes death within a few months. Emphasize that in either form of leukemia, treatment can help to prevent such complications as infection, hemorrhage, and pain and to prolong life. In many patients with chronic leukemia, life expectancy may exceed 5 years.

Describe the diagnostic workup
Teach the patient about blood tests to detect leukemia, including a complete blood count and blood urea nitrogen (BUN) and creatinine analyses. Explain that an elevated WBC count may indicate leukemia or infection. Elevated BUN and creatinine levels suggest that leukemia cells have invaded the kidney and caused renal insufficiency.

Inform the patient about other tests to confirm the diagnosis, including cerebrospinal fluid (CSF) analysis, computed tomography (CT) scan, and bone marrow aspiration or biopsy.

CSF analysis
Explain that this test, which detects abnormal WBC invasion of the CNS, involves removing and analyzing spinal fluid. Tell the patient who will perform the test and where, and that it takes about 15 minutes. Inform him that he'll feel some pressure during the procedure as the doctor inserts the needle into the lumbar area.

Before the test, tell the patient that he'll be seated with his head bent toward his knees, or that he'll lie on the edge of a bed or table with his knees drawn up to his abdomen and his chin resting on his chest. The doctor will clean the spinal area and then numb it with a local anesthetic. Instruct the patient to report any tingling or sharp pain.

Explain that during the test, the doctor will insert a hollow needle into the space surrounding the spinal cord to obtain a CSF sample. Tell the patient to remain still to avoid dislodging the needle. Also inform him that he may be asked to breathe deeply or to straighten his legs.

After the test, the doctor will remove the needle and bandage the area. Instruct the patient to lie flat for 4 to 24 hours to prevent a headache. His head should be even with or below hip level. Remind him that although he mustn't raise his head, he can turn it from side to side. Also advise him to increase fluid intake for the rest of the day to help replenish CSF and prevent a headache.

CT scan
Explain that this advanced imaging technique uses a computer and X-rays to show subtle differences in tissue density, which allows the doctor to identify the organs affected by leukemia. Tell the

Bone marrow aspiration and biopsy sites

To ease the patient's anxiety and ensure his cooperation, explain beforehand which bone marrow site has been selected and how the test will proceed.

Posterior superior iliac crest
With no vital organs or vessels nearby, the posterior superior iliac crest becomes the preferred site for bone marrow biopsy. The doctor positions the patient laterally with one leg flexed.

Spinous process
This is the preferred site if multiple punctures must be made or if other sites are without marrow. The patient sits on the edge of the bed and leans forward over a bedside stand. If necessary, he may lie prone with a support to secure his position.

Tibia
For infants under age 1, this is the site of choice. The child lies prone with a sandbag under his leg. The doctor tapes the child's foot to the table, or an assistant holds the leg still.

Sternum
Seldom selected because of its proximity to the heart and major vessels, the sternal site requires the patient to lie supine with a pillow under his shoulders to elevate his chest and lower his head.

patient who will perform the 30- to 60-minute test and where. Inform him that the test causes no discomfort, but he may feel cold because the equipment requires a cool environment. If the doctor will use a contrast medium, tell the patient to restrict food and fluids for 4 hours before the test.

Explain that during the test, a technician will position the patient on an X-ray table and place a strap across the body part to be scanned, to restrict any movement. Then the table will slide into the scanner's circular opening. If a contrast medium is ordered, the patient will receive it through an I.V. site; the infusion takes about 5 minutes. Instruct the patient to tell the technician immediately if he experiences any discomfort, a feeling of warmth, or itching. (The technician can see and hear him from an adjacent room.) Then describe the loud noises the patient will hear as the scanning mechanism revolves around him.

Reassure the patient that after the test, he can immediately resume his usual activities and diet. If appropriate, advise him to increase his fluid intake to help expel the contrast medium.

Bone marrow aspiration and biopsy

Inform the patient that this procedure helps confirm the diagnosis and identify which WBC type has become cancerous. Explain that it permits microscopic examination of a bone marrow specimen. Tell him who will perform the procedure and where and that it usually takes only 5 to 10 minutes, unless another bone marrow specimen is needed. Test results are usually available in a day. The patient needn't restrict food or fluids before the test.

Suggest that the patient think of his bone marrow as a wet sponge. Aspiration sucks fluid (bone marrow) from the sponge, whereas biopsy involves excision of a small sample of sponge (marrow tissue). For more information, see *Bone marrow aspiration and biopsy sites*. Inform the patient that before the procedure, a blood sample will be drawn for analysis. Then, about 1 hour before the test, he'll receive a mild sedative.

For the biopsy procedure, tell the patient that after the doctor positions him, he must remain as still as possible.

Aspiration. Explain that for this procedure, the doctor will administer a local anesthetic. Next, using a circular motion, he'll insert a needle through the skin into the bone's cortex. After he aspirates 0.2 to 0.5 ml of marrow, he'll withdraw the needle and apply pressure to stop bleeding at the site. Then he'll clean the site and apply a sterile adhesive bandage.

Tissue biopsy. Inform the patient that the doctor will numb the biopsy area with a local anesthetic before inserting a needle through the skin into the bone marrow. Next, he'll insert another needle inside the first needle, directing the inner needle into the marrow cavity by alternate clockwise and counterclockwise rotations. This will enable him to obtain a tissue plug. After withdrawing the needles, he will clean the site and apply a sterile bandage.

After either procedure, advise the patient to rest quietly for several hours and to report any bleeding.

Teach about treatments

Inform the patient that chemotherapy—the cornerstone of leukemia treatment—aims to induce remission by killing leukemic cells and restoring normal blood cell production. Other treatments include radiation therapy and, possibly, bone marrow transplantation. During treatment, the patient may have activity restrictions and dietary changes.

Activity

Advise the patient to limit activities and to plan rest periods throughout the day. Explain that fatigue may result from stress related to his leukemia or to such treatments as chemotherapy or radiation therapy. Suggest that he sleep at least 8 hours at night and take naps during the day, if possible. Tell him that he may need to shorten his workday or to stop working during treatment.

Diet

Encourage the patient to eat foods high in calories and protein to help him maintain his strength and prevent body tissues from breaking down. If he loses his appetite, suggest that he eat frequent, small meals. If he complains of a bitter or metallic taste, advise him to drink more fluids, such as apple juice, water, or tea, or to eat foods that leave their own taste, such as fresh fruit or sugarless hard candy.

Because the patient is at risk for developing mouth ulcers, advise him to eliminate alcohol, extremely hot or spicy foods, and acidic beverages, such as orange or tomato juice, from his diet. Suggest that he eat soft, bland foods, such as soft-boiled or poached eggs and oatmeal. Encourage him to eat soothing foods, such as ice pops or pudding. If the patient's WBC count is below normal, instruct him to avoid fresh, unpeeled fruit, salads, unwashed vegetables, raw meat, and uncooked eggs to prevent infection.

Medication

Explain that drug therapy is tailored to the patient's leukemia type. A combination of drugs is usually necessary to control the disorder. Inform him that he may receive different drugs during various treatment stages (see *Teaching about drug therapy for leukemia,* pages 350 and 351).

If the patient has ALL, explain that chemotherapeutic agents may include asparaginase, vincristine, prednisone, methotrexate, cytarabine, and mercaptopurine. Inform him that he may also receive a prophylactic antibiotic to prevent infection, such as *Pneumocystis carinii* pneumonia, because treatment will lower his resistance.

If the patient has AML, explain that standard therapy includes daunorubicin, cytarabine, and thioguanine. Mention that after treatment achieves remission, the same drugs may be continued, but in different dosages.

If the patient has CML, explain that busulfan is the most commonly used drug. Other frequently prescribed drugs include

Teaching about drug therapy for leukemia

DRUG	ADVERSE REACTIONS	TEACHING POINTS
Adrenocorticoid		
prednisone (Orasone)	• Watch for abdominal pain, acne, back or rib pain, bloody or tarry stools, easy bruising, fever, hypertension, leg swelling, menstrual irregularity, extreme personality changes, purple striae, sore throat, unusual fatigue, vomiting, weakness, significant weight gain, and wounds that won't heal. • Other reactions include unusual appetite, diaphoresis, dizziness, euphoria or feeling of well-being, headache, indigestion, insomnia, mild mood swings, mild nausea, nervousness, restlessness, and slight weight gain.	• Inform the patient that this drug helps to diminish the number of WBCs in his body. • Instruct him not to change his dosage or discontinue the drug without his doctor's approval. Make sure he understands that withdrawal can be life-threatening. • Warn him about cushingoid symptoms (such as edema, weight gain, facial or vision changes, humpback, and easy bruising). Tell him to notify the doctor if these signs or symptoms occur. • Instruct him to take the drug with milk or food to reduce gastric irritation. • Advise against taking the drug with alcohol to avoid GI ulceration. • Instruct him not to take over-the-counter (OTC) drugs that contain aspirin, unless the doctor specifically recommends them. Aspirin may increase the risk of GI ulceration. • Tell him to avoid OTC drugs and foods that contain sodium to reduce the risk of fluid retention.
Alkylating agents		
busulfan (Myleran) **chlorambucil** (Leukeran) **cyclophosphamide** (Cytoxan)	• Watch for prolonged bleeding, easy bruising, chills, fever, hair loss, nausea, pain or redness at the injection site, sore throat, and vomiting. • Other reactions include anxiety, flank or joint pain, swelling of feet or lower legs, and rash.	• Explain that this drug interferes with the growth of leukemic cells. • Warn the patient to avoid exposure to people with infections because chemotherapy diminishes his resistance. Tell him to notify his doctor immediately if infection develops. • Instruct him in proper oral hygiene, including caution when using a toothbrush, dental floss, and toothpicks. • Tell him to complete any dental work before therapy whenever possible, or to delay it until his blood counts are normal. • Warn him that he may bruise easily because of the drug's effect on his blood.
Antibiotic antineoplastics		
daunorubicin hydrochloride (Cerubidine) **plicamycin** (Mithracin)	• Watch for chills, confusion, diarrhea, fever, hair loss, nausea, pain or redness at the injection site, and vomiting. • Other reactions include anxiety, appetite loss, bleeding syndrome (epistaxis to generalized hemorrhage), facial flushing, flank or joint pain, and swelling of feet or lower legs.	• Explain that this drug blocks the division of leukemic cells. • Instruct the patient to avoid exposure to people with infections because chemotherapy diminishes his resistance. Tell him to notify the doctor immediately if infection develops. • Advise him to use proper hygiene and caution when using a toothbrush, dental floss, and toothpicks. Chemotherapy can result in an increased incidence of microbial infection, delayed healing, and bleeding gums. • Tell him to complete dental work before therapy whenever possible, or to delay it until his blood counts return to normal. • Warn him that he may bruise easily because of the drug's effects on his blood. • Tell him to notify the doctor or nurse immediately if redness, pain, or swelling occurs at the injection site. Local tissue injury and scarring may result if I.V. medication infiltrates tissue.

continued

Teaching about drug therapy for leukemia—*continued*

DRUG	ADVERSE REACTIONS	TEACHING POINTS
Antimetabolites		
cytarabine (ara-C) **cytosine arabinoside** (Cytosar-U) **hydroxyurea** (Hydrea) **mercaptopurine** (Purinethol) **methotrexate** (Folex, Mexate) **thioguanine** (Lanvis)	• Watch for easy bruising, chills, diarrhea, fever, hair loss, and pain or redness at injection site. • Other reactions include anxiety, appetite loss, flank or joint pain, rash, and swelling of feet or lower legs.	• Explain that this drug interferes with leukemic cell growth. • Instruct the patient in proper oral hygiene, including caution when using a toothbrush, dental floss, and toothpicks. Chemotherapy can increase the incidence of microbial infection, delayed healing, and bleeding gums. • Tell him to complete dental work before therapy whenever possible, or to delay it until his blood counts return to normal. • Warn him that he may bruise easily because of the drug's effect on his blood. • Warn him to avoid close contact with people who have recently taken oral poliovirus vaccine. • Caution him to avoid crowds and exposure to people with infections because chemotherapy diminishes his resistance. Instruct him to notify the doctor immediately if infection develops.
Miscellaneous antineoplastics		
asparaginase (Elspar)	• Watch for agitation, anaphylaxis, prolonged bleeding, easy bruising, confusion, nausea, and vomiting. • Other reactions include appetite loss, headache, severe skin infection, stomatitis, tremors, and weight loss.	• Inform the patient that this drug interferes with leukemic cell growth. • Encourage him to increase his fluid intake to decrease the risk of some adverse reactions. • Tell him that drowsiness may occur during therapy or for several weeks after it. • Caution him to avoid hazardous activities that require mental alertness.
vincristine sulfate (Oncovin)	• Watch for hair loss, headache, hoarseness, jaw pain, nausea, "pins and needles" sensation, visual disturbances, vomiting, weakness, and wrist or foot drop or both. • Other reactions include abdominal cramps, appetite loss, constipation, difficulty swallowing, and double vision.	• Explain that this drug is used to stop abnormal cell growth in acute leukemia. • Tell him to notify the doctor or nurse immediately if redness, pain, or swelling occur at the infusion site. Local tissue injury and scarring may result from drug infiltration at the site. • Instruct the patient to increase his fluid intake to reduce the risk of some adverse reactions. • Tell him to ask his doctor before using laxatives if he is constipated or has abdominal cramps. • Advise him to avoid crowds and to take other precautions against infection. • If he loses his hair, assure him that hair growth should resume after treatment.

hydroxyurea, mercaptopurine, and thioguanine. If his disorder is in an advanced stage, he may receive a combination of plicamycin and hydroxyurea.

If the patient has CLL, expain that the drugs of choice include chlorambucil and cyclophosphamide. These may be given with prednisone.

Procedures

For some patients, radiation therapy and leukapheresis may be used as ancillary treatments.

Radiation therapy. Inform the patient with ALL that treatment may call for brain irradiation for 2 to 3 weeks. Radiation

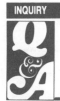

Questions bone marrow donors ask

What determines whether I can be a donor?
Tissue compatibility, for one thing. Poorly matched marrow could make the recipient gravely sick by triggering a rejection reaction in his immune system. Before you can donate marrow, a sample of your blood cells will be mixed and grown in a special solution with a sample of blood cells from the recipient. If cell destruction results, your tissues are not compatible. If the cells remain healthy, they are compatible, indicating that you may be a suitable donor.

Is the procedure risky?
The risk of serious complications is quite small. And no irreversible complications or deaths have been reported among bone marrow donors. To protect yourself from a blood-borne disease, you may want to bank 1 or 2 units of your own blood. These could be used in the unlikely event of complications.

Will I have any bone marrow left?
Yes. In fact, the doctor removes only about 5% of your bone marrow cells. Your body also makes marrow cells quickly, so the amount you donate will be replaced within a few weeks. Just a few days after the procedure, however, you should feel like your old self again.

Will the procedure hurt?
You'll probably feel some stiffness and tenderness for a day or two, but you'll receive medications to relieve it.

usually coincides with a phase of chemotherapy to treat the CNS. Inform the patient that he'll need to lie immobile on a table in the radiation therapy department while a large machine, usually overhead, directs radiation to the brain for a prescribed amount of time. Afterward, he can return to his room or go home.

Local radiation also may be used to treat chronic leukemias. It attempts to shrink organs that have become enlarged or impaired by leukemic cells.

Leukapheresis. A supportive measure used to treat CML, leukapheresis involves removing and separating abnormal or excessive WBCs. Inform the patient that his blood will go through a cell sorter that removes abnormal cells. Then his filtered blood will be reinfused into him.

Surgery

Inform the patient undergoing bone marrow transplantation that this procedure replaces diseased marrow with healthy cells. The new bone marrow may come from a donor or from the patient (after treatment to eliminate cancer cells). Tell him that healthy bone marrow is essential to life because blood cells are formed in the marrow.

Types of bone marrow transplants. Review the three types of bone marrow transplants with the patient. In an autologous transplant, the patient receives his own marrow. In a syngeneic transplant, bone marrow comes from a twin with identical tissue. In an allogeneic transplant, the most common procedure, the patient receives marrow from a fully or partially matched donor, such as a sibling, parent, or unrelated donor.

Take the time to teach the bone marrow donor about his part in the procedure (see *Questions bone marrow donors ask*). Give him a copy of the teaching aid *Your role as a bone marrow donor*, page 355.

Before and during transplantation. Tell the patient that beforehand, he may receive chemotherapy and total-body radiation to remove all traces of leukemia and prevent rejection of the new bone marrow. Explain that the new bone marrow will be infused through a central venous catheter or an I.V. line. The transplanted cells will circulate in his bloodstream and eventually lodge in his bone marrow space. Once there, they'll grow and make healthy blood cells in 2 to 4 weeks.

After transplantation. Inform the patient that he'll receive antibiotics. Then he'll be placed in a sterile environment or a room with laminar airflow to reduce the risk of infection. For 3 to 4 weeks after the transplant he may need packed RBC transfusions to prevent anemia and platelet transfusions to prevent bleeding. Tell him that he may be discharged after 5 to 6 weeks. Then he'll receive outpatient treatment. Explain that his immune system will need a long time to recover. Advise him to plan to return to work or school between 9 months and 1 year after the transplantation.

Make sure the patient understands the risks involved in bone marrow transplantation. Explain that the most serious complica-

Teaching about graft-versus-host disease

If your patient is undergoing a bone marrow transplant, make sure he understands the risk of developing graft-versus-host disease (GVHD). Explain that this immune system disease occurs when white blood cells attack and destroy foreign bone marrow cells from a donor. GVHD affects the skin, liver, intestinal mucosa, and lymph system. It may be acute or chronic.

Acute GVHD
Tell the patient to report any signs or symptoms immediately because GVHD can occur as soon as 1 week after transplantation or, more commonly, between 30 and 50 days after transplantation. An erythematous rash appears first, followed by green, watery diarrhea, abdominal cramps, and, in severe disease, right upper quadrant pain, hepatosplenomegaly, jaundice, and enlarged lymph nodes. With severe infection, mortality is 85%.

Inform the patient that the doctor may order a skin biopsy and blood tests to detect elevated liver enzyme and bilirubin levels.

Explain that treatment includes high-dose corticosteroids, lymphocyte immune globulin, or cyclosporine. Experimental treatment involves monoclonal antibodies to destroy donor T lymphocytes.

Chronic GVHD
The patient can experience chronic GVHD without first having acute GVHD. Signs and symptoms appear about 100 days after transplantation and resemble autoimmune collagen vascular disorders, such as systemic lupus erythematosus. It's characterized by scleroderma-like skin fibrosis and sicca syndrome, in which the mucosa and tear ducts become abnormally dry. In addition, chronic GVHD causes pulmonary changes and muscle wasting.

Explain that skin and mucosal tissue biopsies confirm chronic GVHD.

Tell the patient that localized skin involvement may resolve without therapy. Early systemic involvement is usually treated with immunosuppressive drug combinations, which are still investigational.

Prevention
Inform the patient that he may undergo GVHD preventive therapy. Immunosuppressive therapy against donor T lymphocytes is one preventive measure. However, the most common treatment is methotrexate, an antimetabolite that inhibits DNA synthesis and has a cytotoxic effect on rapidly dividing cells. Irradiation of blood products before they're administered may also help prevent T-lymphocyte replication.

Still experimental is the removal of T lymphocytes from the marrow before it's transplanted. This is done by treating the marrow with monoclonal antibodies or by binding the T lymphocytes to plant substances called lectins.

Teaching tips
If your patient already has GVHD, teach him ways to prevent infection. Also advise him that drinking plenty of fluids and eating a well-balanced diet will help to counter fluid and electrolyte losses caused by diarrhea and vomiting. If he has thrombocytopenia, urge him to report signs of gastrointestinal blood loss, such as bloody vomit or black, tarry stools. Tell the patient to notify his doctor or nurse if he has sore skin lesions, abdominal cramps, or other unusual or persistent symptoms.

tion is graft-versus-host disease (see *Teaching about graft-versus-host disease,* page 353). Urge the patient to report any signs of infection, such as fever, dry cough, difficulty breathing, and fatigue. Also instruct him to notify his doctor if he notices any bleeding—for example, from his nose or gums.

Other care measures
Inform the patient that because of his lowered resistance to disease, he must take special care to prevent infection. Advise him to avoid contact with pet or human feces. Mention that he should avoid cleaning cat-litter boxes and fish tanks. Direct him to call his doctor if he has chills, fever, or a nonhealing wound with drainage, redness, and tenderness. To help him remember, give him a copy of the teaching aid *How to avoid infection,* page 356.

Also explain that he must take care to prevent bleeding because his blood may not have enough platelets for proper clotting. Urge him to report excessive bleeding or bruising to his doctor immediately. Of course, he should avoid rough or hazardous activities, such as football or carpentry. Caution him to be extra careful while gardening or handling pets that might scratch or bite. Suggest other precautions, such as using a soft toothbrush, and an electric shaver instead of a razor. Advise him not to wear tight clothing, which could impair his circulation.

Sources of information and support
American Cancer Society (ACS)
90 Park Avenue, New York, N.Y. 10016
212-599-8200

Leukemia Society of America
733 Third Avenue, New York, N.Y. 10017
212-573-8484

National Leukemia Association
585 Stewart Avenue, Suite 536, Garden City, N.Y. 11530
516-222-1944

Further readings
Gurevich, I., et al. "The Compromised Host: Deficit-specific Infection and the Spectrum of Prevention," *Cancer Nursing* 9(5):263-75, October 1986.
Lakhani, A.K. "Current Management of Acute Leukemia," *Nursing* (London) 3(20):755-58, August 1987.
Lange, B.J., et al. "Home Care Involving Methotrexate Infusions for Children with Acute Lymphoblastic Leukemia,"*Journal of Pediatrics* 112(3):492-95, March 1988.
Peckham, V.C., et al. "Educational Late Effects in Long-term Survivors of Childhood Acute Lymphocytic Leukemia," *Pediatrics* 81(1):127-33, January 1988.
Sherman, D.W., et al. "Shalom, Melissa: Comforting the Terminally Ill Leukemic Patient," *Nursing88* 18(6):52-57, June 1988.

Your role as a bone marrow donor

Dear Donor:

As a donor, your healthy bone marrow cells will replace diseased marrow in a patient with leukemia. Here's what to expect.

Before the procedure

To make sure you're in the best possible health to donate bone marrow, the doctor will schedule:
- a complete physical examination. The nurse or doctor will also question you thoroughly about your health history.
- blood and urine tests
- a chest X-ray
- an electrocardiogram to check your heart.

The night before the procedure, you'll shower using antiseptic soap. This

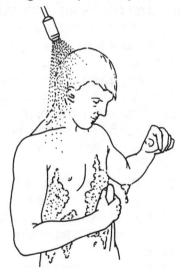

reduces the risk of infection developing during the procedure. Remember, don't eat or drink anything after midnight

because your stomach must be empty before you get an anesthetic.

Shortly before the procedure, an intravenous line will be inserted into your hand or arm to provide you with fluids during the procedure. You'll also receive some medicine to make you relax. You'll probably feel sleepy.

During the procedure

Next, you'll be taken to an operating room, where you'll probably receive a general anesthetic. After you're asleep, the doctor will collect about 5% of your marrow cells by placing a needle in your front and back hip bone. The marrow will be filtered to remove fat and bone particles and then prepared for transplantation.

While you're in the operating room, you may receive a unit of blood to help rebuild your bone marrow. The entire procedure takes about 2 to 3 hours. Once it's finished, a pressure dressing is applied over the area.

After the procedure

From the operating room, you'll be moved to the recovery room. When you awaken, you can expect to feel some pain, but you'll receive medicine to relieve it. Your hip area will be covered with tight bandages for about a day. When they're removed, the nurse will teach you to keep the area clean and covered for about 3 more days.

In 1 or 2 days, you'll probably be discharged from the hospital. Then you can return to your usual activities.

How to avoid infection

Dear Patient:

As your doctor and nurse have explained, you have an increased risk of of getting an infection. Here are some simple steps you can take to protect yourself.

Follow your doctor's directions
• Be sure to take all medications exactly as prescribed. Don't discontinue your medication unless your doctor tells you to do so.
• Keep all medical appointments so that your doctor can monitor your progress and the drug's effects.
• If you need to go to another doctor or to a dentist, be sure to explain that you're receiving an immunosuppressant drug.
• Wear a Medic Alert tag identifying you as taking an immunosuppressant drug.

Avoid sources of infection
• To minimize your exposure to infections, avoid crowds and people who have colds, flu, chicken pox, shingles, or other contagious illnesses.
• Don't receive any immunizations without checking with your doctor, especially live-virus vaccines, such as poliovirus vaccines. These contain weakened but living viruses that can cause illness in anyone who's taking an immunosuppressant drug. Similarly, avoid contact with anyone who has recently been vaccinated.
• Examine your mouth and skin daily for lesions, cuts, or rashes.

• Wash your hands thoroughly before preparing food. To avoid ingesting harmful organisms, thoroughly wash and cook all food before you eat it.

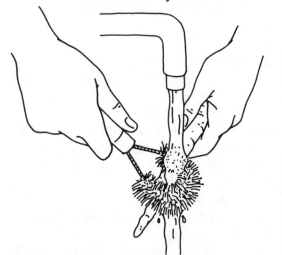

Recognize hazards
• Learn to recognize the early signs and symptoms of infection: sore throat, fever, chills, or a tired or sluggish feeling. Call your doctor *immediately* if you think you're coming down with an infection.
• Treat minor skin injuries with triple antibiotic ointment. If the injury's a deep one, or if it becomes swollen, red, or tender, call your doctor at once.

Perform routine hygiene
• Practice good oral and personal hygiene, especially hand washing. Report any mouth sores or ulcerations to your doctor.
• Don't use commercial mouthwashes because their high alcohol and sugar content may irritate your mouth and provide a medium for bacterial growth.

Breast cancer

This disease strikes about 9% of all women. Although all women are vulnerable, several factors, such as a family history of breast cancer, increase the risk for some. What's more, mortality for breast cancer hasn't changed in more than 30 years. Nevertheless, earlier detection, more accurate staging, improved treatment, and better long-term follow-up care have lengthened disease-free periods.

Teaching about breast cancer can save or lengthen lives. If your patient suspects breast cancer, your first teaching priority may involve helping her to voice her concerns about the disease and its treatment. Other priorities will include informing her about the disease, correcting misconceptions, and providing emotional support.

Specifically, you'll outline a diagnostic workup that may include mammography, biopsy, and a body scan. If test results confirm breast cancer, you'll explain treatment options and recommend ways to reduce or eliminate the side effects of treatments. Finally, because the patient's at risk for recurrent breast cancer and for metastasis, you'll emphasize the benefits of complying with follow-up care, performing breast self-examination, and recognizing the signs and symptoms of cancer elsewhere in the body. Throughout your teaching, you'll be challenged to reduce the patient's anxiety and to maintain a positive focus.

Discuss the disorder

Explain that the cause of breast cancer is unknown but that some women have a statistically higher risk for the disease. Risk factors include a history of breast cancer; a close relative with breast cancer (mother, sister, grandmother, aunt); early menarche (before age 12) or late menopause (after age 50); nulliparity or first childbirth after age 30; a high-fat diet after menopause; and benign breast disease (such as fibrocystic disease). Mention, though, that 75% of women who develop breast cancer have no significant risk factors.

Describe normal breast anatomy, including lobes, lobules, acini, and ducts. Also discuss possible tumor sites (see *Explaining breast structure and tumor sites,* page 358).

Review cancer's warning signs: any breast lump or mass; a change in breast symmetry or size; a change in breast skin, such as thickening, dimpling, swelling, ulceration, reddening, or warm-

Valerie Woebkenberg, RN,C, MSN, OCN, a nurse practitioner at Temple University Hospital, Philadelphia, wrote this chapter.

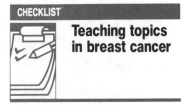

CHECKLIST

Teaching topics in breast cancer

☐ Risk factors and warning signs
☐ A description of breast structure and tumor sites
☐ Breast cancer stages
☐ Diagnostic tests, such as blood tests, mammography, and biopsy
☐ Chemotherapy, hormonal therapy, and radiation, including how to combat side effects
☐ Types of breast cancer surgery and perioperative considerations, such as preparation for surgery, pain after surgery, and coping with emotional distress
☐ Breast prosthesis and reconstruction
☐ After mastectomy, infection prevention, strengthening exercises, and tips for dressing
☐ Caring for a Jackson-Pratt drain at home
☐ Cancer screening guidelines
☐ Sources of information and support

Explaining breast structure and tumor sites

Once the doctor diagnoses breast cancer, help the patient understand the disease by describing breast structure, supporting structures and related lymph nodes, and the area affected by her tumor.

Breast structures
Explain that the breast is a glandular organ composed of lobes, lobules, acini, and ducts. These structures are arranged like spokes on a wheel, with the lobes (15 to 20 in each breast) branching into lobules and terminating in the acini where milk is produced. The ducts direct the milk toward the lactiferous sinuses in the nipple. These sinuses have external openings through which the milk flows.

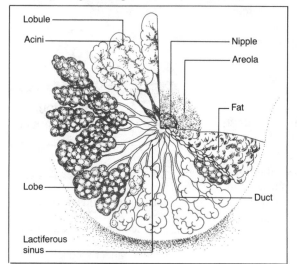

Supporting structures
Composed mostly of fat (adipose tissue), the breast is enclosed by a membrane of fascia and supported by ligaments. Ligaments lie over the pectoral muscles, which cover the ribs and aid in arm movement.

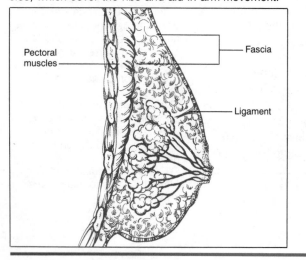

Lymphatics
Each breast has an elaborate lymphatic system that drains primarily into the axilla. Lymph nodes also lie within the breast, between the pectoral muscles, and above and below the clavicle. All these nodes may be sites for metastasis. The preponderance of axillary lymph nodes, however, accounts for the axillary node enlargement common in breast cancer.

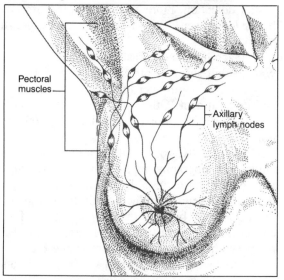

Tumor sources and sites
Tell the patient that about 90% of breast tumors arise from the epithelial cells that line the ducts. About half of all breast cancers develop in the breast's upper outer quadrant—the section containing the most glandular tissue. The second most common cancer site is the nipple, where all the breast ducts converge. The next most common site is the upper inner quadrant, followed by the lower outer quadrant and then the lower inner quadrant.

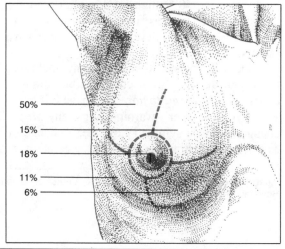

ing in spots; nipple discharge in a nonlactating woman; or nipple itching, burning, erosion, or retraction. Remember to allow time to respond to the patient's questions that result from your discussions.

Complications
Inform the patient that cancer in one breast increases her risk of cancer developing in the other breast or spreading to another site. Be discreet in deciding when and how to teach about potential complications, and try not to increase her anxiety. Stress that early detection of cancer recurrence carries a greater chance for control or cure.

Describe the diagnostic workup
Tell the patient that she may undergo extensive testing to help confirm cancer, select and monitor treatment, predict prognosis, and check for recurrence.

Understandably, the patient may feel fearful and powerless as she endures these tests and awaits the results. Your teaching can support her through this difficult time. Help her maintain a sense of control by clearly explaining the test procedures and encouraging her to voice her questions and concerns. Finally, support her efforts to make informed decisions based on diagnostic findings (for more information, see *Staging breast cancer,* page 360).

Testing may begin with blood studies and mammography. Other tests include a chest X-ray, a needle or excisional biopsy, and a bone, brain, or liver scan.

Blood tests
Tell the patient that blood chemistry studies to check electrolyte balance and kidney function, and a complete blood count to check for anemia and infection are routinely performed in suspected breast disease. In addition, an arterial blood gas analysis is performed to check for blood oxygenation, and prothrombin time and partial thromboplastin time are used to check clotting times. Also explain that specialized blood tests, such as radioimmunoassays to detect tumor markers, provide important information about the extent of malignant disease and treatment effectiveness.

Mammography
Inform the patient that mammography is an essential test for breast cancer. This radiographic study detects a tumor when it's too tiny to feel—at its most treatable stage.

If the patient hasn't undergone mammography before, tell her that she'll undress from the waist up, remove any jewelry from her neck and chest, and also remove her underarm deodorant. (Many deodorants have a metallic base, which can cause false-positive test results.)

Inform the patient that she'll rest one breast at a time on a flat imaging plate. Another plate will gently compress her breast from the top. Then an X-ray picture will be taken. Repeating these steps, the technician will compress the breast from the side

Staging breast cancer

Explain that cancer staging helps form a prognosis and treatment plan. A stage includes data on primary tumor (T) size and fixation, lymph node (N) involvement, and metastasis (M) to sites beyond the tumor. Tumor, node, and metastasis classes follow:

Tumor classifications
$T0$: No evidence of primary tumor
T_x: Tumor cannot be assessed
$T1_s$: Paget's disease of the nipple with no demonstrable tumor. *Note:* Paget's disease with a demonstrable tumor is classified by tumor size
$T1$: Tumor 2 cm or less in its greatest dimension
$T1_a$: Tumor not fixed to pectoral tissue or muscle
$T1_b$: Tumor fixed to underlying pectoral fascia or muscle (I, 0.5 cm; II, 0.6 to 1.0 cm; III, 1.0 cm)
$T2$: Tumor more than 2 cm but not more than 5 cm in its greatest dimension
$T2_a$: Tumor not fixed to pectoral tissue or muscle
$T2_b$: Tumor fixed to pectoral tissue or muscle
$T3$: Tumor more than 5 cm in its greatest dimension
$T3_a$: Tumor not fixed to pectoral tissue or muscle
$T3_b$: Tumor fixed to pectoral tissue or muscle
$T4$: Tumor of any size extending to chest wall or skin (Chest wall includes ribs, intercostal muscles, and serratus anterior muscle, but not pectoral muscle.)
$T4_a$: Tumor fixed to chest wall
$T4_b$: Edema (including *peau d'orange*), ulceration of breast skin, or satellite skin nodules on same breast.
$T4_c$: Both of the above

Lymph node classifications
For diagnosis:
N_x: Regional lymph nodes can't be assessed

$N0$: No nodal involvement
$N1$: Movable ipsilateral axillary nodal involvement
$N2$: Ipsilateral axillary nodal involvement with nodes extending to one another or to nearby structures
$N3$: Ipsilateral supraclavicular or infraclavicular nodal involvement or edema of the arm, which may be caused by lymphatic obstruction, making lymph nodes nonpalpable
For surgical evaluation and postoperative care:
N_x: Regional lymph nodes can't be assessed (not removed for study or previously removed)
$N0$: No evidence of ipsilateral axillary nodal metastasis
$N1$: Metastasis to movable ipsilateral axillary nodes
$N1_a$: Micrometastasis 0.2 cm in lymph nodes
$N1_b$: Gross metastasis in lymph nodes
$N1_{bi}$: Metastasis more than 0.2 cm, but less than 2.0 cm in one to three lymph nodes
$N1_{bii}$: Metastasis more than 0.2 cm, but less than 2.0 cm in four or more nodes
$N1_{biii}$: Extension of metastasis beyond lymph node capsule (less than 2.0 cm in dimension)
$N1_{biv}$: Metastasis in lymph node 2.0 cm or more in dimension
$N2$: Metastasis to ipsilateral axillary lymph nodes fixed to each other or to other structures
$N3$: Metastasis to ipsilateral supraclavicular or infraclavicular lymph nodes

Distant metastases
M_x: Not assessed
$M0$: No known distant metastasis
$M1$: Distant metastasis present

Staging categories
Cancer's stages progress from mild to severe as follows:

Stage $T1_s$
In situ.

Stage X
Cancer can't be assessed.

Stage I
The tumor is smaller than 2 cm (about 1"). It may or may not extend into the pectoral fascia and muscle. No nodes are positive for cancer, and no evidence of distant metastasis exists. Stage I includes:

$T1_{ai}$, N0, M0	$T1_{bi}$, N0, M0
$T1_{aii}$, N0, M0	$T1_{bii}$, N0, M0
$T1_{aiii}$, N0, M0	$T1_{biii}$, N0, M0

Stage II
The tumor is 2 cm to 5 cm (about 2"), with or without extension into pectoral fascia and muscle. As many as three mobile axillary nodes may or may not be positive for cancer. Distant metastasis isn't present.

Stage II includes:

$T0$, $N1_a$ or 1_b, M0	$T2_a$ or 2_b, N0, M0
$T1_a$ or 1_b, $N1_a$ or 1_b, M0	$T2_a$ or 2_b, $N1_a$ or 1_b, M0

Stage III
The tumor exceeds 5 cm (2") and may extend into the pectoral fascia and muscle. Extension of the tumor from the chest wall to the skin may occur. Skin edema, infiltration, or ulceration is present. Four or more fixed axillary nodes are involved. Lymph nodes in the pectoral, supraclavicular, or external mammary areas may be affected. Distant metastasis isn't present. Stage III includes:

$T0$, N2, M0	$T3_a$ or 3_b, N1, M0
$T1_a$ or 1_b, N2, M0	$T3_a$ or 3_b, N2, M0
$T2_a$ or 2_b, N2, M0	Any T, N3, M0
$T3_a$ or 3_b, N0, M0	Any T4, any N, M0

Stage IV
The tumor has spread to other organs, typically the bones, lungs, liver, brain. (Tumor size and number of nodes involved are irrelevant.) Stage IV includes:
Any T, any N, M1

and take an X-ray to obtain another view. Although this process may be uncomfortable, the procedure takes only a few seconds. Tell her that she'll know the test results soon after the doctor interprets the mammogram.

Chest X-ray

Advise the patient that chest X-rays detect breast lesions and can pinpoint metastatic disease in other chest areas. Explain that she'll need to remove all clothing and jewelry from the waist up. Next she'll stand or sit in front of the X-ray machine. She'll be asked to take a deep breath and hold it briefly while the technician takes the X-ray picture. Describe the rapid-fire clicking sound of the X-ray machine.

Bone, brain, and liver scans

Inform the patient that the doctor may order scans of organs—for example, the bones, brain, or liver—to check for metastasis. Scans may be performed with the initial cancer diagnosis and later during treatment. Common methods include computed tomography (CT) and magnetic resonance imaging (MRI).

Depending on which test the patient will have, describe the procedure and define any pretest restrictions. Make sure to discuss what the patient will see, hear, and feel during the test. Explain that though these tests usually cause no discomfort, the magnitude of the equipment may be unnerving. Describe the appearance of a CT or MRI scanner and the mild burning sensation that accompanies the infusion of a contrast medium.

Needle biopsy

For this histologic test, explain that the doctor uses a needle to obtain a sample of the breast lump. Tell the patient that this simple procedure is commonly performed in the doctor's office. Reassure her that she'll receive a local anesthetic, and that the procedure may take only 5 to 10 minutes.

Describe how the doctor will cleanse the skin with an antibacterial solution. Then he'll insert a needle into the breast lump. Using a syringe, he'll aspirate a tissue or fluid sample, which he'll send to the pathology laboratory for evaluation. Warn the patient that she'll feel some pressure during the procedure and that once the anesthetic wears off, her breast may feel sore or tender for a while. Advise her that the doctor will recommend a mild analgesic for pain relief. Tell her when she'll know the test results.

Excisional biopsy

If the patient's having an excisional biopsy rather than a needle biopsy, explain that this test may be curative. The procedure involves removing the entire breast lump and marginal tissue. Tell her that the surgeon usually performs this procedure in the hospital's short-procedure unit, so she'll be home in a few hours. Advise her to arrange for someone to accompany her home because she may be groggy or unsteady after the procedure.

Inform the patient that she'll receive a local anesthetic and medication to help her relax. When the breast area's numb, the surgeon removes the entire lesion with a scalpel or a special needle and sutures the wound closed. Then he sends the excised tissue to the pathology laboratory for analysis. Mention that test results should be available in a few days. Also tell her that 80% of lumps evaluated by excisional biopsy are benign.

Teach about treatments

First, help the patient cope with the breast cancer diagnosis; then help her explore treatment options. Surgery is almost always the initial treatment, with chemotherapy or radiation therapy performed postoperatively, as indicated. Hormonal therapy may be another option if cancer recurs. Emphasize how the patient can participate in posttreatment care by practicing breast self-examination and scheduling regular follow-up examinations and mammograms after surgery.

Medication

Drug treatment for breast cancer falls into two groups: chemotherapy and hormonal therapy.

Chemotherapy. Explain that chemotherapy uses certain drugs or drug combinations to kill cancer cells, to keep them from replicating, or to decrease the tumor's effects. The patient may have chemotherapy postoperatively, she may receive it along with radiation therapy, or it may be her primary therapy. Discuss how and where the patient will receive chemotherapy—in specific cycles and sequences, so that the body can recover during the drug-free period.

Then prepare the patient for possible side effects and discuss ways to manage them. Forewarn her that she may tire easily. Suggest that she pace her activities and rest frequently to help conserve her energy. Also provide nutrition information and tips for appetite stimulation. Give her the patient-teaching aid *How to control the side effects of chemotherapy and radiation therapy,* pages 306 to 309.

Hormonal therapy. If the patient's having hormonal therapy, explain that this treatment decreases levels of estrogen and other hormones suspected of nourishing breast cancer cells. For example, anti-estrogen therapy, specifically tamoxifen, is used in postmenopausal women and is most effective against estrogen-receptor positive tumors. Or the patient may receive anti-androgen therapy (aminoglutethimide) or androgen (fluoxymesterone), estrogen (diethylstilbestrol), or progestin (megestrol acetate) therapy. Discuss drug administration and possible side effects (for more information, see *Teaching about hormonal agents for breast cancer*).

Procedures

Radiation may be used after several types of breast cancer surgery, but it's typically used after lumpectomy and for recurrent

Teaching about hormonal agents for breast cancer

DRUG	ADVERSE REACTIONS	TEACHING POINTS
aminoglutethimide (Cytadren)	• Watch for adrenal insufficiency (signs and symptoms of infection and unusual tiredness or weakness), ataxia, bone marrow suppression (easy bruising and bleeding), dizziness, fever, malaise, and rash. • Other reactions include anorexia, gastric discomfort, hirsutism, hypothyroidism, nausea, periorbital edema, virilization, and vomiting.	• Explain that this drug blocks the effects of adrenal hormones known to stimulate breast tumors. • Reassure the patient that adverse effects are usually dose-related and reversible when aminoglutethimide is discontinued. • Emphasize that she should continue taking the drug even if she has nausea and vomiting. Reassure her that these effects usually subside in about 2 weeks. • Advise her to call the doctor immediately if nausea and vomiting occur shortly after she takes a dose. • Warn her that she may feel drowsy, so she should avoid any activities that require alertness until she builds up a tolerance to the drug. This usually occurs within about a month. • Advise her to stand up slowly, especially at the beginning of therapy when she may feel unsteady. • Tell her to notify the doctor if a rash develops and persists for 5 to 8 days when she begins taking the drug. The doctor may discontinue the drug temporarily until the rash clears. • Warn her to avoid alcohol because it may potentiate the drug's effects. • Tell her to report signs and symptoms of infection, such as persistent fever and sore throat and easy bruising and bleeding. • Because the drug can cause hypothyroidism, instruct her to report signs and symptoms, such as unusual fatigue, unexplained weight gain, cold intolerance, and constipation.
diethylstilbestrol (DES, Stilboestrol)	• Watch for abdominal cramps, depression, embolism, hair loss, headache, hirsutism, jaundice, lethargy, menstrual irregularities, metabolic imbalance, myocardial infarction, nausea, thirst, thrombophlebitis, and vomiting. • Other reactions include constipation, diarrhea, dizziness, intolerance to contact lenses, and vaginal candidiasis.	• Explain that this drug inhibits the growth of hormone-sensitive tissue in breast cancer. • Warn premenopausal women to use an effective form of birth control other than oral contraceptives and to stop the drug immediately if pregnancy occurs. This drug can adversely affect the fetus. • Warn the patient about the risks of smoking while taking this drug; suggest she attend a stop-smoking clinic. • Tell her to discontinue the drug and notify the doctor immediately if she has a sudden severe headache, one-sided weakness or loss of coordination, loss of vision or other dramatic vision changes, unexplained shortness of breath, or severe leg or calf pain.
fluoxymesterone (Android-F, Halotestin, Hysterone, Ora-Testryl)	• Watch for abnormal bleeding, androgenic changes, anxiety, diarrhea, edema, general paresthesias, hypersensitivity reaction, jaundice, menstrual irregularities, mental depression, nausea, and vomiting. • Other reactions include acne, bladder irritability, flushing, headache, sweating, vaginitis, and weight gain.	• Advise the patient that this drug blocks the effects of estrogen on estrogen-stimulated breast tumors. • Warn her that virilization usually occurs, and advise her to report androgenic effects immediately. Although stopping the drug prevents further androgenic changes, it probably won't reverse those already present. • Tell her to report menstrual irregularities to the doctor. He may discontinue the drug depending on what causes the irregularities. • Instruct the patient to take the drug with meals to decrease GI discomfort and to report any persistent GI distress, diarrhea, or jaundice.

continued

Teaching about hormonal agents for breast cancer—*continued*

DRUG	ADVERSE REACTIONS	TEACHING POINTS
megestrol acetate (Megace)	• Watch for fluid retention, hair loss, headaches, menstrual irregularities, skin rash, and weight loss. • Other reactions include nausea, stomach cramps, and vomiting.	• Explain to the patient that this drug blocks the effects of estrogen on estrogen-stimulated breast tumors. • Tell her that GI distress may subside with continued use of the drug. • Explain the importance of having a full physical examination, a gynecologic examination, and a Pap smear every 6 to 12 months while taking this drug. • Because this drug contains progestins, she should follow the same precautions associated with oral contraceptives. • Advise her to discontinue the drug and call the doctor immediately if she has a sudden severe headache, a migraine headache, visual disturbances, or vomiting. • Emphasize the importance of performing regular breast self-examination. • Tell her to check with the doctor promptly if she misses a period or has unusual bleeding. If she suspects pregnancy, she should discontinue the drug immediately and call the doctor. • Tell her to take a missed dose as soon as possible—or to omit it—but not to double-dose.
tamoxifen (Nolvadex)	• Watch for bleeding, bruising, bone and tumor pain, hot flashes, menstrual irregularities, nausea and vomiting, and visual changes. • Other reactions include alopecia, depression, dizziness, headache, peripheral edema, and rash.	• Tell the patient that this drug blocks the effects of estrogen, a hormone that may promote breast tumors. • Reassure her that this drug has relatively few adverse effects and that most patients tolerate it well. • Emphasize that she should continue taking the drug despite nausea and vomiting. She should call the doctor immediately, however, if vomiting occurs shortly after she takes a dose. • Caution her to use an effective form of birth control while she takes this drug; however, warn her not to use oral contraceptives because they may alter her response to the drug.

cancer or for metastatic disease. Let the patient know that before surgery radiation therapy may help to shrink the tumor. After surgery (sometimes along with chemotherapy), radiation may effectively prevent remaining cancer cells from growing, thus preventing recurrent disease. Depending on which type of radiation your patient's receiving (external or internal), describe the procedure and equipment to her.

Then discuss side effects and how to manage them. Explain that radiation therapy, like chemotherapy, may cause the patient to tire easily. Advise her to alternate periods of rest with activity to conserve energy. For more information, provide her with the teaching aid *How to control the side effects of chemotherapy and radiation therapy,* pages 306 to 309.

Surgery
A woman with breast cancer may fear mastectomy—the primary treatment—almost as much as cancer itself, perhaps because mastectomy threatens her self-image more than any other surgery. So

to relieve your patient's fears, you'll need to do considerable teaching before and after surgery.

Preoperative considerations. Discuss the particular operation the surgeon plans (if known), and answer any questions. Most of all, make certain the patient understands exactly what the surgery involves. If she agrees to have curative surgery immediately after unfavorable biopsy results, be sure she clearly understands the possible outcomes.

If the patient's having a *lumpectomy,* explain that the surgeon will remove the breast lump and a margin of normal tissue around it. He may also remove some axillary lymph nodes to screen for disease. In a *simple mastectomy,* he'll remove the entire breast, as well as some of the axillary lymph nodes if cancer has spread beyond the breast. In a *modified radical mastectomy,* he'll remove the breast, the axillary lymph nodes, and the lining over the chest muscles. In a *radical mastectomy,* rarely performed now, the breast, the chest muscles under the breast, and all the axillary lymph nodes are removed, leaving a hollow chest area (see *Options in breast cancer surgery,* page 366).

Inform the patient that shortly before surgery, the breast area may be shaved. Advise her also that she'll be given a sedative to calm her before she goes to the operating room. Once there, she'll receive a general anesthetic. Consider using a drawing or model to show her where the surgeon will make an incision and which tissue portions he'll remove. Describe the dressing and surgical drain she'll have after the operation.

Forewarn her that she'll have some breast-area pain after surgery and that she may also have pain or paresthesias in her shoulder, upper arm, axilla, and other parts of her chest. Mention, too—depending on her operation—that she may have lymphedema and phantom breast pain—a temporary tingling or pins-and-needles sensation in the area of the removed breast tissue. Reassure the patient that she'll receive adequate pain-relief medication.

Postoperative support. Schedule time after the operation to answer questions and discuss new concerns. Encourage the patient to voice her feelings. Discuss available resources for recovering patients, and if she agrees, arrange for her to meet with another breast cancer patient from the American Cancer Society or from the Reach for Recovery Foundation. This type of support can help the patient come to grips with her surgery and emotionally prepare her to look at her wound.

Self-care tips. Point out that effective self-care after surgery can speed recovery and prevent surgical complications, such as infection. If the patient will be discharged with a drain in place, show her how to care for it. Reinforce her efforts with a copy of the patient-teaching aid *How to care for a Jackson-Pratt drain,* page 370.

Stress ways to minimize lymphedema by elevating the affected arm frequently, by avoiding restrictive clothing, and by massaging the affected arm to increase circulation. Because

Options in breast cancer surgery

Every woman with breast cancer dreads breast surgery and its aftermath. Fortunately, because of treatment and technological advances, today's patient may have several satisfactory options. Discuss the options offered by the surgeon.

Lumpectomy

Through a small incision near the nipple, the surgeon removes the tumor, marginal tissue and, possibly, nearby lymph nodes. Typically, the patient will undergo radiation therapy after lumpectomy.

Lumpectomy is used for patients with small, well-defined lesions. Currently, fewer than 20% of breast cancer patients undergo this operation. In some patients, the surgeon will freeze the tumor and then do a lumpectomy using a cryoprobe to freeze the tumor to −292° F. (−180° C.). Then, he thaws the tumor and repeats the procedure four more times. Finally, he refreezes the tumor and performs a lumpectomy. Called a *cryolumpectomy,* this cell-destroying, freezing-thawing procedure is recommended only for small, early primary tumors. Radiation therapy may follow cryolumpectomy. The procedure has few complications and may prevent local recurrence.

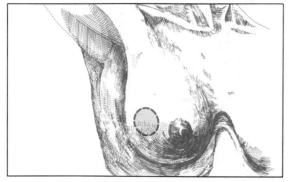

Partial mastectomy

The surgeon removes the tumor along with a wedge of normal tissue, skin, and fascia. He may remove axillary lymph nodes, too. Radiation or chemotherapy usually follows in an effort to kill undetected cancer cells in other breast parts.

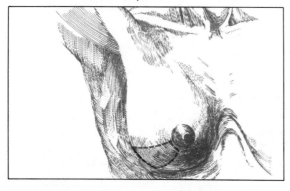

Total mastectomy

Also called a *simple mastectomy,* a total mastectomy involves removal of the entire breast. The surgeon performs this procedure if cancer remains confined to breast tissue and no lymph node involvement exists.

Radiation or chemotherapy may follow total mastectomy.

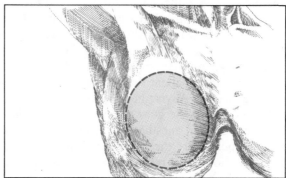

Modified radical mastectomy

In this procedure, the surgeon removes the entire breast, axillary lymph nodes, and the lining that covers the chest muscles.

If the lymph nodes contain cancer cells, radiation or chemotherapy follows the procedure. Modified radical mastectomy differs from *radical mastectomy* in that it preserves the patient's pectoral muscles.

Modified radical mastectomy has replaced radical mastectomy as the most widely used surgical procedure for treating breast cancer.

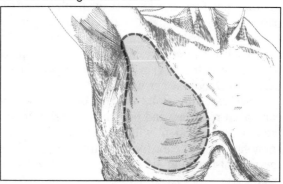

lymphedema makes the patient more susceptible to infection, emphasize measures to avoid infection or injury. (See *Preventing infections after mastectomy,* page 371.)

Exercise guidelines. Discuss postoperative physical activity with the patient. Advise her that ordinarily she can return to her regular activities within several weeks. Urge her to check with the doctor before undertaking strenuous exercise. Instruct her to exercise the arm and shoulder of her affected side. This will prevent muscle shortening, maintain muscle tone, and improve blood and lymph circulation. Once she has permission to start these exercises, show her how to perform them. Offer her the patient-teaching aid *Exercises to strengthen your arm and shoulder,* pages 372 and 373.

Breast prosthesis and breast reconstruction. Assist the patient in dealing with an altered body image. Advise her that after the breast area heals (2 to 6 months after surgery), she can wear a breast prosthesis or explore breast reconstruction possibilities.

If she decides to use a breast prosthesis, describe the temporary, light-weight products available for the immediate postoperative period (4 to 6 weeks). Add that after she heals completely, she can select a ready-made permanent prosthesis or have one custom designed. Offer her the teaching aid *Dressing with confidence after mastectomy,* page 374, to encourage her efforts.

If the patient has questions about breast reconstruction, explain that the surgeon rebuilds the breast using muscle and tissue from the patient's chest, back, and abdomen. In some instances, he may implant a manufactured prosthesis, or he may work with both body tissues and manufactured materials. Inform the patient that the usual waiting period for reconstruction is 6 to 9 months after mastectomy. Depending on the circumstances, however, the procedure may be performed sooner than that or even along with the initial surgery.

Encourage the patient to discuss her reasons for wanting the surgery. Inform her that the reconstructed breast won't be exactly like her natural breast. Add that reconstruction outcomes vary. Urge her to discuss her concerns with the doctor.

Sexual activity. Your patient may voice concerns about sexual activity after mastectomy. Will she feel the same about having sex? Will her partner? Tell her that she may resume sexual activity as soon as she feels ready, but encourage her and her partner to discuss their feelings about the patient's breast surgery. If possible, include the patient's partner in your teaching sessions. If appropriate, refer the couple for counseling to a psychiatrist, clinical specialist, social worker, or social agency. (See *Questions patients ask about mastectomy,* page 368.)

Other care measures

Stress that effective home care and regular follow-up examinations after breast cancer surgery are essential in preventing complications and detecting any new or recurrent cancer. Discuss the benefits of breast self-examination and show the patient how to

Questions patients ask about mastectomy

My doctor has recommended that I undergo a modified radical mastectomy. I think I can deal with the operation, but I'm not sure I can deal with my family and friends. What shall I tell them?
Are you wondering if your diagnosis and treatment will change your close relationships? Keep in mind that your family and friends will probably share many of your concerns and feelings—shock, fear, sadness, guilt, anger, and even embarrassment. Your women friends may begin to express fears about their own health.

Your best bet is to be honest. Give accurate information and answer questions if you want to, but don't dwell on the subject—especially if you begin to feel uncomfortable. With your closest friends and family members, you might want to be more open about your needs and feelings. In most instances, you'll find that gentle candor enhances communication and strengthens relationships.

My illness and mastectomy have put a lot of stress on my husband and me. Will our relationship ever return to normal?
It can. It might even get better, if you both want it to and if you work on it. Together, look at successful ways you've dealt with stress in the past. Consider using some of these methods now. And keep each other's needs in mind. For instance, console each other if you feel loss and grief. Reassure each other if you feel fearful. Keep your lines of communication open, and give yourself time to adapt to the changes in your life. If you still feel your relationship's on shaky ground, don't be afraid to seek professional counseling or advice from a couples' cancer support group.

I'm worried—how will my mastectomy affect my sex life?
It may slow it down for awhile. You'll have less physical energy because your body's under stress from the surgery and from changes occurring in your system. Fatigue can decrease your sex drive. So make sure to rest when you need to. Take naps, and try to schedule sex during your peak energy hours.

Keep in mind that mastectomy can affect your sex life if the surgery alters the way you feel about your sexuality. How comfortable were you and your partner with your sexuality before your surgery? Your answer may predict how comfortable you feel afterwards. Obviously, you and your partner will need to be open and honest about the changes you're experiencing. Share your feelings and needs, and seek counseling, if necessary.

perform it. For example, you can demonstrate the technique on a model and then have the patient demonstrate the technique for you. Urge her to examine her breasts monthly—about 2 or 3 days after her menstrual period. If she's postmenopausal, suggest that she examine her breasts on the same date each month.

Also review the patient's follow-up care schedule. She should see the doctor, for example, every 3 to 4 months for 2 years after surgery; then every 6 months for another 3 years; then yearly thereafter. She'll also need to schedule a yearly mammogram, a chest X-ray, routine blood work, and possibly a bone scan. (See *A schedule for breast cancer screening*.)

Sources of information and support

American Cancer Society
1599 Clifton Road, NE, Atlanta, Ga. 30329
(404) 320-3333

Lumpectomy/Radiation Therapy Information Service
West Coast Cancer Foundation, 50 Francisco Street, Suite 200, San Francisco, Calif. 94133
(415) 981-4590

Office of Cancer Communications, National Cancer Institute (NCI)
Bldg. 31, Room 10A18, 9000 Rockville Pike, Bethesda, Md. 20205
(800) 638-6694

Clinical Research Center, The North Carolina Memorial Hospital
Manning Drive, Chapel Hill, N.C. 27514
(919) 966-1435

Further readings

Clarke, D.E., and Sandler, L.S. "Factors Involved in Nurses Teaching Breast Self-examination," *Cancer Nurse* 12(1):41-46, February 1989.
Crooks, C.E., and Jones, S.D. "Educating Women About the Importance of Breast Screenings: The Nurse's Role," *Cancer Nurse* 12(3):161-64, June 1989.
Dunne, C.F. "Hormonal Therapy for Breast Cancer," *Cancer Nurse* 11(5):288-94, October 1988.
Love, R.R., et al. "Side Effects and Emotional Distress During Cancer Chemotherapy," *Cancer* 63(3):604-12, February 1, 1989.
"Mastectomy (teaching materials)," *Medical Times* 117(3):79-81, March 1989.
McGee, R.F., and White, C.H. "Helping Employees and Families Cope with Breast Cancer Treatment," *American Association of Occupational Health Nurses Journal* 37(5):178-85, 194-96, May 1989.
"The Nurse Can Do Much More to Help Women with Breast Disorders," *MD Nurse* 7(3):2, March 1988.

A schedule for breast cancer screening

Tell the patient that breast cancer can occur in any woman at any age. Inform her that the American Cancer Society recommends breast cancer screening as part of every woman's routine health regimen. Urge her to follow these guidelines.

At any age
See your doctor immediately if you discover a breast lump, notice a discharge from your nipple, or have any other signs of breast cancer. Comply with your doctor's recommendations for follow-up breast examinations and mammograms.

Beginning at age 20
Examine your own breasts monthly if you're over age 20.

Beginning at age 35
Schedule an appointment for a baseline mammogram if you're between ages 35 and 40.

Beginning at age 40
Visit your doctor for a yearly breast examination if you're between ages 40 and 49, and schedule mammography every 1 to 2 years.

Beginning at age 50
Visit your doctor for a yearly breast examination, and have a yearly mammogram.

PATIENT-TEACHING AID

How to care for a Jackson-Pratt drain

Dear Patient:

After surgery, you may notice a bulb-like drain connected to tubing coming from your incision. Called a Jackson-Pratt drain, this little device suctions and collects fluid from your incisional area. The drain promotes healing and reduces the chance of infection.

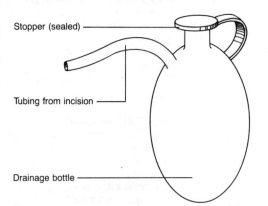

Stopper (sealed)

Tubing from incision

Drainage bottle

You'll have the drain for a few days after surgery. While you're hospitalized, your nurse will care for it. If you go home with the drain in place, you'll have to care for it yourself. The process is easy to learn. Your nurse will show you how.

Remember to empty the drainage bottle every few hours or as often as directed. Use these directions to refresh your memory.

1 First, obtain a measuring cup to collect the fluid. Then wash your hands thoroughly.

2 Unpin the bottle from your dressing or shirt and detach it from the tubing (as your nurse showed you).

3 Remove the rubber stopper from the bottle. Turn the bottle upside down, and squeeze the contents into the measuring cup. Completely empty the bottle. Keep a record of the amount of fluid in the measuring cup.

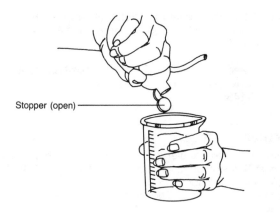

Stopper (open)

Note: To prevent infection, don't let the rubber stopper or top of the bottle touch the measuring cup or any other surface.

4 Now, use one hand to squeeze all of the air from the bottle. With the bottle still compressed, use your other hand to replace the rubber stopper. Do this to make sure the drain suction works well.

5 Last, reconnect the tubing. Then pin the bottle back on your dressing or shirt to avoid pulling it out accidentally. Now, wash your hands again.

Always remember to wash your hands before and after the procedure to reduce the risk of infecting the incisional area.

Preventing infections after mastectomy

Dear Patient:

Because lymph nodes and lymph vessels were removed with your mastectomy, your arm will swell periodically. Called lymphedema, this swelling increases your risk for getting an infection.

Use the suggestions below to help you protect your arm from injury and avoid infection.

Some do's
• Do contact the doctor if your affected arm becomes red, warm, or unusually hard or swollen.
• Do protect the hand and arm on your affected side.
• Do obtain and wear a Medic Alert tag that's engraved: *Caution—lymphedema arm. No tests, no injections.*
• Do use a thimble when you sew.

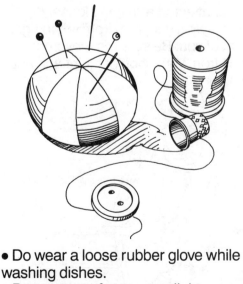

• Do wear a loose rubber glove while washing dishes.
• Do stay out of strong sunlight.

• Do shave with an electric razor if you choose to remove underarm hair.
• Do apply insect repellent to avoid bites or stings.
• Do apply lanolin hand cream several times a day.

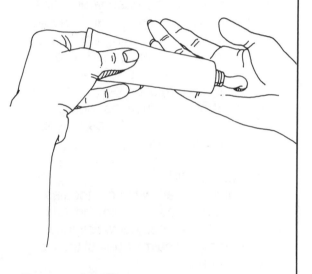

Some don'ts
• Don't cut or pick at your cuticles or hangnails.
• Don't use strong detergents or abrasive cleaning compounds.
• Don't reach into a hot oven with your affected arm.
• Don't dig in the garden or work near thorny bushes.
• Don't allow anyone to draw blood from, give an injection in, or wrap a blood pressure cuff around your affected arm.
• Don't wear tight-fitting bracelets or a wristwatch on that arm.
• Don't carry heavy bags or a heavy purse with the affected arm.
• Don't wear clothing with elastic at the wrists, elbows, or upper arms.

Exercises to strengthen your arm and shoulder

Dear Patient:

After mastectomy, you'll need to strengthen your arm and shoulder muscles. When your doctor gives you the go-ahead, do the exercises below daily. They'll help increase your mobility by preventing your arm and shoulder muscles from stiffening and shortening. Daily exercise will also help maintain your muscle tone and improve your circulation.

Follow these instructions, doing each exercise as many times as your nurse or doctor directs.

The wall climb
Stand facing a wall, with your toes as close to the wall as possible and your feet apart. Bend your elbows slightly. Then place your palms against the wall at shoulder level.

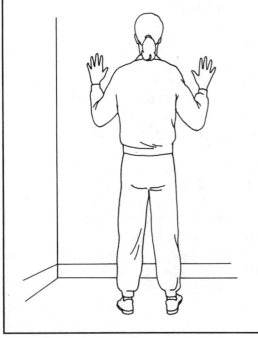

Flexing your fingers, work your hands up the wall until you fully extend your arms. Then, work your hands back down to the starting point.

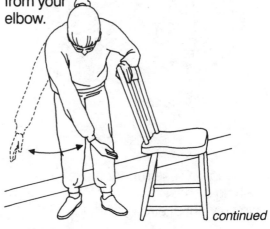

Pendulum swings
Place your unaffected arm on the back of a chair. Bend forward from the waist. Let your affected arm hang loosely.

First, swing your arm from left to right in front of you. Be sure the movement comes from your shoulder joint and not from your elbow.

continued

Exercises to strengthen your arm and shoulder — *continued*

Second, maintaining the same position, trace small circles with your arm. Again, be sure the motion comes from your shoulder joint. (As your arm relaxes, the size of the circle will probably increase.) Then, circle in the opposite direction.

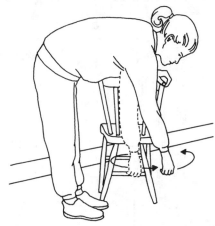

Third, swing your arm forward and backward from your shoulder, within your range of comfort.

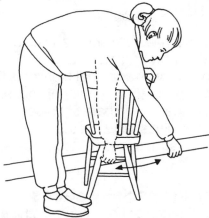

The pulley
Drape a rope over your shower curtain rod (or through an overhead pulley, hook, or loop). Hold the opposite ends of the rope in each hand.

With your arms outstretched, use a seesaw motion to slide the rope back and forth over the rod.

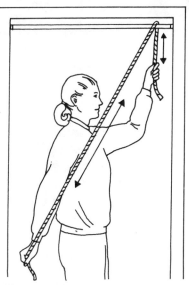

Rope turns
Tie a rope to a doorknob. Then stand facing the door. Hold the rope's free end in the hand of your affected side. Place your other hand on your hip. Extend your affected arm slightly to the side away from your body. Now, turn the rope, making as wide a swing as possible. Start slowly, and increase your speed as your arm grows stronger.

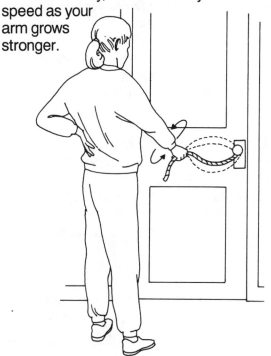

Dressing with confidence after mastectomy

Dear Patient:

Now that your operation's behind you, you can begin dealing with everyday concerns. One concern may be your wardrobe. Your clothes may not fit or look the way they did before your surgery. Don't be discouraged. You can look just as fashionable after a mastectomy as before. Just summon up your creativity—everyone has some—and select a few new styles.

Maybe you'll look for comfort, maybe for flair. Whatever you look for, here are some tips to consider.

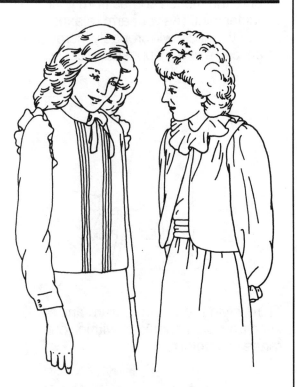

Consider loose, unconstructed styles

• Choose soft, medium-weight fabrics that don't cling.
• Look for textured or patterned materials, which reveal less.
• Soften your line by selecting blouses and dresses with pleats, tucks, and gathers at the shoulder or neckline.
• Avoid form-fitting garments tailored with bust darts.

Divert the fashion focus

• Create an optical illusion with asymmetrical, diagonal, or vertical prints to make differences less obvious.
• Choose necklines that focus attention on your face. Avoid deep "V" or scooped necklines.
• Look for curved lines if you want a more feminine look.
• Select a garment with sleeves that provide comfort but look decorative.

• Accessorize. Add spice and color with scarves, jewelry, and belts.
• Look for swimwear that highlights the waist, hips, or the shoulder of your unaffected side. (Avoid bare shoulders.) High necklines, asymmetrical or wide shoulder straps, and blouson tops add fashion variety.

Shop in specialty stores

Some women's shops carry clothing especially for women who've had mastectomies. Or join the millions of catalog shoppers. Some clothing manufacturers (such as Regenesis, Inc., New York, N.Y., and Camp International, Inc., Jackson, Mich.) make garments especially for women with mastectomies.

Cervical cancer

The best time to teach a woman about cervical cancer is before it's ever diagnosed. Point out to your patient that regular Pap smears can detect this cancer in its earliest stages, before signs and symptoms appear. Explain that the disorder usually can be cured if detected early. If your patient has an abnormal Pap smear, counsel her about the need for further procedures, such as colposcopy, conization, or dilatation and curettage (D&C).

If your patient has invasive cervical cancer, clarify the disorder's stage and recommended treatment. Teach her how to minimize the side effects of therapy, and provide psychological support. Above all, emphasize the need for long-term follow-up care to monitor disease recurrence or progression.

Discuss the disorder

Inform the patient that cervical cancer affects the lower portion of the uterus that protrudes into the vagina. This cancer occurs when normal cells begin to divide and grow at an uncontrolled rate. Although the cancer's cause is unknown, several predisposing factors have been linked to its development. These include intercourse at a young age (under age 18), multiple sexual partners, multiple pregnancies, history of carcinoma in situ, and herpesvirus 2 or other venereal infections. The incidence rises in low socioeconomic groups, but women in all groups are at risk.

Explain that preinvasive carcinoma, the earliest stage of cervical cancer, produces no symptoms or other clinically apparent changes. Untreated, this cancer will progress to invasive cervical cancer with malignant cells spreading beyond the cervical epithelial lining. Discuss the symptoms of early invasive cancer, including spotting after sexual intercourse, bleeding between menstrual periods, or unusually heavy menstrual bleeding. Advancing cancer may cause a yellowish or foul-smelling vaginal discharge (commonly tinged with blood), pelvic pain, rectal bleeding, hematuria, and anemia accompanied by extreme fatigue.

Complications

Emphasize that early treatment may cure the disorder or prevent metastasis. With early treatment, the 5-year survival rate for cervical cancer is 80% to 90%. By the time the disorder produces symptoms, the survival rate drops sharply. With delayed treatment, the survival rate drops still further.

Cathy Mazzone, RN, MS, OCN, who wrote this chapter, is a clinical nurse specialist in medical oncology at the University of Maryland Cancer Center in Baltimore.

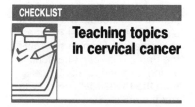

CHECKLIST

Teaching topics in cervical cancer

☐ Explanation of disease and predisposing factors
☐ Importance of Pap smear for early detection
☐ Discussion of staging and diagnostic procedures, such as biopsy, colposcopy, and conization
☐ Review of chemotherapeutic agents and external and internal radiation therapy, including radiation implant
☐ Surgery, such as abdominal hysterectomy or pelvic exenteration
☐ Need for follow-up care to monitor disease recurrence or progression
☐ Sources of information and support

376 Cervical cancer

Who should have a Pap smear?

Inform the patient that a Pap smear, a microscopic study of cervical tissue, can detect cancer cells at a curable stage — quickly and painlessly. Review these National Cancer Institute Pap smear guidelines for who needs a Pap smear.

• All women age 18 or older and all sexually active females under age 18 should have an annual Pap smear and pelvic examination.

After the patient has had three or more consecutive normal examinations, she may have the test less frequently, at her doctor's discretion.

• Women who had a hysterectomy for a nonmalignant disease should have a Pap smear at least every 3 years.

• Mature women (no age limit) should have a Pap smear as often as recommended by the doctor.

For reliable results, direct the patient to schedule the test 5 or 6 days before or after her menstrual period. Remind her that the Pap smear can't be done during a period, because cells from the menstrual flow may falsify the findings.

Also instruct her not to douche or insert any vaginal medicines for 24 hours before the test because these measures also may alter the test results.

Describe the diagnostic workup

Stress that regular Pap smears can detect cervical cancer in its earliest stages (see *Who should have a Pap smear?*). Explain the need for regular pelvic and rectal examinations to detect abnormalities.

If your patient's Pap smear reveals an abnormality, advise her that this doesn't necessarily mean she has cancer. Tell her the Pap smear serves only as an indicator. She'll need to undergo further tests, such as cervical biopsy and colposcopy, conization, D&C, and others. If the patient's scheduled for a conization, offer her a copy of the teaching aid *Understanding conization,* page 384.

Cervical biopsy and colposcopy

If the doctor can see a lesion during the pelvic examination, he may recommend a cervical biopsy. In this procedure, the doctor uses sharp forceps to remove a tiny sample of the cervical lesion. He'll send this specimen to the laboratory for microscopic study. Name who will perform the biopsy and where. Add that the procedure takes about 15 minutes. Before the procedure, instruct the patient to empty her bladder.

Inform the patient that the doctor will insert a speculum into her vagina to view the cervix. Instruct her to take several deep breaths as the doctor advances the instrument. Forewarn her that she may feel mild discomfort during and after this procedure.

If the Pap smear findings were abnormal but the doctor can't see a lesion with his naked eye, prepare the patient to undergo colposcopy. Explain that this procedure allows direct, assisted visualization of the cervix and vagina. Tell her that the doctor will insert the colposcope (an optical device with a light and a magnifier) through the speculum. Using this instrument, he can identify biopsy sites and remove tissue samples for microscopic analysis.

After colposcopy and biopsy, instruct the patient to avoid strenuous activity for 8 to 24 hours. If she's an outpatient, encourage her to rest briefly before leaving the hospital or the doctor's office. Recommend that she have someone accompany her home.

If the doctor inserted a tampon to check any bleeding, instruct the patient to leave it in place for 8 to 24 hours, as ordered. Although she can expect some bleeding, advise her to report bleeding that's heavier than her normal menstrual period. Warn her not to insert tampons herself, which can irritate the cervix and cause more bleeding. Also instruct her to avoid douching and sexual intercourse for about 2 weeks, or as directed. Tell her that she may have a foul-smelling, gray green vaginal discharge for several days after the biopsy. This may persist for about 3 weeks.

Dilatation and curettage

Explain that a D&C can detect whether cancer has spread into the endometrium, the uterine lining. If the patient's having this procedure, instruct her not to eat or drink anything for 8 to 10 hours before the procedure. Review what will occur during the proce-

dure. She'll lie on her back with her feet in stirrups. Then she'll
undergo local or general anesthesia. The doctor will dilate her
cervix and scrape the uterine lining with a curette. He'll send tissue samples to the laboratory for microscopic evaluation. Mention
that the patient can go home about 2 hours after this procedure.
Explain follow-up care and when to call the doctor.

Other tests
If the patient has invasive cancer, inform her that additional tests
may determine whether cancer has spread to other organs. She'll
have blood studies to assess her hemoglobin, white blood cell, and
platelet counts and to evaluate kidney and liver function. Discuss
tests to detect metastasis to the bones, liver, pelvis, abdomen, and
chest.

Explain that the diagnostic workup aims to determine the
cancer's stage—that is, how far it has spread. (See *Staging cervical cancer,* page 378.) Tell the patient that tumor staging helps
direct treatment.

Teach about treatments
Emphasize the need for a joint evaluation between a gynecologist
and an oncologist to determine the best course of treatment. Discuss the need for internal or external radiation therapy. Explain
chemotherapeutic agents, if appropriate, and alert the patient to
possible side effects. Review modifications related to sexual intercourse after therapy. Also discuss douching to reduce foul discharge resulting from treatment.

Medication
If the patient has advanced disease, chemotherapy may be recommended. Explain that chemotherapeutic drugs interfere with the
replication of cancer cells. After checking with the doctor, outline
the type and sequence of drugs the patient will receive. Point out
that no standard chemotherapy regimen has proved more effective
than an individualized regimen for this disease. Review how the
drugs will be administered—intravenously or intra-arterially, for
example—and alert the patient to possible side effects. Give her a
copy of the patient-teaching aid *How to control the side effects of
chemotherapy and radiation therapy,* pages 306 to 309.

If the patient's receiving a vesicant chemotherapeutic agent,
such as doxorubicin or vincristine, instruct her to report burning,
itching, or pain around the I.V. site. Reporting these symptoms
immediately may permit interventions to avoid extravasation and
damage to surrounding tissues.

Procedures
Tell the patient that radiation therapy is the treatment of choice
for cervical cancer. Explain that she may receive external or internal radiation or both. Assure her that this treatment can improve
her quality of life and possibly offer a cure.

Staging cervical cancer

Faced with a battery of diagnostic tests, the patient may not understand the point of her elaborate workup. Tell her that the purpose is to stage her cancer so that the doctor can plan the most effective treatment. Explain that staging determines how far the cancer has spread. In general, the higher the stage, the more invasive the tumor, and the more aggressive the recommended treatment. The International Federation of Gynecology and Obstetrics defines cancer stages as follows:

Stage 0
Carcinoma in situ, intraepithelial carcinoma

Stage I
Cancer confined to the cervix (extension to the corpus should be disregarded)

Stage IA
Preclinical malignant lesions of the cervix (diagnosed only microscopically)

Stage IA1
Minimal microscopically evident stromal invasion

Stage IA2
Lesions detected microscopically, measuring 5 mm or less from the base of the epithelium, either surface or glandular, from which it originates; lesion width shouldn't exceed 7 mm

Stage IB
Lesions measuring more than 5 mm deep and 7 mm wide, whether seen clinically or not (preformed space involvement shouldn't alter the staging but should be recorded for future treatment decisions)

Stage II
Extension beyond the cervix but not to the pelvic wall; the cancer involves the vagina but hasn't spread to the lower third

Stage IIA
No obvious parametrial involvement

Stage IIB
Obvious parametrial involvement

Stage III
Extension to the pelvic wall; on rectal examination, no cancer-free space exists between the tumor and the pelvic wall; the tumor involves the lower third of the vagina; this includes all cases with hydronephrosis or nonfunctioning kidney

Stage IIIA
No extension to the pelvic wall

Stage IIIB
Extension to the pelvic wall and hydronephrosis, or nonfunctioning kidney, or both

Stage IV
Extension beyond the true pelvis or involvement of the bladder or the rectal mucosa

Stage IVA
Spread to adjacent organs

Stage IVB
Spread to distant organs

External radiation. Delivered by a large machine that beams X-rays at the tumor, external radiation destroys cancer cells and some healthy cells. Assure the patient that normal tissues recover quickly. Before therapy begins, explain that the radiation therapist will define the exact treatment areas with a waterproof marking pen. Remind the patient not to remove these markings from her skin until she completes therapy.

Describe the therapy session. The patient will lie flat on her back on a treatment table in the radiation room. Explain that the doctor determines the radiation dose and duration, depending on the cancer stage. Afterward, she may return to her room or to her home, if she's an outpatient.

Because external radiation may dry the skin around the target site, discuss measures to prevent skin breakdown. Instruct the patient to keep her skin clean and dry, especially where the skin creases. If she needs a skin lubricant, ask your hospital's radiation department to recommend a lotion.

Internal radiation. Explain that internal radiation involves placing a radioactive source inside the body in one of two ways. In the *interstitial approach,* the therapist inserts radioactive needle- or bead-like devices into the tumor or surrounding tissues. These devices may remain in place temporarily or permanently. In the *intracavitary approach,* the therapist inserts a special holder containing radioactive substances into the vagina.

Before the patient consents to an intracavitary implant, make sure she understands that she'll be confined to bed for 2 to 3 days. Give her a copy of the patient-teaching aid *Learning about an internal radiation implant,* pages 382 and 383. Inform her that the full benefits of internal or external radiation may not be evident for several months. Support her efforts to cope with long-term side effects—for example, vaginal narrowing caused by scar tissue may be managed by regular sexual intercourse, by dilation, or both. For more information, see *How to use a dilator.*

Also explain that pelvic radiation may decrease female hormone levels, causing infertility and amenorrhea. Diarrhea may result from irritation of the GI tract. Instruct the patient to follow a low-fiber diet to minimize intestinal upset. Advise her to avoid caffeine-containing substances, such as coffee, tea, and cocoa, and to eat small, frequent meals instead of three large ones. Tell her to report persistent diarrhea. If she doesn't experience diarrhea after treatment, advise her to continue her usual diet.

Surgery

Explain that surgery for cervical cancer depends on the stage of cancer. Operations range from total abdominal hysterectomy (with or without lymphadenectomy) to pelvic exenteration.

Abdominal hysterectomy. Inform the patient having an abdominal hysterectomy that her uterus will be removed through an incision in the abdomen. Then discuss the type of hysterectomy she'll have. In a *total hysterectomy,* the surgeon excises the body of the uterus and the cervix, leaving the ovaries and fallopian tubes intact. In a *radical hysterectomy,* the surgeon removes the reproductive organs—including the ovaries and the fallopian tubes. Explore the patient's expectations about her menstrual and reproductive status after surgery. Review the surgical approach, and reinforce what the doctor has told her about the operation. Tell the patient that she'll have a cleansing enema and a douche the evening before surgery. She'll also shower with an antibacterial soap. Explain that because many women commonly retain urine after surgery, she may require an indwelling catheter. If abdominal dis-

How to use a dilator

If the patient needs instructions for using a dilator after she's undergone intracavitary radiation, review these steps with her. Explain that once or twice a day, she'll insert the dilator and leave it in her vagina for about 5 minutes. Advise her to:
• make certain the dilator feels smooth. If the device has any flaws or rough spots, tell her to ask the nurse or doctor for another one.
• wash the dilator with soap and water before and after each use.
• apply a water-soluble lubricant like K-Y Jelly to the tip of the dilator before inserting.
• lie on her back with her knees bent and slightly apart and then insert the dilator tip into the vagina as far as it will go without causing pain.

Forewarn her that she may have mild discomfort and a pink or slightly bloody discharge after using the dilator. She should not, however, have significant bleeding (like a menstrual period). Instruct her to call the doctor if she has further questions.

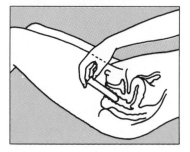

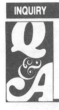

Questions patients ask after cervical cancer biopsy and treatment

I recently had a cone biopsy. The doctor says I'm doing well but I might have difficulty with pregnancy. Does this mean I'll never have a baby?
No. It just means that a cone biopsy—or conization—may interfere with your ability to become pregnant or carry the baby to term. If scar tissue forms after the procedure, the cervical canal may become blocked, preventing sperm from reaching the egg. Or the procedure may weaken the cervix, which can cause miscarriage or premature labor. Bear in mind that these complications seldom occur. However, if you continue to feel concerned, talk with your doctor again.

My doctor feels confident that he removed all of my cancer during the hysterectomy. What are my chances for a complete cure?
If your cancer was diagnosed and treated early before it spread to the lymph nodes or other organs, your chances for full recovery are very good. If the

disease progresses, however, treatment becomes more difficult, and the survival odds dip. The American Cancer Society estimates that the 5-year survival rate for all cervical cancer patients (regardless of detection time) is 66%.

Can I have a normal sex life after treatment?
In most cases, you'll be able to resume sexual relations, but you may need to make some changes. For instance, if you've had radiation therapy, your vagina may not have as much natural lubrication as before. To solve this problem, try using a water-soluble vaginal lubricant, such as K-Y Jelly, available in drug stores. Radiation therapy also may cause scar tissue to form in the vagina, making it narrower. Frequent sexual intercourse will help to widen the vagina. Also talk to the doctor about a dilator, an internal device to expand the vagina. If you've had a hysterectomy or other pelvic surgery, check with the doctor before resuming sexual intercourse.

tention develops, she may have a nasogastric tube or a rectal tube inserted.

Give her postoperative instructions for abdominal surgery. If she's premenopausal, forewarn her that hot flashes, night sweats, vaginal dryness, insomnia, and headaches may result if the surgeon removes the ovaries. Although average recovery time lasts 6 to 8 weeks, suggest that she resume activities at her own pace. Advise her to ask the doctor for instructions about resuming sexual activity and, if appropriate, using tampons or douches. Instruct her to check for fever daily for the first 2 weeks. Advise her to call the doctor if her temperature exceeds 100° F. (37.7° C.). Teach her to inspect the incisional site daily and to call the doctor if she notices infection signs, such as redness, warmth, odor, or drainage.

Pelvic exenteration. If the patient's scheduled for this operation, advise her that the surgeon will remove all reproductive and pelvic structures, including the vagina, urinary bladder, and rectum. Explain ileal conduit, and discuss possible colostomy. Outline the rigorous presurgical bowel and skin preparation she'll undergo to minimize any infection risk. Tell her that for 48 to 72 hours before the operation she'll receive a special diet. Prepare her for postoperative considerations, such as I.V. therapy, a central venous pressure catheter, a blood drainage system, and an unsutured perineal wound with gauze packing.

Other care measures

If the patient has advanced disease, explain that tumor drainage may cause a heavy, foul vaginal discharge. To help control the odor, advise her to douche with a solution of povidone and iodine (Betadine) and water or vinegar and water.

Explore how the patient feels about possible life-style changes resulting from treatment. Also urge the patient to comply with recommended follow-up visits to her gynecologist or oncologist once she completes her initial therapy. Stress the value of follow-up examinations in detecting disease recurrence or controlling progression (see *Questions patients ask after cervical cancer biopsy and treatment*).

Sources of information and support

American Cancer Society
1599 Clifton Road, Atlanta, Ga. 30329
(404) 320-3333

Cancer Connection
H and R Block Building
4410 Main, Kansas City, Mo. 64111
(816) 932-8453

Cancer Information Service
c/o National Cancer Institute
NIH Building 31, Room 10A24, Bethesda, Md. 20892
(800) 4-CANCER

National Cancer Care Foundation
1180 Avenue of the Americas, New York, N.Y. 10036
(212) 221-3300

Further readings

Brenner, P.H. "When the Pap Smear Is Mildly Abnormal," *Patient Care 21* (10):22-26, May 30, 1987.

Garbett, M., et al. "Caring for Julie...A Young Woman Having Inoperable Carcinoma of the Cervix," *Nursing Times* 84(2):25-29, January 13-19, 1988.

Jenkins, B. "Patients' Reports of Sexual Changes After Treatment for Gynecological Cancer," *Oncology Nursing Forum* 15(3):349-54, May-June, 1988.

McCauley, K.M., et al. "Evaluating the Papanicolaou Smear Part 1," *Consultant* 28(12):31-34, 37, 40, December 1988.

Schover, L.R., et al. "Sexual Dysfunction and Treatment for Early Stage Cervical Cancer," *Cancer* 63(1):204-12, January 1, 1989.

Shell, J.A., and Carter, J. "The Gynecological Implant Patient," *Seminars in Oncology Nursing* 3(1):54-66, February 1987.

Skrabanek, P. "Cervical Cancer Screening: The Time for Reappraisal," *Canadian Journal of Public Health* 79(2):86-89, March-April 1988.

Weintraub, N.T., et al. "Cervical Cancer Screening in Women Aged 65 and Over," *Journal of American Geriatrics Society* 35(9):870-74, September 1987.

Learning about an internal radiation implant

Dear Patient:

You're scheduled to have an internal radiation implant. This therapy treats cervical cancer by temporary insertion of a radioisotope (contained inside a special holder) in your vagina. Once in place, the implant will destroy cancer cells in your cervix with X-rays, while at the same time exposing healthy tissues to minimal radiation.

Expect to stay in the hospital about 3 or 4 days, with the implant in place for about 2 or 3 days.

Before the implant procedure
The day before or the morning of the implant procedure, you'll be admitted to the hospital and given a private room. Once the implant is in place, you'll be isolated from other patients and the hospital staff to protect them from unnecessary radiation exposure.

The evening before the procedure you'll have a low-fiber or liquid supper, and the doctor may order an enema to cleanse your bowels. If you'll have a general anesthetic, don't eat or drink after midnight before the procedure.

Before going to the operating room, you may receive a douche with an antiseptic solution.

During the implant procedure
In the operating room, you'll receive a local or general anesthetic—as the doctor directs. You'll also have a catheter placed in your bladder to drain urine.

Next the doctor will implant the holding device for the radioisotope. He'll add packing to secure it in place. This may take 20 minutes. Then X-rays will be taken to confirm that the holder's in the right position. Parts of the holder will be visible outside your vagina.

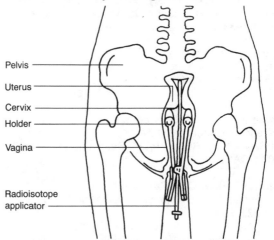

Then you'll go to the recovery room. There, the nurse will check your temperature, blood pressure, heartbeat, and breathing for an hour or two until you recover from the anesthesia.

When you return to your room, the doctor will insert the radioisotope into the holder. This takes a few minutes and doesn't hurt.

The doctor or nurse may draw markings on your inner thighs. They'll check these landmarks periodically to make sure that the implant doesn't move out of place.

Next, the nurse may put support stockings on your legs to improve your circulation while you're confined to bed.

continued

Learning about an internal radiation implant — *continued*

Safety precautions

Once the radioisotope is in the holder, the hospital staff will implement safety measures to avoid exposure to unnecessary radiation. You'll notice that:
• all hospital workers who come into your room will wear a film badge to measure their radiation exposure
• hospital staff members and visitors will limit their time in your room because radiation exposure increases with time
• lead shields may surround your bed to protect the staff from radiation
• staff members may stand some distance away from your bed while talking to you. The farther away they stand, the less radiation they'll receive.

While the implant's in place

For the next 2 or 3 days, you'll lie on your back while the implant does its work. Try not to move around too much — you don't want to risk dislodging it.

The head of your bed may be raised slightly at mealtimes, and you may be served a liquid or a low-fiber diet. This will help prevent you from having gas and bowel movements. You also may take medicine to prevent bowel movements.

Expect some discomfort. Ask the nurse for medicine if you feel sick to your stomach or if you have pain.

Also expect to have vaginal drainage while the implant's in place. The nurse will place pads beneath you and change them frequently to keep you dry and clean. She won't change your bed linens, though, because the movement might dislodge the implant.

Practice breathing deeply and coughing hourly while you're awake. Also exercise your feet and ankles to stimulate your circulation. If you're not sure how to perform these exercises, ask the nurse.

After the implant's removed

You'll probably go home on the day that the doctor removes the implant. The nurse will remove the bladder catheter.

As you recuperate, here are some tips for coping with side effects:
• Try to rest frequently during the day because you may feel tired for several weeks.
• Douche once a day with a solution of 2 tablespoons of vinegar (or Betadine — available at the drugstore) to 1 quart of water. This helps minimize the odor from vaginal discharge, which may last for 2 or more weeks.
• Follow a low-fiber diet. Eat small frequent meals, and avoid coffee, tea, and cocoa. These measures may relieve diarrhea, which may continue for about 2 weeks.
• As comfort permits, resume regular sexual intercourse to counteract a narrowed vagina that may result from scar tissue. Or ask the doctor or the nurse about using a dilator.

When to call the doctor

If you have any of these symptoms, call the doctor right away:
• inability to urinate within 6 to 8 hours of having your catheter removed
• burning when you urinate
• bloody urine
• bowel problems, such as constipation, diarrhea, or rectal bleeding
• extreme nausea or vomiting
• fever over 100° F. (37.7° C.)
• persistent or unusual pain.

PATIENT-TEACHING AID

Understanding conization

Dear Patient:

You're scheduled to undergo a conization. This procedure involves removing a small piece of tissue from your cervix for microscopic study. The doctor may order a conization if previous tests show abnormal cells in your cervix.

The procedure itself takes less than 30 minutes. It's usually done in the hospital, with either a local or spinal anesthetic. Make sure to follow the preoperative instructions your doctor or nurse gave you.

During the procedure

If you're having a spinal anesthetic, you'll receive it before the procedure begins. Then you'll lie on your back on an examination table with your feet in stirrups, just as you would for an internal pelvic examination. The doctor will insert a speculum into your vagina. This instrument will widen your vaginal canal to provide a clear view of your cervix.

If you're having a local anesthetic, you'll receive it at the time of the procedure. The doctor will wait for the anesthetic to take effect. Then he'll proceed to remove a small, cone-shaped tissue sample from your cervix for analysis in the hospital laboratory.

If the doctor suspects cancer in your uterus, he may then perform a D & C to check for cancer cells. (He'll discuss this with you beforehand.)

After these procedures, he'll close and remove the speculum.

After the procedure

The nurse will observe you to make sure you're recuperating. You can go home as soon as the anesthetic wears off, usually in about 30 to 60 minutes. Arrange to have someone transport you in case you feel unsteady.

Expect to feel some mild side effects from the conization. These may include abdominal cramping, some bleeding, and a feeling of fullness in your pelvis—especially if the doctor has inserted some temporary vaginal packing to control bleeding.

Also expect your next two or three menstrual periods to be heavier or longer than usual.

Call the doctor immediately if you notice any of the following symptoms:
• heavy bleeding
• severe or persistent pain
• foul-smelling vaginal discharge
• fever.

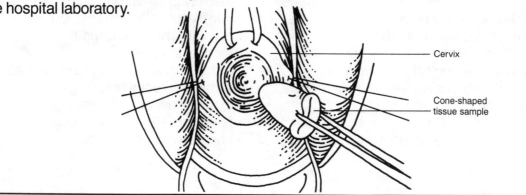

Cervix

Cone-shaped
tissue sample

Bladder cancer

Accounting for more than 40,000 new cancer cases and more than 10,000 deaths annually, bladder cancer ranks 11th in cancer deaths. Because this cancer commonly recurs after treatment, your teaching will emphasize warning signs, risk factors, and regular follow-up evaluations.

Your teaching will also cover the test and treatment procedures used initially and in ongoing care. Of course, you'll individualize your teaching to the patient's cancer stage and his particular need for encouragement and support.

Discuss the disorder

Explain that bladder cancer usually originates in the mucosal tissue that lines the bladder wall. Disease confined to the mucosal layer is *superficial (noninvasive)*. Once rooted in the muscular layer, the cancer is termed *invasive*. From there, it may metastasize—growing and replicating rapidly and erratically and then spreading when the tumor cells break away and enter the blood or lymphatic circulation.

Bladder cancer can mimic other diseases, such as urinary tract infection. The patient may be asymptomatic, or he may experience episodic hematuria and accompanying dysuria, urinary frequency and urgency, tenesmus, nocturia, pelvic pressure, bladder irritability, fatigue, and weight loss. Help the patient understand his symptoms by describing the bladder's location and function (see *Explaining bladder structures and function*, page 386).

Point out that no one knows exactly what causes bladder cancer, but certain risk factors are known. Bladder cancer has a higher incidence in industrialized nations, particularly in urban areas. Elderly patients with chronic obstructive pulmonary disease or bladder calculi are at risk as are patients who have undergone pelvic radiation therapy or drug therapy with cyclophosphamide (Cytoxan). Also at increased risk are hair stylists, metal workers, painters, rubber workers, textile workers, leather finishers, and other laborers exposed to environmental carcinogens.

Other risk factors include cigarette smoking, a diet high in protein and fat, and recurring urinary tract infections associated with indwelling catheterization (see *Questions patients ask about bladder cancer*, page 386, for more information).

Deborah M. Rust, RN, MSN, OCN, who contributed to this chapter, is a liaison oncology clinical nursing specialist at Pittsburgh Cancer Institute, University of Pittsburgh Medical Center, and adjunct instructor, University of Pittsburgh School of Nursing.

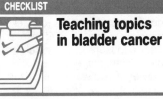

CHECKLIST

Teaching topics in bladder cancer

☐ Where bladder cancer develops
☐ Signs and symptoms of bladder cancer, such as hematuria and dysuria
☐ Risk factors, including industrial exposure to carcinogens, cigarette smoking, and a high-protein, high-fat diet
☐ Complications and the risk of recurrent bladder cancer
☐ Instructions for diagnostic and staging studies, including laboratory tests, excretory urography, retrograde cystography, cystoscopy, bone scan, and ultrasonography
☐ Explanation of treatments, especially chemotherapy, radiation therapy, and surgery, such as transurethral resection of the bladder, cystectomy, and urinary diversion
☐ Management of urinary diversion, if appropriate
☐ Sources of information and support

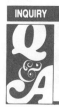
Questions patients ask about bladder cancer

My doctor says smoking contributes to bladder cancer. Is this true?
It's almost certain. Cigarette smokers have a two to three times greater risk of developing bladder cancer than do nonsmokers. Even when a person stops smoking, his risk won't drop to the risk level of a person who never smoked.

I was routinely exposed to chemicals while I was working, but that was years ago. Should I be concerned about bladder cancer?
Probably. Bladder cancer may not develop for years (cancer specialists say 18 to 45 years) after exposure to chemical—or other—carcinogens.

Even if you weren't exposed to industrial carcinogens, you may have used phenacetin, a popular pain reliever, before it was taken off the market by the Food and Drug Administration because it was highly carcinogenic. To be safe, continue to visit your doctor periodically for a cytologic (cell) examination of your urine.

If I have bladder cancer, will the cancer cells show up in a urinalysis?
Not necessarily, although they may be there. If your doctor uses a microscope to detect cancer cells in your urine, he will tell you that this method isn't always definitive—especially if you have blood in your urine. An investigational technique called flow cytometry may give more accurate results. The test instrument has greater magnifying capability, making it easier to identify abnormal cells.

Explaining bladder structures and function

When discussing bladder cancer with your patient, describe the location and function of the bladder. Tell him that the bladder lies in the front portion of the pelvic cavity and is composed of an inner mucosal lining, several layers of muscle, and outer perivesical fat.

Explain that the ureters pipe urine from the kidneys into the bladder. After the bladder fills, the urine leaves the body through another tubelike structure called the urethra.

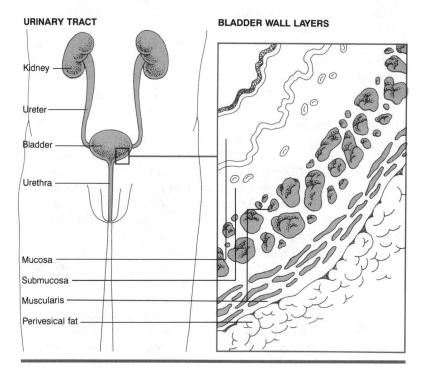

URINARY TRACT

Kidney
Ureter
Bladder
Urethra
Mucosa
Submucosa
Muscularis
Perivesical fat

BLADDER WALL LAYERS

Complications
Despite treatment, the patient with superficial disease has a 30% to 80% chance for recurrent disease. However, only about 10% of superficial bladder cancers develop into invasive disease. With invasive disease, the patient's chances for metastasis increase 40% to 90%. But with treatment, 50% of these patients experience complete remission; 20% have partial remission.

Describe the diagnostic workup
Inform the patient that he'll have a complete physical examination, including a rectal or vaginal examination to search for masses. Then he may undergo a series of tests, ranging from blood and urine tests to excretory urography, retrograde cystography, cystoscopy, and a bone scan. Other diagnostic imaging procedures include a chest X-ray, a computed tomography (CT) scan, magnetic resonance imaging (MRI), and ultrasonography. Explain whether the test will confirm the diagnosis, stage the disease, or monitor the patient's progress with treatment. For more information, see *Staging bladder cancer*.

Staging bladder cancer

Explain to the patient that staging will help to determine the most appropriate treatment for his bladder cancer. One of two staging systems may be used: the tumor-node-metastasis (TNM) system or the Jewett-Strong-Marshall (JSM) system. Note that the JSM system grades cancers O and A through D. Note also that both staging classifications distinguish superficial bladder cancers from invasive bladder cancers, which penetrate bladder muscle and may spread to other sites.

TNM	STAGE	JSM
Superficial cancer		
T0	No tumor	–
TIS	Carcinoma in situ	0
Ta	Papillary tumor; no invasion	0
T1	Lamina propria invaded	A
Invasive cancer		
T2	Infiltrated wall; superficial muscle invasion	B1
T3$_a$	Deep muscle invasion	B2
T3$_b$	Perivesical fat invasion	C
T4$_a$	Contiguous viscera invasion	D1
T4$_b$	Tumor fixed to pelvic or abdominal wall	D1
N0	No lymph node involvement	–
N1	Single, homolateral lymph node involvement	D1
N2	Contralateral, bilateral, or multiple lymph node involvement	D1
N3	Fixed pelvic wall mass separate from primary tumor	D1
N4	Juxtaregional lymph node involvement	D2
M	Distant metastasis	D2

Laboratory tests

Advise the patient that blood will be drawn for a complete blood count and chemistry profile. Explain that test findings can reveal conditions associated with bladder cancer, such as anemia, and also help stage existing disease. For example, elevated alkaline phosphatase levels suggest that the cancer has spread to the bone.

Inform the patient that he'll supply a urine specimen for analysis to detect bacteria, protein, and blood. Additional cytologic studies may reveal cancer cells in the urine.

Excretory urography

Explain that this test (also called intravenous pyelography) evaluates bladder structures. The test can also detect tumors or metastasis elsewhere in the urinary tract. Advise the patient to drink plenty of fluids and then to fast for 8 hours before the test (which takes about 1 hour to complete). Tell him that he may receive a laxative or other bowel preparation before the test.

Inform the patient that during the test he'll lie supine on an X-ray table. A contrast medium will be injected intravenously, and a technician will take X-ray films at specific intervals. Mention that the technician may place a belt around the patient's hips to ensure that the contrast medium remains at a certain level. Also warn him that he may experience a transient burning sensation and metallic taste from the contrast medium. Advise him to report these and any other effects, such as itching, hives, or breathing difficulty.

Retrograde cystography

Inform the patient that this test evaluates bladder structure and integrity and helps to confirm a bladder cancer diagnosis. It takes between 30 minutes and 1 hour to complete. If he will receive a general anesthetic, advise him not to eat or drink anything for 8 hours before the procedure.

Explain that during this test the patient will lie on his back on an X-ray table. Then the doctor will insert a catheter into the bladder and instill a dyelike substance (called a contrast medium). If a local anesthetic is used, forewarn the patient that he may experience some discomfort with insertion of the catheter and instillation of the contrast medium. Films will be taken with the patient in various positions.

After the test, the nurse will monitor his vital signs (blood pressure, heart rate, and respiratory rate) until they're stable. His urine volume and color will also be monitored. Instruct the patient to notify the doctor if blood continues to appear in his urine after the third voiding or if he has chills, fever, or irregular or rapid heartbeats or breathing.

Cystoscopy

Tell the patient that this test involves inserting a flexible, narrow, lighted tube called a cystoscope into the bladder via the urethra. Using this instrument, the doctor can see inside the bladder and obtain a sample of tissue for analysis (biopsy) if necessary. A biopsy is the only definitive way to diagnose bladder cancer. If the patient's scheduled for cystoscopy, give him a copy of the teaching aid *Learning about cystoscopy,* page 396.

Bone scan

Explain that this test can detect disease that spreads to the patient's bones. Performed in the radiology or nuclear medicine department, the test takes about 4 hours. Although the patient needn't fast before the test, advise him to avoid eating a full meal or drinking large amounts of fluid immediately beforehand.

Tell the patient that a tourniquet will be applied to his arm, and the doctor will inject a small dose of a radioactive isotope. Assure him that the isotope emits less radiation than a standard X-ray machine. Inform him that he'll need to wait for 2 or 3 hours while the isotope circulates. During this time, he'll drink four to six glasses of fluid. Then he'll lie supine on an X-ray table beneath a scanner. The scanner will move slowly back and forth, recording images for about 1 hour. Unless the doctor asks the patient to assume various positions, he should lie as still as possible to ensure clear, sharp images of his bones.

Chest X-ray

Inform the patient that no special preparations are needed for a chest X-ray. He'll remove any metal jewelry or objects that can disrupt a clear X-ray image. Then he'll stand before an X-ray film plate while a technician takes films of his chest.

CT scan or magnetic resonance imaging
If the patient is having a CT scan, tell him that this test provides computer-enhanced X-ray images of certain body tissues. If he's having an MRI scan, inform him that this test uses an electromagnetic process to produce images of body organs.

As needed, give him a copy of the patient-teaching aid *Preparing for magnetic resonance imaging,* page 211.

Ultrasonography
Explain that ultrasonography uses high-frequency sound waves and a computer to produce images of body tissues. The sound waves from a transducer pass through tissue and echo back to the transducer, which converts the sound waves into electrical impulses. These impulses are then amplified and displayed on a screen.

Inform the patient that ultrasonography can show whether his disease affects tissues beyond the bladder. The test can also distinguish a bladder cyst from a tumor. Explain that a cyst (filled with fluid) transmits sound very well and shows up clearly on the sonogram; a tumor (a solid mass) appears as a vague image on the sonogram.

Teach about treatments
Explain that treatment for bladder cancer varies, depending on the patient's life-style, any other medical problems, and his mental outlook. As appropriate, teach the patient about chemotherapy, radiation therapy, and surgery, such as transurethral resection of the bladder or cystectomy. For information about experimental treatments, see *Investigational bladder cancer treatments,* page 390.

Activity
Advise the patient to alternate activity with rest periods to conserve his energy, especially while he's undergoing treatment. Encourage him, however, to continue participation in his usual activities of daily living.

Medication
Whether the patient is having systemic chemotherapy, intravesical chemotherapy, or an investigational treatment, such as biotherapy, teach him about its purpose, method of administration, and potential side effects.

Systemic chemotherapy. Typically chosen for locally extensive bladder cancer and metastatic cancer, several drugs may be given intravenously in combination. The most active agent is cisplatin (Platinol). Other active agents include doxorubicin (Adriamycin), methotrexate sodium (Folex), and vinblastine sulfate (Velban). To help the patient cope with the side effects of these drugs, give

Investigational bladder cancer treatments

If your patient asks for information on research programs or investigational bladder cancer treatments, suggest he discuss his concerns in depth with his doctor. Among such investigational treatments are biotherapy, neoadjuvant chemotherapy and radiation therapy, and photodynamic therapy.

Biotherapy
Also known as immunotherapy, this investigational treatment uses the intravesical route to instill interferon-alpha and tumor necrosis factor. These agents may stimulate the patient's immune system to produce natural substances that kill abnormal cells or delay cancer cell growth.

Side effects from interferon-alpha include alopecia, leukopenia, and flulike symptoms such as fever, malaise, and myalgia. Side effects associated with tumor necrosis factor are being studied.

Combination therapy
Patients who have localized bladder tumors judged too extensive for surgical removal may benefit from an experimental combination of radiation and chemotherapy. Considered a neoadjuvant therapy, this treatment shrinks the tumors so that surgery can then effectively remove them or so that the bladder can be retained.

Side effects include those associated with radiation therapy and the particular chemotherapeutic agent used.

Photodynamic therapy
This treatment requires an I.V. injection of a photosensitizing agent called hematoporphyrin derivative (HPD). Malignant tissue appears to have an affinity for HPD, so superficial bladder cancer cells readily absorb the drug. Then the doctor uses a cystoscope to introduce a laser light into the bladder. Exposing HPD-impregnated tumor cells to light kills them.

However, HPD sensitizes not only tumor tissue but also normal body tissue to light. Therefore any patient receiving this treatment must avoid sunlight for about 30 days. Precautions include wearing protective clothing (including gloves and a face mask), drawing heavy curtains at home during the day, scheduling outdoor travel at night, and conducting daily exercises inside (or outside at night) to promote circulation, joint mobility, and muscle activity. After 30 days, the patient can gradually return to daylight activities.

---

him a copy of the teaching aid *How to control the side effects of chemotherapy and radiation therapy,* pages 306 to 309.

Intravesical chemotherapy. Used for treating superficial tumors (especially tumors in many sites) and for preventing tumor recurrence, intravesical chemotherapy directly washes the bladder with anticancer drugs. Explain that the patient will lie horizontally as the drug flows through a catheter into the bladder. Then as directed, he'll turn from side to side and onto his abdomen. Tell him that these motions ensure complete lavage of the inner bladder wall. Commonly used agents include triethylenethiophosphoramide (Thiotepa), doxorubicin (Adriamycin), mitomycin (Mutamycin), and bacillus Calmette-Guérin (BCG). Give him a copy of the patient-teaching aid *Learning about bladder-instilled chemotherapy,* page 397.

Procedures
Inform the patient that radiation therapy destroys the cancer cells' ability to grow and multiply. He'll also need to know that radiation affects normal cells too. Assure him that normal cells usually recover quickly.

Make sure the patient understands when and where he'll receive radiation therapy and who will administer it. Reinforce the doctor's explanations, and answer any questions. Advise him to notify the doctor if side effects persist or become especially troublesome or if fever or unusual pain develops.

Understanding transurethral resection of the bladder

Use this illustration to help your patient understand transurethral resection of the bladder. (Reassure your female patient that gender-related anatomic differences do not affect the essential procedure.) Explain that the doctor will insert a slender device called a cystoscope through the urethra into the bladder to remove small, superficial tumors.

Then explain that during the procedure the patient will lie in the lithotomy position. After administering a local anesthetic, the doctor will introduce a cystoscope into the urethra and advance it into the bladder. Then he'll fill the bladder with a clear, nonconducting irrigant. Next, he'll locate the lesion and position the cystoscope's cutting loop around the bladder tumor. After turning on the electric current (which runs through the cutting loop), he'll cut or cauterize the lesion. Finally, he'll remove the cystoscope.

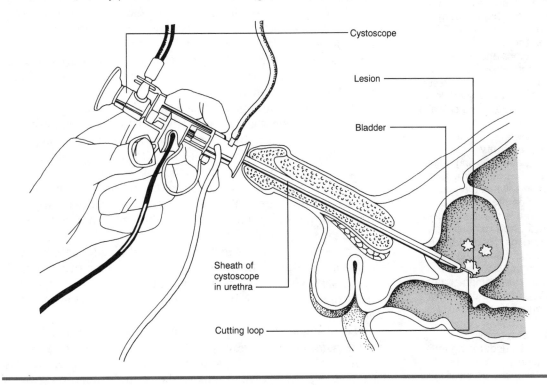

Cystoscope

Lesion

Bladder

Sheath of cystoscope in urethra

Cutting loop

Surgery

Teach the patient about bladder cancer surgery: transurethral resection of the bladder (TURB) or cystectomy.

Transurethral resection of the bladder. Most commonly performed to remove superficial and early bladder cancers, this operation requires the surgeon to insert a cystoscope through the urethra and into the bladder to remove lesions. (See *Understanding transurethral resection of the bladder*.)

Briefly explain the procedure. Inform the patient that he may receive a local anesthetic and be awake during treatment. Reassure him that he should experience little or no discomfort and that postoperative effects, such as hematuria and a burning sensation during urination, should quickly subside. If he experiences additional discomfort with painful bladder spasms, instruct him to request pain-relieving medication. Point out that the operation shouldn't interfere with normal genitourinary function. Potential complications can include hematuria, urine retention, bladder per-

392 Bladder cancer

What happens in cystectomy

Whether your patient's having a partial, simple, or radical cystectomy, he's bound to feel apprehensive. Knowing something about the operation may help him to deal with his fears.

Partial cystectomy
Inform the patient having a partial cystectomy that the surgeon will make a suprapubic incision. He'll open the bladder and remove the tumor and any attached tissue. He'll also excise a small margin of healthy tissue and then close the wound, leaving a surgical drain and catheter in place.

Simple cystectomy
Inform the patient having a simple -- or total -- cystectomy that the surgeon will make an incision and separate the bladder's posterior and lateral connective tissue. Next, he'll remove the bladder and surrounding tissue from near the bladder neck. He'll suture the bladder neck closed, insert a drainage catheter, and redirect the ureters to form a urinary diversion.

Radical cystectomy
If the patient's undergoing radical cystectomy, explain that the surgeon will make an incision from the pubis to the epigastrium on the side opposite the planned urinary diversion. He'll remove any diseased lymph nodes and ligate and divide the ureters deep in the pelvis. Next, he'll remove the bladder and surrounding structures, including the prostate gland and seminal vesicles in men and most reproductive organs in women.

Finally, he'll insert an indwelling urethral catheter to control bleeding from the urogenital diaphragm, position an abdominal drain, and redirect the ureters to form a urinary diversion—most commonly an ileal loop (or ileal conduit).

foration, and urinary tract infection. Reassure him that careful monitoring and catheter care will reduce his risk for complications.

Review care after TURB. Inform the patient that he'll have an indwelling urinary catheter for 1 to 5 days after the surgery to ensure urine drainage. Also tell him that he may need continuous bladder irrigation for 24 hours or more. As ordered, prepare him to undergo further testing to evaluate renal function, rule out tumors elsewhere in the urinary tract, and detect any metastasis.

Advise the patient that slight hematuria may last for several weeks after the resection. However, he should promptly report bleeding or hematuria that lasts longer than several weeks. Instruct him also to report fever, chills, or flank pain, which may signal a urinary tract infection. Encourage him to drink plenty of water—about 10 glasses (80 oz) daily—and to void every 2 to 3 hours. Explain that this reduces the risk of urinary tract infection, clot formation, and urethral obstruction. Stress that he shouldn't ignore the urge to urinate.

To promote healing and reduce the risk of bleeding from increased intra-abdominal pressure, advise the patient to refrain from sexual and other strenuous activity, not to lift anything heavier than 10 lb (4.54 kg), and to continue taking a stool softener or other laxative until the doctor orders otherwise.

Emphasize the importance of regular follow-up examinations to assess the need for further treatments. Point out that early detection and removal of bladder tumors through transurethral resection may prevent the need for cystectomy.

Cystectomy. If the patient has advanced bladder cancer, explain that removal of the bladder and surrounding structures may be necessary. Cystectomy may be partial (segmental), simple (total), or radical (for more information, see *What happens in cystectomy*).

For a single, easily accessible tumor, the patient may have a *partial cystectomy* to remove the diseased portion and preserve bladder function. For multiple tumors or extensive cancer, he may have a *simple cystectomy* to remove the entire bladder, preserve surrounding structures, and create a permanent urinary diversion (see *Teaching about urinary diversions*). For muscle-invasive primary bladder cancer, however, the surgeon may recommend a *radical cystectomy* to remove the bladder and all surrounding diseased tissues and structures and create a permanent urinary diversion.

Provide encouragement and support to the patient having this operation. Radical and simple cystectomy can cause psychological problems related to an altered body image and to loss of sexual or reproductive function. The surgery typically produces impotence in men, although sometimes the surgeon can preserve the nerves needed for ejaculation. In women, the surgery may change the vaginal structure, which may cause discomfort or pain with intercourse.

Reassure the patient that with adequate support services he can continue most of his usual activities. As needed, refer him for psychological and sexual counseling. Also arrange for him to con-

Teaching about urinary diversions

If your patient is scheduled for a simple or radical cystectomy, he'll need a urinary diversion to substitute for his bladder. Teach him about the diversion he'll receive.

Ileal loop or ileal conduit
Also called a ureteroileostomy or urostomy, this is one of the most commonly performed supravesicular urinary diversions. The surgeon first sutures about 6 inches (15 cm) of the ileum closed. Next, he attaches the ureters to the ileum and pulls the ileum through the abdominal wall to form a stoma. Then he reconnects the bowel.

Teaching points. Tell the patient that he'll awaken from surgery with a nasogastric tube in place, and he won't be allowed to eat for several days. He'll also have an ostomy bag in place. This urine-collecting bag won't be changed for several days. Warn him that initially after surgery his urine will contain blood. Also explain that he may see catheters or stents protruding from the stoma and into the urine-collecting bag. These devices, which assist healing, will be removed a few days after surgery. Urge the patient to move carefully to avoid dislodging them.

Possible complications. Review possible problems, such as anuria from edema or obstruction at the ureterointestinal anastomosis; urine or fecal leakage at the anastomosis; abdominal distention or a dusky stoma from vascular infarction of the conduit site; stomal stenosis; pyelonephritis; renal calculi; and skin problems—for example, stomal ulceration.

Ureterosigmoidostomy or ureteroileosigmoidostomy
If the surgeon performs either of these urinary diversion procedures, tell the patient that his ureters will be diverted into his sigmoid colon so that he will void through his anus. He won't need to wear an ostomy bag. This procedure is performed only if the patient has good anal sphincter tone.

Teaching points. Advise the patient to sit or stand frequently after surgery to avoid urine reflux. Also warn him that this diversion may produce urinary incontinence when he passes flatus. Add that choosing a diet low in gas-forming foods may help to allay this problem. Teach the patient to avoid possible electrolyte imbalances related to this diversion by following a diet low in chloride and salt and by taking potassium supplements.

Possible complications. Explain that anuria—resulting from ureteral obstruction, stricture, edema, or fecal matter and mucus—can lead to kidney failure. Also, urine leakage from the anastomosis, pyelonephritis, electrolyte imbalances, and renal calculi may complicate ureterosigmoidostomy.

Ureterostomy
Teach the patient that ureterostomy involves diverting the ureters through an opening on the abdominal wall. Depending on the procedure, one or more stomas will be created. For example, the patient will have one stoma if the surgeon performs a transureteroureterostomy, which directs one ureter into the other so that only one tube opens to the outside. He'll have two stomas if the surgeon performs a double-barrel ureterostomy, which brings the two ureters side by side to the abdominal surface. Because this procedure can be completed quickly, the surgeon may perform it in a patient with low tolerance for anesthesia.

Teaching points. Tell the patient that he will need to wear an ostomy bag—or an external urine-collecting bag—after surgery. However, because the stoma created by this diversion rises very little above skin level, the ostomy bag may adhere poorly. Recommend using an adhesive-backed ostomy bag for better results.

Possible complications. Warn the patient that a dusky (cyanotic) stoma may signal vascular insufficiency, which can lead to stenosis.

Ileal loop
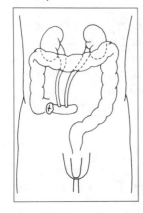

Ureterosigmoidostomy
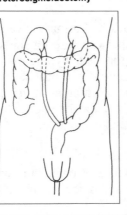

Transureteroureterostomy
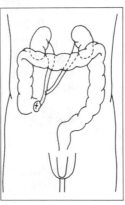

Double-barrel ureterostomy
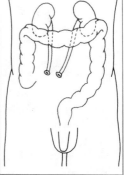

sult an enterostomal therapist, who can provide additional instruction and support.

Review preoperative instructions. Inform the patient that for 4 days before surgery he'll undergo bowel preparation to help prevent infection. For 3 of the 4 days, he'll maintain a low-residue diet; on the day before surgery, he'll receive an infusion of high-calorie fluids. Mention that he'll also receive antibiotics, usually erythromycin (E-Mycin) and neomycin (Mycifradin), for 24 hours before surgery, and inform him that he'll have an enema the night before surgery to flush fecal matter from the bowel. If the patient will need to be cared for in the intensive care unit (ICU), arrange for the patient and his family to visit the ICU before surgery to familiarize them with the unit and meet the staff.

Outline postoperative care. Tell the patient that when he awakens from surgery he'll be in the ICU. Besides a nasogastric tube coming from his nose and a central venous catheter in his upper chest, he may notice a catheter and a drain at the incision site. He won't eat or drink anything until the return of bowel function. He'll be given I.V. fluids during this period. After that, he can resume taking oral fluids and eventually progress to eating solids.

Inform the patient that his vital signs and urine drainage will be monitored, and his stoma and incision will be checked periodically for signs of complications (bleeding and infection). Reassure him that he can request medication to relieve incisional or spasmodic pain. Encourage mobility by advising frequent position changes after surgery. Also teach him coughing and deep-breathing exercises. Tell him that early ambulation after surgery helps to prevent complications.

Before discharge, discuss self-care. Explain that incisional pain and fatigue will probably last for several weeks after discharge. Instruct the patient to notify the doctor if these symptoms persist or worsen. Review possible complications to watch for and report, including urinary tract infection (fever, chills, flank pain, and decreased urine volume) or wound infection (redness, swelling, and purulent drainage at the incision site). Also instruct him to report persistent hematuria, dysuria, and urinary frequency. Caution him to avoid lifting, driving, and strenuous exercise for 4 to 6 weeks. Refer him to his doctor for advice on when he can return to work.

If the patient's had urinary diversion surgery, be sure that he or a family member can care for the stoma and obtain supplies. If needed, arrange for visits by a home care nurse who can reinforce stoma care instructions and provide emotional support. Also give him a copy of the teaching aid *Caring for your urinary stoma*, pages 398 to 400. Refer the patient to a support group, such as the United Ostomy Association.

Other care measures

Stress the importance of complying with follow-up appointments to assess healing and detect recurrent disease. The rate of bladder cancer recurrence is high for patients who retain their bladders. Even those who have undergone cystectomy can still develop metastatic disease.

Advise the patient to report dysuria, frequency, and hematuria to the doctor as soon as possible. Point out that he'll need regular yearly physical examinations and diagnostic tests.

Sources of information and support

American Cancer Society
1599 Clifton Road, NE, Atlanta, Ga. 30329
(404) 320-3333

Cancer Information Service (CIS)
c/o National Cancer Institute
NIH Building 31, Room 10A24, Bethesda, Md. 20892
(800) 4-CANCER

Chemotherapy Foundation
183 Madison Avenue, Room 403, New York, N.Y. 10016
(212) 213-9292

Make Today Count
101½ South Union Street, Alexandria, Va. 22314
(703) 548-9674

United Ostomy Association
36 Executive Park, Suite 120, Irvine, Calif. 92714
(714) 660-8624

Further readings

Ali, N.S., and Khalil, H.Z. "Effect of Psychoeducational Intervention on Anxiety Among Egyptian Bladder Cancer Patients," *Cancer Nursing* 12(4):236-42, August 1989.

Benson, R.C., Jr., et al. "Clues to the Elusive Bladder Cancer," *Patient Care* 22(12):57-60, 65-68, 70-72, July 15, 1988.

Brettschneider, N.R., and Orihuela, E. "Carcinoma of the Bladder," *Urology Nursing* 10(1):14-21, March 1990.

Brixey, M.T. "Chemotherapeutic Agents: Intravesical Instillation," *Urology Nursing* 9(2):4-6, October-December 1988.

Brownson, R.C., et al. "Occupation, Smoking, and Alcohol in the Epidemiology of Bladder Cancer," *American Journal of Public Health* 77(10):1298-1300, October 1987.

Haas, N., and Dalton, J.R. "Perioperative Management of the Continent Right Colon Urinary Pouch: An Experience with Five Cases," *Journal of Enterostomal Therapy* 14(5):188-93, September-October 1987.

Smith, D.B., and Babaian, R.J. "Patient Adjustment to an Ileal Conduit After Radical Cystectomy," *Journal of Enterostomal Therapy* 16(6):244-46, November-December 1989.

Smith, J.A. "Benign and Malignant Diseases of the Bladder: Indications for Laser Therapy," *Journal of Urology Nursing* 7(3):469-74, July-September 1988.

Storrar, M.L. "Urinary Diversion and Bladder Reconstruction," *NATNews: British Journal of Theatre Nursing* 27(1):11-13, January 1990.

Toota, J., and Easterling, A. "P.D.T.: Destroying Malignant Cells with Laser Beams...Photodynamic Therapy," *Nursing89* 19(11):48-49, November 1989.

PATIENT-TEACHING AID

Learning about cystoscopy

Dear Patient:

Your doctor has scheduled you for cystoscopy. During this procedure, he can look inside your bladder through an instrument called a cystoscope. He'll insert the cystoscope through your urethra (the opening through which you urinate).

Cystoscopy allows the doctor to diagnose and, sometimes, treat your urinary disorder. The test may be done in a hospital or the doctor's office. It takes 15 to 45 minutes or more to complete.

What to expect before the test
You may receive a local anesthetic before the procedure. This means that the doctor will numb the area around the urethra before inserting the cystoscope.

Or you may have general anesthesia. In this case, don't eat or drink anything after midnight on the night before the procedure. If the doctor plans to take X-rays of your bladder during the cystoscopy, he may prescribe medication that will clean your bowels to ensure sharper, clearer images.

Just before the procedure begins, you will have an intravenous line inserted in your arm to deliver fluids and medications if you need them. You'll also receive a sedative to help you relax.

What to expect during the test
After the anesthetic takes effect, you'll be positioned on your back. Then the

doctor will insert the cystoscope. Remember to take deep breaths and try to relax. This will allow the test to proceed smoothly.

If you received a local anesthetic, you may feel a strong urge to urinate as the instrument is inserted and removed. If the doctor instills an irrigant into your bladder, you may feel some pressure. Again, try to relax. If you experience any pain or if you feel your heart beating irregularly, let your doctor know.

What to expect after the test
Your condition will be monitored until you're fully alert. If you received a local anesthetic, you'll be awake but you may feel weak; so don't chance walking by yourself. Wait for someone to assist you.

For several days after the cystoscopy, you may void blood-tinged urine. You may also have bladder spasms, a feeling that your bladder's full, or a burning sensation when you urinate. Take aspirin or acetaminophen (Tylenol), drink plenty of fluids, and lie in a tub of warm water to help relieve these possible side effects.

When to call the doctor
Call your doctor if you have heavy bleeding or blood clots in your urine, bladder pain or spasms that aren't relieved by medication, or burning and a frequent urge to urinate that persists for more than 24 hours. Also notify your doctor at once if you can't urinate within 8 hours after the test.

Learning about bladder-instilled chemotherapy

Dear Patient:

The doctor will treat your bladder cancer by instilling medication directly into your bladder. This procedure is called intravesical chemotherapy.

Read the information below to learn what you can expect during your chemotherapy treatments. If you have questions, ask your nurse or doctor for more information.

How does the medication get into my bladder?
The medication reaches your bladder through a very thin tube called a catheter. The catheter will be inserted in your urethra, which is the opening through which you urinate. First, the urethra will be cleaned with a bacteria-fighting solution, such as povidone-iodine. Then the catheter will be inserted, and the urine that's already in your bladder will be drained into a container. Now, you should be ready to receive your treatment medication.

Next, the medication will be instilled through the catheter, and the catheter will remain in place for a certain period of time. During that time, the catheter will be clamped shut so that no medication can escape from the bladder.

Meanwhile, you may be asked to change your position by turning from side to side or walking around. This distributes the medication throughout your bladder.

How is the medication removed?
At the end of the scheduled time, the clamp on the catheter will be released, and the medication will drain out. Then the catheter will be removed. You shouldn't feel any discomfort while this is being done. Try to relax and take a few deep breaths. Afterward, you may wash your genital area.

What about side effects?
The side effects depend on the kind of medication you receive. For example:
● If you're receiving *triethylenethiophosphoramide* (also called Thiotepa), common side effects include fever, chills, a sore throat, hives, itching, bladder spasms, and pain when you urinate.
● If you're receiving *doxorubicin* (also called Adriamycin), you may have pain when you urinate, the sensation of having an urgent need to urinate, and discolored (cherry red) urine.
● If you're receiving *mitomycin* (also called Mutamycin), side effects include pain when you urinate, the sensation of having an urgent need to urinate, and a rash on your palms and buttocks.
● If you're receiving *bacillus Calmette-Guérin* (also called BCG), you may experience pain when you urinate, bladder spasms, blood in your urine, fever, chills, and muscle and joint aches.

Ask your doctor, nurse, or infusion therapist how best to relieve these side effects.

Caring for your urinary stoma

Dear Patient:

The surgeon has constructed a new passageway for your urine. This passageway leads directly to the outside of your body through an opening on your abdomen called a stoma. You'll wear a baglike appliance called an ostomy bag to collect the urine that drains from the stoma.

Learning about your ostomy bag

Most ostomy bags can be worn from 3 to 5 days — sometimes as long as 7 days. To prevent infection, you'll need to change the bag at least weekly. If the bag begins to leak, change it immediately to prevent infection.

To keep the weight of the bag from loosening its seal against the stoma, empty the bag whenever it becomes one-third to one-half full.

At bedtime, consider connecting the bag to a larger urine-collection container. This will keep the urine from stagnating in the bag and will minimize the chance of infection.

Besides, when the urine drains into another container, the weight of the urine won't loosen the bag's seal.

The best time to change the bag is usually in the morning when urine output is less. To control leakage while your bag is off, you may want to insert a thin gauze roll or a tampon into the stoma.

Gathering the equipment

To make changing your ostomy bag easier, gather all the equipment that you'll need. Whether your ostomy bag is permanent, temporary, disposable, or reusable, you'll need the following supplies:
- adhesive tape and scissors
- a skin barrier — either a paste or a solid seal — to protect the skin around your stoma. Skin barrier types include karaya gum, gelatin wafers, or paste.
- ostomy cement or spray adhesive
- an odorproof ostomy bag with an opening at the bottom for draining urine
- a mounting ring (called a faceplate) for

continued

Caring for your urinary stoma — *continued*

attaching the bag
- cleaning supplies, such as soap, vinegar, and water
- gauze pads and a soft, clean towel
- an electric razor (optional).

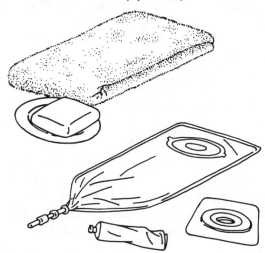

Caring for the stoma

After you remove the ostomy bag, use a vinegar and water solution (one-half vinegar and one-half water) or soap and water to wash off any crystal deposits on or around the stoma.

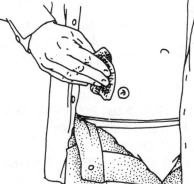

If you use soap, choose a nondrying, nonalkaline soap, such as Basis, Dove, or castile.

Next, rinse the area thoroughly and pat your skin dry with a towel. Any soap or moisture remaining on your skin may keep the ostomy bag from adhering.

If you notice any hairs growing around the stoma, carefully trim them with scissors or an electric razor. Don't risk cutting your skin with a razor blade.

Take meticulous care of your stoma to prevent irritation. Poor skin care may lead to a urinary tract or yeast infection. Avoid changing the ostomy bag too frequently because this can also irritate the skin.

Applying the adhesive

If you use ostomy cement, apply a thin layer around the stoma and allow it to dry.

If you use a spray adhesive, *cover the stoma,* and spray the adhesive onto the surrounding skin. Or you may decide to spray the adhesive onto a gauze pad and then dab the adhesive around the stoma.

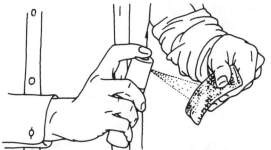

If you use a skin barrier, measure your stoma with the cutting guide found inside the package. Select the flange size that is ¼ inch larger than your stoma.

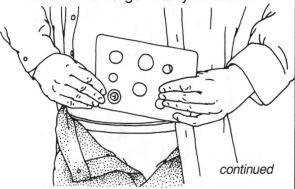

continued

Caring for your urinary stoma — *continued*

Next, trace the right size onto the adhesive paper backing. Now, cut out a skin barrier wafer. Peel off the backing and place the wafer over your stoma. Press the skin barrier wafer against your skin for 30 seconds to form a seal.

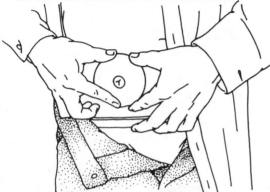

For more security, you may also wish to apply adhesive tape around the barrier.

Attaching the ostomy bag

Remove the gauze roll or the tampon that you placed in your stoma to control leakage.

If you use adhesive, attach the ostomy bag when the adhesive becomes tacky. Center the bag over the stoma and leave a small amount of skin exposed around the stoma.

If you use a skin barrier, attach the ostomy bag by placing the flange on the wafer and pressing firmly. You should feel the flanges snap together.

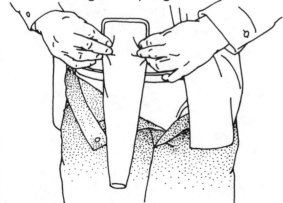

Finally, if you use an adhesive bag system, trace a circle that's ⅛ inch larger than your stoma onto the adhesive backing. Cut around the tracing and remove the backing. Next, check to be sure that the bottom drainage valve is closed.

Now, starting at the bottom, press the adhesive firmly but gently around the stoma. Be careful not to wrinkle the material. You may also wish to apply adhesive tape around the faceplate.

If you want to wear an ostomy belt to further secure the bag, be sure to wear the belt at the level of the stoma. Wear the belt loose enough so it doesn't irritate the skin and leave red marks. (If it's loose enough, you should be able to slip two fingers between your skin and the belt.)

Controlling odor

Besides using vinegar to clean your stoma, try drinking cranberry or apple juice. Or take vitamin C tablets. All of these measures acidify urine and decrease odor.

Also, add a few drops of vinegar or commercially available ostomy deodorizer directly to the ostomy bag to eliminate odors.

Bathing with an ostomy bag

You may take a bath or shower with your ostomy bag on or off, whichever makes you feel most comfortable. With the bag off, of course, urine will flow into the bathwater.

Testicular cancer

Although testicular cancer represents only 1% of all cancers diagnosed in men, it's the leading cause of cancer deaths in men ages 15 to 34. The patient with testicular cancer faces difficult treatment, and he's almost certain to fear sexual impairment and physical disfigurement. In your teaching, you'll be challenged to establish a trusting relationship with the patient, encouraging him to ask questions and express his fears.

Address the patient's concerns as you teach about tests to diagnose and stage testicular cancer and treatments, including surgery to remove the affected testicle and chemotherapy and radiation therapy to arrest the cancer. Reassure him that sterility and impotence aren't inevitable consequences of testicular cancer surgery. As needed, direct him and his family to sources of information and support. Finally, advise him to examine his testicles once a month to detect the possible recurrence of cancer at its earliest, most treatable stage.

Discuss the disorder

Tailor your teaching to the patient's form of testicular cancer—*germinal* or *nongerminal*. Explain that a germinal tumor stems from primitive germ cells; the relatively rare nongerminal tumor arises from interstitial cells. About 60% of the germinal tumors are *seminomas*. Commonly detected before metastasis, these slow-growing cancers are highly curable. Most seminomas respond to radiation therapy. More than 90% of patients with seminomas are disease-free 5 years after diagnosis and treatment.

Nonseminomas include embryonal tumors, teratomas, and choriocarcinomas. Yolk sac-type embryonal tumors, so named because they arise from embryonic cells, may appear in infants and children (although this tumor type also develops in young adults). Nonseminomas, especially teratomas and choriocarcinomas, spread more aggressively than seminomas. About 65% of patients with nonseminomas have metastasis by the time testicular cancer is diagnosed. As a result, survival rates for patients with this type of tumor are lower.

If appropriate, inform the patient that testicular cancer occurs more commonly in White men than in Black men and rarely in Asian, Hispanic, or Native American men. The cause of testicular cancer isn't known; however, 1 of every 10 patients has a history of cryptorchidism (for more information, see *Cryptorchidism and testicular cancer*, page 402). Other risk factors include congenital

Catherine E. Taylor, RN, BSN, who wrote this chapter, is a senior clinical nurse at Johns Hopkins Hospital, Baltimore.

CHECKLIST

Teaching topics in testicular cancer

☐ Explanation of tumor cell types: seminoma or nonseminoma
☐ Risk factors, including cryptorchidism, congenital abnormalities, hormone use, and traumatic injury
☐ Early signs and symptoms, such as a lump in the testicle and swelling or a feeling of heaviness in the scrotum
☐ Signs and symptoms of advanced cancer, such as vague abdominal pain, coughing, and dyspnea
☐ Importance of early detection and treatment to prevent metastasis
☐ Preparation for diagnostic tests, such as blood studies, computed tomography scan, and testicular biopsy
☐ Staging testicular cancer
☐ Chemotherapy and measures to combat side effects
☐ Preparation for radiation therapy or autologous bone marrow transplant
☐ Inguinal orchiectomy and postoperative care
☐ Sexual concerns after orchiectomy
☐ Sources of information and support

Cryptorchidism and testicular cancer

Cryptorchidism—the failure of a testicle to descend into the scrotum—is thought to be a major risk factor for testicular cancer. If you learn that a male patient has an undescended or partially descended testicle, alert him to this association. Mention that testicular tumor development is about 50 times more common in men with an undescended testicle.

Correcting anatomy
Inform the patient that a simple surgical procedure, known as orchiopexy, can restore the testicle to its normal position in the scrotum and reduce the risk of testicular cancer.

Explain that the surgeon makes an incision in the groin and separates the testicle and its blood supply from the surrounding abdominal structures. Then, he creates a "tunnel" into the scrotum to accommodate the testicle.

Stress self-examination
After orchiopexy, urge the patient to examine himself monthly to detect any tumor in its earliest stage. Mention that testicular tumors still occur more commonly in a surgically descended testicle than in a naturally descended one.

Common sites for testicular tumors

Use this illustration of a testicle and surrounding anatomic structures to teach your patient where to look for signs of testicular cancer. Because the testicles lie so close to the retroperitoneal lymph nodes, testicular cancer cells readily spread to these nodes. Instruct the patient to seek medical attention if he finds a firm, painless lump or nodule, usually about the size of a pea.

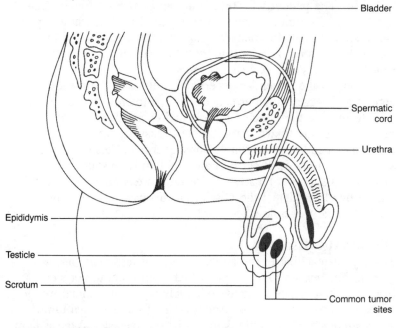

and chromosomal abnormalities, including gonadal aplasia, hermaphroditism, and Klinefelter's syndrome; exposure to diethylstilbestrol or other hormones; and traumatic injury. Viral diseases, such as mumps, may also play a role.

Explain that a small, hard, painless lump in one testicle may be the initial sign of disease (see *Common sites for testicular tumors*). Other signs are swelling or a feeling of heaviness in the scrotum. Pain is unlikely unless infarction or hemorrhage occurs. Gynecomastia and nipple tenderness may result from tumors that secrete human chorionic gonadotropin or estrogens.

Point out the signs and symptoms of late-stage cancer or metastasis: vague abdominal pain, anorexia, behavioral changes, cognitive deficits, coughing, dyspnea, hemoptysis, swelling in the supraclavicular region, and vomiting. Common sites of metastasis include the lungs, liver, bone, and brain.

Complications
Emphasize that early detection and treatment are essential to prevent metastasis. Reiterate how the tumor's proximity to inguinal and abdominal lymph nodes provides cancer cells with easy access to lymphatic circulation and vital organs, such as the lungs and the brain.

Describe the diagnostic workup

Inform the patient that a complete health history and physical examination begin the diagnostic process. Mention that he'll be asked to recall injuries to the scrotum, hormone use, and viral infections, such as mumps. Encourage him to ask questions and to discuss any changes in his sexual ability.

Explain how diagnostic tests, such as computed tomography (CT) and biopsy, can stage the severity of his cancer, based on whether the tumor is confined to the scrotum or has spread to lymph nodes and secondary organs (for more information, see *Staging testicular cancer*). Tell the patient that the prognosis depends on the cancer's cell type and stage. Prepare him for laboratory and radiologic studies to diagnose, stage, and monitor his condition.

Blood tests

Advise the patient that he'll undergo several routine blood tests, including a complete blood count. The doctor will also evaluate beta-subunit human chorionic gonadotropin (hCG) and alpha-fetoprotein (AFP) levels. Explain that elevated levels of these proteins (tumor markers) suggest a testicular tumor. The markers can also differentiate a seminoma from a nonseminoma: Elevated hCG and AFP levels point to a nonseminoma; elevated hCG and normal AFP levels indicate a seminoma.

CT scan

Inform the patient that a CT scan uses three-dimensional X-ray images to examine organs in the abdomen, chest, and head. Explain that this 90-minute test can detect tumors and metastasis.

Instruct the patient to avoid eating or drinking anything after midnight before the test but to continue taking medication as ordered. Explain that during the test he'll lie on a hard X-ray table that will slide into the tubelike CT scanner. Advise him to lie still, relax, breathe normally, and remain quiet to ensure that movement doesn't blur the images and prolong the test. If the doctor orders an I.V. contrast medium, inform the patient that he may experience discomfort from the needle puncture and a localized sensation of warmth when the doctor injects the dyelike substance. Tell the patient to report any hypersensitivity reactions, such as dizziness, headache, hives, nausea, or vomiting. Inform him that he may resume eating after the test.

Other radiologic tests

If necessary, prepare the patient for additional radiologic tests to detect metastasis. For example, excretory urography (intravenous pyelography) may be ordered to detect ureteral displacement caused by metastasis to a para-aortic lymph node. Chest X-rays may reveal pulmonary metastasis, and lymphangiography followed by ultrasonography or magnetic resonance imaging may show other metastases.

Biopsy

Tell the patient that the doctor will perform a biopsy if he finds a testicular mass. He'll make a high inguinal incision, exposing and

---

isolating the spermatic cord. He'll obtain a tissue sample of the affected testicle and the spermatic cord for analysis. Besides confirming and staging the tumor, biopsy findings assist in planning effective therapy.

Teach about treatments

Explain that treatments for testicular cancer include surgery, radiation, and chemotherapy in various combinations. In some cases, treatment may involve autologous bone marrow transplantation. Because treatment usually begins with surgical removal of the affected testicle (orchiectomy), your initial teaching may focus on preparing the patient for surgery. Then, as appropriate, teach about postoperative radiation or chemotherapy.

Medication

Review the purpose, dosage, and possible adverse effects of any prescribed pain medication for testicular cancer.

Prepare the patient for chemotherapy. It's most effective for late-stage seminomas and most stages of nonseminomas when it's used for recurrent testicular cancer after orchiectomy and resection of the retroperitoneal lymph nodes. Emphasize that recent advances in chemotherapy offer improved prognoses for patients with testicular cancer.

Educate the patient about the type and sequence of drugs he'll receive and whether they'll be administered in the hospital or at home. He'll receive combination therapy because different drugs affect cancer cells at various stages of cell division. Inform him that chemotherapy may include cisplatin (Platinol), bleomycin (Blenoxane), vinblastine (Velban), and etoposide (Vepesid). Explain that these drugs are given by mouth or by injection into veins or muscles. They're administered in specific cycles to allow the body time to recover during the drug-free period.

Review the common side effects of the patient's drug regimen. Tell him that side effects occur during chemotherapy because these drugs affect any rapidly growing cells in the body— normal or cancerous. Be sure the patient understands that each person responds differently to chemotherapy. If he expresses concern over severe side effects, reassure him that the doctor can prescribe medications (antiemetics, for example) to relieve his discomfort. Emphasize that most side effects subside before or shortly after the treatment ends. Give the patient a copy of the teaching aid *How to control the side effects of chemotherapy and radiation therapy*, pages 306 to 309.

Bleomycin. Tell the patient that bleomycin (Blenoxane), an antibiotic antineoplastic drug, kills cells by inhibiting the synthesis of deoxyribonucleic acid (DNA) and by severing strands of DNA. Instruct the patient taking this drug to notify the doctor immediately if he has difficulty breathing.

Cisplatin. Explain that cisplatin (Platinol) upsets the balance of cell growth by cross-linking strands of DNA, leading to cell death. Because this drug is especially likely to cause nausea and vomiting, remind the patient to take antiemetic medication as ordered. Inform him that before each dose he'll have blood tests to monitor his kidney function. The drug will be stopped if test results show kidney damage. Instruct him to report any unusual bleeding or bruising, hearing loss, tinnitus, and signs of infection.

Etoposide. If the doctor orders etoposide (Vepesid), explain that this drug blocks cell division. Advise the patient to notify the doctor if he becomes light-headed or dizzy while receiving etoposide. Then tell him that his blood pressure will be monitored and that drug therapy will stop if his systolic blood pressure falls below 90 mm Hg. Point out that hair loss is common, but assure him that his hair should grow back after treatments end.

Vinblastine. Teach the patient that vinblastine (Velban) arrests cell mitosis in metaphase, thereby blocking cell division. Tell him that he'll receive an antiemetic before chemotherapy begins. Explain that the antiemetic should reduce nausea and vomiting. Advise him to notify the doctor immediately if tingling or numbness occurs in his hands or feet.

Procedures

If the patient has a seminoma, postoperative treatment typically involves radiation therapy of the abdominal (and possibly mediastinal) areas. Explain that this form of testicular cancer is especially sensitive to radiation. If the patient's cancer has metastasized to the lymphatic system, he may undergo autologous bone marrow transplantation.

Radiation therapy. Explain that bombarding cancer cells with high-level radiation destroys their ability to grow and multiply. Point out that radiation also affects normal cells but that these cells usually recover quickly. Tell the patient that the doctor will minimize damage to normal cells by calculating the most effective overall dose for the patient and then dividing this dose into several individual treatments.

Inform the patient that a simulated treatment session will be performed before radiation therapy to determine the exact location and size of his tumor. Explain that he'll be asked to lie still on a table while an X-ray machine defines the treatment area. Then the area will be outlined with an ink marker. Warn him not to wash off the ink because it's important to treat the same body area each time.

Describe the treatment session. Stress that radiation therapy is painless and won't make the patient radioactive. Reassure him that special lead shields will protect normal body areas and organs from radiation.

Then, outline standard skin care measures to take after radiation therapy. Instruct the patient not to apply soap, deodorant, lotion, perfume, topical medication, or extreme heat or cold to the treatment area, and to avoid rubbing the skin. Suggest that he wear loose, soft clothing and avoid activities that might irritate the area. Advise him to protect the area from direct exposure to the sun, even after radiation therapy's completed, for as long as the doctor recommends.

Autologous bone marrow transplantation. Explain that this procedure involves high-dose chemotherapy coupled with removal

Sex after testicular cancer surgery

After your patient learns he has testicular cancer, he's bound to feel anxious about his future. And he's probably afraid that he'll lose sexual function after surgery (orchiectomy). To overcome his fears, he'll need your support and a clear explanation of how orchiectomy affects sexual activity.

After unilateral orchiectomy
Inform the patient that unilateral orchiectomy doesn't cause sterility or impotence. Most surgeons remove only the testicle, leaving the scrotum. Consequently, a gel-filled prosthesis, which weighs and feels like a normal testicle, can be implanted in the scrotum. Assure the patient that he can resume sexual activity after the incision heals.

After bilateral orchiectomy
Bilateral testicular cancer is uncommon. However, if surgery will affect both testicles, help the patient come to terms with the resultant sterility. Point out that a loss of fertility doesn't equal a loss of masculinity. Reassure him that the doctor will prescribe synthetic hormones to replace or supplement depleted hormone levels.

and treatment of the patient's bone marrow to kill cancer cells. The remaining processed and healthy marrow cells will be reinjected into the patient to reseed the bone marrow.

Surgery
If the patient will undergo orchiectomy, provide information about the operation and instructions for postoperative care. Address his psychological response to the surgery, and encourage him to express his concerns. Above all, reassure him that unilateral orchiectomy isn't synonymous with castration (see *Sex after testicular cancer surgery*).

Describe the operation, explaining that the surgeon will make an inguinal incision to remove the testicle and the entire spermatic cord. (Using this approach, the surgeon minimizes the chances of metastasis associated with surgical trauma.) The surgeon may also remove retroperitoneal lymph nodes or metastases in distant organs. Sometimes, the patient may have chemotherapy or radiation therapy to shrink the tumor before surgery.

Inform the patient that after surgery he'll have a urinary catheter in place. And if the surgeon plans a retroperitoneal lymphadenectomy, the patient will also have a nasogastric tube. Explain that this will prevent abdominal distention. Otherwise, he'll be able to eat and drink normally as soon as his bowel resumes functioning.

To prevent respiratory complications, show the patient how to cough and breathe deeply at least once every hour. Assure him that he'll receive pain medication as necessary. Mention that he may also wear a scrotal supporter to minimize pain and protect the scrotum.

Before the patient goes home, teach him how to clean and dress his incision. Instruct him to notify the doctor immediately if bleeding occurs or if he develops signs of infection, such as drainage from the incision, fever, pain, redness, or swelling. Reinforce your instructions with a copy of the patient-teaching aid *Recovering from testicular surgery,* page 408.

Other care measures

Because testicular self-examination is the best way to detect a new or recurrent tumor, ensure that the patient knows how to perform this procedure. Urge him to examine himself monthly and to report any changes to the doctor at once. As with all cancers, testicular cancer profoundly affects the patient's emotional well-being and life-style. To help him cope effectively, provide him with the names and telephone numbers of organizations that offer information and support both during and after treatment.

Sources of information and support

American Cancer Society
1599 Clifton Road, NE, Atlanta, Ga. 30329
(404) 320-3333, (800) ACS-2345

Cancer Information Service
c/o National Cancer Institute
NIH Building 31, Room 10A24, Bethesda, Md. 20892
(800) 4-CANCER

Further readings

Barrett, A., and Adams, A. "A Shoulder to Lean On...Canshare...Service for Other Cancer Sufferers," *Nursing Times* 84(39):56-57, September 28-October 4, 1988.

Bell, I. "Testicular Self-examination," *Nursing Times* 86(9):38-40, February 28-March 6, 1990.

Blackmore, C. "The Impact of Orchidectomy upon the Sexuality of the Man with Testicular Cancer," *Cancer Nursing* 11(1):33-40, February 1988.

Faulkenberry, J.E. "Cancer in Men: A Case for Cancer Prevention and Early Detection," *Dimensions of Oncology Nursing* 2(2):17-21, Summer 1988.

Higgs, D.J. "The Patient with Testicular Cancer: Nursing Management of Chemotherapy," *Oncology Nursing Forum* 17(2):243-49, March-April 1990.

Horwich, A. "Testicular Cancer," *Occupational Health* (London) 41(11):326-27, November 1989.

Lasater, S.J. "Testicular Cancer: A Perioperative Challenge," *Association of Operating Room Nurses Journal* 51(2):513, 515-19, 522-23 +, February 1990.

Martin, J.P. "Male Cancer Awareness: Impact of an Employee Education Program," *Oncology Nursing Forum* 17(1):59-64, January-February 1990.

Reno, D.R. "Men's Knowledge and Health Beliefs about Testicular Cancer and Testicular Self-examination," *Cancer Nursing* 11(2):112-17, April 1988.

Rose, M.A. "Health Promotion and Risk Prevention: Applications for Cancer Survivors," *Oncology Nursing Forum* 16(3):335-40, May-June 1989.

Walker, R., et al. "Modeling and Guided Practice as Components Within a Comprehensive Testicular Self-examination Cancer Education Program," *Journal of the American College of Health* 37(5):211-15, March 1989.

Walters, P. "Chemo: A Nurse's Guide to Action, Administration, and Side Effects," *RN* 53(2):52-67, February 1990.

Wilkie, D.J. "Cancer Pain Management: State-of-the-Art Nursing Care," *Nursing Clinics of North America* 25(2):331-43, June 1990.

Recovering from testicular surgery

Dear Patient:

As with most operations, you'll need a few weeks to recover completely from testicular surgery. During this time, follow these guidelines to minimize your discomfort and speed recuperation.

Care for your incision properly

Before you leave the hospital, the nurse will show you how to clean the incisional area and change the dressing. When you go home, refer to the following instructions:

• Keep the incision dry at all times. Change the dressing if it gets wet during bathing or feels damp from perspiration.
• Never reuse cotton-tipped swabs or gauze pads. Discard them after you've changed the dressing.
• If your skin becomes irritated from the adhesive tape, consult the nurse or doctor. They may recommend substituting a protective dressing or using a protective wipe or spray to create a barrier between your skin and the adhesive.
• Call the doctor or nurse at once if the incision opens or bleeds heavily.

Recognize and report infection

Take your temperature three times a day—in the morning, late in the afternoon, and before going to bed. Report a fever above 100.5° F. (38° C.) immediately. Also notify the doctor at once if you have chills, if you notice drainage from the incision, or if your incision becomes painful, red, or swollen.

Special instructions

Wear a scrotal supporter to reduce pain and to protect the scrotum.

Avoid strenuous physical activity until your incision's completely healed. You don't need to stay in bed, however. Walking is a safe way to exercise without overdoing.

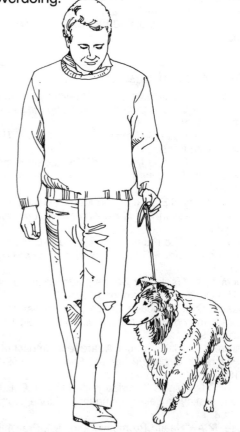

Eat properly and drink plenty of fluids. If you have less of an appetite than usual, try eating small, frequent meals instead of three large meals.

Call the doctor if you still have pain more than 10 days after surgery.

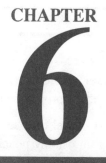

CHAPTER

6

Gastrointestinal Conditions

Contents

Irritable bowel syndrome

To teach your patient how to control this functional syndrome, you'll need to consider his emotional state. Often characterized as tense, rigid, and dependent, the patient commonly experiences irritable bowel syndrome as a reaction to stress. Consequently, he may have trouble changing ingrained responses so that he can relieve the syndrome's symptoms. You'll need to adapt your teaching methods to his personality traits and enlist his cooperation before you can teach about drug therapy or dietary changes to reduce discomfort and life-style changes to reduce stress.

Another challenge will be to counter the patient's confusion and frustration with symptoms that have no organic cause and with treatment that doesn't produce a cure. You'll need to emphasize the positive, helping him learn to cooperate with diagnostic evaluation of his symptoms and to trust the treatment regimen so that he can control his condition—and not let it control him.

Discuss the disorder

Inform the patient that irritable bowel syndrome, also called spastic or irritable colon, is usually chronic and marked by relapses and remissions. In this syndrome, the intestine functions abnormally, producing chronic, excessive spasms.

Tell the patient that normal intestinal contractions and relaxation advance intestinal contents (stool) smoothly and regularly. With irritable bowel syndrome, however, regular motility is impaired. Explain that constipation results from hypomotility. The stool remains in the intestine, where excessive water is absorbed; this delay in movement causes the stool to dry and harden, making passage difficult. Conversely, diarrhea results from hypermotility, when contractions force stool through the intestine so rapidly that too little water is absorbed for the stool to form (see *Understanding irritable bowel syndrome,* page 412). Explain that these abnormal contractions, or spasms, cause cramping and discomfort.

Tell the patient that the exact cause of irritable bowel syndrome remains unknown, but that contributing or aggravating factors include anxiety and stress, diet (including highly seasoned, cold, or laxative foods, fiber, fruits, and alcohol), hormones, laxative abuse, and allergy to certain foods, beverages, and drugs. Initial episodes usually occur early in life; anxiety or stress probably causes most exacerbations (see *Irritable bowel syndrome: The psychological link,* page 413).

Catherine Foran, RN, MSN, and **Nancy Baptie Walrath, RN, BSN, CGC,** wrote this chapter. Ms. Foran, an independent consultant, lives in Cherry Hill, N.J. Ms. Walrath is director of the gastroenterology department at Daniel Freeman Memorial and Marina Hospitals, Inglewood, Calif.

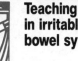

CHECKLIST

Teaching topics in irritable bowel syndrome

☐ Explanation of the disorder and causes of exacerbations
☐ Preparation for tests, such as barium enema and proctosigmoidoscopy, to rule out other disorders
☐ Dietary measures to prevent pain, bloating, constipation, and diarrhea
☐ Drug therapy, including antispasmodics, laxatives, antidiarrheals, and tranquilizers
☐ Other care measures: stress management, cessation of smoking, and a regular bowel routine

Understanding irritable bowel syndrome

Although a patient with irritable bowel syndrome has a normal-appearing GI tract, careful colon examination may reveal functional irritability—an abnormality in colonic smooth muscle function marked by excessive peristalsis and spasms, even during remission.

Intestinal function
Inform the patient that normally, segmental muscle contractions mix intestinal contents while peristalsis propels the contents through the GI tract. Motor activity is most propulsive in the proximal (stomach) and distal (sigmoid) portions of the intestine; activity in the rest of the intestines is slower, permitting nutrient and water absorption.

In irritable bowel syndrome, however, the autonomic nervous system, which innervates the large intestine, fails to produce the alternating contractions and relaxations that propel stool smoothly toward the rectum. This can produce constipation or diarrhea, or both.

Constipation
Some patients have spasmodic intestinal contractions, which sets up a partial obstruction by trapping gas and stool. This causes distention, bloating, gas pain, and constipation.

Diarrhea
Other patients have dramatically increased intestinal motility. Usually triggered by eating or by cholinergic stimulation, the small intestine's contents speed into the large intestine, dumping watery stool and causing mucosal irritation, which results in diarrhea.

Mixed symptoms
If further spasms trap some liquid stool, the intestinal mucosa absorbs water from it, leaving it dry, hard, and difficult to pass. The result: a pattern of alternating diarrhea and constipation.

Complications
Caution the patient that he'll probably experience recurring bouts of irritable bowel syndrome if he doesn't follow prescribed treatment. But assure him that despite being chronic, irritable bowel syndrome doesn't progress to other disorders or affect his life span. Nor is there any evidence linking it to cancer (although constipation may result from a low-fiber diet, which *is* associated with colon cancer and diverticular disease).

Because the patient usually has a history of GI problems, instruct him to note and report any changes, including new or acute symptoms, unexplained weight loss, and hematochezia.

Describe the diagnostic workup
Inform the patient that tests can't specifically diagnose irritable bowel syndrome, but they can rule out other disorders. For example, a stool culture can identify harmful microorganisms. A barium enema study detects intestinal spasms and can rule out inflammatory bowel disease, diverticula, tumors, and polyps. Colonoscopy and proctosigmoidoscopy detect and evaluate lower GI tract inflammation and abnormalities. An upper GI and small-bowel series helps detect motility disorders, abnormal structures, esophageal reflux, pylorospasm, gastric retention, decreased gastric emptying, and small-bowel spasm.

Stool culture
Tell the patient that he'll provide a stool specimen for laboratory analysis. To ensure the best results, instruct him to follow a high-fiber diet and to avoid red meats, poultry, fish, turnips, and horseradish for 48 hours before the collection period and during it. As ordered, instruct him to stop taking medications for this period.

Barium enema study
Explain that this radiologic study uses barium, and sometimes air, to examine the large intestine. The test takes 30 to 45 minutes.

Explain that food or fluid in the GI tract prevents a clear outline of the lower GI tract, so pretest procedures focus on completely cleansing the intestine. Advise the patient to follow a low-residue diet for 1 to 3 days before the test and then a clear-liquid diet for 24 hours before the test. To further cleanse the intestine, the patient will receive a laxative the afternoon before the test and cleansing enemas the evening before or the morning of the test. Or the doctor may order a saline lavage (see *Preparing for saline lavage,* page 414).

Inform the patient that during the test, he'll be secured to a tiltable table and the doctor will take an X-ray of the large intestine to make sure it's empty. Then the patient will lie on his left side while the doctor inserts a small, lubricated tube into his rectum. Once the tube's inserted, the barium slowly fills the bowel while X-rays are being taken. Instruct the patient to keep his anal sphincter tightly contracted against the tube to hold it in position and prevent barium leakage. Stress the importance of retaining the barium because accurate test results depend on adequately coating the large intestine. (Assure him that the barium is easy to retain because it's cool.)

If the doctor also instills air through the tube, tell the patient that the table may be tilted and he'll be assisted into various positions to aid filling. Inform him that if he feels cramps or the urge to move his bowels as the barium or air fills the large intestine, he should breathe slowly and deeply through his mouth to ease the discomfort.

Tell the patient that after the test, he can expel the barium into a bedpan or toilet. Then he'll receive another laxative and an enema to flush any remaining barium from the intestine because barium may harden, causing intestinal obstruction or impaction. Remember to describe how barium makes the stool light in color for 1 to 3 days after the test. Inform the patient that he may resume eating and taking medications, as ordered. Encourage fluid intake to prevent dehydration from bowel preparation and the test. Also, encourage rest because the test is tiring.

Colonoscopy and proctosigmoidoscopy
Explain that these tests allow the doctor to see inside the lower GI tract with an endoscope, a flexible fiber-optic tube inserted into the rectum. The tests take about 30 minutes.

Tell the patient to maintain a clear-liquid diet for up to 48 hours before the test and, as ordered, to fast on the test morning. Advise him, however, to continue his drug regimen, as appropriate. Explain that dietary restrictions and intestinal preparation are essential to clear the lower GI tract for an unobstructed view, so he'll take a laxative the afternoon before the test.

During the test, the patient will lie on an X-ray table as a nurse takes his vital signs. Mention that because the test is uncomfortable, an I.V. line will be inserted into his hand or arm to administer a sedative to help him relax. (If he's having proctosigmoidoscopy or flexible sigmoidoscopy, he probably won't receive I.V. sedation or extensive intestinal preparation.)

Then the doctor will insert a flexible tube into the patient's rectum. Tell the patient that he may feel some lower abdominal discomfort and the urge to move his bowels as the tube advances. To control the urge to defecate and ease the discomfort, instruct him to breathe deeply and slowly through his mouth. Explain that air may be introduced into the intestines through the tube. If he feels the urge to expel some air, tell him not to try to control it. Also tell him that he may hear and feel a suction machine removing any matter that may obscure the doctor's view, but it won't cause any pain.

Inform him that after the test his vital signs will be checked frequently for 8 hours. He can eat after recovering from the sedative, in about 1 hour. If air was introduced into the intestine, he may pass large amounts of gas. Instruct him to report any blood in his stool.

Upper GI and small-bowel series
Instruct the patient to maintain a low-residue diet for 2 to 3 days before the test. Besides discontinuing any medications that retard motility, such as anticholinergics and narcotics (and antacids, if ordered), the day before the test, he'll have to fast and stop smok-

---

Irritable bowel syndrome: The psychological link

To help you individualize your teaching, keep in mind the psychological factors that may be associated with irritable bowel syndrome.

A history of complaints
Some patients' complaints of intestinal problems may be learned behaviors that typically date from childhood. These behaviors commonly result in secondary gain. For example, some people learn that complaints of feeling ill help them get their own way. This reinforces the illness behavior.

If your patient's history reveals this kind of pattern, help him understand that changes in behavior may lead to fewer symptoms.

Avoid stereotyping
Although irritable bowel syndrome is typically associated with stress, you shouldn't automatically label the patient as neurotic and minimize his symptoms. The patient doesn't have to be neurotic, nor does every neurotic patient suffer irritable bowel syndrome.

Is there a correlation?
Studies suggest that sadness and anxiety may lead to diarrhea in irritable bowel syndrome and that angry confrontation may lead to constipation.

However, no findings show a correlation between specific psychological features and severity or chronicity of symptoms.

Keep in mind, too, that the patient's degree of stress and severity of symptoms don't always correlate with irritable bowel syndrome. That is, stressful periods don't always precede symptoms, and tranquil periods aren't always symptom-free.

Preparing for saline lavage

If the doctor orders a saline lavage before a colon examination, help your patient understand that despite its unpleasantness, this bowel preparation effectively removes matter that could obstruct a view of the colon and confuse examination findings.

Tell the patient that he'll drink about 4 liters of a salty solution over a 4-hour period. Inform him that he'll have diarrhea at first. Then, when the colon is clear, he'll eliminate only clear effluent.

Confirm that the salty solution can't be mixed with any other substance or flavoring, but it may be chilled to improve palatability. Emphasize that he'll have to drink the full amount for the preparation to be effective.

Reassure the patient (particularly if he has a cardiac condition) that the intestine doesn't absorb the salt, nor does the preparation cause fluid overload.

If an elderly or debilitated patient has difficulty with the procedure, notify the doctor immediately so that he can provide an alternative preparation.

ing after midnight before the test day. Tell him that he'll receive a cleansing laxative and enema before the test. Suggest that he bring reading material because the test takes up to 6 hours.

Tell the patient that when the test begins, he'll be secured to a tiltable X-ray table. During the test, he'll drink 16 to 20 oz (480 to 600 ml) of a chalky but flavored, milk-shake–thick barium mixture. Then, besides being tilted and turned, positioned and repositioned, he may feel the doctor compressing his abdomen to make sure the mixture thoroughly coats the upper GI tract. He'll hear the X-ray machine clack as it films the structures outlined by the barium mixture.

Assure the patient that he can resume his diet and medications after the test, unless the doctor plans follow-up X-rays. Also tell him that the barium will be flushed from his system by a laxative or an enema. Encourage him to drink lots of fluids, and tell him to expect light-colored stools for 1 to 3 days. Also encourage rest because the test may leave him feeling exhausted.

Teach about treatments
Explain that long-term treatment consists of dietary management. Drug therapy is reserved for severe symptoms and is discontinued as patients make dietary and life-style changes and learn to manage stress.

Diet
Emphasize the positive gains associated with a diet planned to prevent or relieve irritable bowel syndrome: a decrease in the patient's pain, constipation, and diarrhea (see *Managing irritable bowel syndrome with diet*). Then suggest ways to implement the dietary plan.

Establish a schedule. Explain that the GI tract works best on a schedule. And eating three meals daily of about the same volume, and at about the same time, and avoiding between-meal or late-night snacks promote regularity. Advise the patient to eat slowly and carefully to prevent swallowing air and consequent bloating.

Keep a diary. Suggest that the patient keep a daily record of food intake and symptoms. What foods appear to trigger symptoms? Advise him first to note them. Then he can proceed to eliminate them one at a time, thereby discovering which symptoms occur with certain foods. Note that a lactase deficiency can cause symptoms similar to irritable bowel syndrome. If his meals exclude milk products, remind him to include other calcium-rich foods, such as green, leafy vegetables, canned salmon or sardines, and tofu.

Add dietary fiber. Explain that increasing dietary fiber can help relieve both diarrhea and constipation by adding essential soft bulk to stools. Inform the patient that constipation is controlled better by dietary fiber than by laxatives. Identify sources of dietary bulk, such as bran and other whole-grain cereals, fresh fruit, and vegetables. Then propose ways to incorporate fiber into meals. Remind the patient to start a high-fiber diet gradually be-

Managing irritable bowel syndrome with diet

Advise the patient to follow the dietary recommendations listed below to help relieve symptoms of irritable bowel syndrome.

Upper GI symptoms: Pain, reflux, and esophagitis
Instruct the patient to follow a low-fat diet. Explain that fats decrease lower esophageal sphincter pressure. So does alcohol. This permits gastric reflux.

Tell the patient to avoid substances that irritate gastric and esophageal mucosa, including alcohol, caffeinated beverages, chocolate, peppermint, tomatoes, and orange juice.

Diarrhea
Instruct the patient to eliminate, one by one, citrus fruits, coffee, corn, dairy products, tea, and wheat. This will help him to determine if his symptoms result from food intolerance. Caffeine, for instance, may disrupt GI motility.

Warn the patient to avoid sorbitol, an artificial sweetener that may cause diarrhea. Advise him to consume more products that contain bran. Explain

that adding dietary bulk increases the time the stool remains in the bowel, allowing time for stool to form.

Abdominal distention and bloating
Tell the patient to avoid lactose- and sorbitol-containing foods and nonabsorbable carbohydrates, such as beans and cabbage. Explain that these products increase flatulence. For instance, deficiency of the digestive enzyme lactase prevents the body from digesting lactose-containing foods. Unabsorbed lactose causes excessive hydrogen and other gases.

Constipation and abdominal pain
Advise the patient to increase dietary bulk by 15 to 20 g daily, using such sources as wheat bran, oatmeal, oat bran, rye cereals, prunes, dried apricots, and figs. Inform him that the added bulk provided by fiber increases stool weight and may minimize the effect of nonpropulsive colonic contractions that may trap stool or retard its passage, causing abdominal pain. Unless contraindicated, tell him to drink eight glasses of water daily.

---

cause additional fiber may increase bloating and gas. If he can't tolerate bran or other fibrous foods, suggest using stool-bulking agents that contain psyllium, such as Metamucil and Hydrocil.

Balance fluids. Caution the patient to avoid fluids associated with GI discomfort, including carbonated and caffeinated beverages, fruit juice, and alcohol. But advise him to drink 8 to 10 glasses of compatible fluids daily to help regulate the consistency of his stools and promote balanced hydration.

Medication
Inform the patient that drugs are prescribed only to relieve severe symptoms. Anticholinergic, antispasmodic drugs, such as propantheline bromide, may be used to reduce intestinal hypermotility (see *Learning about propantheline bromide,* page 420); antidiarrheal agents and laxatives may be tried as well (see *Teaching patients about drugs for irritable bowel syndrome,* pages 416 and 417). Other possible medication choices include antacids, antiemetics, simethicone, and, occasionally, tranquilizers or antidepressants. Advise your patient always to consult his doctor before treating constipation or diarrhea with over-the-counter medications because many irritate the bowel.

Antacids. In some patients, decreased lower esophageal sphincter pressure may cause reflux of acidic gastric contents onto the esophageal mucosa. If the patient has such dyspeptic symptoms, suggesting involvement of the proximal GI tract, the doctor may advise magnesium-containing antacids (Maalox, Mylanta, Riopan) to help relieve heartburn and acid stomach.

continued on page 418

Teaching patients about drugs for irritable bowel syndrome

DRUG	ADVERSE REACTIONS	TEACHING POINTS
Antispasmodics		
atropine sulfate	• Watch for blurred vision, confusion, dizziness, dyspnea, eye pain, flushing, rash, seizures, tachycardia, unusual fatigue, or weakness. • Other reactions include constipation; decreased sweating; drowsiness; dry mouth, nose, and throat; dysuria; headache; nausea; photophobia; and vomiting.	• Inform the patient that this anticholinergic drug helps relieve stomach cramps and intestinal spasms. • Instruct him to separate doses of atropine from doses of antacids and kaolin- or pectin-containing antidiarrheals. Otherwise, atropine's effectiveness will be diminished. • Tell him to take the drug 30 to 60 minutes before meals, as ordered. • Warn against using alcohol and other CNS depressants when taking atropine because of the heightened risk of adverse reactions. • If he misses a dose, instruct him to take the missed dose as soon as possible. However, if it's almost time for his next dose, he should wait. Tell him never to double the dose. • Advise him to take precautions to avoid heatstroke from hot weather or strenuous exercise because atropine reduces sweating, allowing body temperature to rise. • Explain that atropine may cause photophobia. Suggest wearing sunglasses. • Caution him to ensure that his vision isn't blurred before driving or performing activities that require clear vision. • Suggest using ice chips to relieve dry mouth.
dicyclomine hydrochloride (Bentyl, Dilomine) **methantheline bromide** (Banthine) **propantheline bromide** (Pro-Banthine)	• Watch for constipation, difficult urination, eye pain, rash, and tachycardia. • Other reactions include confusion, decreased sweating, dizziness, drowsiness, dry mouth, fatigue, headache, nausea, photophobia, and vomiting.	• Explain to the patient that this anticholinergic drug relieves stomach cramps, intestinal spasms, and acid stomach. • Advise him that antacids and kaolin- or pectin-containing antidiarrheals may diminish this drug's effectiveness. He should separate doses by at least 1 hour. • Tell him to take the drug 30 to 60 minutes before meals, as ordered. • Advise him to avoid alcohol and other CNS depressants when taking this drug because of the heightened risk of adverse reactions. • If he misses a dose, instruct him to skip the missed dose and resume his schedule. He must never double the dose. • If this drug makes him feel drowsy, caution him to avoid driving, operating machinery, or performing other activities that require alertness. • Explain that this drug may cause photophobia. Suggest wearing sunglasses. • Explain that this drug often reduces sweating, allowing body temperature to rise. To prevent heatstroke, caution the patient to avoid becoming overheated during exercise or hot weather. • Suggest using ice chips to relieve dry mouth.
Antidiarrheals		
difenoxin with atropine sulfate (Motofen) **diphenoxylate hydrochloride with atropine sulfate** (Lomotil)	• Watch for anorexia, bloating, constipation, eye pain, nausea, shortness of breath, stomach pain, tachycardia, and vomiting. • Other reactions include blurred vision, depression, dizziness, drowsiness, dry mouth, dysuria, fever, flushing, headache, and rash.	• Tell the patient to avoid alcohol and cold, allergy, and sleep medications because of the increased risk of adverse reactions. • Explain that this drug controls severe diarrhea by relaxing the intestinal muscles. • If the patient misses a dose and still has diarrhea, instruct him to take the missed dose as soon as possible. Tell him to take any remaining doses for that day at evenly spaced intervals. If he misses a dose and his diarrhea has stopped, tell him to skip the missed dose and to take the next dose on schedule. • Advise him to contact the doctor if he discontinues the drug and then experiences increased sweating, muscle cramps, nausea or vomiting, shivering or trembling, or stomach cramps.
kaolin and pectin (Kaopectate)	• Watch for mild constipation.	• Advise the patient to take doses of this antidiarrheal drug separately from doses of prescription drugs to prevent interactions. • Tell him to shake this liquid drug well before pouring a dose. • Instruct him to take the drug after a loose bowel movement. He doesn't need a regular dosage schedule, but he should consult the doctor for dose-interval instructions. • Advise him to consult the doctor if diarrhea doesn't stop in 1 to 2 days.

continued

Teaching patients about drugs for irritable bowel syndrome — *continued*

DRUG	ADVERSE REACTIONS	TEACHING POINTS
Antidiarrheals — *continued*		
loperamide (Imodium, Imodium A-D)	• Reactions include anorexia, bloating, constipation, dizziness, drowsiness, dry mouth, fever, nausea, rash, stomach cramps, and vomiting.	• Explain that this antidiarrheal drug helps control severe diarrhea by decreasing intestinal motility. • If the patient misses a dose, instruct him to skip the missed dose and to take the next dose on schedule. He must never double the dose. • If this drug makes him feel drowsy, caution him to avoid driving, operating machinery, or performing other activities that require alertness. • Suggest using ice chips to relieve dry mouth.
paregoric	• Watch for abdominal pain, anorexia, constipation, depression, hypertension, nausea, rash, and vomiting. • Other reactions include dizziness, drowsiness, dysuria, increased sweating, and oliguria.	• Explain to the patient that this drug helps control severe diarrhea. • Instruct him to take the drug only as directed; it may become habit-forming. • Advise him to rise slowly from a sitting or lying position to minimize possible dizziness. • If he misses a dose, he should take the missed dose as soon as possible. However, if it's almost time for his next dose, he should wait for the next dose and return to his schedule. Warn him never to double the dose. • Warn him not to drive or operate machinery if the drug makes him drowsy.
Laxatives		
docusate sodium (Colace)	• Possible reactions include bitter taste, diarrhea, mild abdominal cramps, rash, and throat irritation.	• Explain to the patient that this stool-softening laxative allows him to have a bowel movement without straining. The drug helps liquids mix with the stool and form a softer mass. • Inform him that this drug could lose its effectiveness with long-term or excessive use. • Advise him to notify the doctor or pharmacist if the drug fails to relieve his symptoms. • Instruct him to dilute the liquid (but not syrup) dose in juice or another flavored liquid to improve the taste. • If the patient is on a sodium-restricted diet, suggest that he ask his doctor for another stool softener.
lactulose (Cephulac, Chronulac)	• Watch for severe abdominal pain. • Other reactions include abdominal cramping, belching, diarrhea, flatulence, and gaseous distention.	• Reassure the patient that this laxative isn't irritating. • Advise him to drink 8 to 10 glasses of fluid daily. • Suggest that he minimize the drug's sweet taste by diluting it with water or fruit juice or taking it with food.
methylcellulose (Citrucel, Cologel) **psyllium** (Hydrocil Instant, Metamucil)	• Watch for breathing difficulty, diarrhea, itching, nausea or vomiting, rash, and swallowing difficulty.	• Inform the patient that bulk-forming laxatives help relieve constipation or create a formed stool. • Advise him to contact the doctor if he hasn't had a bowel movement after taking the medication for the prescribed time. • Caution against overuse of laxatives. • Instruct him to take tablets with a full glass of water and not to chew them. This prevents the drug from swelling in the esophagus and causing obstruction. • Teach him to mix the powdered form with a full glass of water, milk, fruit juice, or other liquid and to drink it immediately. • Advise him to drink eight glasses of water a day to help prevent impaction. • Inform him that the drug may begin working in 12 hours, but its effects may be delayed for up to 3 days.

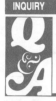

Questions patients ask about irritable bowel syndrome

Why do I have stomach cramps and diarrhea whenever I have too much to do and too little time?

Your body may be reacting to stress. Most people agree that trying to do too many things at one time creates a hectic, stressful atmosphere. In turn, this can overstimulate your nervous system—including the part that controls the bowel—producing cramps and diarrhea.

Try to anticipate stress-filled times. Then find ways to complete tasks ahead of time, or ask your family or friends to help out.

Reduce stress in your life by learning to relax and getting sufficient rest and exercise. Your nurse and doctor can help you learn how.

Besides learning to deal with stress, what else can I do to relieve my symptoms?

Because your symptoms may be linked to diet as well as stress, you'll need to monitor your eating habits. Add more fiber to your diet, and exclude fats and sugar. While no magic cures exist, carefully following your treatment plan is a good bet for controlling your symptoms.

Will I have these symptoms for life, or will I outgrow them?

No one can predict how long your symptoms will last because no one knows why they occur. Although you probably won't outgrow irritable bowel syndrome, you can look forward to periods of remission.

Instruct the patient to watch for anorexia, dizziness, dysuria, headache, irregular heart rate, mood changes, and weakness. Other adverse reactions include diarrhea, nausea, stomach cramps, or vomiting.

Tell the patient to take antacids 1 to 3 hours after meals and at bedtime but not within 2 hours of taking other medications. Advise him to chew the tablet well before swallowing and to follow the dose with a full glass of water. Remind him to shake the liquid form well before pouring. Suggest mixing the tablet and liquid forms with fluids or food if preferred. Instruct him never to double the dose, but to take a missed dose as soon as possible and then resume his schedule. Advise him to consult his doctor before changing his medication regimen. If he experiences diarrhea, the doctor may prescribe an alternate antacid, combination therapy, or a stool softener.

Antiemetics. The doctor may suggest an antiemetic, such as metoclopramide (Reglan), to relieve heartburn, epigastric discomfort, and after-meal fullness. This drug increases upper GI motility, which aids in esophageal clearance and gastric emptying. Instruct the patient to watch for confusion, muscle spasms, severe drowsiness, shuffling, tics, and trembling hands. Mention that other adverse reactions include constipation, depression, diarrhea, dizziness, dry mouth, headache, insomnia, menstrual changes, rash, and unusual tiredness or weakness.

Tell the patient to avoid alcohol and cold, allergy, and sleep medications, which may increase adverse reactions. Explain that for best absorption, he should take this drug 30 minutes before meals. Instruct him to make up a missed dose as soon as possible but not to double the dose. If the drug causes drowsiness, caution him to avoid driving, operating machinery, or performing other activities that require alertness.

Simethicone. Another drug, simethicone (Mylicon, Phazyme), may be used to relieve belching and bloating from gas in the stomach and intestines. For best results, advise the patient to take the drug after meals and at bedtime, as ordered. If he's taking tablets, instruct him to chew them thoroughly.

Tranquilizers. Usually prescribed only for a short term, mild tranquilizers, such as diazepam, may relieve some of the psychological stress associated with irritable bowel syndrome. Instruct the patient that these drugs can cause abdominal discomfort, blurred vision, clumsiness, drowsiness, hangover, lethargy, nausea, rash, slurred speech, tremors, and vomiting. They can also cause breathing difficulties, fainting, slow heartbeat, and transient low blood pressure.

If the patient also takes cimetidine (Tagamet), he may feel even drowsier. As a result, he should avoid activities that require alertness. Caution him that tranquilizers may become habit-forming.

Tricyclic antidepressants. Because depression may result from irritable bowel syndrome or be part of a neurotic syndrome that exacerbates it, the doctor may temporarily prescribe a tricyclic antidepressant, such as amitriptyline. Instruct the patient to watch for anorexia, constipation, dry mouth, nausea, rash, sweating, tachycardia, urination difficulties, and vomiting. Also, he should report confusion, dizziness, drowsiness, excitation, headaches, nervousness, tremors, and weakness.

Explain that using these drugs with barbiturates diminishes their effectiveness. Using them with central nervous system (CNS) stimulants may increase adverse effects. And warn the patient against drinking alcoholic beverages or using other CNS depressants while taking a tricyclic antidepressant.

Advise the patient to take his dose at bedtime, to increase fluid intake, and not to take other medications or over-the-counter drugs before consulting the doctor or pharmacist. Inform him that some of these drugs may slow intestinal motility and worsen constipation. Remind him to follow his diet and drink additional fluids.

Other care measures

Teach the patient that effective treatment may require life-style alterations that emphasize control of emotional tension. Be sure to help him set priorities by pinpointing the activities he enjoys, scheduling more time for rest and relaxation, and, if possible, delegating responsibilities to other family members. If appropriate, encourage him to seek professional counseling for stress management.

Remind the patient that regular physical exercise helps eliminate anxiety and promotes good bowel function. Discourage smoking because it contributes to altered bowel motility. Also help him establish a regular bowel routine.

Stress the need for regular physical examinations. For patients over age 40, emphasize the need for colorectal cancer screening, including annual proctosigmoidoscopy and rectal examinations.

Sources of information and support

Digestive Disease National Coalition
511 Capitol Court, NE, Suite 300, Washington, D.C. 20002
(202) 544-7497

National Digestive Diseases Information Clearinghouse
Box NDDIC, Bethesda, Md. 20892
(301) 468-6344

Further readings

Cerrato, P.L. "A Dietary Remedy for Irritable Bowel Syndrome," *RN* 50(7):65-66, July 1987.

Creed, F., and Guthrie, E. "Psychological Factors in the Irritable Bowel Syndrome," *Gut* 28(10):1307-18, October 1987.

Drossman, D.A. "Irritable Bowel Syndrome: A Multifactorial Disorder," *Hospital Practice* 23(9):119-33, September 15, 1988.

Klein, K.B. "Controlled Treatment Trials in the Irritable Bowel Syndrome: A Critique," *Gastroenterology* 95(1):232-41, July 1988.

Whitehead, W.E., et al. "Symptoms of Psychologic Distress Associated with Irritable Bowel Syndrome: Comparison of Community and Medical Clinic Samples," *Gastroenterology* 95(3):709-14, September 1988.

Learning about propantheline bromide

Dear Patient:

Your doctor has prescribed propantheline bromide (the label may also read Pro-Banthine) to help relieve stomach cramps, spasms, and acid stomach.

Take this medication exactly as the label directs. Take it 30 to 60 minutes before meals. And take your bedtime dose at least 2 hours after your dinner meal. Swallow the tablets whole; don't chew or crush them.

If you forget to take a dose, don't make it up. Just start your schedule all over again with the next dose. *Never* take a double dose.

Report side effects
Call your doctor if you develop difficulty with urinating or swallowing, dizziness, drowsiness, eye pain, headaches, nervousness, rapid heartbeat or palpitations, or rash. Also call him if you have constipation, decreased sweating, heartburn, nausea, or vomiting, or if your eyes are unusually sensitive to strong light.

Watch what you eat and drink
When you're taking this drug, avoid eating spicy or acidic foods. These can upset your stomach. Also avoid alcoholic beverages, but be sure to drink plenty of other fluids.

Be cautious about other drugs
Before you take any other drugs, consult your pharmacist or doctor. And make sure your pharmacist and doctor know all the drugs you're taking (especially if you have more than one pharmacist or doctor).

Special instructions
• Don't drive, operate machinery, or take part in activities that require alertness if the drug makes you feel drowsy.
• Your body sweats less while you're taking this drug. To avoid heatstroke, don't exercise too strenuously or stay outside too long in hot weather.
• If your eyes seem really sensitive to sunlight, protect them by wearing sunglasses or a brimmed hat.

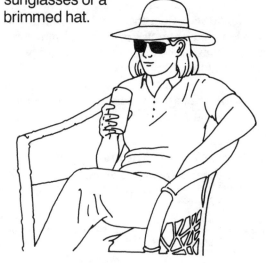

A few reminders
• Store your medication in a cool, dry place.
• Don't let anyone else take your medication. It's intended for your special needs.
• Throw away any propantheline bromide that's unused or several years old.

Inflammatory bowel disease

Whether your patient has ulcerative colitis or Crohn's disease, you'll be challenged to teach him to cope with a chronic disease. Your teaching will also be challenging because most patients are apprehensive about the tests that diagnose and follow these diseases and about the surgery that may be necessary.

Nevertheless, you'll need to prepare the patient for diagnostic tests to help reduce his anxiety and encourage compliance. You'll also need to encourage him to rest during attacks and explain dietary measures that may help diminish his symptoms. What's more, you'll need to teach him about analgesic and anti-inflammatory medications. If surgery is necessary, you may need to provide stoma care directions for an ostomy.

Although interruption of daily activities and possible lifestyle changes may frustrate the patient, emphasize that he can lead a normal life, even after an ostomy. (See *Teaching the patient with progressive inflammatory bowel disease*, page 422.)

Discuss the disorder

Inform the patient that inflammatory bowel disease involves chronic inflammation of the GI tract lining. Explain that this disease has two forms: ulcerative colitis and Crohn's disease (see *Comparing ulcerative colitis and Crohn's disease,* page 423).

Explain that the cause of inflammatory bowel disease is unknown. It may result from an abnormal immune response to bacterial or viral infection (see *What causes inflammatory bowel disease?* page 424). Mention that recent studies refute a psychosomatic origin for inflammatory bowel disease.

Tell the patient with *ulcerative colitis* that inflammation affects the mucosal and submucosal lining of the large bowel and rectum. The disease usually starts in the rectum and spreads upward to involve the colon. It causes an inflamed mucosa, congestion, edema, and small lacerations that ooze blood and eventually develop into abscesses, which may become necrotic and ulcerate.

Inform the patient with *Crohn's disease* that inflammation most commonly affects the terminal ileum but may affect any segment of the GI tract (from mouth to anus). Explain that this disease involves all layers of the bowel wall. Lymphocytes collect throughout the mucosa, submucosa, and serosa. Fissures and ulcerations with granulomas develop in the mucosa, causing ab-

Beverly Folkedahl, RN, BSN, CETN, and **Catherine Foran, RN, MSN,** contributed to this chapter. Ms. Folkedahl is a clinical nursing specialist at the University of Iowa Hospitals and Clinics, Iowa City. Ms. Foran is an independent nursing consultant in Cherry Hill, NJ.

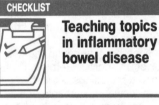

CHECKLIST

Teaching topics in inflammatory bowel disease

☐ Explanation of the type of inflammatory bowel disease: ulcerative colitis or Crohn's disease

☐ Complications, such as nutritional deficiences, anemia, dehydration, and stricture or obstruction

☐ Preparation for diagnostic tests, including barium enema, endoscopy, and other GI studies

☐ Diet, including increased protein, calories, and vitamins

☐ Analgesic and anti-inflammatory drugs

☐ Explanation of surgical procedures, such as colostomy, ileostomy, continent ileostomy, and ileoanal reservoir

☐ Post-ileostomy self-care and life-style alterations, if appropriate

☐ Identification of warning signs of complications

☐ Sources of information and support

Teaching the patient with progressive inflammatory bowel disease

Understandably, the patient with progressive inflammatory bowel disease may be frightened of surgery and the possibility of living with an ostomy. How can you calm your patient's fears yet be certain she understands her treatment options? And how can you help her accept necessary life-style changes?

You can begin by referring to a standard teaching plan to guide your teaching. But you'll also need to customize this standard plan to fit your patient's special needs. Here's how you can do this.

Reviewing the patient's history
Let's say you're caring for Sylvia Levy, a 32-year-old biology teacher and mother of two young children. She was hospitalized several days ago with abdominal pain, 12 to 15 bloody stools daily, anemia, and dehydration. Reviewing her history, you learn that she was diagnosed as having ulcerative colitis 6 years ago. At that time, she responded well to treatment with prednisone and was tapered off the drug after 4 months. Since then, she has suffered minor flareups of colitis, but these haven't hampered her life-style. That is, until now.

Since her first day in the hospital, Sylvia has received I.V. corticosteroids, I.V. hyperalimentation, and blood transfusions. At first, she responded well—with fewer bowel movements and less bleeding. But when she began to eat solid food, the number of bowel movements rose and bleeding increased. Because her disease is worsening, the doctor recommends surgery. He offers Mrs. Levy two options: the permanent ileostomy or the ileoanal reservoir.

What are Mrs. Levy's learning needs?
First, review the standard teaching plan. Then assess Mrs. Levy's knowledge and skills in the standard teaching areas for inflammatory bowel disease. This will tell you which points to add to or delete from the teaching plan, and which ones to modify.

A standard teaching plan includes:
• pathophysiology of the patient's type of inflammatory bowel disease: ulcerative colitis or Crohn's disease
• complications, such as nutritional deficiencies
• tests, such as barium enema and swallow, endoscopic studies, and upper GI series
• surgical options, including traditional ileostomy, continent ileostomy, and ileoanal reservoir
• other treatments, such as activity and diet modifications, drug therapy, and ostomy care.

After reviewing what Mrs. Levy already knows about inflammatory bowel disease, you conclude that she understands the pathology of ulcerative colitis and the purpose and procedures for the GI tests

she's had before. However, she'll need teaching about any new tests, and about complications, surgical options, and life-style changes.

Setting learning outcomes
Consider Mrs. Levy's frame of mind. From talking with her, you know she's worried about how her family will manage while she's in the hospital. She's also discouraged about the course of her disease. Teaching her won't be easy. She lacks the motivation to learn about treatments and life-style changes.

Nevertheless, you outline what you need to teach Mrs. Levy. Reluctantly, she acknowledges that she needs more information to help her combat the disease and resume her normal life-style. So together, you agree on the following learning outcomes. For example, Mrs. Levy will be able to:

```
-explain how her symptoms relate to the complications of ulcerative
colitis
-state the reasons for diagnostic tests (such as upper and lower GI
studies, colonoscopies, and upper GI series)
-state the purpose, advantages, and disadvantages of a permanent
ileostomy and an ileoanal reservoir
-choose the surgical procedure compatible with her life-style
-discuss her feelings about the possible alteration of her body image
-demonstrate how to perform ileostomy care.
```

Selecting teaching techniques and tools
To help Mrs. Levy achieve her learning outcomes, use *short explanations* and *one-on-one* brief discussions to instruct her about complications of ulcerative colitis and pros and cons of surgical options.

Also use *demonstration,* showing her how to care for an ostomy, should she choose a permanent ileostomy or ileoanal reservoir. Show her a *physical model of the GI system,* pointing out the location of the ileoanal reservoir and how it attaches to the rectum. Supplement your teaching with *well-illustrated written materials* that she can read and reread later. If available, show Mrs. Levy a *videotape* of a patient removing, applying, and draining an ostomy pouch.

Evaluating your teaching
Question-and-answer discussion is one way to evaluate your teaching. For example, ask Mrs. Levy to explain why a traditional permanent ileostomy may be used to treat her disease.

Also employ *return demonstration.* Ask Mrs. Levy, for instance, to show you how to apply an ileostomy pouch. Your evaluation will reveal how well she's met her learning outcomes and help redirect your planning and teaching.

Comparing ulcerative colitis and Crohn's disease

Review the information in this chart to help you focus your teaching on the patient's type of inflammatory bowel disease: ulcerative colitis or Crohn's disease.

CHARACTERISTIC	ULCERATIVE COLITIS	CROHN'S DISEASE
Usual site	Colon and rectum	Commonly terminal ileum and right colon. May be anywhere from mouth to anus
Depth of involvement	Mucosal, submucosal	Transmural
Distribution	Continuous	Segmental
Bowel lumen size	Normal	Narrow
Rectal bleeding	Common	May occur
Anorectal fistulas	Rare	Common
Anal abscesses	Rare	Common
Crypt abscesses	Common	Rare
Cobblestoned mucosa	Rare	Common
Inflammatory masses	Rare	Common, extensive
Toxic megacolon	May occur	May occur
Pseudopolyps	Common	Rare
Granulomas	Absent	Common
Strictures	Absent	Common
Bowel shortening	Common	Rare
Mesenteric fat and lymph involvement	Absent	Common
Carcinoma	High risk after 10 years	Slightly increased risk
Diarrhea	Common	Common
Tenesmus	Severe	Rare
Abdominal pain	May occur	Common
Weight loss	Common	Common

What causes inflammatory bowel disease?

Inform the patient that no one knows exactly what causes inflammatory bowel disease. But research does suggest a familial predisposition. Studies postulate that the disease may result from:
• a bacterial or viral infection
• an allergic reaction to food, especially milk or milk products or other substances that release histamine in the bowel
• overproduction of enzymes that break down the mucous membranes
• autoimmune reactions, as occur in arthritis, hemolytic anemia, erythema nodosum, and uveitis.

scesses; the mucosa may take on a cobblestoned look. Since the disease can affect any bowel segment, healthy bowel portions may lie between two diseased segments.

Complications

Emphasize to the patient that certain foods may make symptoms worse and that these foods should be avoided. Vomiting and diarrhea may cause loss of body fluids and electrolytes, and rapid movement of food through the intestines may cause deficiencies of fat, iron, calcium, and vitamins A, B_{12}, C, D, E, and K.

Encourage the patient to report any changes in his condition so that the doctor can tailor the treatment plan most effectively. Tell the patient with ulcerative colitis that he may be at risk for cancer, especially if the disease has persisted more than 10 years or since childhood. Although inflammatory bowel disease doesn't have an emotional origin, warn your patient to avoid excessive stress.

Crohn's disease may lead to complications, such as obstructions, abscess with sepsis, or fistula formation. This disease slightly raises the risk of colon or rectal cancer.

Describe the diagnostic workup

Teach the patient about the various tests that diagnose inflammatory bowel disease and monitor its course. Besides undergoing routine blood, urine, and stool studies, he'll usually have a barium enema, barium swallow, lower and upper GI endoscopy, and an upper GI series. If appropriate, inform the patient that the doctor may schedule a computed tomography (CT) scan to confirm a suspected abscess.

Barium enema

Explain that this radiographic test helps to diagnose inflammatory bowel disease by examining the large intestine after barium enema administration. Tell the patient that the test takes 30 to 45 minutes.

Instruct the patient to maintain a low-residue diet for 1 to 3 days and a clear liquid diet up to 24 hours before the test. The presence of food or fluid may cloud the intestinal outline.

Explain that during the test he'll be secured to a movable table. (Assure him that he'll be adequately draped.) After the doctor X-rays the bowel to make sure it's empty, the patient will lie on his left side, and the doctor will insert a small, lubricated tube into the rectum. Instruct the patient to keep his anal sphincter tightly contracted against the tube to help prevent barium leakage. Stress the importance of retaining the barium, because accurate test results depend on adequately coating the large intestine.

Once the tube's inserted, the barium slowly fills the bowel as X-ray films are taken. If air is also instilled through the tube, tell the patient the table may be tilted and he'll be assisted into various positions to aid in filling. To ease cramping or the urge to defecate as the barium or air fills the large intestine, instruct him to breathe slowly and deeply through his mouth.

Inform the patient that after the test he'll expel the barium into a bedpan or the toilet, and receive a laxative or an enema to clear his bowel of any remaining barium. Stress the importance of barium elimination, because retained barium may harden, causing intestinal obstruction or impaction. Tell him that barium will lightly color his stools for 24 to 72 hours after the test. Mention that he may resume his diet and medications as ordered. Encourage fluids to prevent dehydration from the bowel preparation and test. Also, encourage rest because the test is tiring.

Barium swallow
Explain that a barium swallow (esophagography or upper GI examination) is a 30-minute radiographic test that helps detect Crohn's disease by examining the pharynx and esophagus after the patient swallows barium.

Instruct the patient to restrict antacids (if ordered) for 24 hours and food and fluids after midnight before the test. Tell him to remove jewelry, dentures, and other objects that may obscure details on the X-ray films.

Explain that the patient will lie on an adjustable table and will be asked to swallow barium several times during the test. Describe barium's milkshake consistency and unpleasant, chalky taste. First, he'll swallow a thick mixture, then a thin one. If the doctor wants to accentuate small strictures or demonstrate dysphagia, the patient will swallow a special barium marshmallow (soft white bread soaked in barium). Tell the patient that as the barium outlines his pharynx and esophagus, the table will be adjusted so that the doctor can take films from several angles.

Inform the patient that after the test he may resume his normal diet and medication, as ordered, and will receive a laxative to help expel the barium. Stress the importance of barium elimination, because retained barium may harden, causing obstruction or impaction. The barium will lightly color his stools for 24 to 72 hours after the test.

Lower GI endoscopy
Explain to the patient that lower GI endoscopy (colonoscopy) helps the doctor diagnose the origin of GI bleeding and examine the lower GI tract, using a flexible tube inserted into the rectum. Tell him that the test takes about 30 minutes.

Instruct the patient to maintain a clear liquid diet for 24 hours before the test and, as ordered, to fast after midnight the night before the test. However, he should continue any drug regimen, as ordered. Inform him that he'll receive a laxative the afternoon before the test. Dietary restrictions and bowel preparation are essential to clear the lower GI tract for a better view.

Inform the patient that he'll lie on an X-ray table as a nurse takes his vital signs and inserts an I.V. line into his hand or arm to administer medication. He will be awake during the test, and will be given a sedative to help him relax.

Explain that the doctor will insert a flexible tube into the patient's rectum. Inform the patient that he may feel some lower abdominal discomfort and the urge to defecate as the tube is advanced. To ease the discomfort, instruct the patient to breathe deeply and slowly through his mouth. Explain that air may be introduced into the bowel through the tube. Tell him not to try to control the urge to expel some air. Also, tell him that he may hear and feel a suction machine removing any liquid that may obscure the doctor's view, but that it won't cause any discomfort.

Explain that after the test his vital signs will be checked frequently for 2 hours, and that he can resume his normal diet after recovering from the sedative, in about 1 hour. If air was introduced into the bowel, he may pass large amounts of flatus. Instruct him to report any blood in his bowel movement.

Upper GI endoscopy

Inform the patient that this 1-hour test identifies upper GI abnormalities associated with inflammatory bowel disease. Explain that it examines the esophagus, stomach, and the first part of the small intestine (duodenum), using a flexible tube inserted through the mouth into the intestine.

Instruct the patient to restrict food and fluids after midnight the night before the test. If the test is an emergency procedure, inform him that he'll have his stomach contents suctioned to permit better visualization.

Explain that during the test, the patient will lie on an X-ray table as a nurse takes his vital signs and inserts an I.V. line into his hand or arm to administer medication during the test. Inform the patient that he'll be awake during the test. Mention that he'll receive a sedative to help him relax and relieve discomfort.

Tell the patient that before insertion of the tube, his throat will be sprayed with a local anesthetic. Advise him that the spray may taste unpleasant and will make his mouth feel numb, causing difficulty in swallowing. Instruct him to let the saliva drain from the side of his mouth. Tell him that he'll have a mouthguard to keep him from biting the tube. Assure him that he'll have no difficulty breathing. Explain that as the tube is inserted and advanced, he can expect pressure in his abdomen and some fullness or bloating as air is introduced to inflate the stomach for a better view.

Inform the patient that after the test his vital signs will be checked frequently for 2 hours, and that he can resume eating when his gag reflex returns—usually in about 2 hours. He may have a sore throat for a few days.

Upper GI and small bowel series

Inform the patient that this test helps to diagnose inflammatory bowel disease by radiographically examining the esophagus, stomach, and small intestine after a barium swallow, which clearly outlines the structures. Tell him who will perform the test and where. Inform him that the test requires several films to be taken up to 1 hour apart, so the test may take up to 6 hours. Advise him to bring a book or an activity to help pass the time.

Instruct the patient to maintain a clear liquid diet the day before the test and to restrict food, fluids, and smoking after midnight before the test. As ordered, tell him to stop taking medications for up to 24 hours before the test. He'll also receive a laxative the afternoon before the test. Explain that the presence of food or fluid may obscure details of the structures being studied.

Inform him that he will lie on a movable table and will be asked to swallow small amounts of barium several times during the test. Describe barium's milkshake consistency and chalky taste. Inform him that the doctor may compress the abdomen to ensure proper coating of the stomach and intestinal walls with barium. Also mention that the table will be adjusted to various positions so that the doctor can take films from several angles.

Tell the patient that after the test he may resume his normal diet and medication, as ordered. He'll receive a laxative or enema to help expel barium. Stress the importance of barium elimination, because retained barium may harden, causing intestinal obstruction or impaction. Explain that barium will lightly color his stools for 24 to 72 hours after the test.

Computed tomography (CT) scan
Explain that a CT scan of the intestines can detect abscesses. Tell him that the test takes about 90 minutes. Instruct him to restrict food and fluids after midnight before the test, but to continue any drug regimen as ordered.

Explain to the patient that he will lie on a table while X-rays are taken. Tell him he'll be asked to lie still, relax, breathe normally, and remain quiet, because movement will blur the X-ray picture and prolong the test. If the doctor is using an I.V. contrast medium, inform the patient that he may experience discomfort from the needle puncture and a localized feeling of warmth on injection. Tell him to immediately report any side effects: nausea, vomiting, dizziness, headache, or urticaria. Assure him that such reactions are rare. Inform him that he may resume his normal diet after the test.

Teach about treatments
Explain such measures as rest, dietary restrictions, and drug therapy. Prepare the patient for surgery if his disease progresses.

Activity
Explain the importance of adequate rest to the patient. To decrease intestinal motility during an attack, advise him to reduce physical activity. If his attack is mild, suggest that he rest more during the day.

Urge the hospitalized patient with severe diarrhea to use the call light whenever he needs help going to the bathroom. If he can use the bathroom unassisted, instruct him to tell the nurse when he has a bowel movement so that she can record the number of stools, their consistency, color, and presence of bleeding.

Diet
Explain that dietary changes allow the bowel to heal by decreasing its activity while providing the calories and nutrition necessary for

Reducing inflammation with mesalamine

If ordered, instruct the patient to give himself an enema containing the medication mesalamine (Rowasa). Explain that this drug helps reduce inflammation.

Tell him to give himself the enema at bedtime. He'll retain the contents of one bottle (60 ml) for about 8 hours (preferably overnight).

Instruct him to shake the bottle well first to make sure the suspension is mixed and then to remove the protective sheath from the applicator tip. (Mention that holding the bottle at the neck won't cause any leakage.)

Next, tell him to lie on his left side (to help the medication migrate into the sigmoid colon) with his left leg extended and his right leg flexed forward for balance. Or he can use the knee-chest position.

Advise him to gently insert the applicator tip in the rectum, pointing toward the umbilicus, then to squeeze the bottle steadily to discharge most of the preparation.

healing. Stress the importance of following his prescribed diet to help decrease symptoms. Make sure he understands his prescribed diet—high in protein, calories, and vitamins.

Advise him to avoid foods that irritate his intestines or that require excessive intestinal activity, such as milk products, spicy or fried high-residue foods, raw vegetables and fruits, and whole-grain cereals. Explain that he may need supplemental vitamins to compensate for the bowel's inability to absorb them. Discourage carbonated, caffeinated, and alcoholic beverages because they increase intestinal activity. Also discourage extremely hot or cold food and fluids because they cause gas.

Advise eating small, frequent meals. If anorexia's a problem, reinforce the importance of an adequate diet to promote healing. Suggest snacks, favorite foods if permitted, good mouth care (to enhance taste), and a pleasant dining atmosphere.

Medication

Explain that medications aim to decrease inflammation and control or relieve symptoms. If the doctor orders a corticosteroid, such as prednisone, explain that this drug reduces inflammation, thus relieving such symptoms as diarrhea, bleeding, and pain. Teach the patient to take the drug exactly as prescribed and not to stop taking it abruptly. Stress that after long-term use, stopping the drug suddenly can cause adrenal crisis. Warn about possible adverse effects of corticosteroids, including osteoporosis, increased susceptibility to infection, moon face, fluid retention, and mood swings.

Explain that the doctor may prescribe sulfasalazine to reduce inflammation. This drug breaks down to a sulfa preparation and an aspirin-like drug, mesalamine (see *Reducing inflammation with mesalamine*). If the patient is taking sulfasalazine, tell him to report aching joints and muscles, dizziness, fever, hematuria, itching, jaundice, low back pain, photosensitivity, rash, or unusual bruising or bleeding. Also instruct him to report if he loses weight, feels nauseated, or vomits. The doctor may alter the dose because many of these reactions are dose-related.

Tell the patient that the doctor may order an immunosuppressive drug, such as azathioprine, to alter the body's response to antigens. This drug increases the risk of serious infection by diminishing production of white blood cells and platelets. Advise him to report bleeding tendencies, chills, fever, and sore throat.

If the doctor prescribes metronidazole to treat perianal complications of Crohn's disease, urge the patient to report any numbness or tingling in his extremities to his doctor immediately.

Remind the patient to take antidiarrheals, such as diphenoxylate and atropine, as instructed. Stress that he report increased abdominal pain and distention to the doctor immediately. Antidiarrheal drugs may cause toxic megacolon.

If the doctor orders narcotics, explain that these drugs may control his pain and diarrhea. Warn him to contact the doctor or go to an emergency center immediately if he has difficulty breathing or decreased respirations. Caution him about the risk of addiction with long-term use.

Surgery and procedures

Surgery may be needed if inflammatory bowel disease doesn't respond to treatment, if premalignant or malignant changes appear in the bowel, or if complications become unmanageable. Explain to the patient that surgery for Crohn's disease depends on the affected area and the type of complications. Inform him that surgery may result in resection with a primary anastomosis, or a temporary or permanent colostomy or ileostomy. Tell him that surgery will not cure the disease and the likelihood of its recurrence is high.

Explain to the patient with ulcerative colitis that surgery usually involves removal of the rectum and large bowel, with creation of a permanent ileostomy. Or it may involve creation of a continent ileostomy or an ileoanal reservoir. Reassure the patient that surgery cures the disease. (See *Reviewing types of ostomies*, page 430.)

Colostomy. Tell the patient that a colostomy is a surgically created opening between the colon and the surface of the abdomen, through which he'll excrete body wastes. Show the patient drawings of the colon before and after surgery, and stress how much of the colon remains intact. Mention that the farther down the colon his colostomy is located, the more closely his stools will resemble a normal bowel movement. Inform him that the stoma is normally red, moist, and swollen postoperatively, but that swelling will subside. Explain that the stoma won't hurt when touched because it has no nerve endings capable of detecting sharp pain. Also explain that the stoma has no muscles, so he won't be able to open and close it at will. However, he can learn to control his bowel movements by irrigating the colostomy, if this is not contraindicated because of his Crohn's disease. In the meantime, he'll need to wear a colostomy pouch to collect any wastes that drain from the stoma. Ask a representative of the United Ostomy Association to help the patient adjust to having a colostomy.

After surgery, encourage the patient to look at his stoma and to participate in colostomy care and irrigation as soon as possible. Teach him how to remove, empty, and reapply his colostomy pouch. (See *Questions ostomy patients ask*.) Also, give him a copy of the patient-teaching aids *Removing an ostomy pouch*, page 434, *Applying an ostomy pouch*, page 435, and *Draining an ostomy pouch*, page 436.

Stress the importance of proper skin care, and show him how to keep the skin around the stoma clean, dry, and free from irritation. If he chooses irrigation, demonstrate how to irrigate his colostomy correctly, and supplement this with return demonstration and written instruction. Instruct the patient to notify the doctor or enterostomal therapy nurse if he repeatedly has trouble inserting the irrigation cone or if he develops persistent diarrhea or constipation, bloody or abnormal drainage, unusually colored or foul-smelling stools, or skin irritation around the stoma.

Ileostomy. If the patient's scheduled for an ileostomy, use diagrams to show him what will be removed. Stress that the small bowel remains intact and that his digestion should remain normal.

Inform the patient that preoperative preparation usually is done the day before surgery (or 3 to 4 days before, depending on

INQUIRY

Questions ostomy patients ask

Do I have to eat special foods?
As with any abdominal surgery, you'll be on a liquid diet for a few days after the operation. After that, you'll follow your regular diet. Most people will tolerate the same foods after surgery as before. If certain foods caused gas, they still will. If you were on a special diet, such as a low-sodium one, you'll stay on it.

The doctor may ask you to avoid certain high-roughage foods for 6 to 8 weeks after your surgery so the bowel can heal. These include popcorn, nuts, Chinese vegetables, coconut, fresh fruits, and vegetables. After this period, you may include these foods. Add one new food at a time and in moderation. Remember to eat slowly and chew your food well. Drink plenty of water.

Will I have to wear special clothes?
No. Your pouch shouldn't show under regular clothes. But don't wear a tight belt or undergarment over the stoma to avoid injuring it. You can't rely on an uncomfortable feeling to let you know you've hurt the stoma. That's because the stoma doesn't have nerve endings that detect sharp pain.

Will my sex life suffer?
If your sex life was satisfying before surgery, it should remain so. After all, you're the same person with the same feelings and desires as always. Some people may feel unattractive to their partner right after surgery but with open, honest communication, this feeling will usually go away. If you continue to have problems, though, ask your doctor or enterostomal therapist for advice.

Reviewing types of ostomies

Explain to the patient that an ostomy is the surgical creation of an opening in the bowel that allows elimination of body wastes. A colostomy is an opening in the large bowel; an ileostomy, an opening in the last portion of the small bowel.

Temporary ostomies are used to rest a part of the bowel and allow the inflammation to decrease. Permanent ostomies may be necessary after extensive abdominal surgery. (In Hartman's procedure, an end colostomy is made, but bowel continuity may be restored later if desired.) Explain to the patient that the type of ostomy he'll have — temporary or permanent — depends on the type, location, and extent of his disease.

PERMANENT COLOSTOMY

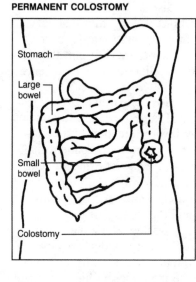

Stomach

Large bowel

Small bowel

Colostomy

DOUBLE-BARREL COLOSTOMY

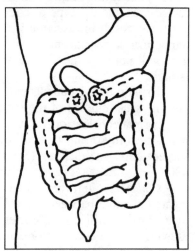

LOOP COLOSTOMY

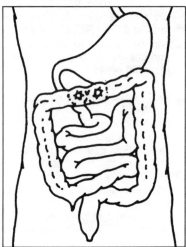

HARTMAN'S PROCEDURE

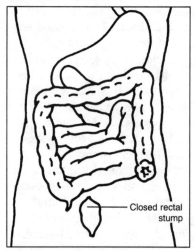

Closed rectal stump

ILEOSTOMY

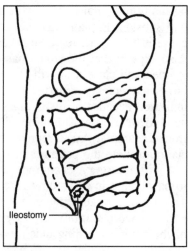

Ileostomy

the disease's severity), and that he'll receive oral laxatives, as well as antibiotics to reduce the risk of postoperative infection. Tell him that his stoma site will be selected and marked. (Assure him that his preference for stoma location will be considered.) Describe the stoma, show him an ostomy pouch, and, if appropriate, ask him to wear it for a short time to ensure proper fit. Also ask a representative of the United Ostomy Association to visit with the patient to help him adjust to having an ileostomy.

Inform the patient that he'll return from surgery with a pouch covering his stoma. The nurse will initially perform stoma care, changing the pouch as necessary, and gradually the patient will learn to do this for himself. Also describe the color and consistency of the drainage, and explain that it will change as his diet changes.

Tell him that he'll have a nasogastric tube in place for several days to prevent distention by draining the GI tract. Also explain that he won't eat for several days after surgery, but that once he resumes his diet, he'll begin with clear liquids and gradually include solid foods. If eating is not permitted for more than a week, he may have I.V. hyperalimentation.

To prevent pulmonary complications, instruct the patient to turn in bed, to cough and deep-breathe at least once every hour, and to use incentive spirometry. Assure him that he'll receive medication if movement and coughing cause pain. To minimize abdominal pain when turning and coughing, show him how to splint his surgical site.

Include a family member in discharge teaching to assist the patient if he cannot care for himself, for example, because of severe viral infection or a broken wrist. Also show the patient how to care for the skin around his stoma site to prevent skin breakdown and infection. Instruct him to contact the doctor or enterostomal therapy nurse if he observes redness, rash, or swelling, or if he experiences itching, warmth, pain, or unusual drainage. Teach him how to manage his ostomy equipment (see *Tips for using ostomy equipment*).

Assure the patient that odor shouldn't be a problem because newer pouches are odor-proof. Instruct him to notify the doctor of any marked decline in ostomy output or spurting or squirting of drainage from the stoma. This may signal stoma stricture and require medical intervention. Also tell him to report any unusually foul odor; it may indicate infection or may be only diet-related. To prevent gas from filling his pouch, advise him to avoid gas-producing foods, such as cabbage and broccoli. Also, he may want to use a pouch with a filter. Inform him that he may wear his pouch when taking a bath or shower, because water won't loosen the pouch seal. He may also remove the pouch if desired because water won't hurt the stoma.

Continent ileostomy. If the patient's scheduled for a continent ileostomy, explain that it consists of an intra-abdominal pouch surgically constructed from the terminal ileum. Solid waste collects in the nipple-valved pouch until the patient drains the pouch through the stoma with a catheter. (See *Continent ileostomy and ileoanal reservoir,* page 432.)

After a continent ileostomy, outline the procedure for emptying the pouch by inserting a lubricated #28 catheter through the stoma. Pouch capacity determines how often it should be drained. Because the pouch will stretch, it will hold only about 70 to 100 ml of fluid right after surgery. Six months later, it will hold about 600 ml and will need emptying only 3 or 4 times a day. Between intubations, instruct the patient to keep his stoma covered with a small gauze pad and to irrigate his pouch weekly—or more often if undigested food causes a drainage block. To prevent blocks, advise him to avoid fibrous foods, such as corn, nuts, lettuce, and celery.

Ileoanal reservoir. If the patient's scheduled for an ileoanal

Tips for using ostomy equipment

If your patient has an ostomy, explain that ostomy pouches are lightweight, odor-proof, and not likely to attract attention. Point out that the pouches can be drained and don't need daily changing.

Reassure him that adhesives on the pouch probably won't irritate his skin. But if his skin is extra-sensitive, advise him how to protect it.

Skin barriers
Explain that he can use a protective film wipe that provides a thin, clear barrier between the adhesive and his skin. Or he can choose a thicker, more protective barrier made from karaya or a pectin-based product. This will fit under any pouch system to help heal irritated skin.

Advise him to contact his enterostomal therapy nurse to show him how to use these products.

Continent ileostomy and ileoanal reservoir

For patients with ulcerative colitis, a continent ileostomy and ileoanal reservoir serve as alternatives to a permanent ileostomy.

Continent ileostomy

The surgeon constructs a nipple valve by intussuscepting several centimeters of terminal ileum into the surgically constructed pouch. After joining the valve's layers with sutures or staples, he sutures the valve flush to the abdominal wall. The illustration below shows the completed procedure.

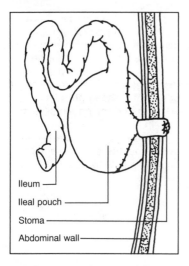

Ileum

Ileal pouch

Stoma

Abdominal wall

Ileoanal reservoir

An ileoanal reservoir can be constructed in either an S shape (by aligning and suturing three loops of ileum together) or a J shape (by suturing a portion of the ileum to the rectal cuff and looping the end upward). In the first stage of the two-stage procedure, a temporary ileostomy is created to allow for stool drainage while the reservoir heals. In the second stage, the ileostomy is reversed and stool then drains into the reservoir.

S-SHAPED ILEOANAL RESERVOIR: FIRST STAGE

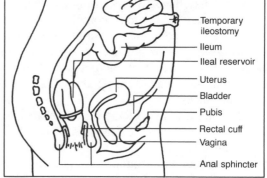

Temporary ileostomy

Ileum

Ileal reservoir

Uterus

Bladder

Pubis

Rectal cuff

Vagina

Anal sphincter

J-SHAPED RESERVOIR: SECOND STAGE

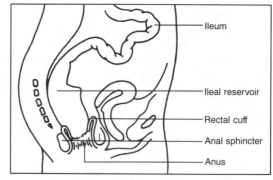

Ileum

Ileal reservoir

Rectal cuff

Anal sphincter

Anus

reservoir, explain that it involves dissection of the rectal area from the submucosa and mucosa. The colon is removed, and the ileum sutured to the rectum by the creation of a J- or S-shaped reservoir pouch. With this procedure, the patient retains the ability to defecate normally through the rectum.

Many patients welcome this newer procedure over a traditional ostomy because the reservoir is internal and preserves the patient's body image. The procedure does have disadvantages, however. It is difficult to perform, and should be done only by a surgeon experienced in the procedure. The patient may also have difficulty differentiating among gases, fluids, and solids in the rectum. In addition, he may experience fecal urgency, nocturnal incontinence, diarrhea, frequent bowel movements, and perianal skin denudation.

Other care measures

Discourage smoking because it contributes to altered bowel motility. If diarrhea's severe, teach the patient proper skin care. Because persistent diarrhea and vomiting may lead to serious metabolic complications, instruct him to report signs of dehydration (confusion, lethargy, dry skin and mucous membranes, dry mouth, weakness, and reduced urine output).

Instruct the patient to notify the doctor if he experiences signs and symptoms of complications: fever, fatigue, weakness, or a rapid heart rate, along with abdominal cramping, vomiting, and acute diarrhea. Abdominal pain and cramping can signal progressive inflammatory bowel disease, indicating stricture or obstruction. Fatigue and weakness, accompanied by pallor and dizziness, can indicate anemia.

If the patient has an ileostomy, tell him to avoid laxatives, enteric-coated pills, and timed-release capsules, because they won't be fully absorbed. Urge him to contact the doctor if he acquires an infection, because diarrhea and vomiting can lead to life-threatening metabolic complications. Also arrange for follow-up examinations by a health care professional. Emphasize the importance of wearing a Medic Alert bracelet or necklace at all times. Advise him to see the doctor regularly for checkups.

Besides teaching the patient about ostomy care, you'll need to help him learn how to adapt his life-style. Be prepared to answer questions on a range of issues.

Refer the patient and his family to the local chapter of the National Foundation for Ileitis and Colitis to provide them with support. Tell the family that many patients feel that their problems are unique. Encourage both patient and family to express their feelings. For the patient with an ostomy, contact the United Ostomy Association to provide guidance and support.

Sources of information and support

International Association for Enterostomal Therapy
2081 Business Center Drive, Suite 290, Irvine, Calif. 92715
(714) 476-0268

National Foundation for Ileitis and Colitis
444 Park Avenue South, New York, N.Y. 10016
(212) 685-3440

United Ostomy Association
36 Executive Park, Suite 120, Irvine, Calif. 92714
(714) 660-8624

Further readings

Bennington, S. "Surgical Treatment of Ulcerative Colitis," *Canadian Operating Room Nursing Journal* 6(2): 20, 22, 24, April 1988.

Brandt, L.J. *Treating IBD: A Patient's Guide to the Medical and Surgical Management of IBD.* New York: Raven Press, 1989.

Farley, D. "Living with Inflammatory Bowel Disease," *FDA Consumer* 22(3): 8-15, April 1988.

Lewis, M.C. "Attributions and Inflammatory Bowel Disease: Patients' Perceptions of Illness Causes and the Effects of These Perceptions on Relationships," *Alberta Association of Registered Nurses Newsletter* 44(5):16-17, May 1988.

Nord, H.J. "Complications of Inflammatory Bowel Disease," *Hospital Practice:* 65-67, 70-72, 75, November 1987.

Prasad, M.L. "Surgical Options for the Patient with Inflammatory Bowel Disease," *Society of Gastrointestinal Assistants Journal* 10(3): 141-44, Winter 1988.

Removing an ostomy pouch

Dear Patient:

Be sure to change your pouch on a regular schedule. This will help prevent skin irritation and leakage.

How often should you change the pouch?

This depends on your type of ostomy, your activities, and the type of pouch you wear. Keep in mind that you may need to change the pouch more often in hot, humid weather. But avoid changing it daily because this can cause skin stripping and irritation. If you think the pouch may need changing daily, contact the enterostomal therapy nurse or your doctor for guidelines.

Removing the pouch

1 Gather a wash cloth, towel or paper towels, adhesive solvent and an eyedropper (if needed), karaya powder or Stomahesive powder, protective film wipes, and karaya or pectin-based skin barriers.

2 Remove your old pouch by gently pulling up on the adhesive with one hand while carefully pushing down on the skin with the other. Most disposable pouches will come off easily without a solvent. If the pouch you're using requires a solvent, follow the product directions. Make sure the solvent is completely removed from your skin before applying the new pouch. If you're using a reusable pouch, set it aside to clean after you apply your new pouch.

3 Wash your skin well with warm water and pat dry. Soap is usually not needed, but if you choose to use it, *rinse your skin thoroughly.* Soap residue will interfere with pouch adhesion and may irritate your skin.

4 Check your skin for redness or irritation. The most common causes of irritation are stool leakage under the seal or an overly large pouch opening, which allows stool to come in contact with the skin and cause irritation. Measure the stoma routinely to ensure that the stomal opening on your pouch is correct.

If your skin is red but intact, use a protective film wipe to provide a clear, thin film between the adhesive and your skin.

If your skin is weeping, dust the affected area lightly with karaya powder or Stomahesive powder. Wipe off any excess powder and then cover the skin with a protective skin barrier. This may be either a karaya or pectin-based wafer cut to fit the stoma. Apply your pouch over this wafer. Many disposable pouches have a protective wafer as part of the system itself.

Skin irritation will usually clear in a few days. If it doesn't, notify your enterostomal therapist or doctor.

Applying an ostomy pouch

Dear Patient:

The nurse will show you how to apply the ostomy pouch. Then you can use this patient-teaching aid to help you remember the steps. Choose a one-piece disposable pouch, a two-piece disposable pouch, or a two-piece reusable pouch.

Applying a one-piece disposable pouch

1 Measure your stoma to determine the correct size of the pouch opening, as shown.

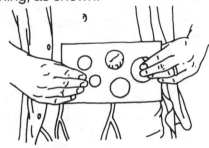

2 If the pouch opening is *precut,* remove the release papers from the pouch, press the pouch to your abdomen, and seal well. Attach the tail closure (a small clip that secures the pouch bottom for later drainage).

If you *custom-cut* your pouch, cut the opening to the correct size, remove the release papers, then apply as above.

Applying a two-piece disposable pouch

1 Measure your stoma to determine the correct size of your faceplate opening.

2 Cut the faceplate to the correct size, remove the release papers, press the faceplate to your abdomen, and seal well. Secure the pouch to the faceplate and attach the tail closure.

Applying a two-piece reusable pouch

1 Measure your stoma to determine the size of your faceplate opening.

2 Follow the manufacturer's directions to apply new adhesive to the faceplate or to your skin with each change. First, peel off one side of the adhesive disk's paper backing. Then center the disk over the faceplate and press firmly to expel any bubbles from between the faceplate and the adhesive.

3 Next, peel the remaining paper backing off the adhesive disk. Center the faceplate over your stoma. Gently press around the stoma so the adhesive sticks to your abdomen.

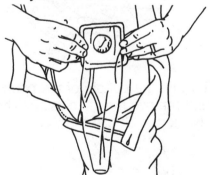

Secure the pouch to the faceplate, attach the supporting O-ring around the faceplate collar, and attach the tail closure.

Draining an ostomy pouch

Dear Patient:

Depending on your type of ostomy, you may need to empty your pouch from 1 to 8 times daily. Empty it when the pouch is about one-third to one-half full.

1 To begin, sit on the toilet and direct the pouch opening into the bowl. To prevent splashing, you may want to place some toilet paper on the surface of the water or flush the toilet as you empty the pouch.

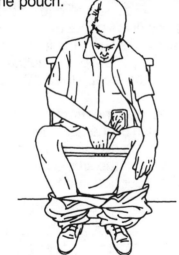

2 Turn up the bottom of the pouch and remove the tail closure. Then empty the pouch into the toilet.

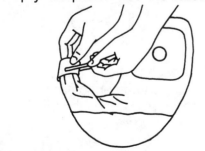

3 Slide your thumb and index finger down the outside of the pouch, squeezing the contents into the toilet.

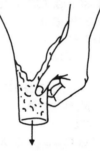

4 Use toilet paper to clean any stool from around and inside the pouch opening.

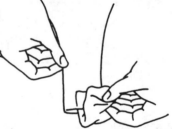

5 If desired, rinse the pouch with cool water. Remember, your pouch is odor-proof, so this step isn't necessary.

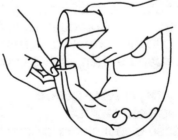

6 Now reattach the pouch's tail closure to complete the procedure.

Cirrhosis

Progression of this life-threatening disorder can be stopped or slowed only by strict compliance with treatment. However, compliance is unlikely if the patient denies his illness and its precipitating factor—alcoholism. As a result, your first goal may well be to establish a trusting relationship with the patient and to encourage him to express his concerns. Only then can you successfully begin to teach about a nutritious diet, use of medications, such as antacids, life-style changes, and, possibly, surgery.

Your teaching should also involve the family, whose relationship with the patient may be strained by his alcoholism. You'll need to pinpoint the family member who's most appropriate for supportive teaching—someone who can be counted on to help the patient adhere to his treatment regimen.

Discuss the disorder

Inform the patient that cirrhosis is a chronic disorder involving irreversible damage to liver cells. Explain that the healthy liver plays a major role in carbohydrate, protein, fat, and steroid metabolism; vitamin storage; blood coagulation; and detoxification. (See *Teaching about liver structure and function,* page 438.) Impairment of these functions results in such problems as nutritional deficiencies, increased susceptibility to infection, and increased potential for bleeding.

Emphasize that once major symptoms occur, cirrhosis can't be cured; in fact, three quarters of the liver can be damaged without causing overt symptoms. Review common symptoms of the disorder. (See *Signs and symptoms of cirrhosis,* page 439.) Inform the patient that although the liver has remarkable regenerative powers if he abstains from alcohol and follows his treatment plan, new tissue doesn't function as effectively. However, with proper treatment, he may experience long-term remission of symptoms.

Explain the causes of cirrhosis to the patient—alcoholism and drug abuse being the most common. (See *Questions patients ask about cirrhosis,* page 440.) Other predisposing factors include viral hepatitis, heart disease, gallbladder disease, and exposure to certain environmental pollutants and chemicals.

Complications

Emphasize that the patient can prevent or relieve complications by strict compliance with treatment. Stress that noncompliance with diet and medication therapy may hasten portal hypertension and hepatic encephalopathy—signaling progressive liver cell damage.

Catherine K. Foran, RN, MSN, and **Brenda I.W. Hagan, RN,C, MSN,** contributed to this chapter. Ms. Foran is an independent nursing consultant in Cherry Hill, N.J. Ms. Hagan is director of clinical services at the Liberty Healthcare Corporation, Inc. in Philadelphia.

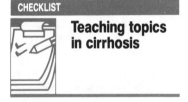

CHECKLIST

Teaching topics in cirrhosis

☐ An explanation of how cirrhosis causes irreversible damage to liver cells
☐ Complications of cirrhosis and their warning signs
☐ Preparation for diagnostic tests, including liver scanning and biopsy, and blood, urine, and stool studies, to confirm or evaluate cirrhosis
☐ Dietary measures and elimination of alcohol
☐ Importance of taking medication as prescribed, because of the liver's impaired ability to detoxify substances
☐ Preparation for portal-systemic shunting, if necessary
☐ Measures to reduce the risk of bleeding and infection
☐ Sources of information and support

Teaching about liver structure and function

Educate the patient about the importance of his liver. Point out that this versatile organ is the body's largest internal organ, performing more than 300 functions. The liver can function even with damage to 90% of its mass. But liver removal or total destruction leads to death within about 10 hours.

Anatomy
Tell the patient that the liver lies on the right side, just under his ribs. An adult's liver weighs about 3 lb (1.36 kg) and is grossly divided into two lobes. The right lobe has three sections; the left lobe, two. Lobules—the liver's functional units—subdivide each lobe section.

To reinforce your teaching, show the patient how to feel the edge of his liver. Instruct him to lie down, take a deep breath, and wrap his fingers over the edge of his lower rib cage. Point out that the normal liver edge is smooth and firm. The lumps or nodules he may feel result from liver damage.

Circulation
The portal vein and hepatic artery supply blood to the liver (about one-third of the heart's output). Tell the patient to imagine about 1½ quarts of blood flowing through his liver each minute. The portal vein delivers nutrient-rich blood from the GI tract, whereas the hepatic artery carries oxygenated blood to hepatic cells. The blood flows through lobular channels called sinusoids, which drain into the central vein.

Explain that the liver also makes bile, a fluid that helps in digestion of fats. Bile flows through canaliculi (small bile ducts between hepatic cell plates), then drains into large hepatic bile ducts.

Hepatic cell function
Teach the patient that hepatocytes are the worker cells of the liver. They work as the following:
• a factory—making chemical compounds, such as blood proteins, bile, and enzymes
• a warehouse—storing glycogen, iron, and vitamins
• a waste disposal plant—breaking down and excreting old red blood cells and urea; detoxifying drugs, poisons, and alcohol
• a power plant—catabolizing carbohydrates, proteins, and fats
• a regulatory agency—maintaining blood glucose concentration; regulating several hormones.

Falciform ligament

Caudate lobe (posterior)

Right lobe

Diaphragm

Triangular ligament

Left lobe

Ligamentum teres

Quadrate lobe

Hepatic artery branch

Portal vein branch

Bile duct

LIVER LOBULE

Canaliculus

Sinusoid

Central vein

Hepatic cells

Explain that portal hypertension can cause esophageal varices. If these varices rupture, massive hemorrhage may occur, requiring emergency treatment. (See *Ruptured esophageal varices: A deadly complication,* page 441.)

In hepatic encephalopathy, inform the patient that the liver can't convert ammonia (the end product of protein breakdown) to urea; consequently, serum ammonia levels rise. Extremely toxic to the brain, elevated ammonia levels produce neurologic changes. Warn the patient that untreated hepatic encephalopathy can ultimately lead to coma and death.

Explain that ascites, a less acute but still ominous complication, results from pathologic changes in the failing liver. Uncontrolled ascites can compromise respiratory and renal function.

Describe the diagnostic workup

Prepare the patient for scheduled diagnostic tests, such as liver scanning and biopsy, to confirm or evaluate cirrhosis. Tell him that blood, urine, and stool samples also may be collected to test liver function. Reassure him that frequent urine and blood testing will monitor the progress of his disease and don't signal worsening of his condition.

Liver biopsy

Explain that a liver biopsy is the definitive test for cirrhosis. It detects destruction and fibrosis of liver tissue. Before the test, give him a copy of the patient-teaching aid *Preparing for a liver biopsy,* page 443.

Liver scan

Inform the patient that this test visualizes his liver with a special scanner or camera. Tell him that the test takes about an hour and causes no discomfort. Explain that during the test he'll receive an injection of a radioactive substance (technetium 99m sulfur colloid) through an I.V. line in his hand or arm to allow better visualization of his liver. Tell him to report immediately any adverse effects: flushing, fever, light-headedness, or difficulty breathing. Assure him that the injection contains only trace amounts of radioactivity and rarely produces adverse effects. If the test uses a rectilinear scanner, he'll hear a soft, irregular, clicking noise as it moves across his abdomen. If the test uses a gamma camera, he'll feel the camera lightly touch his abdomen. Instruct him to lie still, relax, and breathe normally. He may be asked to hold his breath briefly, to ensure good quality pictures.

Teach about treatments

Encourage the patient to change harmful habits that may interfere with his recovery. For example, stress the importance of abstinence from alcohol, and review dietary measures to promote liver regeneration. Teach him to take medications exactly as prescribed, because the liver's ability to detoxify substances is impaired. If necessary, prepare him for portal-systemic shunting to relieve portal hypertension. Discuss how to reduce the risk of GI bleeding and infection.

Signs and symptoms of cirrhosis

Teach your patient that the signs and symptoms of cirrhosis fall into two stages: early and late. In the early stage, his complaints may be vague. He may have a dull abdominal ache and GI problems, such as anorexia, constipation, diarrhea, indigestion, nausea, or vomiting. Later, more severe symptoms develop, resulting from hepatic insufficiency and portal hypertension. These major signs and symptoms include:

• *respiratory*—pleural effusion, limited thoracic expansion due to abdominal ascites, interfering with efficient gas exchange and leading to hypoxia
• *central nervous system*—progressive symptoms of hepatic encephalopathy: lethargy, mental changes, slurred speech, asterixis (flapping tremor), peripheral neuritis, paranoia, hallucinations, extreme obtundation, and coma
• *hematologic*—bleeding tendencies (nosebleeds, easy bruising, bleeding gums), anemia
• *endocrine*—testicular atrophy, menstrual irregularities, gynecomastia, and loss of chest and axillary hair
• *skin*—severe pruritus, extreme dryness, poor tissue turgor, abnormal pigmentation, spider angiomas, palmar erythema, and, possibly, jaundice
• *hepatic*—jaundice, hepatomegaly, ascites, edema of the legs, hepatic encephalopathy, and hepatorenal syndrome
• *miscellaneous*—musty breath, enlarged superficial abdominal veins, muscular atrophy, pain in the upper right abdominal quadrant that worsens when the patient sits up or leans forward, palpable liver or spleen, and temperature of 101° to 103° F. (38.3° to 39.4° C.); bleeding from esophageal varices results from portal hypertension.

INQUIRY

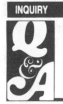

Questions patients ask about cirrhosis

How did alcohol damage my liver?
Drinking large amounts of alcohol over a long time overworks and eventually kills hepatic cells, the liver's worker cells. Scar tissue then fills in, causing changes that interfere with blood flow to the liver, which damages the remaining hepatic cells. Many alcoholics suffer from malnutrition, which also harms the liver.

Will my liver ever recover?
Hepatic cells have a remarkable ability to heal themselves. Be sure to get adequate rest, eat properly, eliminate alcohol, and take care to prevent infection. A damaged liver can regenerate within about 3 weeks and resume normal function within about 4 months. However, cells that die can't be replaced. That means the remaining cells must work harder.

Why is my skin itchy, yellow, and dry? And what can I do about it?
Your symptoms indicate liver damage. One of the liver's jobs is to process and excrete bilirubin, a pigment found in bile. When the liver is damaged, bilirubin can't be processed. As a result, it builds up in the body and accumulates in the skin, where it causes itching and yellowing. Your symptoms should go away in 4 to 6 months, as your liver heals and begins to process bilirubin normally again. In the meantime, to relieve skin discomfort, finish your shower or bath with a cool rinse, then pat—never rub—yourself dry. While your skin is still moist, apply an oil-based moisturizer. (However, don't use bath oil in the tub, which would increase the risk of falling.)

Diet
Because cirrhosis is associated partly with nutritional deficiencies, emphasize the importance of following dietary instructions to achieve remission of symptoms. Give the patient a copy of the teaching aid *Dietary do's and don'ts,* page 444. Tell him that his diet will depend on the severity of the disorder. If he has uncomplicated cirrhosis, tell him that the doctor may prescribe a diet high in calories, carbohydrates, and protein to promote liver regeneration and provide energy for muscle repair and rebuilding. If he has elevated levels of serum ammonia, he'll follow a low-protein diet to minimize the risk of developing uremia. Instruct him to take supplemental vitamins as ordered—A, B complex, D, and K to compensate for the liver's inability to store them, and vitamin B_{12}, folic acid, and thiamine to correct anemia.

Advise the patient to avoid fats if they cause indigestion or diarrhea. Also advise him to restrict sodium to prevent or reduce ascites. Above all, stress abstention from alcohol.

If anorexia's a problem, reinforce the importance of an adequate diet for liver cell regeneration. Advise small, frequent meals, liberal snacking, favorite foods (if allowed), and scrupulous mouth care (especially before meals to encourage adequate intake).

Medication
Instruct the patient to take medications carefully because the liver's ability to detoxify all substances is impaired. Inform him that antiemetics may be prescribed for nausea, diuretics for edema, and antacids for reducing the risk of GI bleeding. Give him guidelines for taking these drugs, and discuss potential adverse effects.

Surgery
If necessary, prepare the patient for portal-systemic shunting to relieve portal hypertension and prevent hemorrhage. Explain that surgery diverts blood flow from the portal vein into another vein that empties directly into the vena cava.

Before surgery. Inform the patient that the preoperative regimen may take 4 to 6 weeks. He'll require rest, a nutritious diet, supplemental vitamins, and adequate protein to relieve ascites and improve liver function. He'll also receive neomycin for 1 week before surgery to cleanse the bowel.

After surgery. Tell the patient that he'll return to the intensive care unit. (If possible, arrange for a preliminary visit.) Mention that he'll have several tubes and drains in place. For example, he'll have a nasogastric tube for 5 to 6 days to prevent distention by draining the GI tract and a drain (or chest tube) at the incisional site for 2 to 3 days to remove accumulated fluid. He'll be connected to a cardiac monitor and also have several hemodynamic monitoring lines—pulmonary artery, arterial, and central venous pressure catheters. Assure him that monitoring of his vital signs is a normal procedure.

Inform the patient that usually he'll resume eating in 5 to 6 days, beginning with clear liquids and gradually progressing to

Ruptured esophageal varices: A deadly complication

If your patient is at risk for portal hypertension, teach him about the danger of ruptured esophageal varices. Explain that esophageal varices are stretched veins whose walls are very thin. Like fragile balloons, they may break without warning, causing profuse bleeding that may be fatal without prompt intervention.

Explain that esophageal varices result from portal hypertension—increased pressure in the portal vein from obstruction in the portal circulation. As blood to the liver backs up, it begins to flow through collateral channels, such as the esophageal veins. The excessive pressure causes these thin-walled veins to be-

come varicose. If the pressure continues, they may rupture. The resulting hemorrhage can lead to hypovolemic shock.

Urge the patient to call the doctor immediately if he detects any signs of GI bleeding, such as dark, tarry stools or vomit that contains blood or looks like coffee grounds.

Teach him about procedures to treat esophageal varices. Electrocoagulation cauterizes the varices. Sclerotherapy, performed after the initial bleeding's controlled, involves injecting a sclerosing agent directly into the esophageal varices. Surgery is the only treatment for portal hypertension.

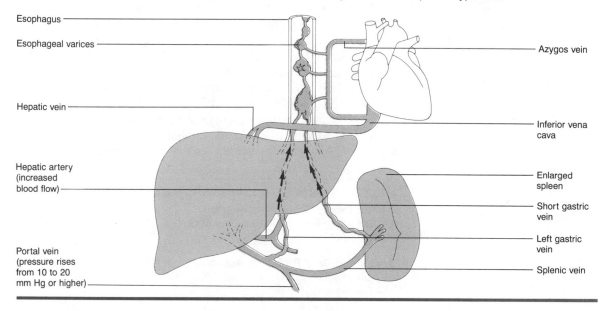

Esophagus

Esophageal varices

Azygos vein

Hepatic vein

Inferior vena cava

Hepatic artery (increased blood flow)

Enlarged spleen

Short gastric vein

Left gastric vein

Portal vein (pressure rises from 10 to 20 mm Hg or higher)

Splenic vein

solid foods. If he's not allowed to eat for more than a week, assure him that he'll receive adequate nourishment through total parenteral nutrition.

Pulmonary complications commonly occur after portal-systemic shunting because the surgical site lies close to the diaphragm. To help prevent them, instruct the patient to turn in bed, to cough and deep-breathe at least once every hour, and to use incentive spirometry. Advise him to ask for medication if moving and coughing cause pain. Show him how to splint his incision to minimize pain.

Discharge instructions. Assure the patient that it's normal to feel tired during the 6- to 8-week recovery period. Explain that the doctor may prescribe a low-protein, low-sodium diet and vitamin supplements. Emphasize the importance of adequate rest to reduce the risk of bleeding and infection. Reinforce the need for strict adherence to the prescribed discharge regimen by pointing out common complications—hepatic encephalopathy, GI bleeding, and ascites. Instruct him to call the doctor if he experiences any symptoms of these complications. Advise him and his family to watch for neurologic alterations, such as confusion, irritability, or lethargy. These symptoms may occur as shunting prevents conversion of ammonia to urea by diverting blood past the portal circulation and into the systemic venous circulation.

Other care measures
Because impaired hepatic production of prothrombin may cause a bleeding tendency, explain the warning signs of bleeding—weakness, hemoptysis, and blood in the stools and urine. Teach the patient to reduce this risk by avoiding aspirin, bruising, and straining during defecation. He should also avoid blowing his nose, sneezing, or coughing vigorously. Also suggest that he use an electric razor and a soft toothbrush.

Teach the patient to avoid contact with people who are ill, obtain adequate rest, and maintain his treatment regimen. Urge him to contact the doctor right away if he becomes ill.

Encourage the patient to seek counseling for alcohol or drug dependency, if appropriate. One of the most successful programs for alcoholism is Alcoholics Anonymous (AA). Provide the patient with the telephone number of the AA group in his area, or offer to arrange a visit from an AA member. Spouses of alcoholics can find support in Al-Anon, another self-help group; children in Alateen. Also explore alcohol rehabilitation programs.

Sources of information and support

Al-Anon Family Group Headquarters
P.O. Box 862, Midtown Station, New York, N.Y. 10018
(212) 302-7240

Alcohol and Drug Problems Association of North America
444 North Capitol Street, NW, Suite 706, Washington, D.C. 20001
(202) 737-4340

Alcoholics Anonymous World Services
P.O. Box 459, Grand Central Station, New York, N.Y. 10163
(212) 686-1100

Further readings

Clark, R.A. "Contrast-Enhancement Strategies in Hepatic CT," *Applied Radiology* 16(2):44-45, 49-50, February 1987.
"Confusion from Portal Occlusion," *Emergency Medicine* 20(17):163, October 15, 1988.
D'Epiro, P. "Acting on Abnormal Liver Findings," *Patient Care* 21(6):50-53, 57-58, March 30, 1987.
D'Epiro, P. "Toxic Liver Disease: Alcohol? Drugs?" *Patient Care* 21(11):153-56, 159, 162, June 15, 1987.
D'Epiro, P. "Which Tests for Liver Disease?" *Patient Care* 21(7):124-27, 131-32, April 15, 1987.
Hennessy, K. "Nutritional Support and Gastrointestinal Disease," *Nursing Clinics of North America* 24(2):373-82, June 1989.
Pimstone, N.R. "Liver Function Tests: Assessing Adequacy of Excretion and Synthesis," *Consultant* 28(8):113-15, 118-20, August 1988.
Pimstone, N.R. "The Spectrum of Alcoholic Liver Disease," *Hospital Medicine,* 22(10): 23-25, 29, 32+, October 1986.

Preparing for a liver biopsy

Dear Patient:

Your doctor wants you to have a liver biopsy. This test helps diagnose cirrhosis and other liver disorders. The test involves removing a small liver sample and studying it under a microscope. Usually, it takes about 15 minutes, and results are available within a day.

Before the test
• Don't eat or drink anything for 4 to 8 hours before the test, as your doctor orders.
• Expect to have a blood test to measure your blood's clotting ability and other factors.
• Just before the test, be sure to empty your bladder.

The procedure
During the test, you'll lie on your back with your right hand under your head. You'll need to remain in this position, and keep as still as you can. The doctor will drape and cleanse an area on your abdomen. He'll then inject a local anesthetic, which may sting and cause brief discomfort.

When you're told, hold your breath and lie still as the doctor inserts the biopsy needle into the liver. Be assured that the needle will remain in your liver for only about 1 second. The needle may cause a sensation of pressure and some discomfort in your right upper back.

After the needle is withdrawn, resume normal breathing. The doctor will apply pressure to the biopsy site to stop any bleeding. Then he'll apply a pressure bandage.

After the test
• You'll be told to lie on your right side for 2 hours, with a small pillow tucked under your side. For the next 24 hours, you should rest in bed. Your vital signs will be checked periodically.
• Tell your doctor or nurse right away if you experience any problems, including chest pain, persistent shoulder pain, or difficulty breathing.
• You can resume your normal diet.

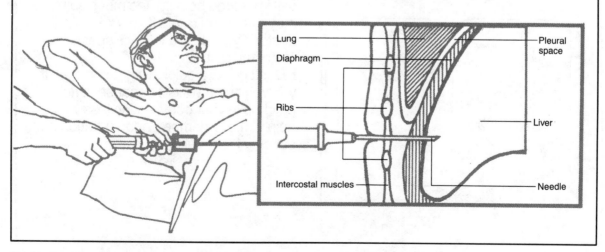

Dietary do's and don'ts

Dear Patient:

Because you have cirrhosis, you need to pay special attention to your diet. Healthful eating habits will help damaged hepatic cells to regenerate and prevent harm to the remaining cells. Follow this list of do's and don'ts when planning your daily meals.

Do's

● Ask your doctor, nurse, or dietitian for help in planning your diet. They can advise you about how many calories you need and how to best meet your nutritional requirements. If you're used to eating fast foods, they can help you choose the most nutritious ones on a fast-food menu.

● Eat small, frequent meals. Instead of the traditional three square meals, try eating five or six lighter ones. This may relieve the bloated or sick feeling that cirrhosis can cause.

● Keep a food diary. After each meal, jot down the foods you ate, the time of day, and how you feel.

After a week, study your food diary for patterns. For example, did certain foods disagree with you? If so, avoid them. What time of day were you hungriest? Plan to eat your biggest meal then. Use the diary to make smarter choices about what and when to eat.

● Weigh yourself daily, and keep a chart. If your weight goes up more than five pounds, call your doctor — you may be retaining fluid.

● Set an attractive table. To perk up your appetite, use nice tableware, add a colorful garnish to your plate, and set an appropriate mood with relaxing music or conversation.

Don'ts

● Avoid drinking alcoholic beverages — even occasionally. Alcohol destroys liver cells, so abstain completely.

● Stay away from coffee or tea. Avoid all caffeine-containing beverages and foods, which can cause indigestion.

● Steer clear of spicy foods, which may upset your stomach.

● Eliminate salt while cooking, and don't salt your food heavily. Too much salt may make you retain fluid. Ask your doctor if you should follow a special salt-restricted diet.

● Don't go on a quick weight-loss diet. If you've gained weight because of fluid build-up in your body, eating less won't help you. Remember, good nutrition is essential to repair your liver.

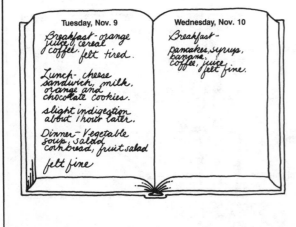

Chronic pancreatitis

The prognosis for chronic pancreatitis is good if the patient complies with his treatment plan—and poor if he doesn't. Yet compliance may be difficult, requiring that the patient—commonly an alcoholic male between the ages of 45 and 60—change years of poor health habits and alcohol abuse. Compliance may also be difficult because family and social support often deteriorates in alcoholism. Your teaching, though, may help the patient begin to accept and control his problems.

You may need to teach the patient slowly and in short sessions because alcoholism can lead to cognitive deficits and slowed comprehension. You'll need to help him understand the relationship between his disorder and alcoholism. You'll also need to prepare him for tests to confirm the disorder or detect complications. And you'll need to teach about treatments—proper diet to reduce gastric secretions and drugs to relieve symptoms and prevent complications—that may allow him to control his disease.

Discuss the disorder

Teach the patient that recurring episodes of inflammation progressively damage the pancreas. Explain that the pancreas normally secretes digestive enzymes. But in chronic pancreatitis, the duct through which these enzymes leave the pancreas becomes blocked. The enzymes back up into the pancreas and eventually begin to destroy pancreatic tissue.

Explain that the term "chronic" means that the disease is of long duration, and damage may have occurred well before the appearance of any signs and symptoms and independently of acute episodes. Tell the patient that continuous or intermittent abdominal pain is the hallmark of the disease, usually with signs of exocrine impairment—diarrhea, steatorrhea, and weight loss.

Point out that long-term, heavy alcohol abuse accounts for most chronic pancreatitis. Scientists theorize that protein precipitates block the pancreatic duct and eventually calcify. Subsequent structural changes lead to fibrosis and glandular atrophy. However, a wide range of other disorders—and some drugs—have been linked to disease development as well (see *Chronic pancreatitis: Causes and effects*, page 446).

Complications

Stress that failure to comply with treatment can cause complications, including the following:

Debra Harris Lillback, RN, BSN, MSN, and **Catherine Kelly Foran, RN, MSN,** contributed to this chapter. Ms. Lillback is a quality assessment coordinator at Crozer-Chester Medical Center in Upland, Pa. Ms. Foran is an independent nursing consultant in Cherry Hill, N.J.

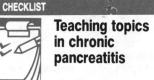

CHECKLIST

Teaching topics in chronic pancreatitis

☐ Explanation of chronic pancreatitis, its causes, and major signs and symptoms
☐ Complications, such as diabetes and variceal bleeding, and their warning signs
☐ Preparation for diagnostic tests, including computed tomography, ultrasonography, endoscopic retrograde cholangiopancreatography, and collection of stool specimens
☐ Dietary measures to decrease the demand for pancreatic enzymes
☐ Drug therapy to reduce gastric acidity, replace pancreatic enzymes, relieve pain, and control hyperglycemia
☐ Preparation for surgery, if necessary
☐ Measures to relieve symptoms and prevent complications, such as avoiding infection, smoking cessation, and abstinence from alcohol
☐ Sources of information and support

Chronic pancreatitis: Causes and effects

Linked to alcohol abuse in over 50% of patients, chronic pancreatitis results from other causes too. Discuss these causes and the signs and symptoms that signal disease as well.

Underlying conditions
Besides alcoholism, the following can cause chronic pancreatitis: cystic fibrosis, Crohn's disease, hyperlipidemia, hyperparathyroidism, lupus erythematosus, malnutrition, penetrating duodenal ulcer, traumatic injury, viral infection, and some drugs.

Drug-related causes
Experts disagree about whether disease or its drug treatment damages the pancreas. They do agree, though, on these drug suspects: anticholinergics, asparaginase, azathioprine, corticosteroids, diazoxide, estrogens, ethacrynic acid, furosemide, isoniazid, opiates, procainamide, salicylates, sulfonamides, tetracyclines, and thiazides.

Signs and symptoms
If your patient's taking any of these drugs or if he has underlying disease, advise him to seek attention for these warnings of chronic pancreatitis:
• anorexia and weight loss
• bluish navel area
• bruising of loin skin
• bulky, foul-smelling stools
• hypotension
• low-grade fever
• nausea and vomiting
• pain (in midepigastrium, left chest, and back—may be constant with acute episodes aggravated by meals and relieved by bending forward)
• tachycardia
• tender, swollen abdomen.

• pseudocysts containing pancreatic enzymes and tissue debris. If these growths become infected, an abscess may result.
• hyperglycemia, leading to diabetes. Teach the patient that damage to the pancreatic islet cells causes this disorder.
• gallbladder disease. Explain that this complication results from compression of the common bile duct as it passes through the pancreas.
• GI bleeding, which may result from peptic ulcers or variceal bleeding. Caution the patient that taking excessive aspirin for pain relief may cause ulcers. Explain that portal or splenic vein thrombosis may cause variceal bleeding.
• steatorrhea. Tell the patient that steatorrhea is a consequence of impaired fat digestion and failure to follow a low-fat diet.
• cancer, a rare complication, which occurs more commonly in hereditary or familial pancreatitis.

Describe the diagnostic workup
Prepare the patient for diagnostic tests to confirm chronic pancreatitis and detect complications. Tests may include: abdominal X-ray or computed tomography (CT) to reveal pancreatic calcification; ultrasonography or CT to evaluate the size of the pancreas and pseudocysts; and endoscopic retrograde cholangiopancreatography (ERCP) to visualize the pancreatic ducts. Also give the patient instructions for collecting stool specimens to evaluate exocrine function.

CT scan
Explain that this test examines the pancreas through computerized X-ray images. Inform the patient that the test is painless, and that it takes about 1½ hours. Instruct him to restrict food and fluids after midnight before the test but to continue any drug regimen as ordered.

Explain that during the test the patient will lie on a table while X-rays are taken. Tell him to lie still, relax, breathe normally, and remain quiet because movement will blur the X-ray picture and prolong the test. If the doctor is using an I.V. contrast medium, inform the patient that he may experience discomfort from the needle puncture and a localized feeling of warmth on injection. Instruct him to report immediately any adverse reactions: nausea, vomiting, dizziness, headache, or urticaria. Assure him that reactions are rare. Tell him that he may resume his normal diet after the test.

Endoscopic retrograde cholangiopancreatography
Teach the patient that ERCP examines the liver, gallbladder, and pancreas through X-ray films. (For details on ERCP procedure, see *Teaching about ERCP*.) Inform him that these films are obtained with a flexible tube passed through the mouth into the intestine. The test takes 30 to 60 minutes. Describe the preparation for the test: he must restrict food and fluids after midnight before the test but should continue any drug regimen as ordered. Tell him that he'll wear a hospital gown and that he should urinate before the test because ERCP can cause urine retention.

Teaching about ERCP

Endoscopic retrograde cholangiopancreatography (ERCP) uses both radiography and endoscopy to examine the pancreatic ducts and hepatobiliary tree.

Teach the patient that the doctor will advance a small side-viewing endoscope through the patient's mouth, esophagus, stomach, and duodenum until he identifies the ampulla of Vater, which is the duodenal end of the drainage systems of the pancreatic and common bile ducts. He then injects a contrast medium by passing a cannula through the endoscope.

Explain that ERCP helps diagnose suspected pancreatic disease. It's also used to locate cysts, calculi, and stenosis in the pancreatic ducts and hepatobiliary tree, particularly when other radiographic studies, such as ultrasonography, computed tomography scans, liver scans, and biliary tract X-rays yield inconclusive findings.

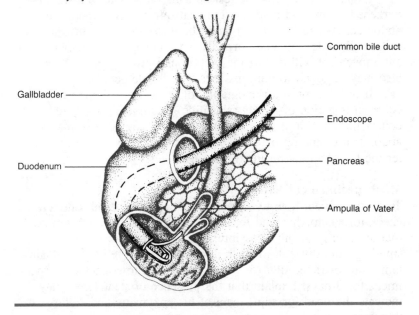

Inform the patient that he'll be awake during the test. Explain that he'll receive a sedative to help him relax because the test is uncomfortable. He'll lie on an X-ray table, and a nurse will take his vital signs and insert an I.V. line into his hand or arm to administer medication.

Before insertion of the tube, the patient's throat will be sprayed with a local anesthetic. Advise him that the spray tastes unpleasant and will make his mouth and throat feel swollen and numb, causing difficulty in swallowing. Instruct him to let the saliva drain from the side of his mouth. Tell him that he'll have a mouthguard to protect his teeth from the tube. Assure him he'll have no difficulty breathing.

After insertion of the tube, he'll receive an anticholinergic or glucagon I.V. to relax the small intestine. Instruct him to report any adverse reactions: dry mouth, thirst, tachycardia, or blurred vision (from the anticholinergic); nausea, vomiting, urticaria, or flushing (from glucagon). Once the small intestine relaxes, he'll be asked to assume various positions to advance the tube to the pancreas and hepatobiliary tree. Inform him that he may experience warmth or flushing with injection of the contrast medium.

Tell the patient that after the test his vital signs will be checked frequently for several hours. Mention that he'll be allowed to eat when his gag reflex returns, usually in about 1 hour. He may have a sore throat for several days.

Ultrasonography

Inform the patient that this procedure uses sound waves to produce images of the pancreas. Tell him that the test takes about 15 to 30 minutes. Instruct him to restrict food and fluids for 8 to 12 hours before the test. If he's having ultrasonography of his gallbladder and biliary system, instruct him to eat a fat-free meal the evening before the test before beginning his fast.

Explain that during the test he'll lie on a table in a slightly darkened room, and he'll feel the transducer moving across his abdomen. Assure him that it won't be uncomfortable. Instruct him to lie still, relax, breathe normally, and remain quiet. Explain that any movement will distort the picture and prolong the test. He also may be asked to hold his breath or inhale deeply.

If he's having ultrasonography of the gallbladder, he may receive an injection of a drug (sincalide) to stimulate gallbladder contraction. Tell him to report immediately any adverse reactions: abdominal cramping, nausea, dizziness, sweating, or flushing. After the test, he may resume his normal diet.

Stool specimen collection

Teach the patient how to collect a stool specimen and routinely check for steatorrhea and fecal blood. Tell him to watch for stools that are greasy or oily (possibly with a silver sheen), foul-smelling, and difficult to flush down the toilet. Tell him to maintain a fat-restricted diet for 2 to 3 days, then to collect stool specimens for 3 days. Explain that the presence of steatorrhea may indicate the need for adjustment of his enzymatic and dietary therapy.

Teach about treatments

Although pancreatic damage cannot be reversed, compliance with treatment will lessen the chance of complications. Teach the patient about the need for pancreatic enzyme replacement and other prescribed medications. Instruct him to rest frequently, follow a fat-restricted diet, and abstain from alcohol. If he has severe pain or complications, discuss his surgical options, if appropriate.

Activity

Explain that the patient may have less energy than usual because of malabsorption of calories and nutrients. Advise him to conserve his energy by resting frequently between periods of activity. Instruct him to rest after meals to aid digestion. Assure him that he may be able to tolerate more activity as his condition improves. However, instruct him to check with the doctor or nutritionist before increasing his activity level.

Diet
Explain that diet therapy aims to reduce gastric secretion. Usually, the doctor prescribes a bland, low-fat, high-carbohydrate, high-protein diet to decrease the demand for pancreatic enzymes. Instruct the patient to avoid rich, fatty foods, which will aggravate his symptoms. Give him a copy of the patient-teaching aid *Combating pancreatitis with a low-fat diet,* page 454.

Encourage the patient to eat small, frequent meals, thereby minimizing the secretion of pancreatic enzymes. Emphasize the importance of eliminating alcohol entirely. If diabetes is a problem, help the patient incorporate the necessary dietary restrictions. If he's malnourished or underweight, explore what foods he likes, so he can increase calories while maintaining his diet.

Medication
Inform the patient that drug treatment relieves symptoms and prevents complications. Prescribed drugs may include antacids, anticholinergics, and cimetidine to decrease gastric acidity; pancreatin or pancrelipase to replace pancreatic enzymes; narcotics to relieve pain; and insulin, glucagon, or oral hypoglycemic agents to control hyperglycemia. (See *Teaching about drugs for chronic pancreatitis,* pages 450 and 451.)

If the patient is taking a narcotic analgesic, such as meperidine (Demerol), tell him to report excessive sleepiness, euphoria, nausea, vomiting, constipation, light-headedness, and fainting. Advise him not to drive or operate machinery, as the drug may cause drowsiness. If he becomes constipated, tell him to check with the doctor about taking a stool softener. Caution him not to take over-the-counter drugs with narcotic analgesics unless his doctor consents.

If the doctor prescribes an anticholinergic, such as atropine, tell the patient to report blurred vision, constipation, or tachycardia. Instruct him to avoid alcohol and other central nervous system depressants because adverse reactions may worsen. Inform him that this drug may reduce sweating, allowing body temperature to rise. To prevent heatstroke, caution him to avoid becoming overheated during exercise or hot weather.

Surgery
Prepare the patient for surgery, if necessary. Explain that surgery aims to relieve chronic pain, treat complications (especially those that are life-threatening), and preserve functioning pancreatic tissue. Surgical options fall into two categories: pancreatic resection and decompression of the ductal system. (See *Chronic pancreatic pain: New surgical approaches,* page 452.) Advise him to question the doctor about the risks and benefits of surgery, and to weigh his decision carefully.

If the patient has an abscess, tell him that it will be lanced and drained. If he has gallbladder disease, inform him that a cholecystectomy may be performed to remove the gallbladder. In sphincter spasm or hypertrophy, explain that a choledochojejunostomy restores free flow of bile into the jejunum by anasto-

continued on page 453

Teaching about drugs for chronic pancreatitis

DRUG	ADVERSE REACTIONS	TEACHING POINTS
Antihypoglycemic agent		
glucagon	• Watch for hypersensitivity (difficulty breathing, dizziness, or rash). • Other reactions include light-headedness, nausea, and vomiting.	• Teach the patient how to mix the medication accurately. Show him how to properly use an appropriate-sized syringe and how to inject the medication at a 90-degree angle. • Recommend that he use medication within 3 months after mixing and store the mixed solution in refrigerator. Instruct him to store any unmixed medication at room temperature. Caution him not to store his medication in the bathroom, which often becomes hot and humid. • Instruct the patient and his family how to administer glucagon accurately and how to recognize characteristic signs and symptoms of hypoglycemia. Urge them to call a doctor immediately in an emergency. • Tell him to expect a response usually within 20 minutes after injection of this medication. Explain that the injection may be repeated if no response occurs. • Instruct him to seek medical assistance if a second injection of medication is needed.
Anti-ulcer agents		
cimetidine (Tagamet) **famotidine** (Pepcid) **nizatidine** (Axid) **ranitidine** (Zantac)	• Watch for confusion, unusual bleeding or bruising, and unusual tiredness or weakness. • Other reactions include decreased sexual ability, diarrhea, dizziness, gynecomastia, headache, muscle cramps or pain, and rash.	• Inform the patient that smoking interferes with the effect of this drug. Advise him to stop smoking. If abstinence is not possible, discourage smoking after taking the evening dose to prevent interference with drug control of nocturnal gastric acid secretion. • If he misses a dose, instruct him to take the missed dose as soon as possible. However, if it's almost time for his next dose, tell him to skip the missed dose and resume his regular schedule. He must never double-dose. • Tell him to take the drug at bedtime if he's taking the drug once a day. • Advise him to separate doses of these drugs and antacids by 1 hour (decreased absorption possible).
Digestants (pancreatic enzymes)		
pancreatin (Pancreatin Enseals) **pancrelipase** (Cotazym, Pancrease, Viokase)	• Watch for diarrhea, hematuria, joint pain, nausea, and swelling of feet. • Other reactions include stomach cramps and stomach pain.	• Tell the patient to follow the doctor's instructions about taking this drug with meals. • Caution him never to chew, break, or crush the tablet form because this destroys the coating and may cause GI irritation. However, he may open the capsule form and gently mix the contents with soft foods. • Instruct him not to inhale the powder, which may result in a stuffy nose, shortness of breath, wheezing, and chest tightness.

continued

Teaching about drugs for chronic pancreatitis — *continued*

DRUG	ADVERSE REACTIONS	TEACHING POINTS
Injectable hypoglycemic		
insulin	• Watch for difficulty breathing, frequent or severe hypoglycemia or hyperglycemia, itching, and skin changes at injection site (such as redness, swelling, stinging, or itching). • Other reactions include mild hypoglycemia or hyperglycemia.	• Explain that insulin helps control blood glucose levels. Emphasize that it's not meant to replace proper diet. • Tell the patient never to adjust the dosage or stop the drug without the doctor's approval: a rapid elevation in blood glucose levels could occur. Also explain the importance of injecting insulin on schedule to avoid extreme fluctuations in blood glucose levels. • Teach him how to administer insulin subcutaneously. Also instruct him how to mix insulin in a syringe. Tell him not to change the order in which he mixes insulins. Stress the importance of administering insulin promptly after mixing to avoid loss in potency. • Advise him to administer insulin at room temperature. Refrigeration isn't necessary unless room temperature is very cold or warm. • Tell him to rotate injection sites. Show him appropriate sites and help him plan rotation. • Teach him to press, not rub, the injection site after withdrawing the needle. Advise him never to change the brand of insulin, syringe, or needle and to use the correct syringe for his type of insulin concentration. • Review blood and urine testing, using the procedure of the patient's choice. Emphasize the importance of monitoring blood glucose levels. • Advise the patient always to wear medical identification, such as a Medic Alert bracelet or necklace stating that he takes insulin to control diabetes. • Tell him to avoid alcohol and aspirin (and other salicylates). Explain that salicylates and alcohol increase insulin's hypoglycemic effect.
Oral hypoglycemics		
acetohexamide (Dymelor) **chlorpropamide** (Diabinese) **glipizide** (Glucotrol) **glyburide** (Micronase) **tolazamide** (Tolinase) **tolbutamide** (Orinase)	• Watch for hypoglycemia and jaundice. • Other reactions include epigastric fullness, facial flushing, headache, heartburn, nausea, rash, and vomiting.	• Explain that this drug helps control blood glucose levels. Emphasize that it's not meant to replace proper diet. • Tell the patient to take the drug exactly as prescribed and not to adjust the dosage or stop taking it without the doctor's approval. • Advise him to avoid alcohol and aspirin (and other salicylates). • Instruct him to take this drug before meals, if possible, for full benefit. • Tell him to monitor his blood glucose levels daily. Show him how to obtain a sample of his blood or urine to check for glucose, using the procedure of his choice. • If he experiences increased stress or illness, tell him to notify the doctor. Explain that a dosage adjustment may be necessary, or he may require insulin.

Chronic pancreatic pain: New surgical approaches

Intractable pain is the primary reason for pancreatic surgery. If your patient's pain is severe enough to warrant narcotic medication, encourage him to discuss his surgical options with the doctor. Point out, however, that no single operation works for all patients, and none of the procedures consistently achieves the desired results.

Unfortunately, though pancreatic resection often provides excellent pain relief, it may cause immediate diabetes mellitus and other major complications. An alternative procedure is decompression of the ductal system. However, this operation isn't feasible for many patients, whose ducts are too small, and it may not relieve pain. To overcome these problems, three new operations have been devised.

Duodenum-preserving resection of the pancreatic head

This procedure controls pain by removing diseased tissue from the head of the pancreas, while allowing secretions from the duodenal rim of pancreatic tissue to drain into the jejunum. A loop of jejunum is interposed between the left side of the resected pancreas and the cored-out pancreatic head.

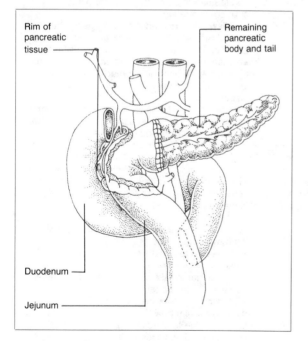

Longitudinal pancreaticojejunostomy

Combined with removal of diseased tissue from the pancreatic head, this operation allows secretions from the remainder of the pancreatic head and most of the main pancreatic duct to drain into a loop of jejunum. This procedure permits effective drainage of

the diseased head, even when it contains obstructed ducts and pseudocysts. It also provides decompression of the main duct throughout the body and tail.

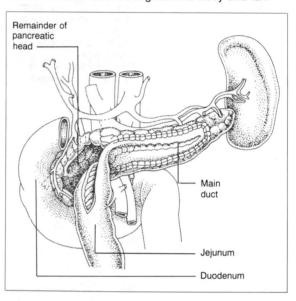

Near-total excision of the pancreatic head

This operation leaves a small amount of tissue on the inner part of the duodenum, and the denervated body and tail remain attached to the splenic circulation. The pancreatic ducts then drain into the jejunum. This procedure provides effective pain relief. However, the remaining pancreatic tissue provides a site for abscess and fistula formation.

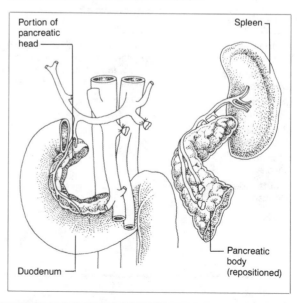

mosing the common bile duct to the jejunum. A sphincterotomy enlarges the pancreatic sphincter, which has been narrowed by fibrosis, and a vagotomy may relax the sphincter and decrease pancreatic secretion. If the patient's pain is severe, a splanchnic resection controls pain, but doesn't change or prevent attacks.

Other care measures

Instruct the patient to reduce his risk of infection by proper hand washing, getting adequate rest, and avoiding crowds and people with known infections. Tell him to contact the doctor immediately if he becomes ill.

Teach the patient relaxation techniques to manage pain before he requires narcotic analgesics, to minimize the risk of addiction. If he develops diabetes or a peptic ulcer, teach him what he needs to know about the disorder.

Discourage smoking. Explain that smoking changes pancreatic secretions that neutralize gastric acid in the duodenum. If the patient needs help abstaining from alcohol, encourage him to seek help from Alcoholics Anonymous.

Sources of information and support

Alcoholics Anonymous World Services
P.O. Box 459, Grand Central Station, New York, N.Y. 10163
(212) 686-1100

American Diabetes Association
National Service Center, P.O. Box 25757, 1660 Duke Street, Alexandria, Va. 22314
(704) 549-1500

Nutrition Education Association
P.O. Box 20301, 3647 Glen Haven, Houston, Texas 77225
(713) 665-2946

Further readings

Banks, P.A., et al. "The Spectrum of Chronic Pancreatitis," *Patient Care* 23(9):163-65, 168, 170+, May 15, 1989.
Hennessy, K. "Nutritional Support and Gastrointestinal Disease," *Nursing Clinics of North America* 24(2):373-82, June 1989.
Holm, A., and Aldrete, J.S. "The Patient Undergoing Pancreatic Surgery," *Current Reviews for Post Anesthesia Care Nurses* 9(1):2-8, 1987.
Mills, A.S. "Pancreatitis: Disruption in Structure and Function," *Gastroenterology Nursing* 12(1):63-65, Summer 1989.
"Pancreatitis From Acne Medication," *Hospital Medicine* 23(9):43, 46, 49, September 1987.
"Recurrent Pancreatitis Linked to Metronidazole," *Nurses Drug Alert* 13(2):13, February 1989.

Combating pancreatitis with a low-fat diet

Dear Patient:

Because you have chronic pancreatitis, the doctor wants you to eat less fat. You should eat no more than 2 teaspoons of fat daily, including fat used in cooking. And you should avoid fatty foods, such as nuts, cream sauces, gravy, peanut butter, french fries, and potato chips. Your new, low-fat diet is high in protein and carbohydrates.

Normally, the pancreas secretes enzymes into the digestive tract, where they help to break down food. In chronic pancreatitis, the duct through which these enzymes leave the pancreas is blocked. As a result, your digestive system has trouble changing food into the nutrients and energy your body needs. By following the list of foods to eat or avoid, you may find relief from your symptoms.

Foods to eat	Foods to avoid
Fruits and vegetables Fruit juices, most fruits, white or sweet potatoes, all other vegetables that don't cause discomfort	Avocado (unless well tolerated), apples, melon, broccoli, brussels sprouts, cabbage, cauliflower, cucumbers, garlic, dried peas or beans, onions, green peppers, rutabaga, sauerkraut, turnips
High-protein foods, such as meat About 6 ounces daily of lean meat, fish, poultry (baked, broiled, roasted, or stewed); fat-free, broth-based soups (such as chicken noodle) or soups made with skim milk	Highly seasoned or fatty meats, such as ham, hot dogs, sausage, bacon, cold cuts, corned beef, goose, duck, poultry skin, spareribs, regular ground beef, tuna packed in oil, all cheeses not made from skim milk, commercial soups or any soup made with milk or cream
Milk and dairy products Skim milk, buttermilk made from skim milk, one whole egg daily (including that used in cooking), egg whites (prepared without fat), low-fat cottage cheese or cheese made from skim milk	Ice cream, whole milk, 2% milk, beverages made from cream
Grains and cereals Pasta, rice, enriched white and whole-grain bread, graham crackers, saltines, cereals	Quick breads, muffins, biscuits, high-fat or sweet breads and rolls, party crackers, 100% bran cereal (unless well tolerated)
Sweets and beverages Angel food cake, sherbet, gelatin desserts, fruit whips, sugar, honey, jam, jelly, syrup, molasses, plain sugar candies, desserts made from skim milk or egg whites	Candy; commercial desserts; desserts made with nuts, chocolate, cream, coconut, or lots of fat; alcoholic beverages; caffeine-containing drinks, such as coffee, tea, breakfast cocoa, and regular colas

Hiatal hernia

Even in its mildest form, hiatal hernia can disrupt the patient's life, forcing him to cope with recurring malaise and persistent dysphagia. To control his condition, your teaching will need to emphasize the direct relationship between the patient's symptoms and his meals, activities, and medications. He'll need to integrate the necessary restrictions into his life-style.

However, because the patient is usually over age 50 and has developed lifelong habits, he may resist your instructions. By helping him understand the need and the methods for preventing extended contact between stomach contents and the esophagus, you can help him reduce the number of painful episodes he experiences.

You'll have to warn him, though, that compliance doesn't guarantee that damage to the stomach or esophageal mucosa won't occur. Complications, such as esophagitis, are common, even if the patient has followed the doctor's instructions to the letter. If this happens, it's important that you discourage him from blaming himself or the doctor.

Discuss the disorder

Prevent confusion by informing the patient that "esophageal," "hiatus," "hiatal," and "diaphragmatic" hernia are all names for the same condition. Explain that a hiatal hernia results from a weakening or enlargement of the diaphragm opening that encircles the distal esophagus. This defect allows part of the stomach to protrude into the chest cavity when intra-abdominal pressure rises—for example, with coughing or bending from the waist. Tell the patient that with these pressure changes, stomach contents and secretions push upward into the esophagus, causing gas or heartburn. (See *What happens in hiatal hernia,* page 456.) The reflux of secretions can also erode the lining of the esophagus.

Inform the patient that muscle weakening, causing insufficient closure of the opening, may result from congenital weakness, abdominal or chest injury, or a loss of muscle tone from aging, pregnancy, or obesity.

Complications

Warn the patient that neglecting his treatment plan will increase his chances of suffering reflux (regurgitation) and heartburn and developing complications, such as irritation of the esophageal mucosa, leading to esophagitis or ulceration, and respiratory distress,

Catherine K. Foran, RN, MSN, and **Brenda L. W. Hagan, RN,C, MSN,** contributed to this chapter. Ms. Foran is an independent nursing consultant in Cherry Hill, NJ. Ms. Hagan is director of clinical services for Liberty Healthcare Corporation in Philadelphia.

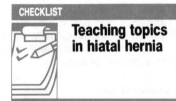

CHECKLIST

Teaching topics in hiatal hernia

☐ Explanation of hiatal hernia as muscle weakness of the diaphragm opening that encircles the distal esophagus and stomach
☐ Possible complications: esophagitis and ulceration, respiratory distress, aspiration pneumonia, cardiac dysfunction, and mucosal erosion
☐ Preparation for tests to confirm hiatal hernia, such as barium swallow, endoscopy, and esophageal manometry
☐ Meal scheduling, size, and contents
☐ Use of antacids, cholinergics, and other drugs to relieve symptoms and prevent complications
☐ Preoperative instruction for hernia repair, if necessary
☐ Positioning, cessation of smoking, and avoidance of activities that increase intra-abdominal pressure

What happens in hiatal hernia

Hiatal hernia includes two classic types: sliding and rolling or paraesophageal.

Two types

In *sliding* hernia (which accounts for over 90% of adult hernias), the stomach slips upward into the chest cavity, displacing organs and causing esophageal spasm when the patient lies down or when activities, such as bending or sneezing, increase intra-abdominal pressure. When he stands or the pressure subsides, the stomach usually slides back into the abdomen. In *rolling* hernia, the stomach sphincter remains below the diaphragm, and the fundus rolls up beside the esophagus when intra-abdominal pressure rises or the patient lies down. Some patients have a *combined* hernia, in which both types occur.

Hernia signs and symptoms

Signs and symptoms, especially heartburn, occur in 50% of patients. Belching and bloating may occur, resulting from increased swallowing in an attempt to remove acid from the esophagus. Reflux may cause aspiration pneumonia.

Other possible signs and symptoms include pain, dyspnea, and tachycardia, which result from rising intrathoracic pressure when part of the stomach slides into the thoracic cavity. Accompanying esophageal spasm may cause severe pain radiating to the back, shoulder, or arm.

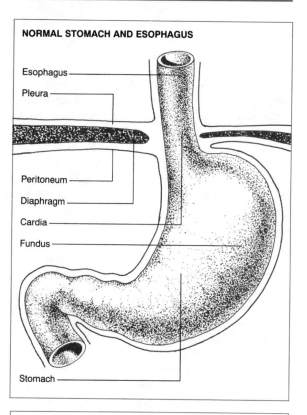

NORMAL STOMACH AND ESOPHAGUS

Esophagus
Pleura
Peritoneum
Diaphragm
Cardia
Fundus
Stomach

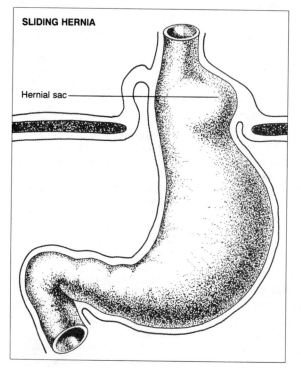

SLIDING HERNIA

Hernial sac

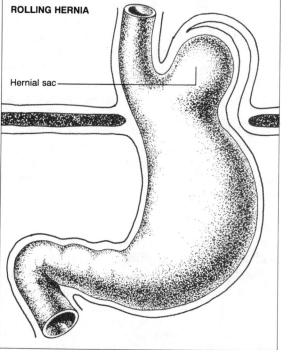

ROLLING HERNIA

Hernial sac

aspiration pneumonia, or cardiac dysfunction from the pressure on his lungs and heart. Tell him that mucosal erosion can result in hemorrhage, peritonitis, and mediastinitis.

Explain that these complications result from the pressure exerted by the stomach bulk pressing upward and the irritation caused by contact between the stomach contents and the esophagus or lungs.

Describe the diagnostic workup

Teach the patient about diagnostic tests used to determine mucosal damage. These tests include a barium swallow, endoscopy, and esophageal manometry.

Barium swallow

Explain that a barium swallow (or upper GI examination) is a radiographic test ordered if the patient has a history of dysphagia and reflux. Tell him that it's used to detect defects in the esophageal pathway and takes about 30 minutes.

Instruct the patient to refrain from eating or drinking for 6 to 8 hours before the test and from smoking the morning of the test. Because enemas increase gastric secretions and motility, they shouldn't be used the evening or morning before the test. Advise him to remove jewelry, dentures, and other objects that may obscure details on the X-ray film.

Inform the patient that during the test a technician will ask him to swallow thick and thin mixtures of barium sulfate. Explain that the barium clearly outlines the esophageal pathway. Describe barium's chalky taste, but also reassure him that it's flavored to make it more palatable. Explain that a series of X-ray films will be taken as the barium progresses to his stomach.

Tell the patient that after the test he'll have chalk-colored stools for 1 to 3 days as the barium passes through the bowel. Advise him to call the doctor if his stools aren't chalky. Stress the importance of barium elimination, explaining that retained barium may become impacted, leading to distention, pain, and perforation of the intestine. Tell the patient that, if needed, additional X-ray films will be taken after he's expelled all of the barium.

Endoscopy and manometry

Inform the patient that endoscopy is used to assess the damage to the esophageal lining. Explain that a flexible rubber tube called an endoscope will be inserted through his mouth and into his stomach. A fiber-optic device within the tube allows the doctor to examine the esophagus. During the procedure, a small brush inserted through the tube may be used to obtain samples of the mucosal lining for cytology. Manometry (measurement of the esophageal sphincter pressure) or a gastric acidity determination may also be performed. The test takes several minutes to half an hour.

Instruct the patient to refrain from eating or drinking for 6 to 12 hours before the test. If he wears dentures, he should remove

Reducing heartburn with histamine₂-receptor antagonists

Histamine is a powerful stimulant of gastric acid secretion. By blocking the action of histamine, cimetidine (Tagamet) and ranitidine (Zantac), for example, decrease gastric acid levels and relieve the heartburn associated with reflux.

Instruct the patient taking a histamine₂-receptor antagonist to report confusion, unusual bleeding or bruising, unusual tiredness, and weakness. He may also experience diarrhea, decreased sexual ability, dizziness, gynecomastia, headache, muscle cramps or pain, and rash.

Tell the patient to take the medication with or immediately after meals. Food delays absorption of these drugs and prolongs their effects. Because antacids can also interfere with drug absorption, advise him to wait at least 1 hour between taking a histamine₂-receptor antagonist and an antacid.

Ideally, the patient should quit smoking because smoking reduces the effectiveness of histamine₂-receptor antagonists. If abstinence isn't possible, discourage him from smoking after the evening dose to prevent interference with drug control of nocturnal gastric acid secretion.

If the patient misses a dose, instruct him to take the missed dose as soon as possible. However, if it's almost time for his next dose, tell him to skip the missed dose and then resume his regular schedule. Caution him never to double-dose.

them before the test. Tell him that about an hour before the test he'll receive a sedative to help him relax and medication to reduce secretions.

Tell the patient that before the tube is inserted, he'll be given a gargle or throat spray containing a local anesthetic to keep him from gagging. The doctor will then ask him to swallow the endoscope tube. To reduce the discomfort, instruct him to breathe through his mouth with a panting motion while swallowing. If the doctor will be examining the stomach and duodenum, the patient will be asked to lie on his side. Emphasize the importance of remaining still to prevent perforation. Explain that during the test a suction machine will keep his mouth and throat free of secretions. Describe the sound made by this machine.

Inform the patient that after the test he may have a sore throat for several days. Suggest that he use a throat spray or lozenges. He may also cough up a small amount of blood during the first day. Instruct him to call the doctor if he has difficulty swallowing, as this may be a sign of laryngeal or pharyngeal swelling. Tell him also to notify the doctor if he vomits, particularly if the vomit contains blood, or if he develops a fever, shoulder or substernal pain, or shortness of breath.

Teach about treatments

Teach the patient and his family about treatment measures, including modifications in diet and activity and medication to control stomach bulk and acidity. If these measures prove ineffective, you'll need to prepare the patient for surgery to reduce the hernia and return the stomach to its normal position.

Diet

Teach the patient to modify the timing, size, and content of his meals. This will control both the amount of acid secreted during digestion and stomach bulk. Instruct him to avoid beverages and foods that may intensify his symptoms, and give him tips to prevent reflux. If the patient is overweight, urge him to lose weight. Tell him the two best ways to do this are to limit food intake and to exercise. Help him formulate an effective weight-loss program. Give him a copy of the patient-teaching aid *Relieving reflux and heartburn with diet,* page 462.

Medication

Teach the patient about medications used to treat the symptoms of hiatal hernia. Explain that antacids, which neutralize gastric acid, or cholinergics, which increase esophageal sphincter pressure, may be prescribed to relieve reflux. The doctor may also prescribe a histamine₂-receptor antagonist (see *Reducing heartburn with histamine₂-receptor antagonists*). Stool softeners prevent straining during bowel movements, and antiemetics prevent vomiting; both of these actions increase intra-abdominal pressure. Antiemetics also promote gastric emptying. Inform the patient that he'll need medications for hiatal hernia indefinitely, even after surgical repair.

Antacids. Tell the patient that antacids taste better cold, and, if needed, he should keep chewable antacids handy. Instruct him to shake a liquid antacid well before taking it. If he's taking the tablet form, advise him to chew it well before swallowing and to follow the dose with a full glass of water. Suggest mixing both liquid and tablet forms with fluids or food if preferred. If he misses a dose, tell him to take the missed dose as soon as possible, then resume his schedule. Caution him never to double-dose. Advise him to check with the doctor before making any changes in the way he takes his medicine.

If the patient experiences diarrhea or constipation, explain that the doctor may prescribe a different antacid, a combination therapy, or a stool softener.

Cholinergics. Bethanecol chloride (Urecholine) is the cholinergic most frequently prescribed for hiatal hernia. Tell the patient to report shortness of breath, wheezing or chest tightness, and excessive dizziness or faintness. Other reactions include excessive salivation, sweating, flushing, and urinary frequency.

If the patient experiences nausea, suggest that he take the drug 1 hour before or 2 hours after meals. Because cholinergics can cause dizziness, light-headedness, or fainting, advise him to get up slowly from a sitting or a lying position.

Antiemetics. Tell the patient taking an antiemetic, such as metoclopramide hydrochloride (Reglan), to report confusion, muscle spasms, severe drowsiness, shuffling gait, tics, or hand tremors. Other reactions include changes in menstruation, constipation, depression, diarrhea, dizziness, drowsiness, dry mouth, headache, insomnia, rash, or weakness.

Instruct the patient to avoid alcohol and cold, allergy, and sleep medications. These substances can increase the possibility of adverse reactions. Tell him that the drug is most effectively absorbed if it's taken 30 minutes before meals. If the medication makes him feel drowsy, caution him to avoid driving, operating machinery, or performing other activities that require alertness.

Medication taken for other purposes may also affect the symptoms of hiatal hernia. Cough suppressants, for example, are often helpful because they decrease the intra-abdominal pressure associated with coughing. However, other medications, such as salicylates and anticholinergics, irritate the gastric mucosa and increase gastric emptying time.

Surgery

If medication and changes in activity and diet fail to relieve the patient's symptoms, the doctor may recommend surgery to repair the hiatal hernia. Severe stricture and ulcerative esophagitis, hemorrhage, and pulmonary aspiration of gastric contents are also indications for surgery. Inform the patient that surgery will restore the stomach to its normal position, reducing the hernia. It also strengthens the lower esophageal sphincter. Tell him to expect laxatives and enemas the evening before the surgery to cleanse the bowel and prevent postoperative complications.

Repairing a hiatal hernia

Tell the patient that fundoplication is the most common procedure for repair of a hiatal hernia. Then use the diagrams and the information below to aid your explanation of this procedure.

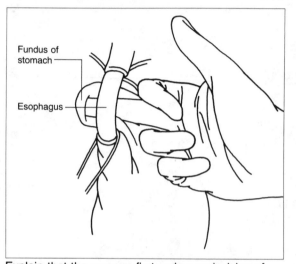

Explain that the surgeon first makes an incision of the skin and muscles overlying the junction of the stomach and esophagus. He retracts a section of the distal esophagus and gently pushes the fundus through this opening.

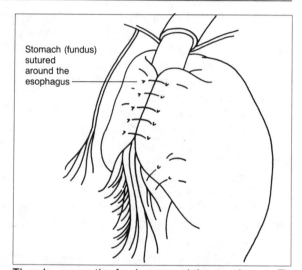

Then he wraps the fundus around the esophagus. Finally, he sutures the fundus to the gastric wall, creating a loose cuff of stomach around the esophagus. Note that the stomach is not incised.

Explain that the doctor will choose one of several procedures to anchor the stomach below the diaphragmatic opening. The most common procedure, known as a fundoplication, is illustrated in *Repairing a hiatal hernia.*

Inform the patient that after surgery he'll have a sore throat related to the placement of a rubber tube down his esophagus to guide the surgeon. He'll also have a nasogastric tube for 2 or 3 days to prevent gas by draining the GI tract. If the abdominal approach is used, he'll have a drain at the incision site to remove accumulated fluid for 1 or 2 days. If the thoracic approach is used, he'll have chest tubes. Explain that his intake may be limited to fluids for the first 24 hours. Then, he'll gradually resume his diet, starting on clear liquids and advancing to solid foods. Tell him to expect smaller, more frequent meals because the surgery reduces the storage capacity of the stomach. He may be asked to keep a record of his intake and output to evaluate the return of proper bowel function.

Stress the patient's susceptibility to pulmonary complications and his role in prevention. He should expect prophylactic antibiotics for 5 to 10 days. Assure him that he'll receive medication if he experiences pain with coughing and movement. Show him how to minimize abdominal pain by splinting his incision.

Explain that after surgery he may experience bloating. To relieve gas pain, teach him to turn from side to side in bed, and advise early ambulation. Inform him that he'll be discharged about 1 week after surgery and will probably resume his normal activities in 2 to 4 weeks. Warn him to avoid exertion or heavy lifting for several months.

Explain that postoperative complications are rare but do occur. Complications generally involve the gastric pouch and include erosion, ulcers, bleeding, pressure on the left lung due to size or placement of the pouch, and production of a volvulus. Advise the patient to notify the doctor immediately if he experiences difficulty swallowing or reflux. If he's overweight, stress the need for weight reduction to prevent complications and recurrence of the hernia.

Other care measures

Advise the patient to restrict activities that increase intra-abdominal pressure, such as strenuous exercise, heavy lifting, bending, and coughing, and to avoid wearing constrictive clothing, such as a long-line bra or a girdle. Recommend methods to avoid straining with bowel movements, such as modifying the diet to include natural laxatives (high-fiber foods, citrus fruits) and, if prescribed, taking laxatives or stool softeners.

Discuss stress-reduction techniques, such as walking, yoga, and deep-breathing exercises.

To relieve symptoms of heartburn, advise the patient to elevate his head with two or three pillows or to place 8" to 10" blocks under the head of his bed. Also suggest that he sleep on his right side. Discourage smoking because it alters pancreatic secretions that neutralize gastric acid in the duodenum.

Emphasize the warning symptoms of complications. Instruct the patient to contact the doctor immediately if he has symptoms of esophagitis, such as difficulty swallowing, chest pain, and bloody sputum; symptoms of gastritis, such as abdominal pain, belching, and nausea and vomiting; or symptoms of aspiration pneumonia, such as fever, difficulty breathing, rapid respirations, and pain with inspiration.

Further readings

Ament, M.E., et al. "Reflux Therapy: A Plan of Attack," *Patient Care* 23(15):30-39, September 30, 1989.

Benjamin, S.B., et al. "Chest Pain: Cardiac or Esophageal?" *Patient Care* 21(12):116-18, 120, 122+, July 15, 1987.

Castell, D.O. "Chest Pain from the Esophagus," *Emergency Medicine* 20(21):92-96, 98, 100+, December 15, 1988.

Dalton, C.B., et al. "Prolonged Ambulatory Esophageal pH Monitoring," *Gastroenterology Nursing* 11(4):221-26, Spring 1989.

Slaughter, R.L. "The Disabled Esophagus," *Emergency Medicine* 20(15): 99-102, 107-08, September 15, 1988.

Relieving reflux and heartburn with diet

Dear Patient:

A change in the timing, size, and content of your meals can help relieve the reflux and heartburn symptoms of hiatal hernia.

Keeping your weight within normal range can help, too. Being overweight not only contributes to the development of a hiatal hernia, but also aggravates the condition. That's because extra body fat means more weight to push upward when you're sitting, lying down, or bending.

Follow the guidelines below to prevent reflux and heartburn or to help make them less severe.

Eat small, frequent meals

This means four to six small meals daily. Eating *frequently* prevents the stomach from becoming totally empty, thereby decreasing the acid it secretes during digestion. Eating *small meals* reduces stomach bulk, which also helps relieve your symptoms.

Prevent reflux

Eat slowly to reduce stomach secretions. And sit up while you're eating. Keep in mind that while you're sitting up, gravity helps drain acid back into the stomach if it refluxes. But gravity can't help if you're lying down.

To decrease nighttime distress, eat your evening meal (a small one) at least 3 hours before bedtime. Also drink water after eating to cleanse the esophagus.

Avoid certain foods

Don't drink beverages that may intensify your symptoms — acidic juice (for example, orange juice), caffeinated coffee or tea, alcohol, and carbonated beverages.

Eliminate raw fruits and highly seasoned foods (such as chili) from your diet. Also avoid foods high in fat (such as fatty meats, eggs, and potato chips) or high in carbohydrates (such as beans).

Instead, consume easily digested foods, such as skim milk rather than whole milk, or broiled chicken with the skin removed instead of fried chicken.

Stay away from extremely hot or cold foods and fluids because they can cause gas.

Keep track of what you eat. Then avoid those foods that seem to cause discomfort.

Lose weight (if you need to)

If you're overweight, ask your doctor about an appropriate weight-loss program. If he doesn't recommend a special diet, ask about following the 1,400-calorie American Diabetic Association food plan used by Weight Watchers. Food exchanges provide for more balanced meals than calorie counting.

If you've ever gone on a diet before, think about what strategies worked best for you. Also ask yourself what strategies and diets didn't work.

Losing weight isn't easy. But it's worth the effort. Losing weight will help you feel better — and look better, too.

Constipation

Seldom serious but always uncomfortable, constipation can disrupt your patient's daily activities and general well-being. What's more, because it typically results from improper diet, physical inactivity, and poor bowel habits, constipation tends to recur. Helping the patient identify and control contributing factors should be your chief teaching goals.

To begin, you'll define constipation, explain how it develops, and identify possible complications. You'll follow up by discussing conservative treatment measures, involving diet and exercise, or more aggressive ones, including laxatives, enemas, and manual disimpaction.

Discuss the disorder

Start your teaching by reviewing normal bowel habits. Inform the patient that the normal defecation pattern varies considerably. One person may have one or two bowel movements a day, whereas another may have one bowel movement a week. Emphasize that these patterns are normal as long as defecation occurs easily and painlessly. Constipation, in contrast, refers to bowel movements that are difficult or painful and less frequent than normal. Other signs and symptoms of constipation include a sensation of rectal fullness with a frequent urge to defecate (tenesmus), belching, dyspepsia, mild abdominal discomfort, and nausea.

Explain that constipation typically starts when the patient suppresses the urge to defecate or when the movement of fluid waste (feces) through the intestines is reduced or slowed. When this happens, excessive fluid is absorbed from the retained feces, leaving them dry, hard, and difficult to pass.

Inform the patient that many other factors can increase intestinal transit time and produce constipation. (For more information, see *What causes constipation?* page 464, *How life-style can contribute to constipation,* page 465, and *Questions patients ask about constipation,* page 465.) Caution the patient not to ignore a sudden change in bowel habits, abdominal distention, pain, weight loss, fatigue, or constipation that recurs frequently or doesn't respond to treatment. All are warning signs of underlying disorders, such as structural lesions and colorectal cancer.

Complications

Stress the importance of complying with treatment to break the constipation cycle. Warn the patient that passage of rough, hard

June E. Breit, RN, CDP, who wrote this chapter, is a health systems consultant in Philadelphia.

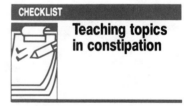

CHECKLIST

Teaching topics in constipation

☐ How constipation differs from normal bowel elimination
☐ How constipation develops
☐ Causes, such as life-style factors and medical conditions, and complications, such as fecal impaction
☐ Diagnosis by medical history
☐ Importance of regular exercise
☐ Dietary modifications to increase fluid and fiber intake
☐ Using laxatives properly
☐ Procedures, such as rectal suppositories, enemas, and manual disimpaction, to relieve constipation
☐ Establishing and maintaining regular bowel habits
☐ Sources of information and support

What causes constipation?

Tell your patient that constipation has many causes, among them medical conditions, life-style factors, drugs, and some tests and treatments. Review some of the most common causes with your patient. Emphasize that knowing the underlying cause will help him find the best ways to relieve constipation and prevent its recurrence.

Medical conditions
GI disorders, such as anal fissure, anorectal abscess, Crohn's disease, diverticulitis, irritable bowel syndrome, hemorrhoids, intestinal obstruction, ulcerative colitis, and proctitis, typically cause constipation.

Because the autonomic nervous system controls bowel movements by sensing rectal distention and stimulating the external sphincter, constipation can result from neurologic disorders, such as diabetic neuropathy, multiple sclerosis, tabes dorsalis, and spinal cord injury.

Cirrhosis, hepatic porphyria, endocrinopathies (such as hypothyroidism and hypercalcemia), and mesenteric artery ischemia also can produce constipation.

Life-style factors
Poor bowel habits, inactivity, inadequate fluid intake, and a diet that's low in fiber are common causes of constipation. Other contributing factors include stress and anxiety.

Drugs
Constipation often goes hand in hand with use of certain drugs. For instance, it occurs with use of antacids (Tums); anticholinergics (Cogentin); narcotic analgesics, such as codeine, meperidine (Demerol), and morphine; vinca alkaloids (Oncovin); and sodium polystyrene sulfonate (Kayexalate).

Tests and treatments
Barium retention (after certain GI studies), anorectal surgery (which traumatizes nerves), and abdominal irradiation (which may cause intestinal stricture) can produce constipation.

---

stools can chafe and irritate sensitive rectal tissues. And repeated straining can produce hemorrhoids or aggravate existing ones. Besides, ensuing pain may lead him to suppress the urge to defecate, causing constipation to persist or recur. Emphasize that protracted retention of hardened feces may ultimately end in fecal impaction.

If the patient has a cardiac, pulmonary, or ophthalmic disorder, caution him that straining during defecation can dangerously increase intrathoracic or intraocular pressure, possibly precipitating myocardial infarction ("bathroom coronary"), cerebrovascular accident, respiratory distress, or retinal detachment.

Describe the diagnostic workup
Tell the patient that constipation is usually diagnosed from a medical history. He'll need to describe the size, consistency, and frequency of his bowel movements. Have his symptoms developed recently or been persistent? Has he had any other symptoms, such as weight loss, unusual fatigue, or bloating? Point out that the doctor will also ask about the patient's diet and life-style, medica-

How life-style can contribute to constipation

Improper diet, inadequate exercise, poor bowel habits, stress, and chronic anxiety top the list of constipation's causes. The chart below represents how these life-style factors can interfere with normal elimination.

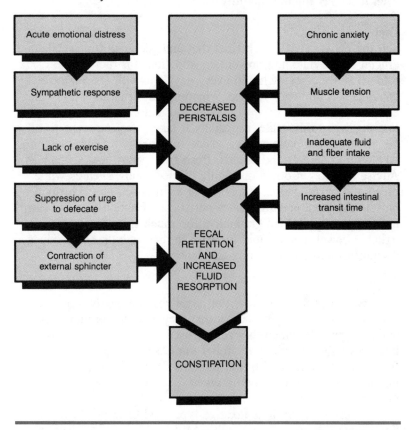

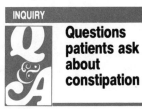

Questions patients ask about constipation

When I was younger, constipation was never a problem, but now I seem to be constipated all the time. Why is that?
Chronic constipation, known as an inactive or "lazy" colon, commonly affects older persons. It usually results from too little bulk in the diet and too little – or no – exercise. Because many people lose the sensation of being thirsty as they get older, insufficient fluid intake is another common cause.

Can constipation cause blood poisoning?
No. It's a myth that unexpelled waste products are reabsorbed into the bloodstream. Although retained stools can produce uncomfortable abdominal distention, gas, and loss of appetite, these symptoms aren't usually serious and should subside once you have a bowel movement.

Why has my daughter developed constipation now that she's pregnant?
During pregnancy, the enlarged uterus may press against the lower colon and rectum, delaying stool passage. Also during pregnancy, elevated levels of the hormone progesterone cause relaxation of the intestinal muscles, decreasing GI motility.

tion regimen, and existing medical conditions. This information will help determine constipation's cause. Inform him that the doctor will probably perform a physical examination and test for fecal occult blood.

If the doctor suspects that constipation stems from another disorder, explain that he may recommend additional tests, such as a barium enema, proctosigmoidoscopy, colonoscopy, or a computed tomography scan. If appropriate, discuss the purpose for these tests, how to prepare for them, and what to expect during and after them.

Teach about treatments
Inform the patient that dietary changes and increased exercise usually can correct constipation. Laxatives may be prescribed to initiate temporary relief. Severe constipation or fecal impaction may require such procedures as enemas or manual disimpaction. For lasting relief from constipation, teach the patient how to establish and maintain regular bowel habits. Provide a copy of the teaching aid *Breaking the constipation habit,* page 470.

Activity

Encourage the patient to exercise. Explain that regular exercise promotes peristalsis. Then help him to plan a program around an activity that he enjoys. Suggest an exercise or sport that's easy to incorporate into his daily routine—walking, for example. Reassure him that a daily exercise program can be tailored to his needs even if he has limited mobility.

Diet

Tell the patient that a high-fiber diet and adequate fluid intake are crucial to alleviate and prevent constipation. Instruct him to drink 8 to 10 full glasses of liquid every day. This will keep intestinal contents soft and easy to pass. Mention that drinking warm beverages, such as coffee or warm water and lemon juice, may stimulate the urge to defecate, especially if taken after a meal.

Instruct the patient to eat plenty of fiber-rich foods, such as whole grain cereals and breads, fresh fruits, nuts, and vegetables. Advise him to cut down on highly refined foods, such as white bread and baked goods. Explain that a fiber-rich diet contributes bulk to the stool and stimulates peristalsis. Caution him, though, to increase fiber intake gradually. Too much fiber can lead to an irritable bowel, and a rapid increase in dietary bulk can produce discomfort and embarrassing flatulence.

Medication

Your patient probably knows that laxatives commonly relieve constipation. But he may not know that they also can promote constipation, especially when they're overused. Suggest that he take laxatives only for temporary relief until exercise and dietary modifications restore normal bowel patterns. Warn him against depending on laxatives (see *Teaching about laxatives for constipation* for more information).

Describe the various laxative types and their modes of action. Some, like magnesium salts (Milk of Magnesia), glycerin suppositories (Fleet Babylax), and lactulose (Cephulac), act by osmosis, drawing water into the intestine to soften the stool and promote peristalsis. Methylcellulose (Cologel) and other bulk-forming laxatives absorb water and expand to increase fecal bulk, stimulating intestinal motility. Stimulant laxatives, such as castor oil, cascara sagrada, and bisacodyl (Dulcolax), are thought to affect peristalsis directly, either by irritating the intestinal musculature or by stimulating the colonic intramural plexus. Stool softeners, such as docusate (Colace), have a detergent effect on feces, and mineral oil acts mainly on the colon, lubricating the intestine and retarding colonic fluid absorption.

Tell the patient that common adverse reactions to all laxatives include bloating, cramping, flatulence, and nausea. Reassure him that these effects are usually transient. Occasionally, however, laxative overuse or overdose causes diarrhea. To prevent a subsequent fluid and electrolyte imbalance, instruct the patient to stop taking the laxative and notify the doctor if diarrhea develops.

Teaching about laxatives for constipation

DRUG	ADVERSE REACTIONS	TEACHING POINTS
Bulk-forming laxatives		
methylcellulose (Cologel) **psyllium** (Metamucil)	• Watch for breathing difficulty, diarrhea, itching, rash, swallowing difficulty, and vomiting. • Other reactions include nausea.	• Advise the patient to contact the doctor if a bowel movement doesn't occur after taking the drug for the prescribed time. • Instruct him to swallow tablets with a full glass of water and not to chew them. This prevents the drug from swelling in the esophagus and causing obstruction. • Advise him to mix the powder form with a full glass of water, milk, fruit juice, or other liquid and to drink it immediately. • Tell him to drink eight glasses of water a day to help prevent impaction. • Inform him that the drug may work in 12 hours, or its effects may be delayed for up to 3 days.
Emollient laxatives		
docusate calcium (Surfak) **docusate potassium** (Dialose) **docusate sodium** (Colace)	• Watch for rash. • Other reactions include mild abdominal cramps, nausea, and throat irritation (with liquid form).	• Tell the patient to take the drug only for the prescribed time. • Advise him that drinking between six and eight full glasses of fluid a day while taking this drug will help soften stools. • Inform him that the liquid drug has a bitter taste. To improve the flavor, suggest adding the drug to milk or fruit juice. • Tell him to expect results usually 1 to 2 days after the first dose; however, results may take up to 5 days. • Instruct him to avoid mineral oil while taking the drug (increased mineral oil absorption and toxicity are possible).
Hyperosmotic laxatives		
magnesium salts (Magnesium Citrate, Milk of Magnesia)	• Watch for confusion, dizziness, irregular heart rate, and unusual tiredness or weakness. • Other reactions include abdominal cramps and diarrhea.	• Advise contacting the doctor if the patient doesn't have a bowel movement after he's taken the drug for the prescribed time. • Suggest mixing the drug with a full glass of water or fruit juice to improve the drug's flavor. • Tell the patient that the drug works in about 2 to 6 hours; advise him to time his dose for convenience. • For best results, tell him to take this drug 1 hour before or 3 hours after meals. • Caution him that the drug's laxative effect may last for up to 4 days.
Lubricant laxatives		
mineral oil (Agoral Plain, Kondremul Plain)	• Watch for abdominal pain, nausea, and vomiting. • Other reactions include irritation of rectal tissues.	• Advise the patient to contact the doctor if he doesn't have a bowel movement after he's taken the medication for the prescribed time. • Instruct him to take the drug with a full glass of water, fruit juice, or carbonated beverage. • Tell him that drinking between six and eight full glasses of fluid a day while taking this drug will help to soften stools. • Suggest taking the drug at bedtime because the drug works in about 6 to 8 hours. • Warn him that with excessive dosages, this drug may leak from the anal sphincter. Suggest wearing a sanitary pad or an incontinence brief. • Inform him that mineral oil may impair absorption of fat-soluble vitamins A, D, E, and K. Tell him not to take mineral oil within 2 hours of meals to prevent decreased absorption of vitamins and other nutrients.

continued

Teaching about laxatives for constipation — *continued*

DRUG	ADVERSE REACTIONS	TEACHING POINTS
Stimulant laxatives		
bisacodyl (Dulcolax) **cascara sagrada** **castor oil** **phenolphthalein** (Ex-Lax) **senna** (Senokot)	• Watch for burning sensation when urinating, confusion, headache, irregular heart rate, irritability, mood or mental status changes, muscle spasm, and rash. • Other reactions include diarrhea, discolored urine, nausea, and stomach cramps.	• Inform the patient that this drug begins to act within 6 to 12 hours of administration (except castor oil, which works within 2 to 6 hours, and bisacodyl suppositories, which work in 10 minutes to 2 hours). Advise him to schedule doses for convenience. • Instruct him to drink six to eight full glasses of fluid a day with this drug to help soften stools. • Warn him that cascara sagrada, phenolphthalein, and senna may color his urine a harmless pinkish red or violet. • Tell the patient to contact the doctor if a bowel movement fails to occur after he's taken the drug for the prescribed time. • If he's taking the drug in suppository form, provide appropriate instructions. • Caution him never to chew, break, or crush bisacodyl tablets because this destroys the coating and may cause gastric irritation. • For best results, tell him to take the drug 1 hour before or 3 hours after meals. • Caution against taking bisacodyl with milk to prevent gastric irritation and cramping.

Procedures

Teach the patient or his caregiver how to use suppositories or enemas, if ordered. Warn him to avoid substituting soap slivers (a common home remedy) for suppositories recommended by the doctor. Point out that bar soaps may contain irritating perfumes or antibacterial agents and that the sharp edges of a soap sliver can further injure rectal tissue already chafed by hard stools. If fecal impaction occurs, inform the patient about manual disimpaction.

Enemas. Advise the patient that an over-the-counter, premixed sodium biphosphate enema (Fleet Enema) may relieve constipation. Explain that this easy-to-administer enema uses a hypertonic solution to draw water into the bowel by osmotic pressure. The resulting distention promotes an urge to defecate. If the patient's a child, advise parents to check with the doctor before administering a Fleet Enema because it can cause fluid and electrolyte imbalances in children.

If the doctor orders a cleansing enema for severe constipation, tell the patient that this type of enema introduces tap water, normal saline solution, or tap water with soapsuds into the bowel. This produces distention and an urge to defecate. Caution parents against using a cleansing enema to relieve a child's constipation. The procedure can cause fluid and electrolyte imbalances.

If the patient has a fecal impaction, explain that the doctor may order two types of enemas: an oil retention enema to soften the stool, then a cleansing enema to purge it. Emphasize that the patient will need to retain the initial oil solution for at least 1 hour.

Manual disimpaction. Tell the patient with a fecal impaction that the nurse may dislodge impacted feces manually. Explain that as the patient lies on his left side (to permit access to the rectum and lower sigmoid colon), the nurse will gently insert one or two gloved, lubricated fingers into his rectum to break up the hardened feces. Acknowledge that the procedure will cause discomfort. But reassure the patient that he'll feel rapid relief with the fecal mass removed.

Other care measures

Assist the patient to establish a bowel routine. Suggest that he schedule a certain time for bowel movements, and advise him to respond promptly to the urge to defecate. Help him to plan for and adjust to interruptions in his routine, such as travel or a busy work schedule. Because stress and interruptions inhibit defecation, underscore the need for privacy and a relaxed atmosphere while he's having a bowel movement. If he has trouble bearing down during defecation, recommend that he lift his feet onto a low footstool positioned at the toilet's base. This will increase thigh flexion.

An invalid or an infirm elderly patient may suppress the urge to defecate for fear of soiling himself. Suggest wearing panty liners or an adult incontinence brief as a precaution. Also recommend using a bedside commode if a bathroom's not nearby or easily accessible.

Sources of information and support

American Digestive Disease Society
60 East 42nd Street, Room 411, New York, N.Y. 10165
(212) 687-4185

National Digestive Diseases Information Clearinghouse
Box NDDIC, Bethesda, Md. 20892
(301) 468-6344

Further readings

Bennett, M. "The Fibre Squad...High-Fibre Diet," *Nursing Times* 84(4):49, January 27-February 2, 1988.

Cerrato, P.L. "Is America Really Constipated?" *RN* 52(5):81-82, 84, 86, May 1989.

"Constipation from Aspirin," *Nurses Drug Alert* 12(11):82, November 1988.

McMillan, S.C., and Williams, F.A. "Validity and Reliability of the Constipation Assessment Scale," *Cancer Nursing* 12(3):183-88, June 1989.

McShane, R.E., and McLane, A.M. "Constipation: Impact of Etiological Factors," *Journal of Gerontology Nursing* 14(4):31-34, 46-47, April 1988.

Osis, M. "Laxatives: Are We Making the Best Choice?" *Gerontion* 2(3):5-7, Fall 1987.

Swartz, M.L. "Citrucel," *Gastroenterology Nursing* 12(1):50-52, Summer 1989.

Yen, P.K. "Nature's Laxative: Fiber," *Geriatric Nursing* 9(6):361-62, November-December 1988.

Breaking the constipation habit

Dear Patient:

You can overcome constipation — even if you've been constipated frequently for many years. Follow these guidelines to break the constipation habit.

Develop good bowel habits

Schedule a regular time for bowel movements. Choose a time when you won't be rushed or interrupted. Many people find that the best time is shortly after a meal.

Anticipate events, such as travel or social plans, that may disrupt your normal routine. That way, you can plan ahead.

Don't ignore the urge to have a bowel movement, even if you're busy or it's inconvenient.

Watch your diet

Cut down on refined, starchy foods. Instead, choose foods like whole grain cereals, pasta, and bread; nuts; and fresh fruits and vegetables. These foods add fiber to your diet. If you get constipated when you're away from home, carry a supply of dried prunes with you to your destination.

Watch your intake of fatty foods, such as butter, cooking oils, cream, and bacon, too. Although these foods can help soften your stools, they may work too well, causing diarrhea.

Drink at least 8 to 10 glasses of fluid every day to keep your stools soft and easy to pass. Prune juice or a hot beverage, like coffee or warm lemonade, may

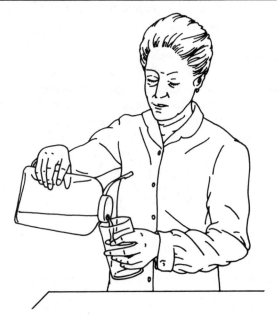

stimulate the urge to have a bowel movement.

Learn to relax

If you're tense, having a bowel movement will be more difficult. Reading or listening to music while you're in the bathroom may help you to relax. Remember that a daily bowel movement isn't essential for everyone.

Other tips

● Develop a daily exercise program. If you've been inactive for a long time, walking is a simple and effective way to get started.
● Get at least 6 hours of rest each night.
● Consult your doctor or nurse before using laxatives, especially if you're pregnant. Remember that *overusing* these medications can cause constipation rather than relieve it.

Fecal incontinence

Although fecal incontinence usually isn't a sign of severe illness, this condition can cause anxiety, shame, and loss of self-esteem. Many patients who are unable to control bowel movements withdraw from society to the point of reclusiveness.

Fecal incontinence is sometimes temporary—as in severe gastroenteritis or after certain types of surgery. But the condition can also be permanent—for example, in spinal cord disease. If the patient must learn to live with this condition for the rest of his life, your emotional support and intensive teaching are especially critical. And because patients with permanent fecal incontinence typically can't care for themselves, teaching the family is also important.

You'll first review how the body normally controls defecation. Then you'll explain the cause of your patient's fecal incontinence. You'll discuss treatments, including exercise, proper diet, and adequate fluids, to help correct the condition, and you'll emphasize good perineal hygiene. Even if the patient's incontinence is permanent, you can boost his self-image and offer new hope for bowel control by explaining a bowel retraining program.

Discuss the disorder

Define fecal incontinence as a loss of control over contraction and relaxation of the external anal sphincter, causing involuntary expulsion of feces. Then describe the neurologic mechanisms that regulate normal defecation. (See *How normal defecation occurs,* page 472.)

Explain that fecal incontinence—temporary or permanent—has several possible causes. Focus on the patient's particular problem. For example, incontinence can result from cerebrovascular accident, dementias, or traumatic injury to the head. These disorders can permanently or temporarily compromise the voluntary and involuntary brain centers that control defecation. Incontinence can also result from traumatic injury to the anal sphincter, from rectal prolapse, or from anorectal diseases, such as cancer. Diarrhea-producing conditions, including gastroenteritis, influenza, and inflammatory bowel disease, can cause temporary incontinence when the amount of feces and the force of peristalsis overwhelm the sphincter. Abdominal, rectal, or prostate surgery can also produce temporary incontinence.

June E. Breit, RN, CDP, and **Marlene Ciranowicz, RN, MSN,** wrote this chapter. Ms. Breit is a health systems consultant in Philadelphia, and Ms. Ciranowicz is an independent nurse-consultant in Dresher, Pa. Both authors are also free-lance clinical editors for Springhouse Corporation.

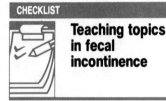

CHECKLIST

Teaching topics in fecal incontinence

☐ Explanation of neurologic control of defecation
☐ Causes of fecal incontinence
☐ Possible complications, such as fluid and electrolyte imbalance and urinary tract infections
☐ Diagnosing fecal incontinence and assessing sphincter control
☐ Activity to maintain intestinal motility and tonicity
☐ High-fiber diet and adequate fluids to aid peristalsis and promote regularity
☐ Bowel retraining program, including the use of rectal suppositories, digital stimulation, and enemas
☐ How to perform perineal care
☐ Source of information and support

How normal defecation occurs

To help your patient understand why he has fecal incontinence and how he can control it, first teach him how normal defecation occurs.

Explain that defecation is regulated by three neurologic mechanisms: the intrinsic defecation reflex in the colon, the parasympathetic defecation reflex involving sacral segments of the spinal cord, and voluntary control, a function of the cerebral cortex. Here's how these reflexes work together.

Fecal distention of the rectum activates the intrinsic reflex, causing afferent nerve impulses to spread through the intestines, initiating peristalsis in the descending and sigmoid colons and in the rectum. Subsequent movement of feces toward the anus causes relaxation of the internal anal sphincter.

To ensure defecation, the parasympathetic reflex magnifies the intrinsic reflex, stimulating nerves in the wall of the rectum. This sends impulses through the spinal cord and back to the descending and sigmoid colons, rectum, and anus to intensify peristalsis. However, fecal movement and internal sphincter relaxation trigger an immediate contraction of the external sphincter and temporary fecal retention.

At this point, a person with normal bowel function either prevents or permits defecation by consciously controlling his external sphincter. This voluntary mechanism (absent in a person with fecal incontinence) further contracts the sphincter, preventing defecation at inappropriate times, or relaxes the sphincter, allowing defecation to occur.

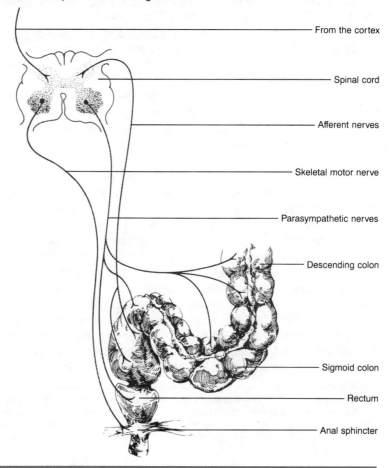

From the cortex

Spinal cord

Afferent nerves

Skeletal motor nerve

Parasympathetic nerves

Descending colon

Sigmoid colon

Rectum

Anal sphincter

Other causes include fecal impaction, which causes liquid feces to leak around the obstruction; neuromuscular disorders, such as multiple sclerosis; and spinal cord injuries, which disrupt neuromuscular control by compressing or transecting the sensorimotor spinal tracts. In addition, aging can cause varying degrees of fecal incontinence from loss of sphincter tone, changes in intestinal motility, and impaired brain function.

Complications
Inform the patient and his family that patients with severe, persistent diarrhea are at risk for fluid and electrolyte imbalance. Urinary tract infections are also common. Because the urinary meatus is so close to the rectum, fecal bacteria can easily contaminate the urinary tract. Improper cleaning after episodes of incontinence can also cause irritated and excoriated skin in the perineal and sacral areas.

Describe the diagnostic workup
Explain that a diagnosis of fecal incontinence is based on observation and a patient history. Prepare the patient and his family for the doctor's questions, including how often the patient has a bowel movement, the nature of the stool, whether he's aware of the need to defecate, and whether he can contract his abdominal or perineal muscles. If the cause of the incontinence is uncertain, the doctor may order tests to determine the underlying problem.

If the patient will undergo anorectal manometry, inform him that this test assesses sphincter control. Explain that a balloon, which is attached to a metering device, is inserted into the rectum and then inflated. The patient contracts his sphincter against the inflated balloon, and the meter measures the amount of sphincter pressure.

Teach about treatments
Instruct the patient and his family that temporary fecal incontinence can usually be corrected through a high-fiber diet, adequate fluid intake, and exercise. Permanent incontinence can be managed by following these same measures in addition to a bowel retraining program. Such a program may involve the use of suppositories, digital stimulation, and enemas. Also review the importance of good perineal hygiene.

Activity
Explain that daily exercise helps stimulate intestinal motility and improve intestinal muscle tone. Tell the patient that walking outdoors is the ideal exercise; however, even walking around his room, walking to the bathroom, or sitting up in a chair can help.

If the patient has neuromuscular problems and can't walk, point out that the physical therapist will develop an exercise program to fit his level of functioning.

Inform the patient who has temporary or intermittent fecal incontinence that abdominal and perirectal strengthening exercises, called Kegel exercises, may help restore muscle tone and bowel control. Teach him how to perform these exercises. To back up your directions, provide a copy of the patient-teaching aid *How to exercise your pelvic muscles*, page 572.

Diet

Instruct the patient to drink 2 to 3 quarts of fluid every day unless the doctor advises otherwise. Explain that drinking adequate fluids will aid peristalsis and soften the stool so it's easier to pass. (Hard stool can cause constipation, fecal impaction, and fecal incontinence.) Also encourage him to consume a high-fiber diet that emphasizes whole-grain breads and cereals, nuts, and raw fruits and vegetables. Explain that fiber increases fecal bulk and promotes regularity.

Medication

If the patient is starting a bowel retraining program, inform him that glycerin or bisacodyl (Dulcolax) suppositories are used initially to stimulate defecation at a desired time and establish a regular pattern of defecation. If appropriate, teach your patient how to insert a suppository. Give him a copy of the patient-teaching aid *How to insert a rectal suppository*, page 476. However, warn him not to use these laxatives routinely because they may foster dependency.

Procedures

Besides a high-fiber diet, adequate fluids, and exercise, a bowel retraining program consists of rectal suppositories, digital stimulation, and enemas. Tell the patient that digital stimulation is used after the suppository has been in for the recommended amount of time. Teach him or the caregiver to insert a gloved, lubricated finger into the rectum, then gently rotate the finger to relax the anal sphincter and stimulate a bowel movement. Offer him the patient-teaching aid *How to perform bowel stimulation*, page 477.

Also teach the patient or the caregiver how to administer an enema, explaining that this procedure is used during bowel retraining if suppositories and digital stimulation aren't successful. Give him or the caregiver the patient-teaching aid *How to give yourself an enema*, page 478.

Advise the patient to set a specific time for having a bowel movement—for example, once a day or once every other day about 30 minutes after a meal (usually breakfast). Tell him to be flexible, though. If he feels the urge to have a bowel movement at another time of day, he shouldn't ignore it. He should use a toilet or a portable commode—not a bedpan—if possible. This way, he'll be sitting upright so gravity can assist the muscles that control bowel movements. Placing his feet on a footstool and leaning forward while sitting on the toilet can also help. Tell him not to rush—he should stay on the toilet for at least 10 to 15 minutes. He shouldn't be discouraged if accidents occur. Reassure him that this is normal and doesn't mean that his efforts have failed. Tell him that retraining takes time. If necessary, suggest that he wear incontinence briefs for protection until he's retrained his bowels.

Other care measures
As part of the patient's bowel retraining program, advise him to accurately record his food and fluid intake and the time, amount, and consistency of his bowel movements. This way, he'll see what foods agree or don't agree with him and what foods keep him most regular. He'll also be able to monitor his progress.

Inform the patient that thoroughly washing and drying the perineal area after each episode of incontinence helps prevent odor, infection, and skin irritation from feces. Needless to say, he'll also feel more comfortable. Teach the patient or caregiver how to perform perineal care. Reinforce your teaching with a copy of the patient-teaching aid *Giving perineal care to a woman*, page 479, or *Giving perineal care to a man*, page 480.

Source of information and support
Digestive Disease National Coalition
511 Capitol Court, NE, Suite 300, Washington, D.C. 20002
(202) 544-7499

Further readings
Achkar, E. "Fecal Incontinence: Relief for the 'Unvoiced Symptom,' " *Consultant* 28(8):43-45, 48, 50, August 1988.

Ashervath, J., and Kizakipunner, K. "Achieving Continence in the Confused Elderly," *Advancing Clinical Care* 5(4):37-40, July-August 1990.

Hanauer, S.B. "Fecal Incontinence in the Elderly," *Hospital Practice* 23(3):105-08, 111-12, March 30, 1988.

Jay, P. "Community Patients' Toilet Needs," *Nursing* (London) 3(35):28-30, March 1989.

Jenkins, G. "Clothed for Continence," *Geriatric Nursing Home Care* 7(9): 11-13, September 1987.

Lara, L.L., et al. "The Risk of Urinary Tract Infection in Bowel Incontinent Men," *Journal of Gerontology Nursing* 16(5):24-26, 40-41, May 1990.

Lincoln, R., and Roberts, R. "Continence Issues in Acute Care," *Nursing Clinics of North America* 24(3):741-54, September 1989.

Norton, C. "Coping with Incontinence," *Geriatric Nursing Home Care* 7(9):16-19, September 1987.

Sprague-McRae, J.M. "Encopresis: Developmental, Behavioral and Physiological Considerations for Treatment," *Nurse Practitioner* 15(6):8, 11-12, 14-16, June 1990.

Stephany, T. "Home Care Hospice Bowel Regimen," *Home Healthcare Nurse* 6(4):40-41, July-August 1988.

Tulloch, G.J. "The Incontinency Taboo," *Geriatric Nursing* 10(1):19, January-February 1989.

Turner, A. "Promoting Continence: The Role of the Continence Advisor," *Senior Nurse* 8(3):15, March 1988.

Turner, A.F. "Continence Promotion in the Community," *Midwife Health Visitor Community Nurse* 23(12):543-44, December 1987.

PATIENT-TEACHING AID

How to insert a rectal suppository

Dear Patient:

The doctor has ordered a rectal suppository to help you stimulate regular bowel movements at the desired time.

Caution: Unless your doctor orders otherwise, don't use rectal suppositories or other laxatives routinely because you can become dependent on them.

You can learn to insert a rectal suppository quickly and easily by following these steps:

1 Wash your hands. Then gather the items you'll need: the suppository, a disposable glove, and a tube of water-soluble lubricating gel.

2 Put the glove on your right hand (or on your left hand if you're left-handed). Now remove the foil wrapper on the suppository.

If you have trouble doing this, the suppository may be too soft to insert. Hold it under cold running water until it becomes firm, or put it in the freezer for a minute or two before inserting it—just don't let it get too cold and hard. Better yet, store your suppositories in the refrigerator.

3 Once you've removed the foil wrapper, put a generous dab of lubricating gel on the rounded end of the suppository, as shown at the top of the next column. Hold the lubricated suppository in your gloved hand.

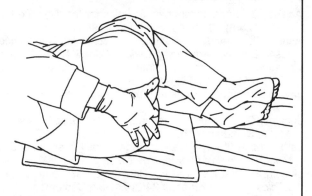

4 Now lie on your side with your knees raised toward your chest. Take a deep breath as you gently insert the suppository—rounded end first—into the anus with your gloved hand. Push the suppository in as far as your finger will go to keep the suppository from coming back out.

5 Once the suppository's in place, you'll feel an immediate urge to have a bowel movement. Resist the urge by lying still and breathing deeply a few times.

Try to retain the suppository for at least 20 minutes, so your body has time to absorb it and get the maximum effect from the medication. After you have a bowel movement, discard the glove and wash your hands.

How to perform bowel stimulation

Dear Patient:

Manual bowel stimulation is an important part of a bowel retraining program. It's done about 30 minutes after inserting a glycerin or bisacodyl (Dulcolax) suppository.

    Although you may feel hesitant about performing this procedure at first, you'll feel more comfortable once you learn how. If the doctor orders bowel stimulation, follow these steps:

1 Wash your hands with soap and water and dry them, using a clean terry towel or a disposable paper towel. Then gather the equipment you'll need: a disposable glove, water-soluble lubricant, and a towel or linen-saver pad.

2 Place the towel or linen-saver pad on your bed.

3 Put a disposable glove on your right hand (or on your left hand if you're left-handed), and lubricate your gloved index finger with a water-soluble lubricant.

4 Then lie on your left side on the towel or pad, keeping your left leg straight and your right knee drawn up toward your chest.
    Note: If you're left-handed, reverse these instructions by lying on your right side with your right leg straight and your left knee drawn up.

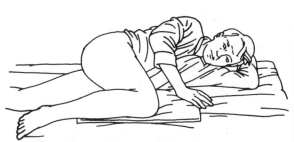

5 Insert the index finger ½ inch to 1 inch into your rectum. Rotate it to stimulate the bowel.

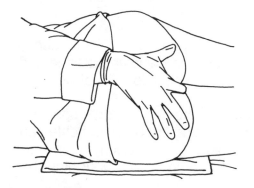

6 Then, if possible, use the toilet—not a bedpan. That way you'll be able to assume a sitting position. This position lets gravity help the muscles control a bowel movement.

7 Allow 15 minutes for your bowels to empty. If this doesn't occur, wait 24 hours before repeating the procedure. If any bleeding occurs, stop immediately and notify the doctor.

8 After the procedure, remove the glove and discard it. Then wash your hands with soap and water and dry them.

How to give yourself an enema

Dear Patient:

If the doctor orders an enema for you, he'll tell you what brand of commercial enema to buy. Giving yourself an enema is a bit awkward, but it really isn't difficult.

Just be sure you're close to a toilet, and if possible, have the enema in the morning, so you won't need to use the bathroom during the night. Here's what to do:

1 Wash your hands. Then open the disposable enema package and read the instructions carefully.

2 Hold the enema bottle upright, grasping the grooved bottle cap with your fingers. Gently remove the protective shield with your other hand.

3 Now lie on your left side with your right knee bent. This position helps the enema solution flow into your colon. Be sure to place a linen-saver pad under your buttocks to keep the bed dry.

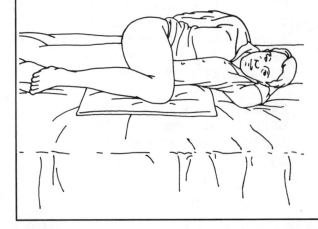

4 Or you can lie in the knee-chest position.

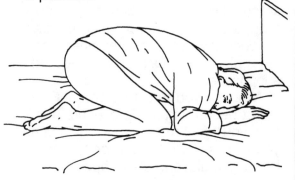

5 Gently insert the tip of the enema bottle about 4 inches into your rectum.

Take slow, deep breaths as you slowly squeeze the bottle to deposit the solution in your rectum. When the bottle is empty, remove the tip from your rectum.

6 Because your colon is full, you'll feel an immediate urge to have a bowel movement.

Try to resist the urge, holding the solution in for 2 to 5 minutes for a cleansing enema and for as long as you can tolerate for an oil retention enema. Then expel the solution into the toilet.

7 After moving your bowels, clean the perineum carefully. Then put the used enema bottle in its original box. Discard the box, the linen-saver pad, and other disposable articles.

Giving perineal care to a woman

Dear Caregiver:

Cleaning the perineum—the area between the thighs, including the genitals and anus—is a must after episodes of bowel incontinence. Besides making the patient more comfortable, cleaning removes excretions that can cause irritation, skin breakdown, infection, and odor. Follow these steps:

1 First, assemble your equipment: several washcloths, a clean basin, mild soap, a linen-saver pad, a bath towel, prescribed ointment or cream, toilet tissue or disposable wipes, and a trash bag.

2 Fill the basin two-thirds full with warm water. Then place it next to the patient's bed, along with the other items.

3 Wash your hands thoroughly. Then help the patient to lie on her back, and place a linen-saver pad under her buttocks.

4 Ask the patient to bend her knees slightly and spread her legs. First, clean the vaginal area.

After applying soap to the washcloth, separate her labia—the outer lips of the vagina—with one hand, and with the other hand, use gentle downward strokes to wash from front to back. Use a clean section of the washcloth for each stroke. Avoid touching the rectal area with the washcloth.

5 Rinse the vaginal area thoroughly with a clean washcloth to remove soap residue that can cause skin irritation.

Pat the skin dry, paying special attention to skin folds. (Don't use powder—it may become caked.)

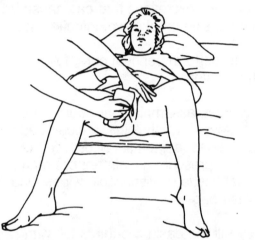

6 Now clean the rectal area. Help the patient turn onto her left side with her right knee raised to expose the rectum. Remove excess feces with toilet tissue or disposable wipes. Then clean, rinse, and dry the area, wiping from front to back. Use a clean section of the washcloth for each stroke.

7 If the doctor orders it, apply ointment or cream to prevent skin breakdown or to heal irritation. Then tuck a pad between the buttocks to absorb oozing feces. Remove the linen-saver pad, then reposition the patient, straightening the bed linens to make her comfortable. Clean the basin for future use, and dispose of soiled articles.

Giving perineal care to a man

Dear Caregiver:

Cleaning the perineum—the area between the thighs, including the genitals and anus—is a must after episodes of bowel incontinence. Besides making the patient more comfortable, cleaning removes excretions that can cause irritation, skin breakdown, infection, and odor.

To perform perineal care, follow these steps:

1 First, assemble your equipment: several washcloths, a clean basin, mild soap, a linen-saver pad, a bath towel, prescribed ointment or cream, toilet tissue or disposable wipes, and a trash bag.

2 Fill the basin two-thirds full with warm water. Then place it next to the patient's bed, along with the other items.

3 Wash your hands thoroughly. Then help the patient to lie on his back, and place a linen-saver pad under his buttocks.

4 Have the patient spread his legs and slightly bend his knees. After applying soap to the washcloth, hold the shaft of his penis with one hand and clean with the other. Begin at the tip of the penis and work in a circular motion from the center outward. Use a clean section of washcloth for each stroke. Rinse thoroughly with a circular motion.

If the man is uncircumcised, gently retract the foreskin and wash underneath it. Rinse well, but don't dry because moisture prevents friction when replacing the foreskin.

5 Wash the rest of the penis, stroking downward toward the scrotum. Rinse well and pat dry. Then gently clean, rinse, and pat dry the scrotum.

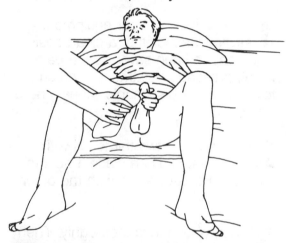

6 Next, help the patient turn onto his left side. Remove excess feces with toilet paper or a disposable wipe.

Then clean, rinse, and pat dry the rectal area.

7 If the doctor orders it, apply ointment or cream to prevent skin breakdown or to heal irritation. Then tuck a pad between the buttocks to absorb oozing feces. Remove the linen-saver pad, then reposition the patient, straightening the bed linens to make him comfortable.

Clean the basin for future use, and dispose of soiled articles.

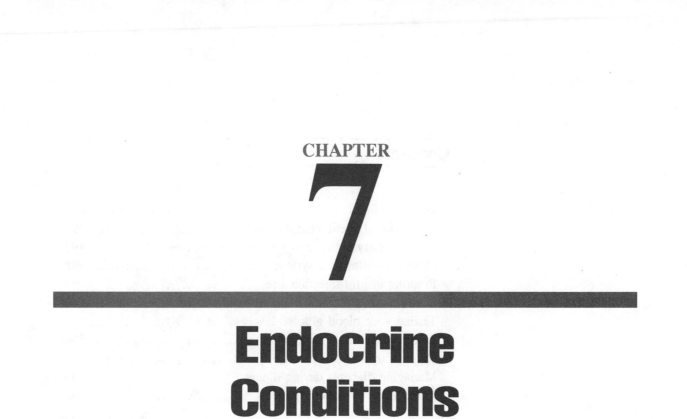

CHAPTER

7

Endocrine Conditions

Contents

Diabetes mellitus

Practically no other disorder requires a greater degree of compliance with prescribed treatment than diabetes mellitus. That's because diabetic control and prevention of complications hinge on successful treatment. And because such treatment usually involves major and permanent life-style changes, the diabetic patient must be highly motivated to comply.

Your teaching will help the patient understand the complexity of his chronic disorder and recognize the benefits of following measures that control blood glucose levels. You'll also need to enlist the family's cooperation.

Obviously, what a diabetic patient needs to learn can't be taught in a few hours. You'll need to encourage him and his family to ask questions and watch them demonstrate various techniques, such as testing blood for glucose and urine for ketones, and drawing up, mixing, and injecting insulin, if appropriate. You'll also need to discuss complications, diagnostic tests, and treatments, such as exercise, diet, and medication. What's more, you'll need to stress preventive health care, such as sick-day and travel precautions and eye and foot care. (See *Teaching the newly diagnosed diabetic patient,* page 484.)

Discuss the disorder

Inform the patient that diabetes mellitus is a chronic disorder in which the pancreas fails to produce enough insulin to control blood glucose levels, or the body cells fail to use the insulin produced efficiently. Two common forms of diabetes mellitus are Type I, or insulin-dependent diabetes mellitus, and Type II, or non-insulin–dependent diabetes mellitus.

Tell the patient with Type I diabetes that his pancreas doesn't produce any insulin in response to elevated blood glucose levels. This type of diabetes, most common in children, accounts for about 10% of all cases. Tell the patient with Type II diabetes that elevated blood glucose levels result from one of two problems: either his pancreas produces too little insulin to control glucose levels, or insulin release is delayed in response to abnormal glucose levels. Moreover, the peripheral cells don't use insulin efficiently. This causes insulin resistance, which is most common in obese people over age 40, accounting for about 90% of all cases.

Complications

To help ensure compliance with treatment, point out to the patient that hypoglycemia and other severe complications can result from

Marlene Ciranowicz, RN, MSN, CDE, who wrote this chapter, is a diabetes clinical nurse specialist at Hahnemann University Hospital, Philadelphia.

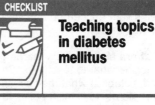

CHECKLIST

Teaching topics in diabetes mellitus

☐ The pathology underlying Type I or Type II diabetes
☐ Complications from untreated or poorly controlled diabetes
☐ Preparation for the oral glucose tolerance test and other diagnostic tests
☐ Role of exercise, including exercise precautions
☐ Role of diet, including meal planning and timing, exchange lists, and insulin injections
☐ Medication, such as insulin, oral hypoglycemics, and glucagon, and how to administer it properly
☐ Techniques for obtaining and testing blood for glucose levels
☐ Techniques for testing urine ketone levels
☐ Preventing or reducing long-term complications by observing proper foot and eye care, sick-day precautions, and travel tips
☐ Sources of information and support

Teaching the newly diagnosed diabetic patient

Patients with diabetes need exhaustive teaching. So a standard teaching plan can really help you save time and organize topics. Of course, you'll modify the plan to fit your patient's needs. Here's how.

Reviewing the patient's history
Let's say you're caring for Marian Stone, age 57, who's just been diagnosed with Type II diabetes mellitus. The first thing you notice about Mrs. Stone is her obesity—at 5 feet 2 inches, she weighs 170 pounds. She tells you that she always feels tired and can't seem to quench her thirst, even though she drinks about 4 quarts of water and soda daily. She also complains of frequent urination, even at night, and of dry, itchy skin and blurred vision.

Mrs. Stone says that her brother also has diabetes and that he's not doing well. She admits to being frightened and tells you, "I feel like I've lost control of my life." But she emphasizes that she'll do whatever is necessary to help herself. Her husband, Carl, also seems very concerned and says that he'll help in any way he can.

What are Mrs. Stone's learning needs?
To decide what to teach Mrs. Stone and her husband, establish what they already know about diabetes. To decide which points to cover, refer to the standard teaching plan, which includes:
• a definition of diabetes mellitus
• pathophysiology of the disease
• types of diabetes and signs and symptoms
• diagnostic tests, such as the fasting plasma glucose test
• treatments, including meal planning; medication (insulin, oral hypoglycemics, and glucagon); exercise; self-monitoring (blood glucose levels and ketone tests); preventing, recognizing, and treating hypoglycemia and hyperglycemia; sick-day guidelines; and preventive health care.

After assessing what the Stones know, you decide that they need education in all areas on the standard teaching plan. Your ultimate aim: to have Mrs. Stone achieve and maintain blood glucose levels as close to normal as possible. But reaching this goal requires scrupulous compliance and a major overhaul in lifestyle for Mrs. Stone. So her husband's cooperation is more important than ever.

Recalling that Mrs. Stone told you that having diabetes makes her feel out of control, you may encourage compliance by demonstrating how maintaining normal blood glucose levels will help her regain control. Describe how losing weight, following a diabetic diet, exercising, and other self-care measures will help her feel more like her old self.

What outcomes should you hope to achieve?
Using the standard teaching plan, you and Mrs. Stone choose suitable learning outcomes. Specifically, she'll be able to:

```
-describe what happens to the body when it's defi-
cient in insulin
-identify her type of diabetes and its symptoms
-state the purpose of diagnostic tests
-identify the normal range for blood glucose levels
-describe an appropriate exercise program, includ-
ing safety guidelines
-use an exchange list to plan her daily meals and
to stay within 1,200 calories a day
-list adverse reactions to insulin, oral hypo-
glycemic agents, and glucagon that she'll report
to the doctor
-demonstrate how to test her blood glucose levels
-show how to give a subcutaneous insulin injection
-list the signs, symptoms, causes, and treatments
for hypoglycemia and hyperglycemia
-explain sick-day guidelines
-list preventive health care guidelines to reduce
the risk of complications.
```

What teaching techniques and tools will you use?
Choose discussion and explanation to teach about insulin deficiency and insulin's relation to blood glucose levels; exercise; meal planning; drug therapy and its adverse effects; hypoglycemia and hyperglycemia; sick-day guidelines; and preventive health care.

Use demonstration to teach techniques, such as blood glucose testing and insulin injection. Enhance your teaching with booklets, posters, flip charts, films, and other visual aids. These tools will reinforce your teaching and make learning easier for Mrs. Stone.

How much information can Mrs. Stone absorb at one teaching session? The answer will influence your teaching strategy. She admits that she's frightened, so don't overwhelm her with too much information at once. Be guided by her response to your discussion. Give her lots of time to ask questions, and arrange for follow-up by a visiting nurse after discharge. Encourage the Stones to keep abreast of new developments in diabetes care by joining the American Diabetes Association as well as joining a support group for diabetics and their families.

How will you evaluate your teaching?
Appropriate evaluation methods include direct observation, discussion (sometimes using questions and answers), and simulation. For example, how would Mrs. Stone handle a typical problem, such as hypoglycemia? Return demonstration can help you evaluate how she tests blood glucose levels, administers insulin, and plans menus.

untreated or poorly managed diabetes. Two of these complications — diabetic ketoacidosis (DKA) and hyperglycemic hyperosmolar nonketotic coma (HHNC) — can be fatal without prompt treatment.

DKA results from extremely high blood glucose levels. Glucose-deprived cells use an alternate energy source that produces glycerol (a glucose substance) and ketones (waste chemicals). The accumulation of ketones causes metabolic acidosis. In HHNC, blood glucose levels quickly and mysteriously exceed 800 mg/dl, producing profound dehydration.

Emphasize that hypoglycemia, another acute complication, usually results from an error in diabetic management—for example, excessive exercise or insulin, or insufficient food intake. Untreated, it can cause seizures, brain damage, coma, and death.

Explain that chronic complications include retinopathy, neuropathy, kidney disease, cardiovascular disease, and infections. Why these complications develop isn't clearly understood, but diabetes experts think that inadequate blood glucose control may be the cause. Stress that by testing blood glucose levels daily, the patient may be able to stabilize the disease and prevent complications. Offer him a copy of the patient-teaching aid *Preventing diabetic complications,* page 496.

Describe the diagnostic workup

The diagnostic tests ordered for a patient with suspected diabetes will depend on his signs and symptoms. Tell the patient, however, that he can count on having tests to measure blood glucose levels, necessitating several blood samples. Describe what he can expect from venipuncture, and discuss such typical tests as the fasting plasma glucose test, the random plasma glucose test, the oral glucose tolerance test, and the glycosylated hemoglobin test.

Fasting plasma glucose test

Instruct the patient not to eat or drink anything except water for 12 hours before the test. Explain that glucose levels exceeding 140 mg/dl on two or more occasions confirm diabetes.

Random plasma glucose test

Advise the patient that fasting isn't necessary for this test, which measures his glucose level at the time of the test. Diabetes is confirmed if his blood glucose level measures 200 mg/dl or above, and if his symptoms include polyuria, polyphagia, polydipsia, weight loss, and fatigue.

Oral glucose tolerance test

Tell the patient that this test evaluates his body's response to ingested glucose. Explain that for 3 days before the test he'll follow a diet that ensures a daily intake of 150 to 300 g of carbohydrates. (Give him a copy of the patient-teaching aid *Getting ready for an oral glucose tolerance test,* page 497.) Then he won't be allowed food or fluids for 12 hours before the test. Tell him to avoid caffeine, alcohol, strenuous exercise, and smoking during the fasting and testing periods because these factors can cause misleading test results. Discuss any medications that must be withheld during the test period.

Inform him that he'll be given a sweet solution to drink at the start of the test—urge him to drink it all. If his blood glucose levels exceed 200 mg/dl before 2 hours have elapsed and at the 2-hour mark, diabetes is confirmed. Mention that the test can take up to 5 hours.

Glycosylated hemoglobin test
Performed about every 3 months, this test monitors the patient's blood glucose control during the previous 2 months. Explain that persistently elevated glycosylated hemoglobin levels predict a greater risk for developing chronic complications.

Teach about treatments
Emphasize the patient's strict compliance with all treatment measures, including medication, controlled activity and diet, blood and urine testing, and other self-care measures.

Activity
Teach the patient that a balanced program of exercise and rest will help stabilize his blood glucose levels and reduce insulin requirements. However, caution him to gear the amount of exercise to his food and medication consumption and to follow his doctor's exercise guidelines to the letter.

Inform the patient that aerobic exercise, such as walking, running, cycling, and swimming, can decrease blood glucose levels. Anaerobic exercise, such as weight lifting, can build muscle mass but can also increase blood glucose levels and, therefore, should be avoided.

Exercise in phases. Instruct the patient to exercise regularly, every other day, for 40 to 60 minutes at a time, to achieve maximum benefits. During the warm-up phase, he should stretch his muscles and slowly increase his heart rate for 5 to 10 minutes. During the conditioning phase, he should reach his target heart rate and maintain it for 20 to 30 minutes. Tell him to ask the doctor how high his heart rate can safely go during this most intense part of the workout. During cool-down, he should walk slowly or do other activities for 10 to 15 minutes to gradually return his body systems to normal. Instruct him to monitor his heart rate by taking his pulse before, during, and after exercise. Give him a copy of the patient-teaching aid *How to take your pulse,* page 26.

Take precautions. Warn the patient always to carry a source of simple carbohydrates and an identification tag that gives his name, condition, and medications, just in case he becomes hypoglycemic while exercising. Also advise him to eat a snack before exercising, if appropriate.

If the patient is taking insulin, advise him not to inject it into a part of his body that he'll use during exercise. Instruct him to avoid exercising at the peak of insulin activity or before meals, and to refrain from drinking alcohol before exercise. Also instruct him never to exercise alone.

Caution the patient to stop exercising immediately if he experiences chest pain, severe dyspnea, palpitations, dizziness, weakness, or nausea. If any of these symptoms persist, he should see his doctor at once.

Diet

Stress the importance of carefully following the prescribed diet to prevent rapid changes in blood glucose levels. Make sure the patient understands his specific meal plan, and urge him to stick to it. Advise him to eat about the same number of calories each day and to spread out his meals and snacks evenly. If appropriate, discuss investigative diet therapy to help control blood glucose levels (see *What's new in diabetes treatments*).

Limit calories. Stress that controlling caloric intake is a key factor in regulating blood glucose levels. Encourage the overweight patient to cut down on the amount he eats. But remember, the less drastic the change in his eating habits, the better the chances he'll comply.

What's new in diabetes treatments

After you discuss conventional diabetes treatment with your patient, give him encouraging news about investigative treatments that aim to refine the monitoring and control of blood glucose levels.

Glycemic index
This diet therapy links blood glucose fluctuations with specific foods and identifies low-fat, starchy foods that diabetic patients can eat to increase carbohydrate intake without triggering high postprandial blood glucose levels. A patient must comply with therapy by determining his blood glucose level after every meal and snack.

Pancreas islet cell grafts
Grafted islet cells may help control blood glucose metabolism and prevent or resolve microangiopathic complications. However, this therapy requires pure, undamaged pancreas islet cells for grafting, and they're hard to obtain. Another obstacle: isolated islet cells are more likely to be rejected than islet-cell grafts in an intact pancreas.

Pancreas transplants
Because of the high rejection risk, patients receiving pancreas transplants need immunosuppressive drug therapy. Unfortunately, long-term immunosuppression can cause more problems, including hepatotoxicity, nephrotoxicity, and infection. Consequently, most patients currently selected for a pancreas transplant are already receiving immunosuppressive drugs for a previous transplant; they also face a greater risk to life from diabetic complications than from long-term immunosuppression.

Implantable probes and pumps
Designed to monitor blood glucose levels and automatically deliver the correct insulin dose, implantable probes and pumps offer the potential for more exact blood glucose control. However, problems with clogging and unreliable insulin secretion remain unresolved.

Cyclosporine therapy
A promising treatment for Type I diabetes, cyclosporine therapy aims to prevent islet beta-cell destruction. Cyclosporine's immunosuppressive action may prevent circulating serum islet-cell antibodies from attacking islet cells. However, the drug can also cause nephrotoxicity and hepatotoxicity.

Fast facts on oral hypoglycemics

Tell the patient why it's important to adhere strictly to his drug regimen. Because blood glucose levels change with time and other variables, the patient needs to know how long it takes for his drug to act (onset) and how long the drug effect lasts (duration). Before you discuss dosage recommendations, review the following sulfonylureas—the most commonly prescribed oral hypoglycemic agents.

DRUG	ONSET (hours)	DURATION (hours)
acetohexamide (Dymelor)	1	8 to 24
chlorpropamide (Diabinese)	1	24 to 72
glipizide (Glucotrol)	1 to 1½	6 to 24
glyburide (Micronase)	2 to 4	16 to 24
tolazamide (Tolinase)	4 to 6	10 to 18
tolbutamide (Orinase)	1	6 to 12

Ask the patient where he usually eats his meals. Does he eat most of them in restaurants? If so, he'll need special instructions. Emphasize that no matter how large the servings are at a restaurant, he must eat only the amount specified in his meal plan.

Discuss which foods the patient likes. Then help him to understand his meal plan by having him write preferred foods on index cards. Assist him to color-code the index cards by food groups. Next, explain how many foods per color group he may have for each meal.

Coordinate meals and insulin needs. If the patient is taking insulin, instruct him to time and limit his meals to match the amount of insulin he injects each day. Explain that this may help prevent abrupt shifts in blood glucose levels and possible complications. If he's using food exchange lists in his diet regimen, help him to use them to plan meals. Instruct him to avoid foods high in sugar, saturated fats, and cholesterol. His doctor can tell him whether he should abstain from drinking alcohol.

If the patient has Type II diabetes, explain that diet alone may control his blood glucose levels. Simply eating less will lower the amount of glucose he produces and thus the amount of insulin he needs to control blood glucose levels. If he's overweight, however, emphasize the importance of weight reduction. Explain that an obese person needs to produce more insulin to control his glucose levels than does a person whose weight falls within a normal range. Discuss ways to help the overweight Type-II diabetic decrease his caloric intake.

Medication

Depending on his condition, your patient may be taking insulin or an oral hypoglycemic (see *Fast facts on oral hypoglycemics*). The doctor may also prescribe glucagon for emergencies. Teach your patient about the purpose, administration, and possible adverse effects of his medications.

Insulin. If the patient will be taking insulin after his discharge, explain that this drug helps control blood glucose levels. But emphasize that it's not meant to replace a proper diet. Then outline the types of insulin available: rapid-acting, intermediate-acting, and long-acting. Discuss in more detail the type or types of insulin the patient will be taking (see *Comparing insulin preparations,* pages 490 and 491).

Next, teach the patient how to administer insulin. If he'll be taking two different kinds, show him how to mix them together in a syringe. Give him a copy of the patient-teaching aid *Mixing insulins in a syringe,* page 498. Then show him how to draw up insulin in a syringe and how to give himself a subcutaneous injection. Provide a copy of the patient-teaching aid *Giving yourself a subcutaneous insulin injection,* pages 500 and 501. If he'll be administering his insulin with a mechanical device, or if he'll be wearing an insulin pump, explain how to use this equipment. (See *Understanding insulin pumps,* page 492.) Also teach him how to rotate injection sites. Give him a copy of *Rotating insulin injection sites,* page 499.

Impress upon the patient the importance of adhering to his prescribed medication regimen. Tell him always to take his insulin on schedule and never to adjust his insulin dosage or stop taking the drug without his doctor's approval—his blood glucose level could rise rapidly. Also caution him always to use the same brand of insulin, syringe, and needle and to be sure the syringe corresponds with his insulin concentration.

Warn him also to avoid alcohol, explaining that alcohol increases insulin's hypoglycemic effect. Add that changing his food or fluid intake or taking over-the-counter drugs can affect his insulin requirements. Finally, tell him to report these adverse reactions to insulin to the doctor: difficulty breathing; frequent or severe hypoglycemic or hyperglycemic symptoms; generalized itching; or redness, swelling, stinging, or itching at injection sites.

Oral hypoglycemic agents. If the patient's taking an oral hypo-

Comparing insulin preparations

Once the doctor determines the insulin regimen, your teaching can help the patient understand and follow it precisely. Inform him that insulins come in a wide variety of types. Point out that they also have varying times of onset and peak effect and varying durations of action. The doctor may prescribe any of the insulins shown below for your patient, or he may prescribe a mixture of them.

PREPARATION	ONSET (hours)	PEAK EFFECT (hours)	DURATION OF ACTION (hours)
Rapid-acting insulins			
Insulin injection (regular, crystalline zinc)			
Regular Iletin I	½ to 1	2 to 4	6 to 8
Regular Insulin	½	2½ to 5	8
Pork Regular Iletin II	½ to 1	2 to 4	6 to 8
Regular (concentrated) Iletin II	½	1 to 5	24
Velosulin	½	1 to 3	8
Purified Pork Insulin	½	2½ to 5	8
Humulin R	½ to 1	2 to 4	6 to 8
Novolin R	½	2½ to 5	8
Prompt insulin zinc suspension (semilente)			
Semilente Iletin I	1 to 3	3 to 8	10 to 16
Semilente Insulin	1½	5 to 10	16
Semilente Purified Pork Prompt Insulin	1½	5 to 10	16
Intermediate-acting insulins			
Isophane insulin suspension (NPH)			
NPH Iletin I	2	6 to 12	18 to 26
NPH Insulin	1½	4 to 12	24
Beef NPH Iletin II	2	6 to 12	18 to 26
Pork NPH Iletin II	2	6 to 12	18 to 26
NPH Purified Pork Isophane Insulin	1½	4 to 12	24
Insulatard NPH	1½	4 to 12	24
Humulin N	1 to 2	6 to 12	18 to 24
Novolin N	1½	4 to 12	24
Isophane (NPH) 70%, regular insulin 30%			
Mixtard	½	4 to 8	24

continued

Comparing insulin preparations — *continued*

PREPARATION	ONSET (hours)	PEAK EFFECT (hours)	DURATION OF ACTION (hours)
Intermediate-acting insulins *(continued)*			
Insulin zinc suspension (lente)			
Lente Iletin I	2 to 4	6 to 12	18 to 26
Lente Insulin	2½	7 to 15	24
Beef Lente Iletin II	2 to 4	6 to 12	18 to 26
Pork Lente Iletin II	2 to 4	6 to 12	18 to 26
Lente Purified Pork Insulin	2½	7 to 15	22
Humulin L	1 to 3	6 to 12	18 to 21
Novolin L	2½	7 to 15	22
Long-acting insulins			
Protamine zinc insulin suspension			
Protamine Zinc & Iletin I	4 to 8	14 to 24	28 to 36
Beef Protamine Zinc & Iletin II	4 to 8	14 to 24	28 to 36
Pork Protamine Zinc & Iletin II	4 to 8	14 to 24	28 to 36
Extended insulin zinc suspension (ultralente)			
Ultralente Iletin I	4 to 8	14 to 24	28 to 36
Ultralente Insulin	4	10 to 30	36
Ultralente Purified Beef Insulin	4	10 to 30	36

glycemic drug, explain that this drug helps regulate his blood glucose levels by increasing insulin secretion and decreasing cellular insulin resistance. Emphasize that the drug augments diet therapy and doesn't replace it. Then caution him never to adjust the dosage or stop taking the drug without his doctor's approval.

Warn the patient to avoid alcohol because it may cause a disulfiram reaction (severe nausea, vomiting, and sweating) or a hypoglycemic reaction. Advise him to take the oral hypoglycemic before meals, to avoid possible GI upset, and to call the doctor if he has any other adverse reactions, such as epigastric fullness, facial flushing, headache, heartburn, nausea, rash, vomiting, and jaundice. He should also notify the doctor if he's ill or under increased stress because these conditions may increase his insulin needs. The doctor may adjust the dosage accordingly or prescribe insulin.

If the patient takes insulin *and* oral hypoglycemics, make

Understanding insulin pumps

If your patient needs long-term insulin therapy, the doctor might recommend an insulin pump instead of injections. If so, tell the patient how these pumps work, and discuss their advantages and disadvantages.

Closed-loop system
A closed-loop pump detects and responds to changing blood glucose levels. At present, only one closed-loop system is available. It's used only in hospitals because it's large and it withdraws blood and infuses insulin intravenously. A smaller version is being developed for implantation under the skin.

Open-loop system
Open-loop pumps infuse insulin but can't respond to blood glucose level changes. They're offered by various manufacturers for home use. Also called continuous subcutaneous insulin infusers, these pumps continuously deliver insulin in small (basal) doses. They may be set manually to deliver bolus doses when blood glucose levels rise, such as with meals.

An open-loop system consists of a reservoir containing regular insulin; a small pump; an infusion rate selector, allowing insulin release adjustments; a battery; and a plastic catheter with an attached needle leading from the syringe to the subcutaneous injection site.

The patient fastens the pump to his belt or waistband. He must change the syringe daily and the needle, catheter, and injection site every other day.

Pros and cons
An open-loop pump may be more convenient than insulin injections, and the delivery system more closely matches the body's natural insulin-release pattern. However, insulin pumps also have some disadvantages, including possible infection at injection sites, catheter clogging, and insulin loss from a loose reservoir-catheter connection.

Not for everyone
Patients who benefit most from an insulin pump are those with widely fluctuating blood glucose levels despite optimal insulin and dietary regimens, those whose job or life-style prevents regular meals, and pregnant women.

The doctor probably won't order an insulin pump for patients who won't comply with prescribed regimens or keep scheduled medical appointments; for those who can't recognize the symptoms of hypoglycemia; or for those with diabetic complications, such as advanced renal disease, proliferative retinopathy, or severe autonomic neuropathy.

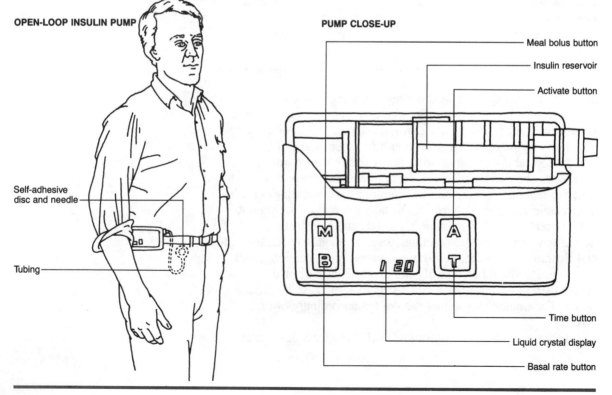

OPEN-LOOP INSULIN PUMP

Self-adhesive disc and needle

Tubing

PUMP CLOSE-UP

Meal bolus button

Insulin reservoir

Activate button

Time button

Liquid crystal display

Basal rate button

sure he understands the purpose of combining these therapies (see *Helping the patient understand insulin and oral hypoglycemic therapy*).

Glucagon. Explain to the patient and his family that glucagon, a drug administered to treat hypoglycemic crisis, raises blood glucose levels when the patient cannot take oral glucose.

Teach the family how to administer glucagon subcutaneously, and stress the importance of calling the doctor at once if hypoglycemia doesn't improve. Tell them that once it's reconstituted, glucagon may be stored in the refrigerator for up to 3 months. They should check the expiration date regularly and keep the correct type of syringes available.

Warn the family that nausea and vomiting may occur after taking this drug. But if the patient has difficulty breathing, if a rash develops, or if the patient doesn't respond to glucagon, the family should call the doctor immediately.

Procedures

Stress that checking blood glucose levels every day is crucial in managing diabetes. Show him how to collect a blood sample and test it for glucose levels (see *Testing your blood glucose levels*, pages 502 and 503). If appropriate, inform him how to use a computerized blood glucose meter to check his glucose levels. Tell him where he can obtain one, and teach him how to use it. Also teach him how to test his urine for ketones when he's hyper-

Helping the patient understand insulin and oral hypoglycemic therapy

The better your patient understands how insulin and oral hypoglycemic agents work, the better he'll comply with his prescribed regimen. Explain that oral hypoglycemic agents were first used nearly 50 years ago to treat Type II diabetes. They were found to lower blood glucose levels, presumably by stimulating the pancreas to produce more insulin.

Recent findings

Recent research shows that these agents act principally by enhancing peripheral cell sensitivity to insulin; their stimulating effect on the pancreas declines within a few months. This explains why after initial success, these drugs often fail to sustain blood glucose control in Type-II diabetics.

Combined therapy

Today, some doctors prescribe both oral hypoglycemics and insulin to regulate blood glucose levels and to combat the insulin deficiency and peripheral resistance to insulin common in Type-II diabetics.

Patients take a daily, supplemental dose, usually of an intermediate or long-acting insulin, to correct their insulin deficiency. Then they take an oral hypoglycemic agent, usually a sulfonylurea, to correct peripheral insulin resistance. Usually, they take the oral hypoglycemic agent 30 minutes before meals and the insulin as a small dose before bedtime.

This timing takes advantage of increased peripheral cell receptivity resulting from the effects of the oral hypoglycemic agent used during the day.

Who benefits most?

Combined therapy works best for Type-II diabetics who fail to respond to oral agents alone or who require large doses of insulin (more than 100 units a day). Because the oral hypoglycemic agent increases cellular sensitivity to insulin, the insulin dosage can then be reduced. This therapy doesn't help Type-I diabetics who characteristically have total insulin deficiency, not insulin resistance.

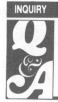

Questions patients ask about gestational diabetes

My obstetrician says I have gestational diabetes. Why did this happen to me?
Pregnancy increases the body's need for insulin. So some pregnant women (1% or 2%) develop diabetes temporarily because their pancreas can't produce the extra insulin required to keep their blood glucose level normal.

Will I have to take insulin from now on?
No. You'll need to take insulin only until your child's born. When you're no longer pregnant, your insulin requirements will drop, and your own pancreas will produce enough insulin to meet your body's needs. Later in life, you may develop diabetes.

Why does my doctor say that I'll have a big baby?
During pregnancy, the fetus relies on maternal glucose as a primary energy source. So elevated blood glucose levels cause the fetus to be overnourished and gain more weight than normal.

My grandmother takes pills for her diabetes. Can I take them, too?
No. During pregnancy, never take pills to stimulate insulin production or oral hypoglycemic agents. Their effect on the fetus isn't known.

glycemic or ill (see *Testing your urine for ketones,* page 504). Then teach him how to interpret the results and what to do if they're abnormal.

Other care measures
Educate the patient about preventive health care measures and ways to deal with special problems.

Hypoglycemia. Make sure the patient knows the symptoms of hypoglycemia (weakness, headache, anxiety, sweating, and vision changes) and how to prevent it by avoiding overexertion, inadequate food, and excessive insulin.

Infection. Advise the patient to avoid extreme temperature changes to reduce the risk of infection, especially in the respiratory tract. Also teach him to perform meticulous skin and foot care. Warn him that some diabetics develop neuropathies, typically in the legs. To prevent problems from developing, teach him how to care for his skin and feet. For example, tell him not to use a hot-water bottle or heating pad; he may burn himself because of reduced sensation. Also teach him the signs and symptoms of impaired circulation, such as dependent edema, pallor, numbness and tingling (paresthesia), and hair loss on the affected limb.

Instruct the patient to be especially careful to avoid accidents. If the patient works, discuss possible job hazards. If he's likely to cut or bruise himself at work, advise him to wear sturdy clothing and shoes and to be extremely cautious. Teach him how to treat cuts or bruises if they do occur. Even a relatively minor injury—such as a stubbed toe—can be serious for a diabetic; he could develop an infection from impaired circulation. Emphasize the need to be careful. Give him a copy of the patient-teaching aid *Taking care of your feet,* page 505. Also recommend using a night-light or a flashlight if he habitually goes to the bathroom in the middle of the night.

Vision problems. If your patient has diabetic retinopathy with vision loss, be sure the booklets and other teaching aids you give him have large type. Explain that he should read with a strong light behind him and that he should be examined regularly by an ophthalmologist.

Illness. Advise the patient of measures to take during illness. Reinforce your instruction with the patient-teaching aid *Managing diabetes during illness,* pages 506 and 507.

Sexual concerns and pregnancy. Mention that diabetic patients, particularly men, may experience sexual dysfunction, such as impotence. Encourage the patient to discuss any sexual problems he may be having. Also discuss problems of pregnancy with female diabetics. If your patient is already pregnant, refer her to a specialist who cares for diabetics of childbearing age. (See *Questions patients ask about gestational diabetes.*)

Travel precautions. Tell the patient who travels for business or vacation to make plans for meals and medication beforehand. He should also pack his insulin and syringes separately, and adjust his insulin schedule accordingly if he crosses time zones. (See *Travel tips for diabetic patients,* page 508.)

Living alone. If the patient lives alone, spend a little extra time with him; he may find it more difficult to comply with therapy than someone who has a spouse or other family member to encourage him. Ask him how he deals with stress. Many people overeat when they're frustrated or anxious. A diabetic who tries to cope with stress in this way won't be able to control his blood glucose levels.

Sources of information and support

American Diabetes Association
1660 Duke Street, Alexandria, Va. 22314
(703) 549-1500

Juvenile Diabetes Foundation International
432 Park Avenue South, New York, N.Y. 10016-8013
(800) 533-2873

Further readings

"1989 Buyer's Guide to Diabetes Products," *Diabetes Forecast* 41(10):39-79, October 1988.

Beller, B., et al. "Brushing Up on Dental Health," *Diabetes Self-Management* 5(5):4-6, September-October 1988.

Franz, M. "Exercise: Its Role in Diabetes Management," *Diabetes Spectrum* 1(4):217-52, September-October 1988.

Freinkel, R. "Caring for Your Skin," *Diabetes Forecast* 41(7):76-81, July 1988.

Genuth, S. "Treatment Times Two," *Diabetes Forecast* 41(8):40-45, August 1988.

"How to Use...Novolin Pen." Princeton, N.J.: Squibb-Novo, Inc., 1988.

Jette, D. "Warming Up to Exercise," *Diabetes Forecast* 41(5):58-63, May 1988.

Lewitt, M.S., et al. "Effects of Combined Insulin-Sulfonylurea Therapy in Type II Patients," *Diabetes Care* 12(6):379-83, June 1989.

Narins, V. "Site Rotation on Target," *Diabetes Forecast* 39(7):21, October 1986.

Physician's Guide to Insulin-Dependent (Type I) Diabetes: Diagnosis and Treatment. Alexandria, Va.: American Diabetes Association, 1988.

Physician's Guide to Non-Insulin–Dependent (Type II) Diabetes: Diagnosis and Treatment, 2nd ed. Alexandria, Va.: American Diabetes Association, 1988.

Robertson, C. "The New Challenges of Insulin Therapy," *RN* 52(5):34-38, May 1989.

Service, F.J. "Hypoglycemias: Their Etiologies and Diagnosis," *Clinical Diabetes* 7(2):25, 27, 30-32, 37-39, March-April 1989.

PATIENT-TEACHING AID

Preventing diabetic complications

Dear Patient:

There's no way around it. Controlling your diabetes means checking your blood glucose levels daily and making the following good health habits a way of life.

Care for your heart
Because diabetes raises your risk of heart disease, take care of your heart by following these American Heart Association guidelines:
• Maintain your normal weight.
• Exercise regularly, following your doctor's recommendations.
• Help control your blood pressure and cholesterol levels by eating a low-fat, high-fiber diet, as your doctor prescribes.

Care for your eyes
Have your eyes examined by an ophthalmologist at least once a year. He may detect any damage, which can cause blindness, before symptoms appear. Early treatment may prevent further damage.

Care for your teeth
Schedule regular dental check-ups and follow good home care to minimize dental problems, such as gum disease and abscesses, that may occur with diabetes. If you experience any bleeding, pain, or soreness in your gums or teeth, report this to the dentist immediately. Brush your teeth after every meal and floss daily. If you wear dentures, clean them thoroughly every day, and be sure they fit properly.

Care for your skin
Breaks in your skin can increase your risk of infection. So check your skin daily for cuts and irritated areas, and see your doctor, if necessary. Bathe daily with warm water and a mild soap, and apply a lanolin-based lotion afterward to prevent dryness. Pat your skin dry thoroughly, taking extra care between your toes and in any other areas where skin surfaces touch. Always wear cotton underwear to allow moisture to evaporate and help prevent skin breakdown.

Care for your feet
Diabetes can reduce blood flow to your feet and dull their ability to feel heat, cold, or pain. Follow your nurse's instructions on daily foot care and necessary precautions to prevent foot problems.

Check your urine
Because symptoms of kidney disease usually don't appear until the problem is advanced, your doctor will check your urine routinely for protein, which can signal kidney disease. And don't delay telling your doctor if you have symptoms of a urinary tract infection (burning, painful, or difficult urination, or blood or pus in the urine).

Have regular checkups
See your doctor regularly so that he can detect early signs of complications and start treatment promptly.

Getting ready for an oral glucose tolerance test

Dear Patient:

To prepare for an oral glucose tolerance test and to ensure accurate results, you need to follow a high-carbohydrate diet for 3 days before the test. Below you'll find a sample diet you can use. If you find it too restrictive, follow your regular diet, but eat 12 additional slices of bread each day.

Breakfast
1 serving fruit
Eggs, as desired
5 bread exchanges
1 cup milk
Butter or margarine
Coffee or tea, if desired

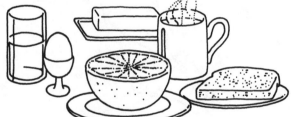

Lunch and dinner
Meat, as desired
5 bread exchanges
2 vegetables
1 serving fruit
1 cup milk
Butter or margarine
Coffee or tea, if desired

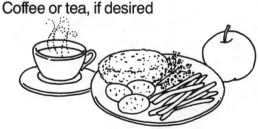

What are bread exchanges?
One of the following equals one bread exchange:
1 slice bread, white or whole wheat
1½-inch cube of corn bread
½ hamburger or hot dog roll
½ cup cooked cereal
¾ cup dry cereal (avoid sugar-coated varieties)
½ cup noodles, spaghetti, or macaroni
½ cup cooked dried beans or peas
⅓ cup corn or ½ small ear of corn
1 biscuit
½ corn muffin
1 roll
5 saltine crackers
2 graham crackers
½ cup grits or rice
1 small white potato
½ cup mashed potato
¼ cup sweet potato
¼ cup baked beans
¼ cup pork and beans

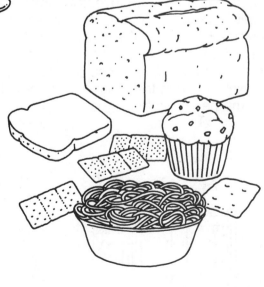

NPH — then Reg —

Mixing insulins in a syringe

Dear Patient:

Your doctor has prescribed regular and either intermediate or long-acting insulin to control your diabetes. To avoid giving yourself separate injections, you can mix these two types of insulin in a syringe and administer them together. Here's what to do.

1 Wash your hands. Then prepare the mixture in a clean area. Make sure you have alcohol swabs, both types of insulin, and the proper syringe for your prescribed insulin concentration. Then mix the contents of the intermediate or long-acting insulin by rolling it gently between your palms.

2 Using an alcohol swab, clean the rubber stopper on the vial of intermediate or long-acting insulin. Then draw air into the syringe by pulling the plunger back to the prescribed number of insulin units. Insert the needle into the top of the vial. Make sure the point doesn't touch the insulin (see illustration). Now, push in the plunger, and remove the needle from the vial.

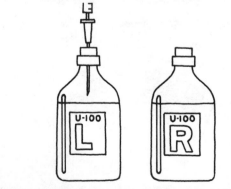

3 Now clean the rubber stopper on the regular insulin vial with an alcohol swab. Then pull back the plunger on the syringe to the prescribed number of insulin units, insert the needle into the top of the vial, and inject air into the vial. With the needle still in the vial, turn the vial upside down and withdraw the prescribed dose of regular insulin.

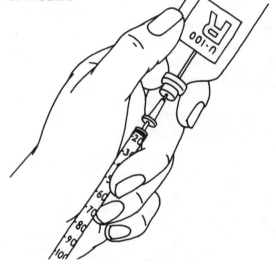

4 Clean the top of the intermediate or long-acting insulin vial. Then insert the needle into it without pushing the plunger down. Invert the vial and withdraw the prescribed number of units for the *total* dose. (For example, if you have 10 units of regular insulin in the syringe and you need 20 units of intermediate or long-acting insulin, pull the plunger back to 30 units.)
 Never change the order in which you mix insulins, and always administer the insulin immediately to prevent loss of potency.

Rotating insulin injection sites

Dear Patient:

Whether you administer your insulin by needle or by an insulin pump, you need to rotate the injection sites.

Why rotate sites?

Rotating the site for injecting insulin reduces injury to the skin and underlying fatty tissue. It prevents a buildup of scar tissue and swelling and lumps.

It can also minimize a slow insulin absorption rate. This can result from repeated injections in one spot, which can cause fibrous tissue growth and decreased blood supply in that area.

Site rotation can also offset changes that exercise causes in insulin absorption. Exercise increases blood flow to the body part being exercised, thereby increasing the insulin absorption rate. So don't inject yourself in an area about to be exercised. (For example, don't inject yourself in the thigh before you go walking or bike riding.)

Where can I inject insulin?

You can inject insulin into these areas:
• the outer part of both upper arms
• your right and left stomach, just above and below your waist (except for a 2-inch circle around your navel)
• your right and left back below the waist, just behind your hip bone
• the front and outsides of both thighs, from 4 inches below the top of your thigh to 4 inches above your knee.

Keep in mind that different parts of the body absorb insulin at different rates.

The stomach absorbs insulin best, then the upper arm, and last, the thighs. Use this approach:
• Inject into the same body area for 1 to 2 weeks, depending on the number of injections you need daily. For example, if you need four injections a day, use one area for only about 5 days.
• Cover the entire area within an injection site, but don't inject into the same spot.
• Don't inject into spots where you can't easily grasp fatty tissue.
• Have a family member give you injections in hard-to-reach areas.
• Check with your doctor if a site becomes especially painful, or if swelling or lumps appear.

INJECTION SITES

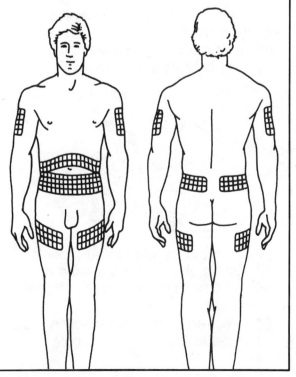

Giving yourself a subcutaneous insulin injection

Dear Patient:

Before you can administer your insulin, you must transfer the correct amount from the medication vial to the syringe. Follow these guidelines.

1 Wash your hands. Then assemble this equipment in a clean area: a sterile syringe and needle, insulin, and alcohol swabs or wipes (or rubbing alcohol and cotton balls).

2 Check the labels on the syringe and insulin to be sure they match. If you're using U-100 insulin, you must use a U-100 syringe. Also check that you have the correct type of insulin, such as NPH or Lente.

3 If your insulin is the cloudy-looking type, roll the bottle between your hands to mix it. Mix gently to prevent large air bubbles in the insulin.

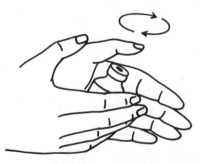

4 Clean the top of the insulin bottle with an alcohol swab or wipe or with a cotton ball and rubbing alcohol.

5 Select an appropriate injection site. (Refer to the guide your nurse gave you, showing you how to rotate your injection sites correctly. Keep a record of which sites you use and when you use them.)

Pull the skin taut; then, using a circular motion, clean the skin with an alcohol swab or wipe or a cotton ball soaked in alcohol.

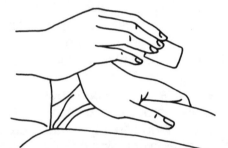

6 Remove the needle cover. *To prevent possible infection, don't touch the needle.* Touch only the barrel and plunger of the syringe. Pull back the plunger to the prescribed number of insulin units. This draws air into the syringe.

Insert the needle into the rubber stopper on the insulin bottle, and push in the plunger. This pushes air into the bottle and prevents a vacuum.

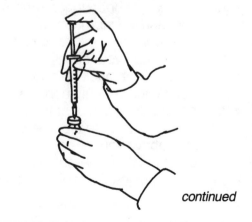

continued

Giving yourself a subcutaneous insulin injection — *continued*

7 Hold the bottle and syringe together in one hand, then turn them upside down so the bottle is on top. You can hold the bottle between your thumb and forefinger and the syringe between your ring finger and little finger, against your palm. Or you can hold the bottle between your forefinger and middle finger, while holding the syringe between your thumb and little finger.

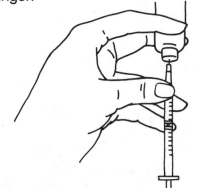

8 Pull back on the plunger until the top, black portion of the barrel corresponds to the line that indicates you have withdrawn your correct insulin dose. Remove the needle from the bottle.

9 If air bubbles appear in the syringe after you fill it with insulin, tap the syringe and push lightly on the plunger to remove them. Draw up more insulin, if necessary.

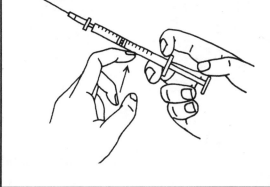

10 Using your thumb and forefinger, pinch the skin at the injection site. Then quickly plunge the needle (up to its hub) into the subcutaneous tissue at a 90-degree angle. Push down the plunger to inject the insulin.

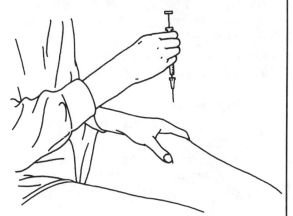

11 Place an alcohol swab or cotton ball over the injection site; then press down on it lightly as you withdraw the needle. Don't rub the injection site when withdrawing the needle.

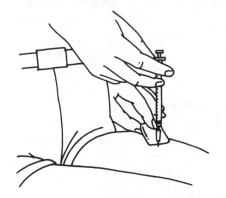

Snap the needle off the syringe, and dispose of both needle and syringe.

Important: If you travel, keep a bottle of insulin and a syringe with you at all times. Keep insulin at room temperature. Don't refrigerate it or place it near heat (above 90° F).

Testing your blood glucose levels

Dear Patient:

Testing blood glucose levels daily will tell you whether your diabetes is under control. Follow these steps to learn how to obtain blood for testing and how to perform the test.

Getting ready
1 Begin by assembling the necessary equipment: a lancet, a mechanical device to draw blood (optional), a vial with reagent strips, cotton balls, a watch or a clock with a second hand, and a pen.

2 Remove a reagent strip from its vial. Then replace the cap, making sure it's tight. Two types of reagent strips are commonly used to test blood glucose levels visually: Chemstrip bG and Visidex II. (You can also use a glucose meter to measure levels. If you do, be sure to follow the manufacturer's directions precisely.)

Obtaining blood
1 Choose a site on the end or side of any fingertip. Wash your hands thoroughly and dry them. To enhance blood flow, hold your finger under warm water for a minute or two.

2 Hold your hand below your heart, and milk the blood toward the fingertip you plan to pierce. Squeeze that fingertip with the thumb of the same hand. Place your fingertip (with your thumb still pressed against it) on a firm surface, such as a table.

3 If you're using a lancet manually, twist off the protective cap. Then grasp the lancet and quickly pierce your fingertip just to the side of the finger pad where you have more blood vessels and fewer nerve endings.

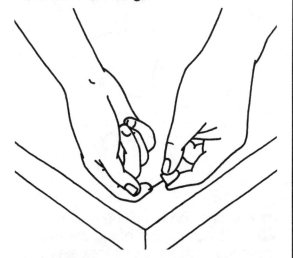

4 Remove your thumb from your fingertip to permit blood flow. Then milk your finger gently until you get a hanging drop of blood that looks large enough to cover the reagent area of the test strip. Be patient. If blood doesn't flow immediately from the puncture site, keep milking your finger before trying another site.

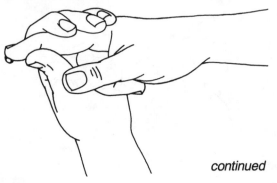

continued

PATIENT-TEACHING AID

Testing your blood glucose levels — *continued*

5 If you're using a mechanical device, follow the manufacturer's instructions precisely. To prevent a deep puncture, don't press the device too deeply into the skin surface.

Testing blood

1 Carefully lift the reagent strip to the drop of blood. (The strip has a shiny, slippery undersurface; the blood will roll off if you don't place it on the strip correctly.) Let the blood completely cover the reagent area without rubbing or smearing it. If the blood smears, start over with a new strip.

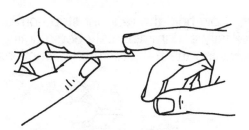

2 As you put the drop of blood on the reagent area, look at your watch or a clock. Begin timing according to the manufacturer's directions. Make sure you keep the strip level.

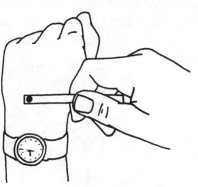

3 When the recommended time has elapsed, gently wipe all the blood off the strip with a clean, dry cotton ball.

Wipe the strip three times, using a clean side of the cotton ball each time. Then wait the recommended time.

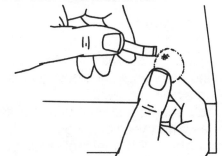

4 Now determine your blood glucose level by holding the reagent strip next to the area of color blocks on the vial. Then match the colors that have appeared on the strip with the two color blocks on the vial. Example: If both colors match the block labeled 180, your blood glucose level is about 180 mg/dl.

If the colors fall between two blocks, take the average of the two numbers. Example: If the colors fall between the two blocks labeled 120 and 180, your blood glucose level is about 150 mg/dl.

Note: The reagent strip and vial shown below don't appear in their actual colors.

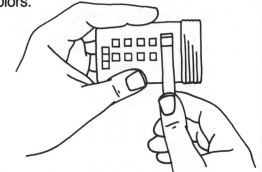

5 Write the date, time, and your initials on the reagent strip and store it in an empty vial. Make sure the cap is tight. The colors on the reagent area will last for up to a week.

Testing your urine for ketones

Dear Patient:

If your urine contains waste chemicals called ketones, your blood glucose levels may be too high.

You should test your urine for ketones when your blood glucose level rises above 240 mg/dl or when you're ill. Even a minor illness can dramatically affect your blood glucose levels.

Your doctor will probably recommend testing every 4 hours until your blood glucose levels have stabilized or until your illness is over. To test your urine for ketones, follow these steps.

1 First, gather a clean container (a small plastic cup will do), a bottle of reagent strips, and a wristwatch or a clock with a second hand.

2 Collect a urine specimen in the container.

3 Remove one reagent strip from the bottle and replace the cap. Hold the strip so the test blocks face up, but don't touch the blocks.

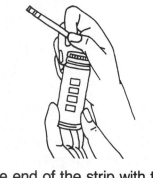

4 Dip the end of the strip with the test blocks into the urine for about

2 seconds. Then remove the strip and shake off excess urine. (Or you can perform the test while you urinate by simply holding the strip under the urine stream for about 2 seconds.)

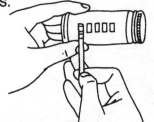

5 Now hold the reagent strip horizontally and immediately begin timing, following the manufacturer's directions.

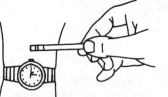

6 After waiting the recommended time, compare the ketone test block with the ketone color chart on the bottle label.

Note: The reagent strip and vial shown below don't appear in their actual colors.

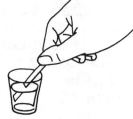

7 Keep a record of your tests, listing the date, the time, the results, and any other pertinent information. Call the doctor if your urine is positive for ketones.

Taking care of your feet

Dear Patient:

Because you have diabetes, your feet require meticulous daily care. Why? Diabetes can reduce blood supply to your feet, so normally minor foot injuries, such as an ingrown toenail or a blister, can lead to dangerous infection. Because diabetes also reduces sensation in your feet, you can burn or chill them without feeling it. To prevent foot problems, follow these instructions.

Routine care
● Wash your feet in warm, soapy water every day. To prevent burns, use a thermometer to check the water temperature before immersing your feet.
● Dry your feet thoroughly by blotting them with a towel. Be sure to dry between the toes.
● Apply oil or lotion to your feet immediately after drying, to prevent evaporating water from drying your skin. Lotion will keep your skin soft. But don't put lotion between your toes.
● If your feet perspire heavily, use a mild foot powder. Sprinkle it lightly between your toes and in your socks and shoes.
● File your nails even with the end of your toes. Don't cut them. And don't corner nails or file them shorter than the ends of your toes. If your nails are too thick, tough, or misshapen to file, consult a podiatrist. Also, don't dig under toenails or around cuticles.
● Exercise your feet daily to improve circulation. Sitting on the edge of the bed, point your toes upward, then downward, 10 times. Then make a circle with each foot 10 times.

Special precautions
● Make sure your shoes fit properly. Buy only leather shoes (because *only* leather allows air in and out), and break in new shoes gradually, increasing wearing time by half an hour each day. Check worn shoes frequently for rough spots in the lining.
● Wear clean cotton socks daily. Don't wear socks with holes or darns that have rough, irritating seams.
● Consult a podiatrist for treatment of corns and calluses. Self-treatment or application of caustic agents may be harmful.
● If your feet are cold, wear warm socks or slippers and use extra blankets in bed. Avoid using heating pads and hot-water bottles. These devices may cause burns.
● Check the skin of your feet daily for cuts, cracks, blisters, or red, swollen areas.
● If you cut your foot, no matter how slightly, contact the doctor. Meanwhile, wash the cut thoroughly and apply a mild antiseptic. Avoid harsh antiseptics, such as iodine, which can cause tissue damage.
● Don't wear tight-fitting garments or engage in activities that can decrease circulation. Especially avoid wearing elastic garters, sitting with knees crossed, picking at sores or rough spots on your feet, walking barefoot, or applying adhesive tape to the skin of your feet.

Managing diabetes during illness

Dear Patient:

Minor illnesses—a cold, flu, infection, or upset stomach—can drastically alter your ability to control your blood glucose levels. As your body attempts to compensate for the stress of an illness, your blood glucose levels may rise. To prevent this, maintain your usual insulin schedule and pattern of meals and snacks, if possible, and follow these guidelines:

• Check your blood glucose levels every 4 hours.
• Test your urine for ketones every 4 hours.
• *Never* skip an insulin injection.
• Call the doctor if you can't eat or keep any food or liquids down, if you can't eat normally for more than 24 hours, or if you have a fever.
• If you live alone, arrange for someone to check on you several times daily.

In addition, you can use this list of foods and liquids to guide you through the different stages of an illness. Just follow the instructions for your stage of illness. You don't have to start with stage 1 and progress through the remaining stages. You could, for instance, start with stage 3, depending on your symptoms.

Also, if your symptoms get worse and you can't tolerate recommended foods, you can drop back one stage until you feel better.

Stage 1

Your symptoms: severe nausea and vomiting, severe diarrhea, fever

Allowable foods and beverages: orange, grapefruit, or tomato juice; soup; broth; tea; coffee; cola

Special instructions: Sip a teaspoon of liquid every 10 to 15 minutes. If you can't tolerate this, call your doctor. Advance to stage 2 when nausea and diarrhea stop (or almost stop) and you're no longer vomiting.

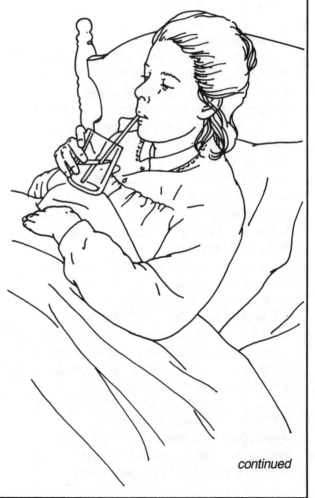

continued

Managing diabetes during illness — *continued*

Stage 2

Your symptoms: little or no appetite, occasional diarrhea, fatigue, fever

Allowable foods and beverages: creamed soup, mashed potatoes, cooked cereal, plain yogurt, bananas, fruit-flavored gelatins, juice, broth, regular soft drinks

Special instructions: Take ½ to 1 cup of food or beverage every 1 to 2 hours. Because fever causes you to perspire and lose body fluids, you should also continue to sip an unsweetened beverage (tea or coffee without sugar, water, or diet soft drinks, for example) every 10 or 15 minutes.

You're ready to advance to stage 3 when you've consumed the suggested amount of food and liquids several times, and your symptoms are improving.

Stage 3

Your symptoms: limited appetite, small meals tolerated, sluggishness, slight fever, able to sit up or walk

Allowable foods and beverages: Use your diabetic meal plan to guide you through this stage of your illness. (If you don't have one, talk to a diet counselor.) You can skip the protein and fat groups listed on your meal plan.

• Milk list: You can eat one of these foods instead of drinking 1 cup of milk — ½ cup of eggnog or sweetened custard; or 1 cup of creamed soup or plain yogurt.

• Bread and cereal list: You can eat one of the following foods instead of one bread or starch serving — ¼ cup of sherbet; ½ cup of cooked cereal, mashed potatoes, ice cream, or fruit-

flavored gelatin; ¾ cup of regular soft drink; 1 cup of noodle soup; or five salted crackers.

• Vegetable list: You can eat ½ serving from the bread and cereal serving list in your meal plan.

• Fruit list: You can eat any of these foods instead of one fruit serving — ¼ cup of grape or prune juice; ⅓ cup of apple juice; ½ cup of unsweetened applesauce, regular soft drink, or orange or grapefruit juice; ½ of a banana or an ice pop; or 2 teaspoons of honey.

Special instructions: Eat as many meals and snacks as your meal plan calls for.

Advance to stage 4 when your appetite increases and you can follow your diabetic meal plan without any problems. If you still have a fever, drink several extra glasses of water, tea or coffee without sugar, or diet soft drink each day.

Stage 4

Your symptoms: general sick feeling, stomach upset by heavy or spicy foods

Allowable foods and beverages: Use food lists on your regular meal plan. Choose foods that don't give you problems. For protein, you might want to try cottage cheese, broiled fish, or baked chicken. Eat fruit, vegetables, starch, and protein in moderation.

Special instructions: Eat at regular meal and snack times. Use your regular diabetic meal plan if you have no problems with the easier-to-digest foods for a day.

Travel tips for diabetic patients

Dear Patient:

If you enjoy traveling, having diabetes won't cramp your style—as long as you plan ahead and make the following adjustments.

Before you go

Visit your doctor for a general checkup, travel guidelines, and prescriptions (for example, for antidiarrheal medication). Ask for a note describing your condition, the type of medications you're taking, and any allergies you have.

Unless you're traveling by car, pack your diabetic supplies in a carry-on bag, in case your luggage is lost or delayed. Be sure to pack enough insulin, syringes, and other supplies to last for the entire trip. In some states, insulin and syringes can't be purchased over the counter. And in some countries, only U-40 and U-80 insulin are available.

If you're traveling by boat or plane, ask your doctor if you can take an antiemetic (a medication that prevents nausea or vomiting), such as Dramamine. Take the medication 4 hours before departure and as often as needed thereafter.

If your insulin dosage will need adjusting when you cross time zones, ask your doctor about the exact amount of insulin to take. Remember to ask him for guidelines for the return trip, too.

If you're visiting a country where English isn't spoken, learn how to say the following sentences, or write them on a card:

- I am a diabetic.
- Please get me a doctor.
- Sugar or orange juice, please.

During your trip

Continue to follow your diabetic diet while en route. If you're traveling by boat or plane, call ahead and request special diabetic meals. After boarding, identify yourself to the steward, and explain what time you must eat so your meals and snacks can be ready.

Regardless of how you're traveling, always carry some simple carbohydrate snacks, such as sugar cubes, hard candy, an apple, or an orange, in case a meal or snack is delayed or you have an unexpected hypoglycemic reaction. If you're traveling by car and can't stop every couple hours for a snack or a meal, carry food with you.

Some precautions

Wear sturdy, comfortable shoes to avoid foot injury—don't wear new shoes or open-toed sandals.

Plan your activities carefully—excessive exercise can cause your blood glucose level to fall dangerously low. Be sure to monitor your blood glucose levels daily. Always carry a simple carbohydrate snack.

Wear a Medic Alert bracelet or carry a card that identifies you as a diabetic and lists your medications. And be sure your traveling companions know you're a diabetic and know how to treat you for low blood glucose levels in case you should become unconscious.

Bon voyage!

Hyperthyroidism

Although chronic, hyperthyroidism can be a relatively benign condition if the patient complies with therapy. To encourage compliance, you'll need to explain that thyroid hormone overproduction can be curbed by medication or other treatments. What's more, you'll need to emphasize that such measures will allow the patient to lead a nearly normal life.

Discuss the disorder

Explain that hyperthyroidism results from excessive production of thyroid hormone. Point out that this hormone is produced by the thyroid, a butterfly-shaped gland in the anterior portion of the lower neck. Overproduction of thyroid hormone accelerates all bodily functions and activities.

Explain that hyperthyroidism's exact cause is unknown. Mention that the condition has several forms. The most common, Graves' disease, may be related to an immune defect that causes formation of abnormal antibodies. Apparently, these antibodies stimulate production of thyroid hormone regardless of whether the body needs it, causing elevated serum levels.

Inform the patient that elevated thyroid hormone levels increase the rate at which the body uses energy. This can lead to symptoms that affect all body systems. (See *Reviewing clinical features of hyperthyroidism,* page 510.) Cardiovascular effects, for instance, include hypertension and tachycardia, which can lead to flushing, palpitations, and congestive heart failure. Central nervous system effects include emotional instability, irritability, difficulty concentrating, and insomnia. Other effects are fine hand tremors, weight loss, and fatigue.

Complications

Encourage compliance with the treatment regimen by pointing out that untreated or poorly managed hyperthyroidism can lead to severe complications. For example, thyroid storm, an acute complication, can be fatal without prompt treatment. In thyroid storm, the patient's metabolic rate rapidly accelerates. The functions of all body systems become severely taxed. Body temperature may rise as high as 106° F. (41° C.); both heart and respiratory rates rise dramatically. Total systemic collapse becomes imminent.

Explain to the patient that compliance can also forestall common chronic complications of hyperthyroidism, such as cardiac dysfunction, weight loss, and GI problems.

Marlene M. Ciranowicz, RN, MSN, CDE, and **Susan Zemble, RN, MaEd, JD,** contributed to this chapter. Ms. Ciranowicz is a diabetes educator in the outpatient department of Hahnemann University Hospital, Philadelphia. Ms. Zemble, former coordinator of patient and community health education at Memorial Hospital, Philadelphia, is an associate with the law firm of O'Brien and Ryan.

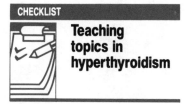

CHECKLIST

Teaching topics in hyperthyroidism

☐ Explanation of hyperthyroidism

☐ Complications, such as thyroid storm

☐ Blood and X-ray tests to evaluate thyroid function

☐ Activity restrictions to help counteract increased metabolic rate

☐ Dietary measures to ensure sufficient caloric intake

☐ Medications and their administration

☐ Radioactive iodine therapy, if indicated

☐ Subtotal thyroidectomy, if indicated, and possible need for lifelong hormonal replacement therapy

☐ Relation of stress to hormonal balance

☐ Eye care, if exophthalmos or visual changes occur

Reviewing clinical features of hyperthyroidism

When discussing the signs and symptoms of hyperthyroidism with the patient and her family, tell them to be alert for the following:
- weight loss
- muscle wasting
- muscle weakness and tremors
- fatigue
- dyspnea
- breast enlargement
- palpitations
- increased appetite
- irritability and nervousness
- exophthalmos, lid lag
- profuse sweating
- heat intolerance
- fine, straight hair.

Graves' disease—a common form of hyperthyroidism—produces three characteristic signs:
- a uniformly enlarged thyroid gland (goiter)
- infiltrative ophthalmopathy
- infiltrative dermopathy.
(*Note:* All three signs may not appear in every patient.)

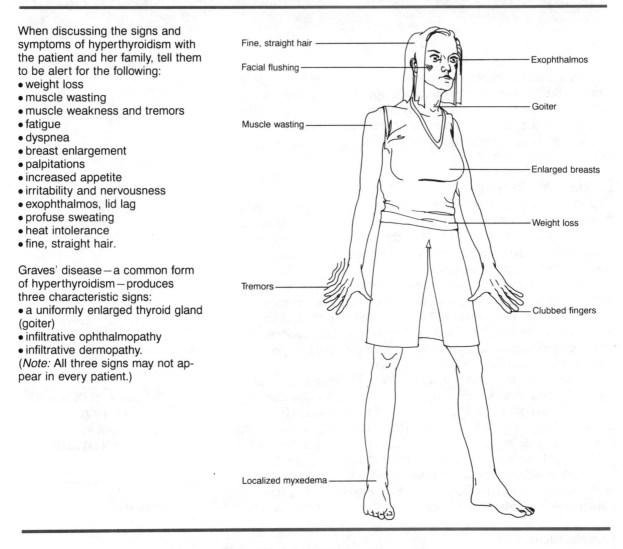

Fine, straight hair

Facial flushing

Exophthalmos

Goiter

Muscle wasting

Enlarged breasts

Weight loss

Tremors

Clubbed fingers

Localized myxedema

Describe the diagnostic workup
You'll need to teach the patient about the tests commonly used to evaluate thyroid function. Explain that blood tests can measure levels of circulating thyroid hormone. A thyroid scan or ultrasonography can evaluate the gland's structure and position. Another diagnostic procedure, the radioactive iodine uptake test, measures the gland's ability to accumulate iodine, which is a precursor in the production of thyroid hormone.

Blood tests
Explain that these tests require a small blood sample drawn by venipuncture at regular intervals. Studies will be done on thyroid hormone itself or on its by-products found in the blood.
    Serum thyroxine (T_4). Levels of circulating T_4 are used to

screen for hyperthyroidism. Elevated levels confirm the disease.

Serum long-acting thyroid stimulator. This test may be ordered to determine if the abnormal antibody thought to be responsible for Graves' disease is present. If it is, the hyperthyroidism is attributed to Graves' disease.

T_3 (triiodothyronine) resin uptake. Occasionally, this test is ordered to further evaluate thyroid function. An elevated T_3 level strengthens a diagnosis of hyperthyroidism. A thyroid scan may also be ordered to aid diagnosis.

Thyrotropin releasing hormone (TRH) stimulation. This test may be ordered if only an eye abnormality, such as exophthalmos, suggests Graves' disease. It involves injection of the TRH, followed by a series of blood samples drawn periodically over the next hour.

Thyroid scan

Tell the patient that this painless, 30-minute test allows visualization of the thyroid gland by a gamma camera after administration of radioactive iodine. Stress that the test will not expose him to dangerous radiation levels. Tell him who will perform the scan and where. Advise him to follow his doctor's guidelines for discontinuing medications before the test. Usually, the patient mustn't take any medications (particularly multivitamins and cough syrups) for at least 3 days before the test. Also instruct him to avoid iodized salt, iodinated salt substitutes, and seafood for 3 days before the test.

Explain what takes place during the test. First, the patient will be given a radioisotope either orally or intravenously. If he receives the oral radioisotope, tell him that his thyroid gland will be X-rayed 24 hours later. If he's given the I.V. form, the gland will be scanned within 20 to 30 minutes. Before the X-ray, instruct him to remove dentures and jewelry. Explain that he'll lie on his back with his neck extended. A special X-ray machine called a gamma camera will then be positioned over his throat to visualize the thyroid gland.

Ultrasonography

Inform the patient that this painless, 30-minute test visualizes his thyroid gland. Explain that this is done using a transducer to direct high-frequency sound waves at his thyroid. Once these waves strike the thyroid, they're reflected back to the transducer and converted to images on an oscilloscope screen.

Tell the patient what to expect: During the test, he'll lie on his back, with a pillow placed under his shoulder blades to hyperextend his neck. Explain that the skin over his thyroid will be coated with a water-soluble gel. Then the technician will move the transducer over the area to study the gland.

Radioactive iodine uptake test

Explain that this test assesses thyroid function by measuring the gland's ability to accumulate iodine. It may be used with other

INQUIRY

Questions patients ask about thyroidectomy

I know the thyroid gland is located near my voice box. Will removing my thyroid change my voice?
It shouldn't. After surgery, you may notice some slight hoarseness for a few days. However, there is a small chance that surgery may injure the recurrent laryngeal nerve. This could cause a permanent change in your voice. Be assured this risk is slight.

Are there other risks?
Very few. You should know how to recognize them, however, so that they can be promptly corrected. After surgery, the main risks are bleeding, infection, and breathing difficulty. There's also a slight chance that surgery may injure the nearby parathyroid glands, which help to control your body's calcium supply.

After my thyroid is removed, will I have to keep taking medication?
That depends. If your surgeon removes all or most of your thyroid gland, you may need to take thyroid hormone medication to replace what your body can no longer make. On the other hand, if you have enough healthy thyroid gland remaining, you won't need this medication.

tests to help distinguish between primary and secondary thyroid disorders. Instruct the patient not to eat anything after midnight before the test.

Describe what will happen during the test. First, the patient will be given either a radioactive iodine capsule or liquid. After 2, 6, and 24 hours, his thyroid gland will be scanned in the X-ray department to determine how much iodine remains in it. Reassure him that the amount of radioactivity involved is extremely small and harmless.

Teach about treatments
Tell your patient that he'll probably be able to live a nearly normal life if he follows the treatment regimen. Warn him not to overdo physical activity, which may aggravate his disease. Encourage him to eat a well-balanced diet to prevent vitamin deficiencies. Point out the benefits and risks of major treatments, including drugs, radioactive iodine therapy, and thyroidectomy.

Activity
Explain to the patient that excessive exertion will increase his symptoms. Encourage him to engage instead in less strenuous activities and to rest frequently. Keep in mind that this may be difficult because of the patient's accelerated metabolic rate.

Diet
Stress the importance of following the prescribed diet to prevent nutritional deficiencies, such as vitamin A and B deficiencies. Advise the patient to eat well-balanced meals each day, plus snacks, so that his caloric intake can keep pace with his rapid caloric expenditures. Caution him to avoid caffeine, yellow and red food dyes, and artificial preservatives because these substances may make him more irritable. If necessary, arrange for nutritional counseling.

Medication
If prescribed, teach the patient about thyroid hormone antagonists and propranolol, which may be given to control cardiac effects. (See *Teaching about drugs for hyperthyroidism.*) Also teach him about other prescribed drugs, such as tranquilizers to control irritability and hyperactivity. Warn him to avoid taking aspirin and any aspirin-containing drugs because they increase the metabolic rate.

Procedures
Radioactive iodine therapy may be called for if thyroid hormone antagonists prove ineffective. If the patient is scheduled for this treatment, explain that it reduces thyroid hormone production by destroying thyroid tissue. Reassure him that the procedure is painless and won't harm other body tissues. Be sure he understands the risk of hypothyroidism, which can result from excessive de-

Teaching about drugs for hyperthyroidism

DRUG	ADVERSE REACTIONS	TEACHING POINTS
Thyroid hormone antagonists		
methimazole (Tapazole) **propylthioura-cil (PTU)**	• Be alert for severe diarrhea, fever, jaundice, mouth sores, severe nausea or vomiting, pruritic rash, and sore throat. • Other reactions include mild diarrhea, dizziness, loss of taste, mild nausea, and skin discoloration or rash.	• Explain to the patient that this drug will correct his hyperthyroidism. Tell him the drug prevents the thyroid gland from producing excessive thyroid hormone. Advise him not to adjust the dosage or discontinue the drug without his doctor's approval. • Tell him to avoid over-the-counter drugs that contain potassium iodide or other forms of iodine. Also tell him to ask his doctor about eating shellfish and using iodized salt during treatment. • Advise him to take his medication at the same time every day for uniform absorption. • Tell him to take the drug with meals to reduce GI adverse reactions. • Instruct him to store the drug in its original container. • Teach him the symptoms of hypothyroidism (such as cold intolerance, edema, and depression) and to report them if they occur. A dosage adjustment may be necessary.
potassium iodide (SSKI)	• Watch for rash and salivary gland swelling or tenderness. • Other reactions include bloody or black, tarry stools; confusion; diarrhea; fever; irregular heartbeat; nausea and vomiting; numbness, tingling, pain, or weakness in hands or feet; stomach pain; swelling of neck or throat; unusual fatigue; and weakness or heaviness in the legs.	• Explain that this drug corrects hyperthyroidism by blocking hormone production and release. It also may be used to protect the thyroid gland from exposure to radioactive forms of iodine. • Advise taking this drug with water or after meals to mask its salty taste, to prevent GI irritation, and to ensure hydration. • Warn the patient not to stop taking the drug. Doing so may precipitate thyroid storm. • To prevent tooth discoloration, suggest drinking the medication through a straw. • Tell the patient to ask his doctor about using iodized salt or eating shellfish during treatment. Iodized foods may not be permitted. • Advise him to store the drug in its original light-resistant container.
Beta-adrenergic blocking agent		
propranolol (Inderal)	• Be alert for bradycardia, depression, dizziness, dyspnea, rash, and wheezing. • Other reactions include decreased libido, diarrhea, fatigue, headache, insomnia, nasal stuffiness, nausea and vomiting, and vivid dreams or nightmares.	• Explain that this drug helps to counteract some effects of hyperthyroidism by lowering blood pressure, controlling rapid heart rate, and reducing hand tremors. • Advise taking this drug with foods to increase drug absorption. • If the drug is to be taken daily, missed doses should be made up within 8 hours. If it's to be taken more often, missed doses should be made up as soon as possible. However, instruct the patient not to double the dose. Also, warn him that severe cardiovascular complications may develop if he stops taking the drug suddenly rather than tapers the dosage. • Tell him to make sure he has enough medication on hand to get through weekends and vacations. • Instruct him to take his pulse rate before taking the drug and to notify the doctor if it is below 60 beats/minute. • If the patient experiences insomnia, suggest that he take the drug no later than 2 hours before bedtime.

struction of thyroid tissue and may occur several months to 1 year after treatment. Assure the patient that exposure to this small amount of radioactivity doesn't cause cancer. (See *Precautions after radioactive iodine therapy*, page 516.)

Inform the patient that symptoms of hyperthyroidism should subside after radioactive iodine therapy. If they don't, the patient may need a second round of therapy.

Preventing neck strain after thyroidectomy

After thyroidectomy, show the patient how to prevent strain on her neck muscles when rising to a sitting position. Instruct her to support her head with a pillow and to put her hands together behind her neck, as shown here.

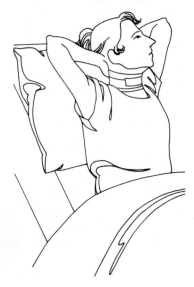

Surgery

In a subtotal thyroidectomy, more than 80% of the thyroid is removed, significantly reducing the gland's ability to produce thyroid hormone. If the patient is scheduled for subtotal thyroidectomy, instruct him to increase his caloric intake before surgery to regain weight. (Surgery may have to be delayed until he gains back any weight he lost.) If a special preoperative diet (such as a high-protein diet) has been ordered, explain its purpose and urge strict compliance. Remind the patient to avoid caffeine and other stimulants, which will aggravate his condition.

Explain the purpose of preoperative thyroid medication—to suppress secretion of thyroid hormone so that an excessive amount isn't released during surgery. Iodine preparations may also be ordered to diminish blood flow to the thyroid, thereby minimizing bleeding during surgery.

Before surgery, review preoperative and postoperative procedures. Explain preoperative preparation of the incision site. Tell the patient that the incision will be made in the lower neck.

Show the patient how to avoid putting stress on his incision postoperatively by placing his hands behind his neck for support whenever he wants to turn his head. When rising to a sitting position, he should support his head with a pillow and put his hands together behind his head (see *Preventing neck strain after thyroidectomy*). If the patient has difficulty swallowing, he should report it immediately. This may indicate hemorrhage or swelling, which could interfere with the patient's breathing. Mention that cold drinks and ice will help relieve discomfort and that he'll be on a soft diet temporarily.

Tell the patient that his voice will be checked periodically for hoarseness after surgery. Advise him to talk as little as possible during the first few days postoperatively. If he has difficulty breathing, he should report it at once. Oxygen may have to be administered. He can expect to be out of bed on the lst day after surgery.

Reassure the patient that he'll receive pain medication postoperatively. Inform him that sutures or surgical clips are usually removed on the 2nd postoperative day, just before discharge.

To prepare the patient for discharge, teach him how to take care of his incision at home. Make sure that he understands the importance of getting adequate rest and nutrition during his recovery. Tell him to promptly report any signs of infection and hypothyroidism to his doctor.

Other care measures

Advise the patient to avoid stressful situations, which can exacerbate his irritability. Recommend keeping environmental stimulation to a minimum. For example, the patient should avoid watching television programs or movies that may cause him to become excited or upset. Reassure the patient and his family that behavioral changes, such as irritability, anxiety, lack of concentration, and fatigue, stem from hyperthyroidism and will subside with treatment.

If ophthalmopathy is present, teach the patient the essentials of good eye care. Advise him to wear sunglasses and to avoid irritating his eyes. If eyedrops are ordered, show him how to instill them. Instruct him to limit his fluid and salt intake to minimize fluid retention. Such retention will worsen exophthalmos.

Suggest that the patient sleep with his head elevated to prevent fluid accumulation behind the eyes. Instruct him to notify his doctor at once if visual changes, such as blurring, occur. Advise him to visit an ophthalmologist regularly.

Sources of information and support

American Thyroid Association
Mayo Clinic, 200 First Street, SW, Rochester, Minn. 55905
(507) 284-4738

National Institutes of Health
Institute of Diabetes, Digestive, and Kidney Disorders
9000 Rockville Pike, Bethesda, Md. 20892
(301) 496-3583

Further readings

Bybee, D.E. "Saving Lives in Thyroid Crises," *Emergency Medicine* 19(16):20-23, 27, 31, September 30, 1987.
Kerlikowske, K., et al. "Euthyroid Sick or 'Hyperthyroid Sick'?" *Hospital Practice* 22(10):113, 115-18, October 30, 1987.
O'Neil, J.R. "Action STAT! Thyroid Crisis," *Nursing* 17(11):33, November 1987.
Papazoglou, N., et al. "Vasospastic Angina with Hyperthyroidism," *Heart and Lung* 16(4):437-438, July 1987.
Sarsany, S.L. "Thyroid Storm," *RN* 51(7):46-48, July 1988.
Szollar, S.M., et al. "Neuroleptic Complications of Thyrotoxicosis: Case Report," *Archives of Physical Medicine and Rehabilitation* 69(1):41-43, January 1988.

PATIENT-TEACHING AID

Precautions after radioactive iodine therapy

Dear Patient:

You've received a dose of radioactive iodine to help treat your thyroid condition. This treatment won't affect your other body tissues. Although this is a safe treatment, you'll need to follow these instructions to prevent any harm to you or others.

Eating and drinking
You can eat what you like, but be sure to use disposable plates, cups, and utensils for the next 48 hours. Drink plenty of fluids (about 2 quarts, or liters) for the next 48 hours to help remove the radioactive iodine from your body.

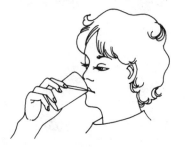

Using the bathroom
All your urine, feces, saliva, and perspiration will be slightly radioactive for 48 hours after therapy. You may use your family bathroom to urinate or defecate, but flush the toilet three times to make certain all waste is discarded. Wash your hands thoroughly afterward.

Washing yourself
If you take a shower or bath within 48 hours after treatment, remember to rinse the shower stall or tub after each use. Wash your clothes, towels, and washcloths separately from those of your family.

You can brush your teeth and resume any other normal mouth care. Just make sure you rinse and drain the sink when you've finished.

Living arrangements
Avoid close contact with infants, children, and pregnant women for 1 week after therapy. For safety's sake, sleep alone and avoid kissing or sexual intimacy for 48 hours after your treatment. After that, you may resume your normal relationship unless your doctor gives you other instructions.

If you're breast-feeding, you must stop. Your doctor will tell you when you can start again.

When to call your doctor
If you vomit within 12 hours after therapy, call your doctor immediately. Flush the vomit down the toilet and, if possible, wear gloves while cleaning up. (Discard the gloves in a plastic bag after use.) Discourage other people from coming in contact with the vomit. If they do, however, tell them to wash their hands thoroughly.

If you get a fever and feel restless or upset within 48 hours of therapy, call your doctor right away. Also call him if your neck feels tender. He may prescribe medicine to make you more comfortable.

Hypothyroidism

If left untreated or managed improperly, hypothyroidism can have devastating effects. Both acute and chronic complications may occur, affecting the quality of the patient's life and possibly even shortening his life span. That's why it's important for you to teach the patient about his disorder's chronicity. Most important, you'll need to stress the need for his compliance with lifelong thyroid hormone replacement therapy. Other areas you'll need to cover include dietary and activity precautions and possible adjunctive care measures.

Discuss the disorder

Inform the patient that hypothyroidism is a chronic disorder in which the thyroid gland fails to secrete sufficient thyroid hormone. Explain his type of hypothyroidism: primary or secondary.

Primary hypothyroidism results from gradual destruction of vital thyroid tissue. In the absence of goiter, its most common cause is radioactive iodine therapy or surgery. When goiter is present, its most common cause is Hashimoto's thyroiditis, in which lymphocytes mistake normal thyroid cells for foreign cells and destroy them.

Secondary hypothyroidism, which seldom occurs, results from the destruction of pituitary tissue responsible for producing thyroid-stimulating hormone (TSH), or thyrotropin. Without TSH stimulation, the thyroid gland cannot produce thyroid hormone.

Explain to the patient how hypothyroidism affects the body. For example, explain that thyroid hormone deficiency causes a significant decrease in the body's ability to use energy. As a result, cells don't function effectively and use up what little energy is available to them. This causes the patient to tire easily.

Besides fatigue, early symptoms include forgetfulness, sensitivity to cold, and constipation. The patient also may gain weight, even though his caloric intake is unchanged (see *Reviewing clinical features of hypothyroidism,* page 518).

Complications

To underscore the importance of complying with therapy, point out to the patient the complications that might occur if hypothyroidism is poorly managed or left untreated. Myxedema, for example, may develop gradually. In early stages, it produces generalized symptoms, such as fatigue and lethargy. Later, it

Marlene M. Ciranowicz, RN, MSN, CDE, and **Susan Zemble, RN, MaEd, JD,** contributed to this chapter. Ms. Ciranowicz is a diabetes educator in the outpatient department of Hahnemann University Hospital, Philadelphia. Ms. Zemble, former coordinator of patient and community health education at Memorial Hospital, Philadelphia, is an associate with the law firm of O'Brien and Ryan.

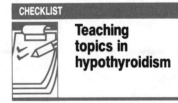

CHECKLIST

Teaching topics in hypothyroidism

☐ Explanation of the patient's type of hypothyroidism: primary or secondary
☐ Symptoms of hypothyroidism
☐ Complications
☐ Preparation for diagnostic tests to evaluate thyroid function
☐ Activity restrictions
☐ Dietary guidelines for ensuring adequate nutrition
☐ Importance of lifelong thyroid hormone replacement therapy
☐ Symptoms of hyperthyroidism (in accidental thyroid hormone overdose)

Reviewing clinical features of hypothyroidism

To help the patient and her family understand hypothyroidism, describe its characteristic effects:
- lethargy
- cold intolerance
- constipation
- muscle aches and weakness
- rough, thick, scaly skin
- dry, coarse, brittle hair
- facial edema, blank facial expression
- thick tongue, slow speech

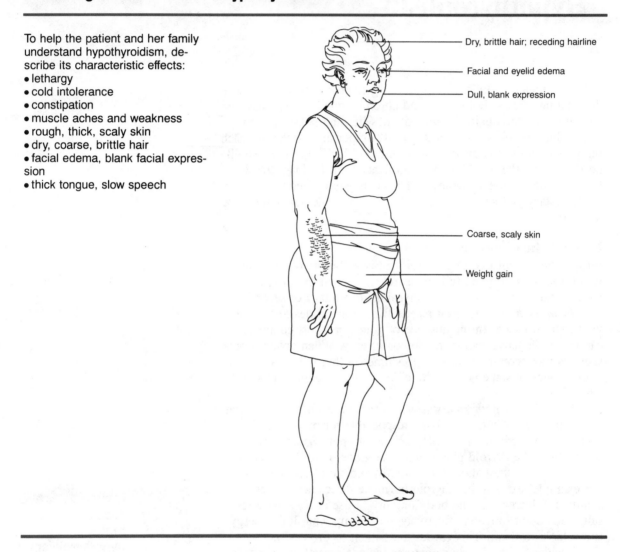

Dry, brittle hair; receding hairline

Facial and eyelid edema

Dull, blank expression

Coarse, scaly skin

Weight gain

causes cool, dry skin; decreased sweat and oil production; thinning of scalp hair; and loss of body hair.

The patient with myxedema may also develop menstrual irregularities, hearing loss, ataxia, dependent edema, and congestive heart failure. Muscles may increase in bulk but decline in strength, and the patient may have muscle cramps.

Impaired muscle function from myxedema predisposes the patient to constipation and urinary tract infection. Decreased lung expansion heightens the risk of respiratory infection. As myxedema worsens, profound hypotension, bradycardia, hypoventilation, and hypothermia may develop. The patient must understand that without prompt treatment, myxedema can be fatal or it can lead to other life-threatening conditions, such as coma.

Other chronic complications of uncontrolled hypothyroidism arise from the accumulation of fatty substances in interstitial tissues and decreased metabolism. Atherosclerosis is one such complication.

Describe the diagnostic workup

Explain that thyroid hormone deficiency is easily confirmed by measuring serum levels of thyroxine and protein-bound iodine. Additional blood studies will be necessary to see if the pituitary gland is producing enough thyrotropin to stimulate the thyroid. An elevated thyrotropin level confirms primary hypothyroidism.

The thyrotropin releasing hormone (TRH) infusion test may be ordered to measure the pituitary's thyrotropin reserve if the patient's thyrotropin level is normal or borderline. Explain to the patient that this procedure requires the insertion of an I.V. catheter and the infusion of synthetic TRH through it. Tell him that several blood samples will be drawn over about an hour and that the catheter will be removed after the last sample has been collected. If the pituitary responds to the TRH infusion by releasing an excessive amount of TSH, primary hypothyroidism is indicated; a blunted response indicates secondary hypothyroidism.

Additional tests may include a thyroid scan or ultrasonography to evaluate the thyroid's size and structure and a radioactive iodine uptake test to assess gland function. For patient-teaching points, see pages 510 to 512.

Teach about treatments

Discuss treatments for hypothyroidism, including guidelines for safely increasing activity, dietary restrictions, and thyroid hormone replacement therapy. Also teach the patient to recognize possible complications of this lifelong disorder.

Activity

Because hypothyroid patients have so little energy, they tend to be sedentary. As a result, you'll need to encourage your patient to increase his activity level. But caution him to do so gradually because he risks pain and impaired muscle function from myxedema. Discuss activities he enjoys and can fit into his life-style. (His doctor will have to provide guidelines for all such activities.)

Warn him to stop any activity and to notify his doctor immediately if he feels chest pain or tightness or experiences severe dyspnea or palpitations.

Diet

Stress the importance of following dietary restrictions to minimize weight gain, reduce cholesterol intake, and alleviate constipation. Remind the patient that thyroid hormone deficiency decreases his body's ability to use sugars and carbohydrates as sources of energy. It will also cause him to store fats.

Advise the patient to avoid foods high in saturated fats and cholesterol. Suggest that he talk with his doctor about whether he can drink alcohol. Explore ways to help him adhere to a calorie-restricted diet. If appropriate, encourage him to join a support group.

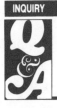

Questions patients ask about thyroid hormone replacement

Why should I tell my other doctors and my pharmacist that I have hypothyroidism?
Because hypothyroidism slows down your metabolism, prolonging the effects of any medications you take. This increases your risk of having a serious drug reaction. To prevent this, your doctor (or dentist) may have to reduce the dosage of your other medications.

Thyroid hormone may also change the effectiveness of certain medications you take. Again, your doctor may need to adjust the dosage of these medications.

Why do I feel nervous and restless now after taking medication when I was tired and slow-moving before?
You may be taking too much thyroid hormone. Tell your doctor about these symptoms. Also tell him if your hands become shaky, you have trouble sleeping, or you develop palpitations, unexplained weight loss, rash, or a change in appetite or bowel habits.

These symptoms could also mean that your dosage needs to be adjusted.

Be patient. It will take time until your doctor finds the right medication dosage for you.

Will taking thyroid hormone medication affect my other health problems?
Possibly. If you have heart disease, taking thyroid hormone may put added stress on your heart. Also, thyroid hormone treatment may interfere with successful therapy for diabetes or Addison's disease. If you have any of these disorders, be sure your doctor knows about them. Ask him what special precautions, if any, you should take. Your doctor will closely monitor your condition, so you don't have to worry.

How long will I need to take thyroid hormone medication?
In order for your body to function properly and for you to feel well, you'll need to take it for the rest of your life.

Teach the patient how to increase the fiber content in his diet. If he has nonpitting edema, advise him to reduce fluid intake by one to two glasses daily, as prescribed.

Medication
Inform the patient that thyroid hormone replacement is the primary treatment for hypothyroidism and will help him to achieve a normal metabolic rate and energy level. Explain that therapy will be tailored to meet his individual requirements and that he'll need to take thyroid hormone replacement for the rest of his life. The dosage will depend on the severity of his hypothyroidism. (See *Questions patients ask about thyroid hormone replacement*.)

Explain to the patient that finding just the right dosage for him is a gradual process. This will allow his body to adjust slowly to the changes resulting from the medication, thus preventing complications.

If the patient is taking a thyroid hormone replacement, such as levothyroxine (Levothroid, Levoxine, or Synthroid), liothyronine (Cytomel), or thyroid USP, tell him to take the drug exactly as prescribed and not to adjust the dosage or discontinue the drug without his doctor's approval. Advise him to take this drug at the same time every day for uniform absorption. Tell him to store his medication in the original container.

Instruct the patient to watch for adverse reactions, including a change in appetite, abnormal bleeding or bruising, chest pain, diarrhea, fever, severe headache, heat intolerance, insomnia, leg cramps, nervousness, palpitations, shortness of breath, rash, sweating, tremors, and weight loss. Mention that constipation, drowsiness, dry skin, headache, menstrual irregularities, nausea, and temporary hair loss may occur. If he's taking levothyroxine, provide a copy of the patient-teaching aid *Learning about levothyroxine,* page 522, for additional tips on safe usage.

Warn the patient never to take nonprescription drugs without his doctor's approval. Explain that hypothyroidism slows down his metabolism and thus prolongs drug effects, creating the risk of drug toxicity. Advise him to inform all health care providers of his hypothyroidism so that any prescribed medications (especially narcotics, barbiturates, and digoxin) may be chosen carefully and the dosage reduced appropriately.

Other care measures

Review the symptoms of hypothyroidism with the patient. Tell him to be especially alert for increased lethargy, sensitivity to cold, weight gain, facial and hand puffiness, changes in his skin or hair, and muscle cramps. Instruct him to report any of these changes immediately to his doctor.

At the same time, make sure he's familiar with the symptoms of hyperthyroidism, which would develop if his thyroid hormone dosage were too high. These include heat intolerance, increased sweating, nervous activity, difficulty concentrating, frequent defecation, skin changes, apprehensiveness, and irritability.

Because hypothyroidism is a chronic disorder, encourage the patient to see his doctor regularly for blood tests and physical examinations. Tell him to report any symptoms of infection, such as fever, malaise, diarrhea, and muscle pain. Remind the patient that hypothyroidism makes him vulnerable to infections.

Sources of information and support

American Thyroid Association
Mayo Clinic, 200 First Street, SW, Rochester, Minn. 55905
(507) 284-4738

National Institutes of Health
Institute of Diabetes, Digestive, and Kidney Disorders
9000 Rockville Pike, Bethesda, Md. 20892
(301) 496-3583

Further readings

Bybee, D.E. "Saving Lives in Thyroid Crises," *Emergency Medicine* 19(16):20-23, 27, 31, September 30, 1987.
"Hypothyroidism on the Horizon," *Emergency Medicine* 19(21):47, 50, December 15, 1987.
McMillan, J.Y. "Preventing Myxedema Coma in the Hypothyroid Patient," *Dimensions of Critical Care Nursing* 7(3):136-145, May-June, 1988.

Learning about levothyroxine

Dear Patient:

The medication you're taking is called levothyroxine. (The label may also read Levothroid, Levoxine, or Synthroid.) Your doctor has prescribed it to correct your thyroid hormone deficiency.

Taking your medication
Take levothyroxine exactly as your doctor prescribes. Don't take more or less than prescribed, and don't take it more or less frequently than prescribed. Also, don't stop taking it without your doctor's approval.

Take levothyroxine at the same time each day to keep a constant level of the medication in your body. The best time to take levothyroxine is in the morning. Otherwise, it may keep you awake at night.

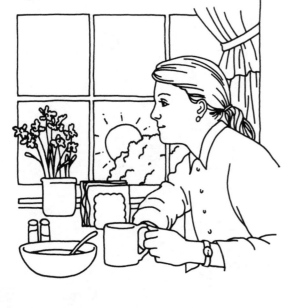

Once you've started taking one brand of levothyroxine, don't switch to another brand without asking your doctor. This is important because other brands may not have the same effectiveness.

When to call your doctor
Call your doctor right away if you feel chest pain or experience shortness of breath, or if your heart starts to pound or beat rapidly or irregularly. Also call him if you develop any of these problems: hair loss, headache, heat intolerance, nervousness, leg cramps, rash, sweating, tremors, menstrual irregularities, or weight loss.

Special instructions
Take it easy on hot days. Don't overexert yourself because levothyroxine increases your risk of heatstroke.

If you notice some hair loss while taking this drug, don't worry—it's only temporary.

Reminders
Be sure to tell your other doctors, including your dentist, that you're taking levothyroxine.

Don't let anyone else take your medication, and don't try any of theirs. The doctor's prescription is intended for your specific needs.

Store the drug in its original container in a cool, dry, and dark place, away from excessive heat and humidity. Avoid the bathroom medicine cabinet.

CHAPTER

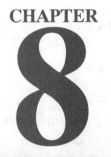

Renal and Urologic Conditions

Contents

Chronic renal failure

Thanks to dialysis and kidney transplantation, patients with chronic renal failure are surviving longer than ever before. As a result, you'll have more opportunities to teach the patient how to manage this life-threatening disorder. Above all, you'll be challenged to convince him that complying with prescribed treatment really *can* improve his quality of life despite the disorder's irreversible and progressive course.

To promote compliance, you'll need to provide thorough teaching about regular exercise, dietary changes, medications, and such therapies as hemodialysis, peritoneal dialysis, and kidney transplantation. You'll also need to provide emotional support to help the patient cope with life-style changes, frequent hospitalizations, long-term complications, and the prospect of a shortened life.

Discuss the disorder

Tell the patient how the disorder results from progressive, irreversible damage to the nephrons—the kidneys' structural and functional units. Explain that in the earliest stage of renal disease, called *reduced renal reserve,* about 50% of renal tissue has already been damaged but that no signs or symptoms occur. During this stage, too, the effects of other conditions (such as hypertension), dehydration, or the effects of nephrotoxic drugs may cause rapid, sometimes irreversible renal failure.

In the second stage, *renal insufficiency,* up to 80% of renal tissue is destroyed. With the kidneys unable to concentrate urine, the patient may experience dehydration and anemia. In the third stage, *chronic renal failure,* more than 80% of renal tissue is damaged. The patient experiences increasing fatigue, anorexia, weakness, decreased attention span, weight loss, and behavioral changes. In *end-stage renal disease,* more than 90% of renal tissue is damaged, and dialysis or transplantation becomes necessary to maintain life. The patient's signs and symptoms worsen and may include nausea, vomiting, dyspnea, drowsiness, and increased edema.

Complications

Stress that failure to comply with prescribed therapy can hasten the progression of renal disease, increase the risk and severity of complications, and shorten the patient's life. Discuss potential complications, such as anemia, hyperkalemia, hypertension, peri-

---

Betty Dale, RN, BSN, and **Elaine M. Musial, RN, MSN, CS,** contributed to this chapter. Ms. Dale is a former head operating room nurse at Abbott-Northwestern Hospital in Minneapolis. Ms. Musial is a clinical nurse specialist, dialysis program, at Thomas Jefferson University Hospital, Philadelphia.

CHECKLIST

Teaching topics in chronic renal failure

☐ Explanation of the disorder and the extent of nephron damage
☐ Importance of treatment to delay onset of end-stage renal disease and to prevent complications
☐ Preparation for blood and urine tests and for other scheduled diagnostic studies, such as radiography and renal ultrasonography, biopsy, and bone X-rays
☐ Prescribed exercise, diet, and fluid restrictions
☐ Drugs and their administration
☐ Explanation of hemodialysis (if ordered), including access site care
☐ Explanation of peritoneal dialysis (if ordered), including solution exchanges and tips for preventing peritonitis
☐ Preparation for kidney transplantation or nephrectomy, if indicated
☐ Symptom management, depression, and sexual concerns
☐ Sources of information and support

carditis, fluid overload, coronary artery disease, and bone disease (see *Teaching about complications of chronic renal failure*).

Describe the diagnostic workup
Prepare the patient for routine blood and urine tests to evaluate renal function, detect complications, and monitor treatment; radiologic tests to visualize abnormalities; and renal biopsy to permit histologic examination of tissue.

Blood and urine studies
Tell the patient that blood studies include a complete blood count (CBC) and electrolyte, creatinine, blood urea nitrogen (BUN), and periodically, calcium and phosphorus analyses. Urine studies include a urinalysis with microscopic study, creatinine clearance and protein loss determinations, and cultures, if infection is suspected.

For a *clean-catch midstream specimen,* instruct the patient to cleanse the area around the urinary opening before voiding into the bedpan, urinal, or toilet because the urinary stream washes bacteria from the urethra and urinary meatus. Then, tell him to void directly into the sterile container, collecting about 30 to 50 ml at the midstream portion of voiding. He can then finish voiding into the bedpan, urinal, or toilet. Emphasize that the first and

Teaching about complications of chronic renal failure

Explaining possible complications of chronic renal failure to the patient will help you underscore the need for compliance.

Short-term complications
These include anemia, hyperkalemia, hypertension, fluid overload, and pericarditis.
• *Anemia.* Tell the patient that anemia causes fatigue, diminished exercise tolerance, and pallor. Explain that it results from the kidney's inability to produce erythropoietin, a hormone that stimulates the bone marrow production of red blood cells (RBCs). In addition, RBCs have a shortened life span related to uremia, and they're lost because of easy bruising, clotting abnormalities, and frequent blood studies.
• *Hyperkalemia.* Explain that hyperkalemia results when excessive potassium—an electrolyte that's normally excreted by the kidneys—accumulates in the blood. Warn the patient that this electrolyte imbalance can lead to cardiac arrest. Instruct him to report weakness, malaise, and abdominal cramps.
• *Hypertension.* Tell the patient that this common complication, if uncontrolled, can lead to cardiac disease, cerebrovascular accident, and worsening renal function.
• *Fluid overload.* Explain that fluid overload can result

from the diseased kidney's inability to remove excess fluid. If not managed through fluid restriction, it can cause arm and leg edema, hypertension, congestive heart failure, and if severe, pulmonary edema.
• *Pericarditis.* Inform the patient that pericarditis—an inflammation of the sac that surrounds the heart—can interfere with the heart's normal pumping action. It most commonly occurs with end-stage renal failure. Instruct the patient to report any sudden chest pain or dyspnea.

Long-term complications
These include bone and coronary artery disease.
• *Bone disease.* Explain that the patient risks developing bone disease because renal failure depresses serum calcium levels (related to decreased vitamin D activation) and increases serum phosphorus levels (resulting from the failing kidney's inability to excrete phosphorus). To compensate for decreased calcium, the parathyroid gland is stimulated, resulting in resorption of calcium from bone tissue to increase the calcium level. Aluminum hydroxide gels, given to reduce phosphate, also contribute to bone disease.
• *Coronary artery disease.* Inform the patient that he's at an increased risk for developing coronary artery disease. Tell him to avoid smoking and to follow a low-fat diet.

the last portions of the voiding are discarded. If his urine output must be measured, tell him to pour these portions into a graduated container. Remind him to include the amount in the specimen container when recording the total amount voided.

For a *24-hour urine specimen,* instruct the patient to save all urine during the collection period, to notify you after each voiding, and to avoid contaminating the urine with stool or toilet tissue. Explain any dietary or drug restrictions. When he's ready to start the collection period, tell him to void. Then, remind him to discard this urine so he starts the collection time with an empty bladder. Tell him to record the time. After pouring the first urine specimen into the collection bottle, instruct him to add the required preservative. Then, refrigerate the bottle or keep it on ice until the next voiding.

Remind the patient to collect *all* urine voided during the 24-hour period. Warn that if he accidentally discards a specimen during the collection period, he must start over or discuss a possible shortened collection time with the doctor. Instruct him to void just before the collection period ends and to add this last specimen to the container.

Radiologic tests

Prepare the patient for radiologic studies, such as kidney-ureter-bladder (KUB) radiography and renal ultrasonography, to determine kidney size and to detect cystic disease. If appropriate, prepare him for a chest X-ray to assess heart size and identify pulmonary edema. Explain that he'll have bone and skeletal X-rays, usually annually, to detect the presence or progression of bone disease. Stress the importance of returning for follow-up studies.

Biopsies

Tell the patient that renal biopsy, a 15-minute test, helps determine the cause of his condition. Mention that the biopsy needle remains in the kidney for only a few seconds. Instruct him to restrict food and fluids for 8 hours before the test. Inform him that he'll receive a mild sedative beforehand to help him relax.

Explain that during the biopsy he'll be placed in a prone position with a sandbag positioned under his abdomen. After the biopsy site is numbed with a local anesthetic, he'll be asked to hold his breath as the biopsy needle is inserted through his back into the kidney. Warn him that he may feel a pinching pain during needle insertion.

Inform the patient that after the test, pressure will be applied to the biopsy site to stop bleeding; then a pressure dressing will be applied. Instruct him to lie flat on his back without moving for at least 12 hours to prevent bleeding. Tell him to expect frequent monitoring of his blood pressure, heart rate, and respirations. Advise him also that he may notice blood in his urine, which should stop within 1 or 2 days.

If the patient has bone pain, inform him that he may undergo a *bone biopsy.* Tell him what to expect before, during, and after the procedure.

Teach about treatments

Describe treatments for chronic renal failure, such as dietary modifications and drug therapy. If the patient has end-stage renal disease, describe treatment options, such as hemodialysis and peritoneal dialysis. If appropriate, prepare him for a kidney transplantation or for nephrectomy. Teach him how to manage symptoms of renal failure, such as dry skin, bad breath, and muscle cramps; and discuss sexual difficulties.

Activity

Emphasize the need for regular exercise to maintain muscle strength and mobility and to prevent bone demineralization. Caution the patient to protect his dialysis access site during exercise. Advise him to avoid excessive fatigue and to conserve energy, for example, by resting after periods of activity.

Diet

With the help of the doctor and dietitian, teach the patient about dietary restrictions. Inform him that a diet high in calories but low in protein, sodium, potassium, and phosphorus helps avoid taxing the kidneys and may even slow progression of renal disease. Explain that his dietary needs will change as his disease progresses and that he may need to restrict fluids to prevent fluid overload (see *Key dietary goals*).

Medication

Tell the patient that the doctor may prescribe drugs to help control the disorder's effects and relieve symptoms. Explain that vitamin supplements provide nutrients that are necessary because of dietary restrictions. He'll also need extra iron to replace what's lost from bleeding (caused by bruising or a clotting disorder) and frequent blood studies. Warn him iron deficiency may worsen his anemia.

Inform the patient that he may receive recombinant human erythropoietin or epoetin alfa (Epogen) to treat anemia associated with renal disease. Tell him that the drug increases red blood cell (RBC) production and, as his energy levels improve, may enhance his sense of well-being. Instruct him to carefully monitor his blood pressure and weight. Advise him that he will be monitored for adverse reactions, such as hypertension, clotting at the access site, and seizures.

Explain that the doctor may alternatively prescribe anabolic steroids to stimulate RBC production. Warn the female patient that her facial hair may proliferate and her voice deepen. Mention that acne commonly occurs. Depending on the patient's response, dosage adjustments may be necessary.

If the patient requires an antihypertensive drug, inform him that the drug and dosage may change as renal function declines. Point out that compliance is critical to prevent progression of chronic renal failure.

Explain that the doctor will prescribe phosphate binders, either aluminum hydroxide gels or calcium compounds, to reduce

Key dietary goals

Inform the patient that dietary restrictions can significantly slow the progression of renal disease. Explain that these restrictions will change, depending on the disease's stage and whether he's undergoing hemodialysis or peritoneal dialysis. Emphasize three key dietary goals:
• regulation of fluid and sodium intake to control fluid balance
• protein restriction to prevent complications associated with waste product accumulation
• potassium restriction to prevent weakness and cardiac conduction abnormalities.

Fluids and sodium
Explain that early in renal disease the kidneys' ability to concentrate urine may be lost, resulting in excessive sodium losses. As a result, sodium and fluid restrictions may be harmful, resulting in dehydration, which would further damage the renal system. Sodium intake should equal urinary losses (as much as 4 g daily), and fluid intake should be encouraged. Sodium losses may increase if the patient also takes diuretics.

As renal disease progresses, sodium restriction becomes necessary (to about 2 g daily) to prevent fluid retention. Teach the patient about foods that are high in sodium, especially processed foods, such as canned goods and frozen dinner entrees.

Fluid restriction (to 32 to 48 oz [1 to 1½ liters] daily) may be necessary to prevent retention and overload. Tell the patient to use small (4 oz) drinking glasses, which will help him stay within his limits. He may use ice chips to help alleviate thirst, but caution him to account for the ice in his prescribed fluid restriction.

If the patient is undergoing hemodialysis, tell him that fluid and sodium restrictions are necessary to prevent excess fluid accumulation between treatments.

The patient on peritoneal dialysis usually doesn't require sodium and fluid restriction.

Protein
Tell the patient that protein restriction may start early in renal disease (when creatinine clearance is reduced by one-half). Instruct him to eat meat, fish, eggs, and dairy products so that protein intake includes all essential amino acids. Inform him that appropriate protein intake can delay uremia's onset. In nephrotic syndrome, the patient requires increased protein to replace urinary protein losses.

After hemodialysis begins, advise the patient to increase his protein intake. Dialysis effectively removes metabolic wastes, so that protein restrictions can be relaxed. However, caution the hemodialysis patient that excessive protein may worsen his symptoms. Inform the peritoneal dialysis patient that he may increase his protein intake because of additional protein losses through the peritoneal membrane. If the patient develops peritonitis, provide increased protein because of urinary losses.

Keep in mind that safe, effective protein restriction requires adequate intake of fat or carbohydrate calories. Why? Insufficient calories can lead to the use of protein as an energy source, thus reducing the amount available for tissue growth and repair.

Potassium
Because the kidneys play a major role in potassium regulation, restrictions are necessary when the patient has lost more than 90% of renal function. At this point, potassium accumulation can result in hyperkalemia, characterized by weakness and cardiac conduction abnormalities. Tell the patient that foods high in potassium include many fruits, vegetables, and high-protein foods. Inform him that his potassium levels will be monitored carefully. Mention that salt substitutes commonly include potassium. He should check with his doctor before using them.

Tell the hemodialysis patient that potassium restrictions should continue because hyperkalemia can occur between treatments. During peritoneal dialysis, restrictions usually aren't needed.

phosphate levels. Instruct the patient to take them with meals— the largest dose with the largest meal of the day. Advise him to use stool softeners to prevent constipation. If the patient needs laxatives, tell him to avoid ones containing magnesium. He may also receive supplemental vitamin D to enhance calcium absorption.

Instruct the patient to inform other health professionals (such as his dentist) that he has chronic renal disease, so that any prescribed medications will be appropriate. Suggest that he have all his prescriptions filled by the same pharmacy to ensure an accurate record of his medications. Tell him not to take over-the-counter drugs unless his doctor approves their use.

Procedures

If the patient requires dialysis, explain its purpose and discuss the two types: hemodialysis and peritoneal dialysis.

Hemodialysis. If the patient selects hemodialysis, tell him that he'll undergo surgery to create a vascular access called a native arteriovenous fistula—a connection between an artery and a vein—or a graft arteriovenous fistula—a synthetic bridge between an artery and a vein. This connection ensures adequate blood flow for hemodialysis (see *Caring for an arteriovenous fistula site*).

Explain that for hemodialysis, two needles will be placed in the fistula or graft. Inform the patient that blood leaves his body via one needle, circulates through the dialyzer (for removal of wastes and excess fluid and electrolytes), and then returns to him through the other needle. The procedure is repeated three times weekly for up to 4 hours each time. Tell him that he'll be awake during each treatment and will have minimal discomfort related to the needle insertion. Instruct him to notify the nurse if he experiences dizziness, hot or cold flashes, and headache or nausea—all possible symptoms of hypotension, a common complication of hemodialysis. Also instruct him to report any other symptoms. Tell him that he's likely to feel tired for several hours after dialysis.

Emphasize to the patient that he'll need to continue hemodialysis for life unless he receives a successful transplant or changes to peritoneal dialysis.

Peritoneal dialysis. This type of dialysis may be performed using an automatic cycler machine (continuous cyclical peritoneal dialysis, or CCPD) or using 4 to 6 fluid exchanges daily (continuous ambulatory peritoneal dialysis, or CAPD). If the patient chooses CCPD or CAPD, inform him that a catheter will be inserted into the peritoneal cavity through a small incision in his abdomen. Explain that after the catheter site heals, dialysate solution will be instilled through the catheter into the peritoneal cavity, where it will remain for a specified time to allow excess fluid and electrolytes and accumulated wastes to pass through the peritoneal membrane into the dialysate. At the end of the prescribed time, the dialysate is drained and new solution instilled. Give the patient a copy of the teaching aid *Tips for preventing peritonitis*, page 535.

If the patient will be using *CCPD*, teach him or a family member how to prepare the equipment, determine the solution to use, and program the infusion, dwell, and drainage durations. Demonstrate how to connect the cycler system to the peritoneal catheter, emphasizing sterile technique. The cycler will automatically perform the entire procedure, usually overnight while the patient sleeps. The last exchange solution will remain in the peritoneal cavity until the procedure is repeated the next night. Demonstrate the disconnection procedure, again emphasizing sterile techniques.

If the patient will be using *CAPD*, teach him how to drain and instill dialysate solution, using a plastic bag that he'll store in

Caring for an arteriovenous fistula site

Inform the patient that the surgeon has created a permanent vascular access site in the forearm to allow hemodialysis. This involves creation of an arteriovenous (A-V) fistula, making a connection between an artery and a vein. The connection can be made directly between an artery and a vein in the forearm (native A-V fistula), or the connection can involve grafting a vein from the forearm or leg or the use of a synthetic blood vessel to bridge the artery and vein (graft A-V fistula). Blood then flows through the artery into the vein. Give the patient guidelines for fistula care.

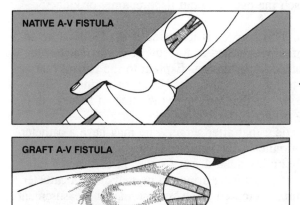

NATIVE A-V FISTULA

GRAFT A-V FISTULA

Postoperative care
If the patient has a *native A-V fistula,* tell him that after his incision heals well, he should do exercises for a few months to help enlarge the vein that will be used for hemodialysis. Tell him to squeeze a tennis ball, soft putty, or a sponge to increase blood flow through the fistula vein, which enlarges it. He should perform the squeezing exercise for 20 minutes, three times daily.

If the patient has a *graft A-V fistula,* tell him to expect swelling around the graft area. Advise him to elevate his arm on pillows to help swelling subside.

With both types, advise the patient to protect his arm from bumping into hard or sharp objects. He should avoid heavy lifting until the incision has healed and the stitches have been removed (10 to 14 days after surgery). If necessary, the doctor may prescribe an analgesic.

Checking for clotting. Instruct the patient to check his fistula at least three times daily for blood flow—in the morning, at noon, and at bedtime. Interrupted flow indicates clotting. Tell him to place his fingers directly over the vein above the incision (or directly over the graft). He can expect a tingling sensation or

wavelike pulsation, called a thrill. Caused by blood rushing through the fistula, the thrill should feel the same every time.

Explain that another way to check the fistula for blood flow is to listen with an ear or a stethoscope directly over the vein or graft segment for the sound of blood flowing. Called a bruit, this sounds like the ocean's roar.

Tell the patient that if the thrill or bruit sounds different or he can't hear it at all, he should contact the doctor. If the doctor discovers a clot, he may remove it so that hemodialysis can continue.

To reduce the risk of clotting, advise the patient to avoid wearing constrictive clothing over or above the fistula. Warn him to never allow anyone to place a tourniquet on or to take a blood pressure in the arm with the fistula. Caution him against sleeping on that arm.

Preventing infection. Tell the patient to check his incision daily for signs of infection and to notify the doctor right away if he notices redness, swelling, tenderness, or drainage. Remind him to keep his arm clean and dry until the wound is healed. He shouldn't let anyone except the dialysis nurse take blood samples from the arm with the fistula.

After hemodialysis
If the patient has a *native A-V fistula,* the vein requires several months to enlarge before the fistula will be usable. If the patient has a *graft A-V fistula,* hemodialysis can begin as soon as swelling subsides, the incision heals, and the patient's body tissues accept the graft. This takes about 2 weeks.

When the fistula is ready for hemodialysis, inform the patient that the dialysis nurse will use a special cleaning procedure to reduce the risk of infection at the access site. After each treatment when the needles are removed, tell the patient to apply pressure to the site for 5 to 10 minutes to ensure that the bleeding has stopped. The nurse will apply an adhesive bandage which the patient should remove after 6 hours. If the bandage remains in place too long, the site may become infected.

Tell the patient to notify the dialysis nurse of any signs of infection (redness, swelling, pus, or drainage). He should check for infection every day until the needle sites heal.

If bleeding from a needle site occurs after the patient leaves the dialysis unit or while he's at home, instruct him to apply pressure until it stops. Then he should apply a clean bandage and keep it in place for 6 hours. Tell him to report the bleeding at the next dialysis session. If the bleeding won't stop easily, he should return to the dialysis unit or go to the hospital emergency department.

a pouch under his clothing. Give him a copy of the teaching aid *Performing a solution exchange,* pages 536 to 539.

The same principles apply to an alternative bagless CAPD system (with this system, the patient doesn't wear the bag and tubing continuously). However, the tubing used to drain and instill the solution is primed with povidone-iodine between exchanges. At the end of the dwell time, an empty bag is attached to the tube to collect the used dialysate. In both CAPD and bagless CAPD, explain to the patient that the tubing used for infusing the dialysate will be connected to the catheter by a specially trained nurse. This tubing is changed at regular intervals or when it becomes contaminated.

Surgery

If appropriate, teach the patient about nephrectomy or kidney transplantation.

Nephrectomy. This surgery is indicated if the kidneys are severely infected, greatly enlarged as a result of cystic disease, or causing renin-induced hypertension. Explain to the patient that nephrectomy refers to the removal of part or all of a kidney. Show him the incision site—in the flank over the affected kidney. Tell him that the surgery takes 2 to 3 hours.

Inform the patient that after surgery, he may have a catheter in his bladder to monitor urine volume. (Whether he has a catheter depends mostly on his renal disease stage. In early renal failure, he'll still be manufacturing urine, so he may have a catheter. In later renal failure, decreased urine volume makes measurement less important than avoiding the infection associated with catheter use, so he probably won't have a catheter.) Mention that he may have a Penrose or Hemovac drain in place to remove fluid from the surgical site and thereby prevent infection. Both the catheter and drain will be removed before the patient goes home. Tell him that full recovery takes 6 to 8 weeks.

Kidney transplantation. This treatment for end-stage renal disease may be performed unless the patient has a recent cancer history, chronic infections, or severe cardiac disease. Tell the transplant candidate that the treatment, if successful, will restore renal function. Stress that he'll need medical follow-up for the rest of his life.

Inform the patient that the donor kidney can come from a healthy family member or from a cadaver. Tell him that before transplantation, he'll have a comprehensive examination and tests to identify and treat any disorders that might complicate recovery. This includes urologic studies, an infectious disease workup, and dental, cardiac, and psychological examinations.

Tell the patient what to expect before surgery. If a cadaver kidney will be used, he'll be notified when a kidney is available, then surgery will be performed immediately. Stress the importance of staying healthy during the waiting period so the surgery can be performed safely on short notice. Explain that he may need dialysis immediately before surgery to ensure satisfactory fluid, electrolyte, and acid base balance and to remove uremic toxins from the blood. Then the surgeon will place the donor kidney in a pocket created in the right or left lower abdomen. The surgery usually takes 3 to 4 hours.

Tell the patient that after surgery he will be monitored closely in an intensive care or transplant unit. He'll have a catheter in his bladder to monitor urine output. He'll also receive immunosuppressive drugs to prevent rejection. Explain that immunosuppressive therapy will continue as long as the transplanted kidney remains in place.

Explain that with a cadaver transplant, the kidney may not function immediately—the result of possible damage to the kidney between removal and transplantation. Reassure the patient that dialysis will continue until renal function is restored.

Before discharge, stress the need for adhering to his immunosuppressive drug regimen. Tell the patient that the regimen may include combinations of prednisone, azathioprine, and cyclosporine. Warn him that these drugs raise the risk of infection. Tell him to report signs of infection immediately, such as chills, fever, and fatigue. Point out that he'll require frequent blood studies (several times weekly right after transplantation, then tapering off if he remains stable) to monitor drug effects and transplant function. If he receives prednisone, tell him about sodium restrictions. Prednisone may also increase his appetite, resulting in weight gain.

Teach the patient to watch for and report immediately signs of transplant rejection: fever, decreased urine output, sudden weight gain, and swelling or tenderness over the transplanted kidney. Explain that rejection doesn't always mean loss of the kidney. The doctor may increase the dosages of the immunosuppressive drugs or give him other drugs to counteract rejection.

Tell the patient that long-term complications of transplantation include recurrence of the original disease in the new kidney, drug-induced diabetes, aseptic necrosis of the hip joints, cancer, muscle wasting, and coronary artery disease.

Other care measures

Teach the patient how to manage signs and symptoms of renal failure. Pruritus, which results from dry skin, calcium and phosphorus imbalances, and uremic toxins, can be relieved by antipruritic drugs, by avoiding daily bathing and deodorant soaps, and by using moisturizing soaps and lotions. Uremic mouth odor can be minimized by good oral hygiene and regular dental visits. Tell the patient to promptly report muscle cramps to the doctor so that he can treat their cause; in some instances, quinine tablets may help.

Recognize that lifelong kidney disease disrupts the patient's normal activities, life-style, and relationships and may trigger serious depression (see the teaching aid *Coping with depression*, page 540, for more information). Also recognize that a major relational problem may be sexual dysfunction. As appropriate, discuss the patient's sexual concerns. Both physiological and psychological problems, which may hamper sexual activity, occur more commonly in hemodialysis patients than in peritoneal dialysis patients.

However, in any patient with chronic renal failure, anemia may cause fatigue and weakness. Medications, especially antihypertensives, can cause impotence. Altered body image, resulting from pallor, discolored skin, uremic mouth odor, or the presence of a vascular access or peritoneal catheter, may all contribute to sexual difficulties, too.

To help the patient deal with his sexual concerns, encourage him to follow his treatment regimen closely. This should improve his feelings of well-being. And although dialysis doesn't completely restore health, it may minimize complications, thus improving the patient's outlook. If antihypertensive drugs cause impotence, advise the patient to discuss with his doctor the option of changing drugs.

Talk frankly with the patient about psychological obstacles. Ask for a sexual history and encourage him to share his feelings. Advise him to pursue sexual activity when he's most energetic— perhaps in the morning or after a rest. Explain that time pressures and stress inhibit sexual pleasure. Because role reversal may affect his relationship with his partner, be sure to include his spouse in your discussion. Reassure them that sexual activity won't damage the patient's health.

If intercourse isn't possible, discuss alternate forms of sexual expression, such as touching, stroking, and caressing. Advise the patient that a close, supportive relationship with his partner is crucial in managing his disorder.

Sources of information and support

American Association of Kidney Patients
211 East 43rd Street, Suite 301, New York, N.Y. 10017
(212) 867-4486

American Kidney Foundation
6110 Executive Boulevard, Suite 1010, Rockville, Md. 20852
(800) 638-8299

National Kidney Foundation
Two Park Avenue, New York, N.Y. 10003
(212) 889-2210

Further readings

Booth, L.S., and Dobberstein, K. "Living Without Kidneys," *American Journal of Nursing* 89(2):270, February 1989.

Danziger, C.H. "Uremic Neuropathy and Treatment with Renal Transplantation," *ANNA Journal* 16(2):67-70, April 1989.

Garfinkel, H., et al. "Renal Failure: Are Drugs the Cause?" *Patient Care* 22(14):71-74, 77, 80, September 15, 1988.

Rorer, B., et al. "Long-term Nurse-Patient Interactions: Factors in Patient Compliance or Noncompliance to the Dietary Regimen," *Health Psychology* 7(1):35-46, 1988.

Stevens, E. "End Stage Renal Failure," *Nursing* (London) 3(28):1034-36, June-July 1988.

Worsman, R. "Haemodialysis: A Fragile Lifeline," *Nursing Times* 84(42):31-32, October 19-25, 1988.

Tips for preventing peritonitis

Dear Patient:

Because you'll be using peritoneal dialysis at home, you must guard against peritonitis—an infection that occurs when harmful bacteria enter the dialysis system. Follow these tips to help prevent peritonitis.

Avoid contamination

• Wash your hands before opening the dialysis system, handling the dialysis solution, or changing the dressing over your catheter.

• Change the dressing over your catheter every day and whenever it becomes wet or soiled.

• Cover your mouth or nose with a surgical mask whenever you open the dialysis system—for example, to perform a solution exchange.

• Perform solution exchanges in a clean, dry room with the doors and windows closed. Don't do them in the bathroom.

• Check dialysate drainage for cloudiness or particles—possible signs of infection.

• Always be sure that you have all the equipment you will need to do the exchange before you get started.

• Ask your family to take care of the telephone and other interruptions while you are doing your exchange, or ignore them until you are through.

• Don't use fresh dialysate solution that has excessive moisture on the outside of the bag. This could indicate a leak in the bag and possible contamination.

• Take showers instead of tub baths to prevent bacteria from entering the dialysis system. Tape a plastic cover over the site to prevent contaminating the connections.

• Follow any other instructions or restrictions recommended by your nurses and doctors.

When to seek help

• Call your CAPD unit or doctor if the skin around the peritoneal catheter becomes red, warm, or painful or if you note any drainage. Also report any leakage around the catheter insertion site.

• Follow the instructions that you were given for care of the dialysate tubing spike should it become contaminated by touching your hand or some other surface. This will necessitate a tubing change, which is usually done in the CAPD unit.

• Notify your CAPD unit or doctor if you detect signs of peritonitis, such as abdominal pain, cloudy dialysate, fever, chills, nausea, vomiting, or diarrhea.

Performing a solution exchange

Dear Patient:

You and your doctor have chosen continuous ambulatory peritoneal dialysis (CAPD) for your dialysis program. CAPD is easier to do at home than other forms of dialysis. But when you perform a CAPD solution exchange at home, you must guard against bacteria entering the dialysis system. The following instructions will tell how to drain the used solution and replace it with a fresh one so you don't contaminate the system.

Gather the equipment

First, gather the prescribed bag of peritoneal dialysate solution of the correct volume and dextrose concentration, two outlet port clamps, and a sterile CAPD prep kit. This kit contains povidone-iodine (Betadine) sponges, 4-inch x 4-inch sterile gauze pads (you can also use a shell clamp on the connection between the solution spike and the dialysate outflow port), nonallergenic tape, and a mask. If you must inject medication into the solution, you'll also need the necessary number of 25G needles, 10-ml syringes, and the medication itself.

Before you begin

If you want to warm the dialysate solution, wrap it in a heating pad for several hours. Warming the solution isn't essential, but it should be done if you feel cramps during infusion. Keep the protective wrap on the bag until it's ready to be used. Remember to wash your hands thoroughly before removing the outer wrap and handling the bag.

Draining the old solution

1 Remove the empty solution bag from inside your clothing. Check to be sure that the shell clamp or povidone-iodine-saturated dressing is still in place. If it has become dislodged, apply a gauze dressing covered with povidone-iodine to the connection and cover it with a dry sterile dressing.

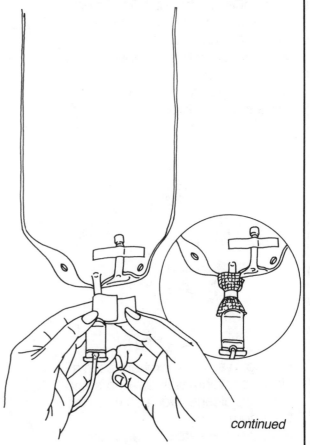

continued

PATIENT-TEACHING AID

Performing a solution exchange — *continued*

2 Now put on your mask and place the bag in the drainage position below your stomach. Open the clamp on the drainage tubing. Allow about 15 to 20 minutes for the solution to drain from your abdomen into the bag.

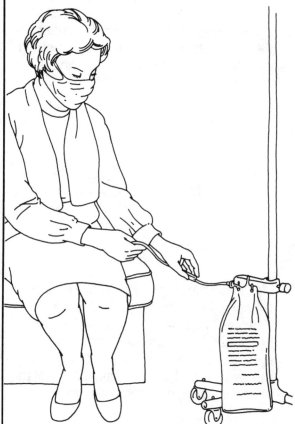

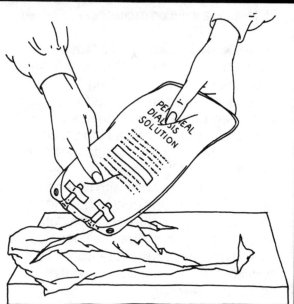

Adding medication
If your doctor has told you to add medication to the new bag, wipe the injection port with a sponge saturated with povidone-iodine and allow the solution to dry for a few minutes. Draw up the prescribed amount of medication. Then insert the needle through the rubber stopper of the injection port, as shown below, and inject the medication. To mix the medication in the solution, turn and squeeze the bag several times. Tape the injection port so it's out of the way.

Checking the new solution bag
Meanwhile, remove the dialysate bag wrapping. Is the solution clear? If it isn't, don't use it. Read the concentration information on the label to make sure you have the right solution, and check the expiration date. Squeeze the bag firmly to test for leaks.

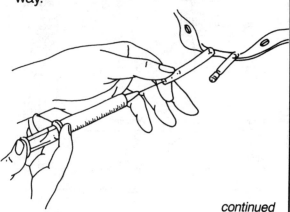

continued

Performing a solution exchange — *continued*

Double-checking the bags

When the solution has finished draining, close the clamp on the tubing and place the drainage bag on a flat surface, next to the new bag. Position the used solution bag with its clear side up, so you can check the fluid for cloudiness or particles.

Position the new bag with its label side up, so you can double-check the concentration and the expiration date. Arrange the bags so that their ends extend over the edge of the work surface. Place a clamp on the outlet port of the new bag.

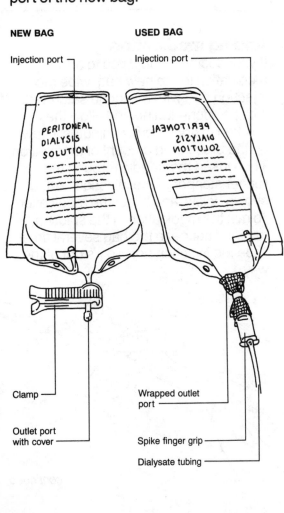

NEW BAG

Injection port

PERITONEAL DIALYSIS SOLUTION

Clamp

Outlet port with cover

USED BAG

Injection port

PERITONEAL DIALYSIS SOLUTION

Wrapped outlet port

Spike finger grip

Dialysate tubing

Setting up the new bag

1 Remove the povidone-iodine dressing or shell clamp from the outlet port tubing junction of the used bag. Clamp the outlet port of the used bag, being sure that it remains a safe distance from the spike junction.

2 Remove the cover from the outlet port of the new bag without touching the port. Now you're ready to transfer the tubing spike.

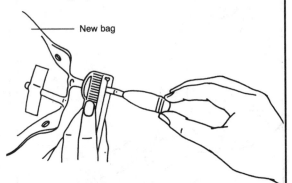

New bag

3 Grasp the finger grip on the tubing spike in the drainage-bag outlet port. With your free hand, hold the clamp on the outlet port of the used bag. Twist and pull the spike of the used bag to remove it from the port. Take care not to touch anything with the spike tip.

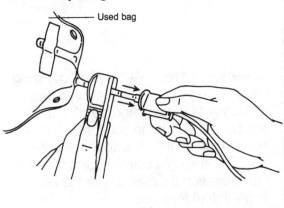

Used bag

continued

Performing a solution exchange — *continued*

4 Immediately insert the spike into the outlet port of the new bag. Apply a shell clamp or povidone-iodine dressing to the junction of the outlet port and tubing. Then remove the outlet port clamp.

5 Hang the new bag on an I.V. pole. Then open the roller clamp on the tubing to allow the solution to drain into

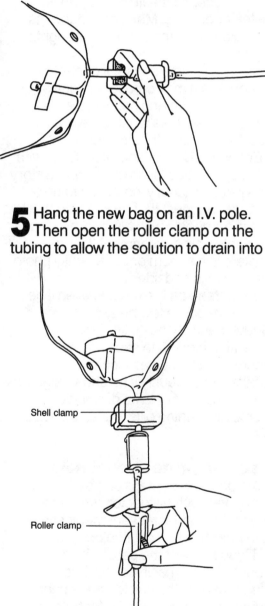

Shell clamp

Roller clamp

your abdomen. After about 5 minutes, when almost all the solution has drained from the bag, close the clamp. Leaving a little fluid in the bag will make it easier to fold.

6 Remove the bag from the pole and place it in front of you. Fold over the connection between the spike and outlet port so it's centered on the bag. Then coil the tubing over this connection. Next, fold the other end of the bag over the connection and tubing and place the bag inside a pouch, if you use one. Put the pouch inside your clothing.

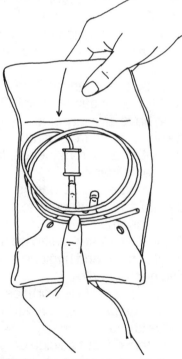

If your doctor has ordered a drainage sample, take the used bag to the hospital laboratory for analysis. Otherwise, carefully empty the used solution into the toilet, and discard the empty bag in a trash can.

PATIENT-TEACHING AID

Coping with depression

Dear Caregiver:

The person in your care may be depressed because his illness keeps him from participating in activities with his family and friends. Although depression is an understandable response to illness, it's not inevitable. With support and counseling, a person can cope with the blues.

Recognizing depression

How can you tell if a person's depressed? If you answer "yes" to some or most of these questions about the person you're caring for, he may well be depressed.
• Has his appetite changed? Has he inexplicably lost or gained weight?
• Does he have difficulty sleeping? Or does he sleep more than usual?
• Has he withdrawn from friends, family, and social activities?
• Is he agitated easily? Does he explode into angry outbursts for no apparent reason?
• Has he lost interest in self-care tasks, such as grooming and hygiene? Has his sex drive decreased?
• Does he feel that life is worthless? Does he act helpless or have an "I'm-in-the-way" attitude?
• Does he think about suicide or harming himself in some other way?

Overcoming depression

Here's how you can help the person you're caring for understand and resolve his depressed feelings:
• Encourage him to express his feelings and to accept himself the way he is. Listen attentively. Make no judgments and allow him time to put his thoughts together.
• Help him gain a sense of control. Encourage him to care for himself as much as he can and make daily decisions, such as what to wear each day. Praise his self-help efforts.
• Encourage him to socialize. Start with simple activities, such as sharing a story or a joke. Gradually, coax him to go on outings. Suggest that he join a support group for people with his disorder.
• Brighten his environment. Hang posters in his room or put a family photo album at his bedside.
• Encourage daily exercise, even if he can move only a few body parts. Regular activity helps lift depression.
• Caution him not to seek relief with depressants, such as alcohol.
• Take him seriously if he shows signs of injuring himself or talks of suicide. Remove sleeping pills, guns, and razor blades.

Seeking professional help

If the person's depression persists, urge him to talk with his doctor, who may prescribe antidepressant medications and refer him to a counselor.

If you suspect the person is thinking about killing himself, call his doctor, clergyman, or the suicide prevention center in your community for help.

Neurogenic bladder

One of your primary goals in neurogenic bladder involves guiding the patient through a lengthy diagnostic workup to identify his bladder dysfunction. Affecting more than 1 million Americans of all ages, neurogenic bladder results from altered bladder innervation and may lead to urinary tract infections, hydronephrosis, and calculi formation.

Fortunately, you can help the patient minimize or prevent these complications by encouraging strict compliance with treatment. However, you'll be challenged to help him overcome anxiety and squeamishness about performing many treatments himself, such as bladder training and intermittent self-catheterization.

What other areas should you cover in your teaching? First, discuss conservative treatment, such as drug and diet therapy. If necessary, explain the use of indwelling urethral catheters, an artificial urinary sphincter implant, or a bladder pacemaker. Discuss major surgery, such as cutaneous ureterostomy and ileal conduit. Of course, besides tests and treatments, your teaching will address background information about the causes, signs and symptoms, and types of neurogenic bladder, and possible complications.

Discuss the disorder

Describe normal bladder function to your patient. Explain that the bladder is a smooth, muscular organ that can hold 250 to 500 ml of urine with little change in pressure. When the bladder fills to 500 ml, the patient experiences the urge to void. During voiding, the detrusor muscle contracts, the urinary sphincter relaxes, and the bladder empties. Afterward, the sphincter closes again.

Explain that neurogenic bladder involves an interruption or delay in normal nerve impulse transmission from the spinal cord to the bladder. This leads to inadequate bladder storage capacity and voiding problems, such as incontinence and incomplete emptying.

Inform the patient that neurogenic bladder is associated with several underlying disorders. (See *What causes neurogenic bladder?* page 542.) Point out that signs and symptoms vary, depending on the cause and its effect on the bladder. Neurogenic bladder is classified as spastic or flaccid.

Spastic neurogenic bladder

Tell the patient that spastic neurogenic bladder, which affects the upper motor neurons, results from spinal cord damage above the S2, S3, or S4 sacral segments. Symptoms include loss of con-

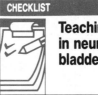

Arlene M. Clarke Coughlin, RN, MSN, who wrote this chapter, is a nursing instructor at Holy Name Hospital School of Nursing and a nursing supervisor and clinical specialist in urology at Holy Name Hospital, Teaneck, N.J.

CHECKLIST

Teaching topics in neurogenic bladder

☐ Comparison of normal and neurogenic bladder function
☐ Causes of neurogenic bladder
☐ Types of neurogenic bladder—spastic and flaccid—and their signs and symptoms
☐ Complications, such as recurrent urinary tract infections, hydronephrosis, and calculi formation
☐ Diagnostic procedures, including excretory urography, cystourethroscopy, cystometry, external sphincter electromyography, uroflometry, retrograde cystography, and voiding cystourethrography
☐ Importance of adequate fluid intake
☐ Prescribed medications and adverse reactions
☐ Role of bladder training and intermittent self-catheterization
☐ Caring for an indwelling catheter, including changing and emptying bags, solving catheter problems, irrigating a blocked catheter, and preventing infection
☐ Use of artificial urinary sphincter implant and bladder pacemaker
☐ Cutaneous ureterostomy and ileal conduit
☐ Sources of information and support

What causes neurogenic bladder?

Once your patient's diagnosed with neurogenic bladder, tell him that this disorder was once thought to result mainly from spinal cord injury. Studies now conclude that it stems from various underlying conditions that can affect bladder innervation.

Diseases of the brain
- amyotrophic lateral sclerosis
- brain tumors
- cerebrovascular accident
- encephalopathy
- multiple sclerosis
- Parkinson's disease

Diseases of peripheral innervation
- diabetes mellitus
- Guillain-Barré syndrome

Diseases of the spinal cord
- myelomeningocele

- spina bifida
- spinal cord trauma
- spinal cord tumors
- spinal stenosis

Other diseases
- alcoholism
- atherosclerosis and other vascular diseases
- herpes zoster
- hypothyroidism, porphyria, and other metabolic disturbances
- systemic lupus erythematosus and other collagen diseases

scious sensation in the bladder, decreased bladder capacity, hypertrophy of the bladder wall, spontaneous detrusor muscle contractions, urinary sphincter spasms, urinary frequency and retention, recurrent urinary tract infections, and lack of urinary control, including stress incontinence.

Flaccid neurogenic bladder

Explain that flaccid neurogenic bladder, which affects the lower motor neurons, results from spinal cord damage, usually traumatic injury at or below the S2, S3, or S4 sacral segments. The bladder becomes flaccid, resulting in overfilling and overdistention, less efficient bladder and detrusor muscle contractions, and a lack of bladder sensation, so the patient doesn't realize when his bladder is full. Other effects include urine retention, urinary tract infections, and overflow incontinence.

Complications

Warn the patient that untreated neurogenic bladder can lead to recurrent urinary tract infections, calculi formation, hydronephrosis, and renal failure, a life-threatening complication.

Describe the diagnostic workup

Inform the patient that the doctor will first take a thorough medical history, emphasizing neurologic and urologic problems. Then he'll order routine laboratory tests, including a urinalysis and a urine culture, to screen for renal or urinary tract disease and urinary tract infection. Explain that he may also order several other diagnostic tests, including excretory urography, cystourethroscopy, urodynamic tests (cystometry, external sphincter electromyography, and uroflometry), retrograde cystography, and voiding cystourethrography.

Excretory urography

Explain that this test (also known as intravenous pyelography) evaluates the kidneys and the urinary tract for abnormalities. Tell the patient that the test takes about 1 hour. Instruct him to drink plenty of water but to stop eating solid food 8 hours before the test. Mention that he may receive a laxative or other bowel preparation. Also, before this test and any other test using a contrast medium, he should inform the doctor if he has an allergy to shellfish or iodine because he may have an allergic reaction to the contrast medium.

Inform the patient that during the test he'll lie supine on an X-ray table. After injection of a contrast medium, X-rays are taken at specific intervals. Warn him that he may experience a transient burning sensation and a metallic taste when the contrast medium is injected. Instruct him to report these and other sensations to the doctor. Tell him that he'll hear loud, clacking sounds as the X-ray machine exposes films. Advise him to report any delayed reactions to the contrast medium, such as hot flashes, rash, itchiness, or difficulty breathing.

Cystourethroscopy

Inform the patient that this 20-minute test permits visualization of the bladder. If a general anesthetic is used, he must fast for 8 hours before the test; if a local anesthetic is used, he may receive a sedative before the test to help him relax.

Tell the patient that he'll lie supine on an X-ray table with his hips and knees flexed. His genitalia will be cleansed with an antiseptic solution, and a drape will be placed over him. The doctor will administer a local anesthetic, if appropriate, then introduce the cystourethroscope through the urethra into the bladder. Next, he'll fill the bladder with an irrigant and rotate the scope to inspect the entire surface of the bladder wall. If the patient is to receive a local anesthetic, warn him that he may feel a burning sensation when the scope passes through the urethra and an urgent need to urinate as his bladder fills with irrigant.

Inform the patient that after the test his vital signs will be monitored every 15 minutes for the first hour, then every hour until he's stable. Instruct him to drink plenty of fluids and to take the prescribed analgesics. He should avoid alcohol for 48 hours. Reassure him that urinary frequency and burning during voiding will soon subside. Tell him to take antibiotics, as ordered, to prevent bacterial infection. Warn him to tell the doctor immediately about any signs of urinary tract infection, such as flank or abdominal pain, chills, fever, or decreased urine output. Also tell him to notify the doctor if he doesn't void within 8 hours after the test or if he continues to see bright red blood after three voidings.

Urodynamic tests

Explain that these tests evaluate the bladder's motor and sensory functioning and voiding efficiency. Tell the patient that these tests provide information on bladder capacity and pressure profiles before and during voiding. The following tests require insertion of a urethral catheter and periodic filling and emptying of the bladder.

Cystometry. Teach the patient that this test evaluates the urgency to void and the ability to suppress voiding by assessing detrusor muscle function and tonicity. The test takes about 40 minutes. Tell him to void just before the test.

Explain that during the test he'll lie supine on an examination table while a catheter is passed into his bladder. As fluid is instilled into the bladder, he'll be asked to report his sensations, such as a strong urge to void, nausea, flushing, or warmth. Warn him that after the test he may experience urinary frequency or transient burning during voiding.

External sphincter electromyography. Tell the patient that this test assesses neuromuscular function of the external urinary sphincter by evaluating how well the bladder and urinary sphincter muscles work together. This test takes from 30 to 60 minutes.

Teach the patient that the skin over his bladder area will be cleansed before placement of skin or needle electrodes. If skin electrodes are used, tell him where they'll be placed and that the area might be shaved first. If needle electrodes are ordered, tell him where they'll be placed and that he'll feel slight discomfort when they're inserted. Explain that both types of electrodes are connected to wires leading to the recording machine that evaluates muscle activity. Reassure him that there's no danger of electric shock. If an anal plug will be used, inform him that only the tip will be inserted into the rectum and that he may feel fullness or an urge to have a bowel movement. But reassure him that this rarely occurs. After the test, advise him to take warm sitz baths to ease discomfort and to drink 2 to 3 liters of fluids daily.

Uroflometry. Teach the patient that this test evaluates his voiding pattern. The test takes about 10 to 15 minutes. Advise him not to void for several hours before the test and to increase his fluid intake so that his bladder is full.

Explain that during the test the patient will be asked to void into a special commode chair with a funnel that measures his urine flow rate and the amount of time he takes to void. Reassure him that he'll have complete privacy during the test. To help ensure accurate results, instruct him to remain as still as possible while voiding.

Retrograde cystography
Tell the patient that this test evaluates bladder structure and integrity. It takes about 30 to 60 minutes. If a general anesthetic is ordered, he must fast for 8 hours before the test.

Explain that during the test the patient lies supine on an X-ray table. A catheter is inserted into his bladder, and then a contrast medium is instilled through the catheter. Films will be taken with the patient in various positions. If a local anesthetic is used, warn him that he may have some discomfort when the catheter's inserted and when the contrast medium is instilled. Also mention that the X-ray machine makes loud, clacking sounds as it exposes the film.

Tell the patient that after the test the nurse will monitor his vital signs frequently until he's stable and will also check his urine volume and color. Instruct him to notify the doctor if he notices blood in his urine after the third voiding or if he develops chills, fever, or an increased pulse or respiration rate.

Voiding cystourethrography
Teach the patient that this test assesses the bladder and urethra for abnormalities. Tell him that the test takes 30 to 45 minutes.

Explain that the patient lies supine on an X-ray table and a catheter is inserted into his bladder. Then a contrast medium is instilled through the catheter. Tell him that he may have a feeling of fullness and an urge to void when the medium is instilled. He'll be asked to assume various positions for X-rays of his bladder and urethra.

Explain that after the test the nurse will record the time, color, and amount of each voiding. The patient should drink plenty of fluids to reduce burning on voiding and to flush out any residual contrast medium. Advise him to report any signs of urinary infection, such as chills and fever, to the doctor immediately.

Teach about treatments
Inform the patient that treatment for neurogenic bladder aims to maintain bladder function, control infection, and prevent incontinence. Explain conservative measures first, such as bladder training techniques, increased fluid intake, medication, and intermittent self-catheterization. If these measures are unsuccessful, teach the patient that the doctor may insert an indwelling catheter temporarily or implant an artificial urinary sphincter or a bladder pacemaker. If all else fails, prepare the patient for urinary diversion surgery.

Diet
Encourage the patient to drink 8 to 10 glasses (at least 64 oz) of fluids a day to flush his urinary system and to reduce the risk of urinary tract infections. He should drink 8 oz every 2 hours and try to void 30 minutes later. Remind him that foods that are liq-

uids at room temperature—such as gelatin, pudding, or ice cream—can be counted as fluids. Advise him to drink cranberry juice daily to help keep the urine acidic, decreasing the risk of urinary tract infections, and to avoid foods rich in calcium and phosphorus, to reduce the risk of developing kidney stones. In addition, the doctor may suggest taking ascorbic acid (vitamin C) to help maintain urine acidity.

Medication
Explain that drug therapy is usually the first-line treatment for neurogenic bladder. Drug therapy corrects incontinence by helping the bladder empty more efficiently and improving coordination between the detrusor muscle and the urethral sphincter. (See *Teaching about drugs for neurogenic bladder*.)

Procedures
Explain to the patient that certain self-care measures can help him empty his bladder and avoid urinary tract infections. These measures include bladder-training techniques—manual stimulation, Credé's method, and Valsalva's maneuver—intermittent self-catheterization, and the use of an indwelling catheter. While he practices any of these methods, instruct him to record what time he voids, the length of time between voidings, and fluid intake and urine output. Teach him the signs and symptoms of a full bladder—discomfort and distention around the bladder, restlessness, and sweating.

Manual stimulation. If the patient has a spastic neurogenic bladder, teach him to activate urination and relax the urethral sphincter by stimulating "trigger areas." Tell him to sit on the toilet and stroke his abdomen or genitalia, then pull gently on the pubic hair. Or he can digitally stimulate the anal sphincter.

Credé's method. If the patient has a flaccid neurogenic bladder, teach him to manually empty the bladder. Tell him to sit on the toilet and apply pressure to his abdomen over the bladder, moving his fingers downward in a "milking" motion.

Valsalva's maneuver. This method is also effective for the patient with a flaccid neurogenic bladder. Instruct him to sit on the toilet, then to forcibly exhale while keeping his mouth closed. This helps the bladder release urine and promotes complete emptying of the bladder.

Intermittent self-catheterization. In conjunction with a bladder training program, this method is especially useful for patients with a flaccid neurogenic bladder. Explain how to perform self-catheterization, using the patient-teaching aids *For women: How to catheterize yourself*, page 215, and *For men: How to catheterize yourself*, page 216.

Indwelling catheterization. Usually this method is reserved for patients who lack the manual dexterity to perform a bladder training program, such as those with multiple sclerosis or other neuro-

Teaching about drugs for neurogenic bladder

DRUG	ADVERSE REACTIONS	TEACHING POINTS
Alpha-adrenergic blocker		
prazosin (Minipress)	• Watch for fainting, persistent lethargy, unusually rapid heart rate, vomiting, and weakness. • Other reactions include dizziness, light-headedness, nausea, pinpoint pupils, postural hypotension, stomach pain, and stuffy nose.	• Teach the patient that this drug should ease bladder contraction, improve voiding, and decrease residual urine in the bladder. • Tell him that the dosage will be increased gradually over several days until he obtains symptomatic relief without adverse effects. Note that mild adverse effects usually disappear after prolonged therapy. • If the patient's being treated for hypertension, advise him that the drug will cause a further drop in his blood pressure. • Because the drug may cause dizziness or light-headedness, caution him to rise slowly from a sitting or a lying position. • Advise him to stop taking the drug immediately if he experiences hypotension, fainting, vomiting, or lethargy. Tell him to lie down with his legs elevated until these symptoms subside. Have him call the doctor if symptoms are severe or don't improve within 24 hours. • Warn a male patient that he may experience retrograde ejaculation.
Anticholinergics		
anisotropine methylbromide (Valpin) **belladonna alkaloids** (Atropine) **dicyclomine hydrochloride** (Bentyl) **glycopyrrolate** (Robinul) **propantheline bromide** (Pro-Banthine)	• Watch for difficult voiding, eye pain, severe constipation, and skin rash. • Other reactions include blurred vision, decreased sweating, drowsiness, dry mouth and throat, mild constipation, and rapid pulse.	• Explain that this drug inhibits bladder contraction, eases bladder spasms, and should increase the patient's bladder capacity. • Caution the patient not to drive or operate machinery while taking the drug. • Because the drug can decrease sweating, tell him not to become overheated to prevent heatstroke. Inform him that hot baths may also make him feel faint or dizzy. • Suggest using sugarless gum, hard candy, or ice chips to relieve dry mouth. • Tell him to avoid over-the-counter products containing antihistamines. • If he's taking antacids and antidiarrhea drugs, tell him to take them at least 1 hour before or 1 hour after he takes his anticholinergic, for best absorption. • Advise against taking the drug with alcohol. • Instruct him to take the drug 30 minutes before meals.
Antispasmodics		
flavoxate hydrochloride (Urispas) **oxybutynin chloride** (Ditropan)	• Watch for confusion, difficult voiding, eye pain, fever, skin rash, and sore throat. • Other reactions include blurred vision, constipation, decreased sweating, dizziness, drowsiness, dry mouth, impotence, nausea, and rapid pulse.	• Explain to the patient that this drug inhibits bladder and detrusor muscle contractions and should relieve urinary discomfort and bladder spasm. Note that it delays the initial desire to void and may increase bladder capacity. • Advise him to take the drug on an empty stomach, 1 hour before or 3 hours after meals, for best absorption. • Because the drug can decrease sweating, tell him not to become overheated to prevent heat stroke. • Instruct him not to drive or operate machinery while taking the drug. • If appropriate, warn the female patient that the drug can suppress lactation. Warn the male patient that it can cause impotence. • Tell the patient to stop taking the drug immediately and to notify the doctor if he develops an allergic reaction. • Suggest using sugarless gum, hard candy, or ice chips to relieve dry mouth.

continued

Teaching about drugs for neurogenic bladder — *continued*

DRUG	ADVERSE REACTIONS	TEACHING POINTS
Cholinergics		
bethanechol chloride (Duvoid, Urecholine) **neostigmine methylsulfate** (Prostigmin)	• Watch for hypotension, shortness of breath, and wheezing or tightness in the chest. • Other reactions include abdominal cramps, dizziness, fainting, headache, nausea, excessive salivation, sweating and skin flushing, and urinary frequency.	• Explain that this drug causes bladder contraction that should stimulate voiding and enhance bladder emptying. • If the patient experiences nausea, tell him to take the drug 1 hour before or 2 hours after meals. • Because the drug may cause dizziness, light-headedness, or fainting, advise him to rise slowly from a sitting or lying position. • If the drug makes him dizzy, tell him not to drive or operate machinery.
External sphincter relaxants		
baclofen (Lioresal)	• Watch for bloody urine, chest pain, fainting, itching, mood changes, skin rash, and tinnitus. • Other reactions include confusion, constipation, dizziness, drowsiness, dry mouth, nausea, urinary frequency, and weakness.	• Explain to the patient that this drug helps treat uninhibited bladder contraction and promote adequate bladder emptying. • Instruct him not to take the drug with other central nervous system depressants, such as antihistamines, or with alcohol. • Warn him not to stop taking the drug abruptly. He must gradually taper the dosage to avoid hallucinations and seizures. • If the drug makes him dizzy or drowsy, tell him not to drive or operate machinery.
dantrolene sodium (Dantrium)	• Watch for black or tarry stools, chest pain, dysuria, severe constipation, severe diarrhea, and yellowing of eyes or skin. • Other reactions include dizziness, drowsiness, mild constipation, mild diarrhea, muscle weakness, nausea, photosensitivity, unusual tiredness, and vomiting.	• Explain to the patient that this drug relaxes certain muscles in his body and should promote adequate emptying of the bladder. • Inform him that because of the risk of hepatotoxicity, he'll need to undergo liver function tests while taking the drug. • Instruct him not to take the drug with alcohol or over-the-counter products that contain antihistamines. • Because the drug may cause dizziness or drowsiness, caution him against driving or operating machinery. • Instruct him to avoid overexposure to sunlight and to use a sunscreen to prevent sunburn.
Tricyclic antidepressant		
imipramine hydrochloride (Tofranil)	• Watch for blurred vision, confusion or hallucinations, constipation, eye pain, fainting, irregular heart rate, and urine retention. • Other reactions include dizziness, drowsiness, dry mouth, fatigue, nausea, and weakness.	• Explain that this drug should help control enuresis, particularly in children age 6 and older, or symptoms of urinary urgency. Note that prolonged use, however, may decrease drug effectiveness. • Advise taking the drug 1 hour before bedtime. To lessen nausea, suggest taking the drug with food. • Warn against taking the drug with systemic decongestants that contain sympathomimetics, such as epinephrine, and to use topical decongestants in moderation. • Advise against taking this drug with alcohol. • Warn against stopping taking the drug suddenly. The patient must taper the dosage gradually to prevent relapse of symptoms or development of withdrawal symptoms, such as headache and nausea. • Because the drug can cause an irregular heart rate, inform the patient (or the parent) that he may need periodic ECGs. • Instruct the patient not to drive or operate machinery while taking the drug.

muscular problems. If your patient has an indwelling catheter, teach him and his family how to care for it at home and how to cope with any problems. Discuss what to do if the catheter becomes blocked and how to recognize signs and symptoms of infection. Urge the patient to contact the doctor or nurse if these problems arise. Give him copies of the patient-teaching aids *Preventing bladder infection from an indwelling catheter*, page 553; *How to care for an indwelling catheter*, pages 554 and 555; *Dealing with a blocked indwelling catheter*, page 556; and *How to irrigate a blocked indwelling catheter*, pages 557 and 558.

Surgery

Inform the patient that the doctor may implant an artificial urinary sphincter or a bladder pacemaker if diet, drug therapy, and bladder training fail to improve his bladder function. If the patient's scheduled for one of these procedures, explain it to him and describe how the device works. (See *Teaching about the artificial urinary sphincter implant*, page 550, and *Restoring bladder function with a pacemaker*, page 551.)

If necessary, the doctor may perform surgery to provide an alternate route for urine excretion. Two such procedures are cutaneous ureterostomy and ileal conduit.

Tell the patient that a *cutaneous ureterostomy* is the simplest type of urinary diversion surgery. In this procedure, one or both ureters are dissected from the bladder and brought through the abdominal skin surface to form one or two stomas. Inform him that the exact stoma site is often chosen during surgery, based on the length of ureter available.

Explain that an *ileal conduit* involves anastomosis of the ureters to a small portion of the ileum excised especially for the procedure, followed by the creation of a stoma from one end of the ileal segment. Explain that the stoma will be located somewhere in the lower abdomen, probably below the waistline.

Preoperative and postoperative considerations. Tell the patient scheduled for one of these procedures that he'll receive a general anesthetic, so he'll have to fast for 8 hours before surgery. He'll also have a nasogastric tube in place after surgery.

Review the enterostomal therapist's explanation of the urine collection device the patient will use after surgery. Encourage the patient to handle the device to help ease his acceptance of it. Reassure him that he'll receive complete training on how to use it after he returns from surgery.

If possible, arrange for a visit by a well-adjusted ostomy patient who can provide a firsthand account of the operation and offer some insight into the realities of ongoing stoma and collection-device care. And, as appropriate, include the patient's family in your preoperative teaching—especially if they'll be providing much of the routine care after discharge.

Tell the patient that after surgery the nurse will monitor his

Teaching about the artificial urinary sphincter implant

An artificial urinary sphincter implant can be a boon for a patient with neurogenic bladder. But using the implant requires a high degree of motivation and compliance and a thorough understanding of how the implant works. Your teaching can help the patient adjust to the implant and use it successfully.

Review criteria for using an implant
Discuss the following:
• incontinence associated with a weak urinary sphincter
• incoordination between the detrusor muscle and the urinary sphincter (if drug therapy is unsuccessful)
• inadequate bladder storage (if intermittent catheterization and drug therapy are unsuccessful).

Explain the implant procedure
Show the patient an implant or a picture of one and explain its parts: the control pump, an occlusive cuff, and a pressure-regulating balloon. Then show him a picture of an implanted device. Point out that the cuff is placed around the bladder neck, and the balloon is placed under the rectus muscle in the abdomen. The balloon holds the fluid that is used to inflate the cuff. If the patient is male, the control pump is placed in the scrotum; if the patient is female, the pump is placed in the labium.

Outline how to use the device
After surgery, instruct the patient to squeeze the bulb when he wants to void. This deflates the cuff and opens the urethra by returning fluid to the balloon. After voiding, the cuff reinflates automatically, sealing the urethra until the patient needs to void again.

Discuss postimplant considerations
Show the patient how to perform intermittent catheterization to check for residual urine in the bladder. Tell him that before discharge he'll have daily urodynamic testing and ultrasonography to check for residual urine after voiding. He'll also have an X-ray to check for kinking or other implant problems. Advise him to avoid sports and strenuous activities for 6 months after surgery, and encourage him to keep all follow-up appointments.

Cover possible complications
Make sure that the patient's aware of complications that can necessitate implant repair or removal. For example, the cuff or balloon can leak (uncommon), or trapped blood or other fluid contaminants can cause problems in the control pump, increasing resistance to fluid passage to and from the cuff. Surgical complications include skin erosion around the bulb or in the bladder neck or the urethra, infection, inadequate occlusion pressures, and kinked tubing.

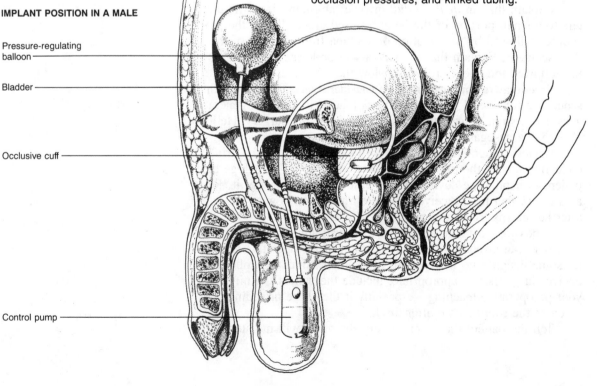

IMPLANT POSITION IN A MALE

Pressure-regulating balloon

Bladder

Occlusive cuff

Control pump

Restoring bladder function with a pacemaker

Is the doctor considering a bladder pacemaker for your patient? If so, inform the patient that this procedure uses electrical stimulation to help restore bladder function.

Who's a candidate?
Explain that a bladder pacemaker is used in patients with spastic neurogenic bladder. Then inform the patient about other factors that help determine suitability for this procedure. They include age, bladder storage capacity, kidney function, sphincter competence, and general neurologic and psychological status. Mention that urodynamic bladder monitoring and sphincter stimulation tests also help to decide eligibility for this procedure.

How does the pacemaker operate?
Tell the patient that the pacemaker consists of these components: electrodes, a receiver, and an external transmitter. The electrodes are implanted on the third and occasionally on the fourth sacral motor nerve roots. When they're stimulated, they trigger detrusor muscle contraction. Electrical stimulation also reduces sphincter hyperreflexia by dividing the sensory component of the same sacral nerve roots and selective branches of the pudendal nerves.

Inform the patient that the electrodes are connected to a receiver, which is placed under the skin. Explain that every 3 to 4 hours he'll use the external transmitter to control bladder continence.

vital signs until he's stable. His dressings will be checked periodically and changed at least once every shift.

Home care. If the patient will be discharged with an indwelling urethral catheter, explain how to care for it and how to handle problems. Make sure that the patient and any caregivers know how to care for the stoma and change the ostomy pouch. Refer them to a support group, such as the United Ostomy Association. Also stress the importance of keeping scheduled follow-up appointments with the doctor and enterostomal therapist to evaluate stoma care and make any necessary changes in equipment. For instance, stoma shrinkage, which normally occurs within 8 weeks after surgery, may require a change in pouch size to ensure a tight fit.

Tell the patient that he should be able to return to work soon after discharge; however, if his job requires heavy lifting, he should talk to his doctor before resuming work. Explain that he can safely participate in most sports, even strenuous ones, but suggest that he avoid contact sports, such as wrestling.

If the patient expresses doubts or insecurity about his sexuality related to the stoma and collection device, refer him for sexual counseling. Also reassure the female patient that pregnancy should pose no special problems. But urge her to consult with her doctor before she becomes pregnant.

Sources of information and support

Continence Restored, Inc.
785 Park Avenue, New York, N.Y. 10021
(212) 879-3131

Help for Incontinent People
P.O. Box 544, Union, S.C. 29379
(803) 585-8789

National Kidney and Urologic Diseases Information Clearinghouse
P.O. Box NKUDIC, Bethesda, Md. 20892
(301) 468-6345

Simon Foundation
Box 815, Wilmette, Ill. 60091
(708) 864-3913

United Ostomy Association
36 Executive Park, Suite 120, Irvine, Calif. 92714
(714) 660-8624

Further readings

Balmaseda, M.T., Jr., et al. "The Value of the Ice Water Test in the Management of the Neurogenic Bladder," *American Journal of Physical Medicine and Rehabilitation* 67(5):225-27, October 1988.

Bisson, D.J. "Sorting Out Spinal Cord Syndromes," *Journal of the American Academy of Physician Assistants* 1(1):4-8, January-February 1988.

Brinkso, V. "Preventing Infection in the Continent Urinary Reservoir," *Journal of Urology Nursing* 8(2):624-25, April-June 1989.

Koch, M.O. "Bladder Substitution with Intestine: Past and Present," *Journal of Urology Nursing* 8(2):610-17, April-June 1989.

Lastnik, A.L. "The Antireflux Pouch: Is It Effective, Is It Functional?" *Journal of Enterostomal Therapy* 16(2):84-85, March-April 1989.

Long, B.W. "Radiography of Cutaneous Urinary Diversions," *Radiology Technology* 60(2):109-20, November-December 1988.

McLean, M.H. "Implanting an Artificial Urinary Sphincter," *Canadian Operating Room Nursing Journal* 7(2):5-6, 9-11, April-May 1989.

Nordstrom, G. "Urostomy Patients: A Strategy for Care," *Nursing Times* 85(18):32-34, May 3-9, 1989.

Shipes, E. "Nursing Care of Patients with CUR: Continent Urinary Reservoir," *Journal of Urology Nursing* 8(2):595-609, April-June 1989.

Smith, C.G. "A Urostomy Patient Visiting Program," Urology Nursing 9(5):10-11, July-September 1989.

Tanagho, E.A., and Schmidt, R.A. "Electrical Stimulation in the Clinical Management of the Neurogenic Bladder," *Journal of Urology* 140(6):1331-39, December 1988.

Preventing bladder infection from an indwelling catheter

Dear Patient:

Your indwelling catheter increases your risk of developing a bladder infection.

However, you can prevent or at least control infection by taking the following precautions.

Report warning signs
Contact the doctor immediately if you have any of the warning signs listed below:
• fever above 100° F. (37.7° C.)
• cloudy urine
• discharge around the catheter
• pain in the bladder area.

Don't give infection a chance
You may not always be able to prevent a bladder infection, but you can reduce your chances for infection by following these guidelines:
• Drink at least eight 8-ounce glasses of fluid a day. Include cranberry juice, which keeps urine acidic.
• Take the medicine prescribed by your doctor.
• Wash the catheter area with soap and water twice a day to keep it from becoming irritated or infected. Also wash your rectal area whenever you have a bowel movement. Dry your skin gently but thoroughly.
• If you're a woman, always wipe from front to back after bowel movements. Do the same when washing and drying the genital area. This prevents contamination of the catheter and urinary tract with germs from the rectum.

• Once a day, wash the drainage tubing and bag with soap and water. Rinse with a solution made from about 1 part white vinegar to 7 parts water.
• Empty your leg drainage bag every 3 or 4 hours. Empty your bedside drainage bag at least every 8 hours.
• Always keep the drainage bag below bladder level.

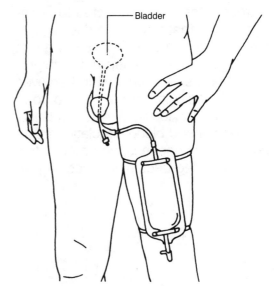

Bladder

• Never pull on the catheter. Disconnect it from the drainage tubing only to clean the bag.
• Contact the doctor immediately if you have urine leakage around the catheter, abdominal pain and fullness, scanty urine flow, or blood or particles in your urine.
• Never try to remove the catheter yourself unless the doctor or nurse has given you instructions.
• Keep your follow-up appointments with the doctor.

How to care for an indwelling catheter

Dear Patient:

Your doctor says your indwelling catheter will have to stay in place for the next few weeks. This latex tube permits continuous urine drainage, so you won't need to use a bedpan or the toilet. A balloon on one end of the tube holds it inside your bladder.

Your catheter is connected to drainage tubing that leads to a drainage bag. During the day, you'll strap a drainage bag to your leg at the thigh level. Make sure to empty this bag every 3 to 4 hours. Also make sure not to secure the bag too tightly—skin irritation and decreased blood circulation could result. If this happens, you may notice your lower leg becoming discolored.

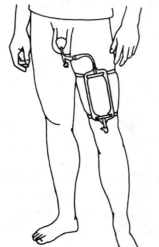

Emptying the leg bag

1 First, wash your hands. Then remove the stopper and drain all the urine, either into the toilet or if the doctor orders it, into a measuring container so you can record the amount. Don't touch the drain tip with your fingers or with the container.

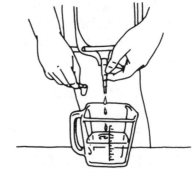

2 After the urine has drained completely, swab the drain tip and the stopper with a povidone-iodine swab. Replace the stopper.

Attaching the bedside drainage bag

Before going to bed, replace the leg bag with a bedside drainage bag. This bag holds more urine, so you can sleep for 8 hours without emptying it.

1 To replace the leg bag, first empty it. Now clamp the catheter and swab the connection between the catheter and the leg bag with povidone-iodine.

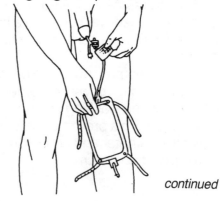

continued

How to care for an indwelling catheter — *continued*

Then disconnect the leg bag, and connect the catheter to the bedside drainage tubing and bag. Finally, unclamp the catheter.

2 Which side of the bed do you want the drainage bag to hang from? Tape the drainage tubing to your thigh on that side, using nonallergenic tape.

Shave your skin in that area, if needed. Leave some slack in the line so that you won't pull on the catheter when you move your leg. If you're a man, tape the drainage tubing to your inner thigh, opposite the base of your penis. If you're a woman, tape the drainage tubing to your inner thigh below the vaginal area.

3 When you get into bed, arrange the drainage tubing so it doesn't kink or loop. Then hang the drainage bag by its hook on the side of the bed. To ensure proper drainage and reduce the infection risk, keep the bag below your bladder level at all times, whether you're lying, sitting, or standing.

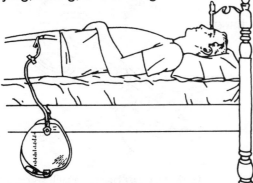

Reattaching the leg bag

1 When you're ready to reattach the leg bag in the morning, empty the bedside drainage bag. To do this, first unclamp the drainage tube and remove it from its sleeve, without touching its tip.

—— Unclamped drainage tube

2 Then let the urine drain into the toilet or into a measuring container, if required. Don't let the drainage tube touch the toilet or container.

3 When the bag is completely empty, swab the end of the drainage tube with povidone-iodine solution. Reclamp the tube and reinsert it into the sleeve of the drainage bag.

Don't let anyone else empty your drainage bag, unless one member of your family performs your catheter care. If your doctor has requested it, record the amount of urine drained.

4 Now repeat the steps you took when connecting the bedside drainage bag, but use the leg bag instead: Clamp the catheter and swab the connection between the catheter and the bedside drainage bag with povidone-iodine, disconnect the bedside drainage bag, and connect the catheter to the drainage tubing and leg bag. Finally, unclamp the catheter.

Cleaning the drainage bags
When you've finished, wash out the bag with soap and water, and rinse it with a solution of 1 part white vinegar and 7 parts water to clean and deodorize it.

Soak leg bags overnight in the vinegar-water solution. You can use both types of drainage bags for up to 1 month before replacing them.

Dealing with a blocked indwelling catheter

Dear Patient:

Learning to care for an indwelling catheter at home takes time and practice. However, even if you're careful, the catheter can still become blocked.

How do I know the catheter's blocked?

Suspect blockage if urine hasn't drained for 2 hours, even though you've been drinking plenty of fluids. Other signs are damp underwear that smells of urine, lower-abdominal pressure, and the urge to urinate.

How do I unblock the catheter?

• First, straighten any kinked tubing.
• Next, try changing position. (Drainage can stop if the catheter lies against the bladder wall. Changing your position can restart the drainage.)
• Or try lowering the drainage bag — it won't drain if it's above bladder level.
• Last, try irrigating the catheter if you've been taught this procedure. If this doesn't help, contact the visiting nurse or doctor.

But don't remove the catheter yourself unless the nurse or doctor tells you to and you've had previous instruction.

How do I remove the catheter?

If the nurse or doctor tells you to remove the catheter, follow these instructions: First, deflate the balloon on the end of the catheter. (Not doing so can injure your bladder and urethra.)

To do this, attach a syringe without a needle to the unattached end of the tubing's Y-shaped portion (inflation port).

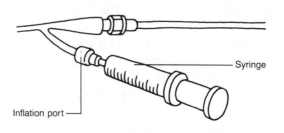

Syringe

Inflation port

If the inflation port doesn't have a special tip that the syringe fits into, put a needle on the syringe and puncture the port.

Gently pull back on the plunger. The water in the balloon will flow into the syringe, deflating the balloon.

If that doesn't work, try this method only as a last resort: Place a small basin under the inflation port to catch the fluid from the balloon. Then cut the catheter in two just above the inflation port.

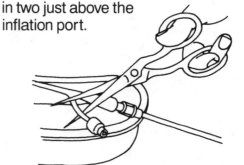

Now the water in the balloon will escape into the basin. When the balloon is deflated, pull gently on the catheter to remove it.

Important: If it doesn't come out easily, don't force it. Instead, call the visiting nurse or doctor for help.

How to irrigate a blocked indwelling catheter

Dear Patient:

If your indwelling catheter becomes blocked for no apparent reason, you can try irrigating it to correct the blockage. Although you probably learned to irrigate a catheter in the hospital, use these instructions as a review.

Getting ready
Assemble the equipment: irrigation solution (as ordered by the doctor), irrigation solution container (not the one you use to collect urine), drainage container, bulb syringe, two alcohol swabs, gloves, a plastic bag (to protect linens), and a 4-by-4-inch gauze pad. Make sure these items are clean.

Note: You can buy prepackaged kits with this equipment. If you're ill or have an infection, you may wear gloves and a face mask.

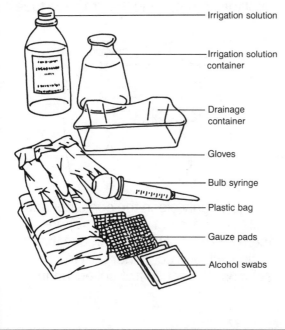

- Irrigation solution
- Irrigation solution container
- Drainage container
- Gloves
- Bulb syringe
- Plastic bag
- Gauze pads
- Alcohol swabs

Preparing the irrigant
Place the plastic bag, covered by a towel, under your buttocks. Expose the indwelling catheter. Open the gauze pad package and place it on the towel without touching the gauze.

Then pour the amount of irrigation solution prescribed by the doctor into the collection container. Draw 30 to 50 ml of the solution into the bulb syringe.

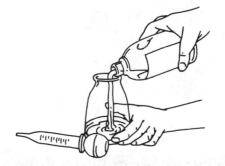

Cleaning the connection
Open the alcohol swab wrapper. Then put on the gloves. To avoid spreading germs, don't let the gloves touch anything other than the clean equipment.

Remove the alcohol swab from its wrapper, and use it to clean the area where the catheter connects with the drainage tube.

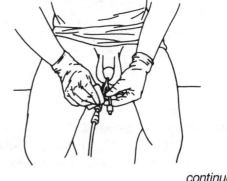

continued

PATIENT-TEACHING AID

PATIENT-TEACHING AID

How to irrigate a blocked indwelling catheter — *continued*

Disconnecting the catheter and drainage tube

Disconnect the catheter and drainage tube by carefully twisting them apart.

Make sure you do this without pulling on the indwelling catheter. Use one hand to place the end of the drainage tube on the gauze pad to keep it clean as you hold the indwelling catheter in the other hand.

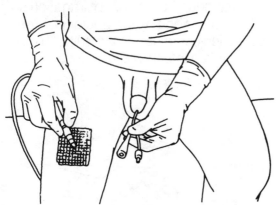

Instilling the irrigation solution

Insert the tip of the bulb syringe into the indwelling catheter. Then gently and slowly squeeze the solution into the catheter. *Note:* Don't apply forceful pressure to squeeze the bulb syringe.

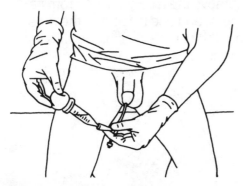

Draining the solution

Remove the syringe and let the solution flow into the drainage container. Don't

let the end of the catheter touch the drainage container. Also don't draw up any of the solution after it's drained into the container.

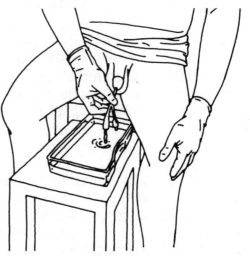

Reconnecting the catheter and drainage tube

After all the solution has drained, wipe the end of the catheter with the unused alcohol swab. Wait a few seconds to let the alcohol evaporate and then reconnect the catheter and the drainage tube.

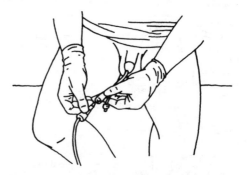

Thoroughly clean the container and bulb syringe in hot water to prepare them for reuse. Remember, use the irrigation solution container only to collect solution. Never use it to collect urine.

Urinary incontinence

You may find yourself teaching about urinary incontinence to people of all ages but mostly to elderly adults. Altogether, nearly 10 million Americans (more women than men) have urinary incontinence. About 30% are elderly people who live at home; about 50% live in nursing homes.

Although urinary incontinence doesn't necessarily signal a serious disease, it *is* an embarrassment. At worst, it leads to depression and reclusive behavior when the incontinent person hesitates to leave home for fear of having an "accident."

Most people don't know what causes urinary incontinence, let alone that the disorder can be treated and possibly reversed. Many people wrongly assume that incontinence is an annoyance of aging to be endured. So before you can teach about managing incontinence, you'll dispel common misconceptions. At the same time, you'll give the patient continued emotional support. Discuss the types and causes of urinary incontinence, and then explain diagnostic studies and recommended treatments, including activity and dietary changes, drug therapy or surgery, and procedures such as self-catheterization or bladder retraining.

Include close relatives and other caregivers in your teaching sessions, especially when the disorder negatively affects the patient's family. Coping with incontinence can become so burdensome that many families seek institutional care for the incontinent member. (In fact, it's a common reason for placing elderly persons in nursing homes.) Your teaching may improve the family's coping skills as well as the patient's quality of life.

Discuss the disorder
Tell the patient and her family that urinary incontinence—the involuntary passage of urine—is a symptom that has many causes. For example, it may result from a nervous system or urinary tract disorder; weak pelvic muscles; pressure on the bladder and urethra caused by a fecal impaction, a tumor, or an enlarged prostate gland; or age-related changes in lower urinary tract function.

Point out that urinary incontinence may be acute or chronic. Typically associated with a severe illness, *acute* urinary incontinence usually subsides with successful treatment of the illness. (See *What causes acute incontinence?* page 560.) *Chronic* incontinence may be classified as stress, urge, overflow, or functional incontinence.

Diane Kaschak Newman, MSN, CRNP, and **Diane A. Smith, MSN, CRNP,** wrote this chapter. Ms. Newman is a continence management specialist and vice-president of Golden Horizons, Inc., Newtown Square, Pa. Ms. Smith is a continence management specialist and president of Golden Horizons.

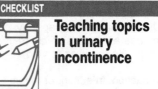

CHECKLIST

Teaching topics in urinary incontinence

☐ Definition of acute and chronic urinary incontinence
☐ Causes of acute urinary incontinence
☐ Causes and types of chronic urinary incontinence
☐ Complications, such as irritation and infection
☐ Diagnostic studies, including post-void residual urine volume, cystometry, urinalysis and urine culture, and uroflometry
☐ How to perform Kegel exercises
☐ Dietary modifications and fluid requirements
☐ Medications and their effects
☐ Devices, such as pessaries and condom catheters, and procedures, such as artificial sphincter implantation and intermittent self-catheterization
☐ Surgery to correct the cause
☐ Other care measures—habit training and bladder retraining, wearing protective pads and garments, and preventing skin breakdown
☐ Sources of information and support

What causes acute incontinence?

Explain the most common causes of acute incontinence to your patient. Prompt your memory with the mnemonic DRIP.

Delirium and disorientation associated with a serious illness, such as myocardial infarction, stroke, or sepsis, can hinder the patient from recognizing an urge to void. And dehydration can cause urine to concentrate, resulting in bladder wall irritation and incontinence.

Retention of urine or restricted mobility may cause incontinence. For instance, an obstruction can cause urine retention and subsequent incontinence. Or a physical handicap may impede a person's timely response to the urge to void.

Impaction, infection, or inflammation also can cause incontinence—an impacted fecal mass by compressing the bladder, a urinary tract infection by producing bladder wall inflammation, and a hormonal deficiency by fostering urinary muscle weakness and inflammation (atrophic vaginitis, for example).

Pharmaceuticals, polyuria, or Paget's disease can contribute to incontinence. For instance, diuretics may increase the bladder's work load, and antihypertensives may relax the urinary sphincter muscle. Hypnotics, sedatives, and anticholinergics can also produce incontinence. Polyuria and glucosuria (from diabetes, for example) can irritate the bladder wall. And hypercalcemia (associated with Paget's disease) leads to incontinence by causing bladder muscle hypertonicity and increased contractility.

In *stress incontinence,* intermittent leakage results from a sudden increase in intra-abdominal pressure, which occurs when laughing, coughing, running, or lifting a heavy object. Weak pelvic muscles or urinary sphincter damage or weakness causes this disorder. Typical patients include mature women who've borne several children, young or middle-aged women who've just experienced a difficult childbirth, and women who've had recurrent pelvic and bladder surgery. Men who sustain urethral damage from a transurethral prostatectomy may also have stress incontinence.

The patient with *urge incontinence* cannot suppress a sudden urge to urinate—for example, when rising from a seat or for no apparent reason. Uncontrolled detrusor (bladder) muscle contractions or detrusor hyperreflexia may cause this incontinence.

The patient with *overflow incontinence* usually doesn't sense bladder fullness; consequently, urine overflows from the bladder. This can happen if a structural abnormality or an obstruction from a urethral stricture, an enlarged prostate, or a stone or tumor impairs normal bladder contraction and blocks normal urine passage. Also, overflow incontinence may result from a neurogenic bladder (interruption of normal bladder innervation), which stems from spinal cord injury, cerebrovascular accident or other neurologic injury, diabetes, or drug-induced atonia from anticholinergics, narcotics, antidepressants, or smooth muscle relaxants.

Functional incontinence is associated with an inability to reach the bathroom in time. Why? The patient may have trouble walking or undressing, or the bathroom may be inaccessible. She may not sense an urge to urinate until the bladder's almost full—and then the urge may be immediate and intense. Because lower urinary tract function deteriorates with age, this type of incontinence affects mostly elderly patients.

Complications
Point out to family members and the patient that untreated or poorly managed urinary incontinence can lead to skin irritation, ulceration, and infection. Urosepsis (septic poisoning from urine retained in the bladder) may also occur. Other complications include possible emotional and social dysfunction, depression, diminished self-esteem, and social isolation.

Describe the diagnostic workup
Inform the patient that the diagnosis will be based on a patient history, a physical examination, a post-void residual (PVR) urine volume test, cystometry, and a urinalysis and urine culture. If needed, the doctor will order uroflometry and more extensive urodynamic tests.

Patient history and physical examination
Tell the patient that the doctor will ask about her medical history, her typical urinary pattern and degree of control, the amount she usually voids, and her daily fluid intake. He may ask her to keep bladder records to determine the degree of her incontinence. He'll

also ask about other urinary problems: Does she have urinary hesitancy, urgency, nocturia, or urinary tract infections?

Inform the patient that during the physical examination, the doctor will inspect the urethral meatus for inflammation or anatomic defects. He'll palpate the abdomen for bladder distention (which signals urine retention) and perform a complete neurologic assessment. He'll also test the pelvic muscles, especially the bladder muscle, for strength and tone. In an older patient, he'll test this during a digital rectal examination by asking the patient to contract her pelvic muscles around his finger.

PVR urine volume test
Explain that this test determines whether the bladder retains urine. After the patient urinates, the doctor inserts a straight catheter into the urethra to measure PVR urine volume. If the residual volume is normal, urine retention isn't the problem, and the patient's incontinence has another cause.

Cystometry
Inform the patient that this test assesses bladder sensation and capacity. The test also detects uninhibited detrusor contractions. Explain that the doctor will instill sterile water into the bladder through a urethral catheter. When the patient reports the urge to void, he'll ask her to breathe slowly and deeply until the urge passes. Then he'll instill more sterile water until she again feels the urge to void. She'll breathe deeply again until the urge subsides. With her bladder full, he'll ask her to cough. If the patient leaks urine around the catheter, the doctor will diagnose stress incontinence.

Urinalysis and urine culture
The doctor may order a urinalysis and a urine culture to rule out a urinary tract infection as the cause of incontinence. Tell the patient that she'll be asked to urinate into a container. The urine will be examined visually and microscopically for signs of infection, such as a cloudy appearance, a foul odor, bacteria, pus, proteins, red and white blood cells, and alkaline pH. If the signs suggest infection, a urine culture can identify the disease-causing agent.

Uroflometry
Explain that the doctor may order a uroflometric test if he suspects an obstruction, possibly from an enlarged prostate or a urethral stricture. This 10- to 15-minute test assesses the urine flow rate. Instruct the patient not to urinate for several hours before the test and to increase her fluid intake so that she'll have a full bladder and a strong urge to void.

When the test begins, direct the patient to urinate into a special commode chair equipped with a funnel device that measures the urine flow rate and voiding time. Reassure her that she'll have complete privacy during the test. Remind her that remaining as still as possible while voiding will help to ensure accurate results.

Other tests

If the patient has asymptomatic hematuria, lower abdominal pain, or recurrent urinary tract infections, the doctor may order various urodynamic tests to document bladder pressure, muscle contractility, urethral length, and sphincter control. These tests detect kidney and bladder stones and tumors, obstructions of the lower urinary tract, and enlarged prostate glands.

Teach about treatments

Treatments for urinary incontinence involve exercises to strengthen pelvic muscles; dietary modifications and fluid restrictions; medications to treat underlying conditions; and procedures and devices, such as habit training, bladder retraining, pessaries, condom catheters, artificial sphincter implantation, and intermittent self-catheterization. Occasionally, treatment may include surgery.

Activity

Tell the patient that strong pelvic muscles can help to prevent incontinence. Describe the pelvic floor musculature and its function. Then teach her how to do Kegel exercises to strengthen muscles that control urine flow. Provide her with a copy of the teaching aid *How to exercise your pelvic muscles*, page 572.

Diet

Inform the patient that she may need to limit or eliminate foods that irritate the bladder and cause urinary frequency—for example, foods and beverages with caffeine, such as coffee, tea, cola, and dark chocolate; alcohol; and the artificial sweetener aspartame (Nutrasweet). Tell her that many prescription and nonprescription medications contain caffeine, including such remedies as Anacin, Excedrin, Midol, and Dristan. Urge her to check food and medication labels carefully.

If the patient's keeping a "bladder record" to document her fluid intake and her voiding and incontinence episodes, advise her to review her record daily. In this way, she can make sure that she's taking in at least 64 oz of fluid each day. Explain that many incontinent patients consciously or unintentionally restrict fluids, which isn't the treatment's aim. If the patient's concerned about nocturia, suggest that she consume most fluids in the daytime and limit evening intake to small sips after 6 p.m.

Because urinary incontinence may stem from pressure on the bladder and urethra from constipation or fecal impaction, recommend a fiber-rich diet to help counter these conditions. High-fiber foods include whole grain breads and cereals, nuts, and raw fruits and vegetables.

For the patient with established bowel problems, suggest eating unprocessed, coarse wheat bran (available in health food stores). Advise her to start with 1 tbs of bran daily and gradually increase the amount until her bowel function returns to normal. (A gradual increase helps prevent flatulence, abdominal bloating, and cramps.) She can start by topping foods with a sprinkle of bran and then increase the amount over time. She also can mix 1 cup of bran and 1 cup of applesauce with ½ cup of prune juice.

Advise her to consume just 2 tbs of the mixture a day at first. Then she can increase her intake by 2 tbs a week until bowel movements resume a normal pattern.

Medication

Identify the medications that the patient may take to treat conditions causing urinary incontinence. They include antibiotics, antispasmodics, and various other preparations. See *Teaching about drugs for urinary incontinence,* pages 564 and 565.

Antibiotic therapy. If urinary incontinence results from an inflammation caused by bacterial infection, explain that the doctor may prescribe an antibiotic—for example, norfloxacin (Noroxin)—that's effective against the disease-causing organism.

Antispasmodic therapy. Tell the patient that various medications may help incontinence from detrusor muscle instability, for example, an anticholinergic drug, such as propantheline (Pro-Banthine), to improve bladder function and treat bladder spasms.

If detrusor hyperreflexia causes incontinence, tell the patient that antispasmodic drugs with anticholinergic properties may help. Examples include oxybutynin (Ditropan) and flavoxate (Urispas). Point out that these drugs directly suppress the bladder's smooth muscle activity. They may also increase bladder capacity and urine retention.

Other drugs. If incontinence results from atrophic vaginitis, explain that the doctor may prescribe estrogen (Premarin, Ogen) in oral, topical, or suppository form on a 1-month trial basis. Estrogen restores urethral mucosal integrity and increases resistance to urine outflow. Depending on the therapy's success, the patient may continue the drug for a longer time.

Or the doctor may order an antidepressant drug to treat stress incontinence or incontinence caused by an unstable bladder. For example, a side effect of the antidepressant imipramine (Tofranil) is increased bladder capacity and improved sphincter tone.

Recently approved for the patient with primary nocturnal enuresis, desmopressin acetate (DDAVP) may be prescribed as a nasal spray. It drastically reduces the amount of urine produced overnight.

Procedures

If appropriate, describe procedures and devices used to improve or manage urinary incontinence. Explain that initial measures include habit training and bladder retraining. Next the patient might use a pessary or a condom (external) catheter. Then, if appropriate, the doctor may recommend artificial sphincter implantation or intermittent self-catheterization.

Habit training. Helpful when the patient has dementia or other types of cognitive impairment, habit training requires maintaining a rigid voiding schedule—usually every 2 to 4 hours. The patient's objective is to void before an accident occurs. Because the habit training schedule relies on the patient's typical voiding-incontinence pattern as determined by her bladder records, make sure to include family members or other caregivers in your teaching. Stress keeping accurate records to help the doctor monitor progress and adjust treatment, if necessary. Direct the patient to

Teaching about drugs for urinary incontinence

DRUG	ADVERSE REACTIONS	TEACHING POINTS
Antibiotic		
norfloxacin (Noroxin)	• Watch for seizures (rare). • Other reactions include abdominal pain, confusion in elderly patients, constipation, diarrhea, dizziness, dry mouth, dyspepsia, erythema, fatigue, fever, flatulence, headache, heartburn, insomnia, rash, and somnolence.	• Advise the patient to take this drug with an 8-oz glass of water either 1 hour before or 2 hours after eating. • If the drug causes nausea or upset stomach, suggest taking it with food. • Caution the patient to avoid activities that require physical coordination or alertness if the drug causes dizziness. • Tell her to increase her fluid intake while she's taking the drug unless the doctor orders otherwise. • Stress that she should finish the prescription, taking all medicine as directed even after she feels better. Stopping the medicine too soon may cause symptoms to recur. • Instruct her to space doses evenly — day and night — and never to skip a dose because the drug works best at a constant level in the body. • Tell her to take a missed dose as soon as possible, but not to double-dose.
Antispasmodics		
flavoxate (Urispas)	• Watch for blurred vision and mental confusion (especially in elderly patients) and dermatoses. • Other reactions include abdominal pain, constipation (with high doses), difficulty concentrating, dizziness, drowsiness, dry mouth and throat, fever, headache, nausea, nervousness, palpitations, tachycardia, urticaria, and vomiting.	• Advise the patient to avoid activities that require alertness if blurred vision, confusion, or drowsiness occurs. • Tell her to contact the doctor if she doesn't respond to the drug.
oxybutynin (Ditropan)	• Watch for blurred vision, cardiac disturbances (palpitations and tachycardia), constipation, drowsiness, dry mouth, and urinary hesitance or urine retention. • Other reactions include bloated feeling, confusion, decreased sweating, dizziness, fever, flushing, hives, impotence, insomnia, mydriasis, nausea, severe allergic skin reactions, suppressed lactation, and vomiting.	• Advise the patient to suck on sugarless hard candy or ice chips or to chew sugarless gum to relieve a dry mouth. • Caution her not to perform any activities that require alertness if blurred vision, dizziness, or drowsiness occurs. • Urge her to exercise caution in hot, humid weather because this drug suppresses sweating, which may trigger fever or heatstroke or aggravate symptoms of hyperthyroidism, coronary artery disease, congestive heart failure, cardiac dysrhythmias, tachycardia, hypertension, or prostatic hypertrophy.
propantheline (Pro-Banthine)	• Watch for blurred vision, confusion, or excitement (in elderly patients); palpitations; and urine retention. • Other reactions include constipation; dizziness; drowsiness; dry mouth, nose, and throat; headache; hives; insomnia; nausea; nervousness; photophobia; reduced sweating; swallowing difficulty; and weakness.	• Advise the patient to take the drug 30 to 60 minutes before meals and at bedtime; the bedtime dose can be larger and taken at least 2 hours after the day's last meal. • Warn her to take the drug cautiously in hot or humid weather because of the risk of drug-induced heat stroke. • Suggest relieving oral dryness by sucking on ice chips or sugarless hard candy or by chewing sugarless gum. • Caution the patient to avoid activities that require coordination, such as driving, if she has blurred vision. • Instruct her to drink plenty of fluids to avoid constipation. • Prepare her for post-void retention urine volume tests to evaluate her progress.

continued

Teaching about drugs for urinary incontinence — *continued*

DRUG	ADVERSE REACTIONS	TEACHING POINTS
Other (for conditions leading to urinary incontinence)		
conjugated estrogen (Premarin) **estropipate** (Ogen)	• Watch for breathing difficulty, chest pain, pain in groin or legs (especially the calf), severe headache, shortness of breath, sudden loss of balance or incoordination, and weakness on one side. • Other reactions include abdominal cramps, anorexia, bloating, breast enlargement and tenderness, depression, diarrhea, dizziness, excessive thirst, headache, increased appetite, leg cramps, libidinal changes, nausea, vision changes, and weight changes.	• If the patient is taking oral estrogen, instruct her to follow the doctor's orders. • If she's taking estrogen in suppository or vaginal form, teach her how to insert the drug according to the manufacturer's directions inserted in the product package. • If she's using suppositories, suggest that she wear a sanitary napkin to protect her clothing from possible leakage. • Instruct a diabetic patient to monitor blood glucose levels closely. She may need adjustments in the dosage of the antidiabetic agent.
imipramine hydrochloride (Tofranil)	• Watch for blurred vision, confusion, constipation, dizziness, drowsiness, sweating, tachycardia, and urine retention. • Other reactions include cardiac (ECG) changes, confusion, dry mouth, headache, orthostatic hypotension, tinnitus, and urticaria.	• Explain that once incontinence improves, the doctor will decrease the dosage to the lowest one effective to control the patient's symptoms. • Warn the patient not to stop taking the drug abruptly and not to perform activities that require alertness until she adapts to the drug. • Tell her to avoid alcohol and not to take other drugs without first checking with the doctor. • Advise her to increase fluids to decrease constipation and to take a stool softener, if needed. • Suggest relieving a dry mouth with sugarless hard candy, ice chips, or sugarless chewing gum. • Direct her to take one of her daily doses at bedtime.

urinate at specified times whether or not she feels the urge. If she needs to urinate at additional times, instruct her to do so immediately. Also advise her to urinate just before going to bed.

Bladder retraining. Tell the patient with full cognitive function that she may benefit from bladder retraining. Explain that this technique gradually restores a normal voiding pattern and normal bladder function. Unlike habit training, which follows a rigid voiding schedule, bladder retraining teaches the patient to resist the urge to void. This gradually increases bladder capacity and the intervals between voiding. As capacity increases, urgency and frequency decrease. Demonstrate how the patient should suppress the urge to void by breathing slowly and deeply. Encourage her to practice this, and provide her with a copy of the teaching aid *Retraining your bladder,* pages 568 and 569.

Pessary. Explain that a pessary may improve incontinence caused by an anatomic abnormality, such as severe uterine prolapse or pelvic relaxation. Tell the patient that she'll wear the pessary internally like a contraceptive diaphragm. Inserted into the vagina, the device stabilizes the bladder's base and the urethra, preventing incontinence during physical strain (for example, laughing, coughing, or sneezing). Teach the patient the correct technique for inserting and positioning the device. Also teach her to remove and clean it according to the doctor's directions. Stress infection-prevention methods.

Condom catheter. Inform your male patient that short-term use of a condom catheter may effectively help him avoid accidents. Caution him that long-term use can lead to urinary tract infections and skin irritation. Teach him how to apply and wear this device, and point out ways to avoid complications, such as contact dermatitis and penile maceration, ischemia, and obstruction. Reinforce your instructions with a copy of the teaching aid *How to use a condom catheter,* pages 570 and 571.

Artificial sphincter implantation. A patient with urinary incontinence from spina bifida, myelomeningocele, spinal cord injury, pelvic traumatic injury, and postradical prostatectomy and a female patient with stress incontinence unresponsive to other treatments may obtain relief with an implanted artificial urinary sphincter. Inform the patient that the implant is made of silicone rubber. It consists of a urethral cuff (placed around the bladder neck in men and in women or around the bulbar urethra in men), a pressure-regulating balloon in the pelvic perivesical space (the balloon holds the fluid that inflates the cuff), and a bulb pump in the scrotum or labium.

Describe how the pump works. As the bladder fills with urine, the pressure-sensitive cuff inflates to prevent urine from leaking around the bladder neck or urethra. Then, by squeezing the bulb pump to move fluid from the cuff into the pressurized balloon, the patient can urinate. After the patient voids, the cuff reinflates automatically, sealing the urethra until voiding is again necessary.

Review preoperative and postoperative instructions, including possible complications that may necessitate implant repair or removal. For example, the cuff or balloon can leak (uncommon), or trapped blood or other fluid contaminants can impair the bulb pump, increasing resistance to fluid passage to and from the cuff. Other complications include tissue erosion around the bulb or in the bladder neck or urethra, infection, inadequate occlusion pressures, and kinked tubing.

Intermittent self-catheterization. This procedure may help the patient who has overflow incontinence from urine retention. Reassure her that although this procedure may seem difficult at first, practice makes it easier to do. Show her (or a caregiver) how to perform the procedure correctly. Illustrate your directions with the patient-teaching aids *For women: How to catheterize yourself* and *For men: How to catheterize yourself,* pages 215 and 216.

Surgery

In women, treatment for stress incontinence may include surgical repair of the anterior vaginal wall or retropubic suspension of the bladder and urethra. Explain that retropubic suspension restores the bladder and urethra to their proper intra-abdominal positions.

Mention that the operation may be effective for only a short time in some women.

In men with urge incontinence resulting from prostatic hypertrophy, treatment may involve transurethral resection of the prostate or open prostatectomy. Add that surgery may remove obstructive lesions that cause urge or overflow incontinence. If your patient's scheduled for one of these operations, explain the surgical procedure and preoperative and postoperative care.

Other care measures

Discuss wearing protective pads and garments to augment habit training and bladder retraining. Mention that these absorbent devices boost comfort and confidence and allow the patient more mobility during treatment for urinary incontinence. Describe the types available. (See *Teaching about protective pads and garments.*)

Preventing skin breakdown. Finally, teach your patient how to prevent skin irritation and breakdown. After each incontinence episode, direct her to wash the skin exposed to urine with mild soap and water. Instruct her to pat the area dry and then to apply a protective barrier cream, such as Sween.

Sources of information and support

Continence Restored, Inc.
785 Park Avenue, New York, N.Y. 10021
(212) 879-3131

Help for Incontinent People
P.O. Box 544, Union, S.C. 29379
(803) 579-7900

Simon Foundation
Box 815, Wilmette, Ill. 60091
(708) 864-3913

Further readings

Black, P.A. "Urinary Incontinence: A Many Faceted Problem," *Professional Nurse* 5(7):378, 380, 382, April 1990.
Blannin, J.P. "The Sooner the Better! Teaching Continence Promotion to Women," *Professional Nurse* 5(3):149-50, 152, December 1989.
Kovach, T. "Skin Care During Incontinency: Containment Is Key," *Provider* 16(4):33-34, April 1990.
Newman, D.K. "The Treatment of Urinary Incontinence in Adults," *Nurse Practitioner* 14(6):21-22, 24, 26, June 1989.
Newman, D.K., and Smith, D.A. "Incontinence: The Problem Patients Won't Talk About," *RN* 52(3):42-45, March 1989.
Suter, F., and Waddell, R. "Focus on Incontinence: Nursing Care," *Australian Nurses Journal* 19(4):11-13, October 1989.
Wells, T. "Conquering Incontinence," *Geriatric Nursing* 11(3):133-35, May-June 1990.

Teaching about protective pads and garments

If your patient is just starting a bladder retraining program, inform her that wearing a protective pad or garment can help her feel more comfortable and secure. She can choose from several types.

Disposables
Explain that disposable pads include thin panty liners and sanitary pads, which can adequately absorb intermittent dribbling. Disposable adult-size diapers have greater absorbency.

To prevent skin irritation and urinary tract infection, remind the patient to change a pad every few hours and a diaper each time it gets wet. Instruct her to wash and dry the perineum gently each time she changes a pad or a diaper. Then she should apply the skin barrier cream recommended by the doctor to protect her skin from urine and to avoid chafing.

Washables
Less expensive than disposable pads and diapers, washable incontinence briefs have a protective outer layer of rubber, plastic, or some other synthetic material. Inform the patient that either a disposable or a washable liner pad fits in the crotch of these briefs and requires changing after each incontinence episode. Briefs come in pull-on or snap styles.

Advise the patient to change the liner pad in washable briefs when it's wet and to wash the perineum and apply ointment. Tell her to wash the briefs and reusable pads daily or as needed.

Retraining your bladder

Dear Patient:

You can "retrain" your bladder—and correct or manage incontinence—by reestablishing a normal urination pattern.

First, you'll keep a careful record of your fluid intake and urination pattern. Then you'll schedule urination at regular intervals and increase the time between urinations gradually. Your goal will be to urinate no more than once every 3 to 4 hours.

Step 1: Keeping a record

Do your accidental urinations follow a pattern? You'll know at a glance by recording your fluid intake, how you urinated (intentionally or by accident), and why you think an accident occurred. Keep a chart (like the one shown) throughout your retraining program. Record exact times and amounts. Make notations.

DATE	10/17			
TIME	FLUID INTAKE	URINATED IN TOILET	SMALL ACCID
6 to 8 a.m.	small glass of orange juice	✓	
8 to 10 a.m.	2 cups of coffee		sma

After a few days, your chart will show when you're most likely to become incontinent—for example, after meals or during the night. Your chart will also help your doctor evaluate your progress and adjust your treatment, if necessary.

Step 2: Scheduling urination

Now schedule specific times to urinate. Practice this technique at home, where you're relaxed and close to the bathroom. Start by urinating every 2 hours, whether or not you feel the need. If you have to urinate sooner, practice "holding" it by relaxing, concentrating, and taking three slow, deep breaths until the urge decreases or goes away.

Wait 5 minutes. Then go to the bathroom and urinate—even if the urge has passed. Otherwise, your next urge may be very strong and difficult to control.

If you have an accident before the 5 minutes are up, shorten your next waiting time to 3 minutes. After a week of training, if waiting 5 minutes is easy, increase your waiting time to 10 minutes.

Using the method above, gradually increase the interval between urinations. Strive for 3- or 4-hour intervals.

Tips for success

- Set an alarm clock to remind you when to use the toilet.
- Make sure you can reach the bathroom or portable toilet easily.
- Walk to the bathroom slowly.
- If possible, urinate in your usual position, sitting or standing.
- Always urinate just before bedtime.
- Drink between eight and ten 8-ounce glasses of fluid every day. This helps to prevent urinary tract infection and constipation, which also can cause incontinence. To prevent nighttime accidents, drink most of your fluids before 6 p.m.

Remember to count foods containing mostly liquid (such as ice cream, soup, and gelatin) as fluids. *continued*

PATIENT-TEACHING AID

Retraining your bladder — *continued*

DATE				
TIME	**FLUID INTAKE**	**URINATED IN TOILET**	**SMALL OR LARGE ACCIDENT**	**REASON FOR ACCIDENT, IF KNOWN**
6 to 8 a.m.				
8 to 10 a.m.				
10 a.m. to noon				
12 to 2 p.m.				
2 to 4 p.m.				
4 to 6 p.m.				
6 to 8 p.m.				
8 to 10 p.m.				
10 to midnight				
12 to 2 a.m.				
2 to 4 a.m.				
4 to 6 a.m.				

How to use a condom catheter

Dear Patient:

Here are some guidelines for wearing a condom catheter temporarily for urinary incontinence. This catheter fits over the penis and connects to a drainage bag that you'll strap on your leg. You'll need to clean the bag about twice a day.

Follow these steps for applying the catheter, connecting the drainage bag, removing the catheter and bag, and solving problems.

Getting started
• Wash your hands. Then gather your equipment: correct-sized condom catheter, double-sided elastic stomal tape, leg drainage bag with tubing, clamp, manicure scissors, soap, washcloth, towel, and protective ointment.

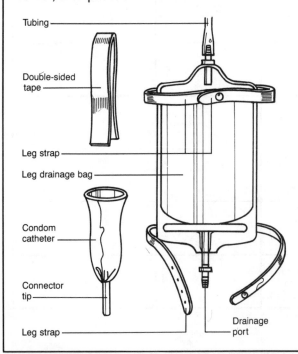

Tubing

Double-sided tape

Leg strap

Leg drainage bag

Condom catheter

Connector tip

Leg strap

Drainage port

• Trim the hairs on the shaft and base of your penis. That way they won't stick to the stomal tape you'll use. Before each catheter change, wash, rinse, and dry your penis. To protect your skin from urine, coat your penis with protective ointment and let the ointment dry (it will feel sticky).

• Now remove the backing from both sides of your tape. Place the side marked "skin side" against your penis. Starting at the penis base, spiral the tape.

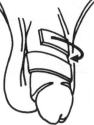

Caution: Don't let the edges of the tape overlap. Don't stretch the tape or you'll wind it too tightly. And never wrap the tape in a circle around your penis — you may cut off circulation.

Applying the catheter
First, tightly roll the condom sheath (balloonlike part) to the edge of the connector tip.

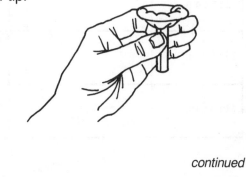

continued

How to use a condom catheter — *continued*

Now place the catheter sheath on the end of your penis, leaving about half an inch of space between the tip of your penis and the connector tip.

Gently stretch your penis as you unroll the condom. When the condom's unrolled, gently press it against your penis, so it sticks to the tape.

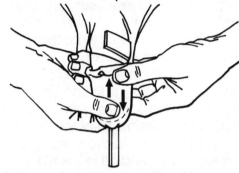

Connecting the drainage bag

Connect one end of the tubing to the connector tip and the other end to the drainage bag. Strap the drainage bag to your thigh.

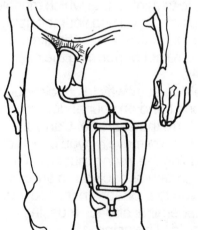

Removing the equipment

To remove the drainage bag, clamp the tube closed. Release the leg straps, and disconnect the extension tubing at the top of the bag. Remove the condom catheter and the tape by rolling them forward.

Special instructions

• If the tape doesn't stick to your skin, make sure that your penis is completely dry and that the protective ointment is completely dry too.

• If the tape pulls away from your skin, you may need to apply more ointment. Also make sure the tape is snug (but not tight).

• If urine leaks when you're wearing the catheter, squeeze the sheath to get a better seal.

• If the catheter sheath wrinkles in contact with the tape, the sheath may be too large. If so, select a smaller size sheath.

• Empty the drainage bag every 3 to 4 hours. Never let it fill completely to the top.

• Wash the drainage bag twice a day with soap and water. Rinse it with a solution of one part vinegar and seven parts water.

• Don't use the same drainage bag any longer than 1 month.

• Use only ointments and adhesives prescribed by your doctor. Don't wash with Betadine — this can irritate your skin.

• Remember to change the condom catheter every 24 hours. Make sure to thoroughly wash and dry the penis between changes.

• Check your penis every 2 hours for swelling or unusual color. If it feels uncomfortable or doesn't look normal, take off the condom catheter and call your doctor.

• Call your doctor if you feel pain or burning when you urinate, have the urge to urinate very frequently, smell an unpleasant odor from your urine, or see blood or pus in your urine.

PATIENT-TEACHING AID

How to exercise your pelvic muscles

Dear Patient:

Exercising your pelvic muscles every day can make them stronger and help to prevent incontinence. The following exercises, called "Kegel exercises," are easy to learn and simple to do.

If you have stress incontinence, try to do these exercises just before a sneeze or a cough. Also try to do a few exercises before you lift something heavy or cumbersome.

By exercising faithfully and correctly, you'll notice an improvement in about 4 weeks. In 3 months, you'll notice an even greater improvement. Here's how to do the exercises:

Finding the right muscle
The muscle you want to strengthen is called the pubococcygeal (PC) muscle. This is the muscle that controls the flow of urine. You can find this muscle in two ways:
• by voluntarily stopping the stream of urine
• by pulling in on your rectal muscle as you would to retain gas.

Once you've mastered these motions, you've mastered the exercises.

Practicing the exercises
Strengthen and tone your PC muscle by performing one of the two motions described above. Hold the muscle tight, working up to 10 seconds. Then relax the muscle for 10 seconds. Do 15 exercises in the morning, 15 in the afternoon, and 20 at night. Or exercise for about 10 minutes, three times a day.

Where and when to exercise
You can do Kegel exercises almost anywhere and at any time. Most people sit in a chair or lie on a bed to do them. You can also do them standing up.

How can you remember to do these exercises? One way is to combine them with an activity you do regularly. For example, if you spend a lot of time in the car, do an exercise at every red light. Or exercise while standing in line at the grocery store or at the newsstand, while waiting for the bus or train, and especially while urinating.

Avoiding mistakes
Take time to think about which muscles you're using. If you find yourself using your abdominal, leg, or buttocks muscles, you're not performing the exercises correctly.

Here's an easy way to check yourself: Place one hand on your abdomen while you perform the exercise. Can you feel your abdomen move? If you can, then you're using the wrong muscles. Or, if your abdomen or back hurts after exercising, you're probably trying too hard or using abdominal or back muscles that you shouldn't be using.

If you get headaches after exercising, be careful not to tense your chest muscles or hold your breath.

Remember: These exercises should feel mild and easy — not strenuous.

Gynecologic Conditions

Contents

Fibrocystic breast changes

In teaching about fibrocystic breast changes, your first priority is to reassure the patient that this condition isn't cancerous. Emphasize to her that the vast majority of women with fibrocystic breast changes have no increased risk of breast cancer. In fact, many medical experts don't consider fibrocystic breast changes a disorder at all. Because of the condition's benign nature, they've dropped the use of pathologic terms, such as "fibrocystic breast disease," to describe it.

Even so, take your patient's symptoms seriously. If she has lumpy breasts, prepare her for diagnostic tests, such as mammography, ultrasonography, and needle aspiration or biopsy. If she has breast discomfort, review treatment measures, including dietary changes and medications.

Although the patient with fibrocystic breasts may be no more prone to breast cancer than other women, her lumpy breasts may make it harder to detect a malignant tumor. Therefore, be sure to emphasize the importance of monthly breast self-examinations. Help her to distinguish normal breast lumpiness from suspicious lumps that require medical evaluation.

Discuss the condition

Tell the patient that fibrocystic breast changes describe various differences in the breasts that occur during the menstrual cycle. Above all, emphasize that the condition is benign. (In fact, it's sometimes called "benign breast disease.") Also stress how common the condition is: About 50% of all women have signs and symptoms of fibrocystic breast changes, and 90% of all women have tissue changes characteristic of the condition.

To help the patient understand fibrocystic breast changes, teach her about breast anatomy. Then discuss cyclical changes in the breast that cause signs and symptoms. (See *Understanding cyclical changes in breast tissue,* page 576.)

Explain that signs and symptoms differ among patients. The most common complaints are lumpy, tender, and painful breasts, but cysts or nipple discharge also may be present. Point out the cyclical nature of most signs and symptoms and their close relationship to the menstrual cycle. Mention that they usually worsen just before the menstrual period and improve after it.

Tell the patient that estrogen levels rise during the menstrual cycle's follicular phase, causing fluid retention and glandular tissue proliferation. As breast tissue stretches to accommodate the excess fluid, she may experience breast discomfort—often de-

Pamela Currie, RN, MSN, CRNP, who wrote this chapter, is a nurse practitioner and health promotion coordinator at CIGNA Corporation in Philadelphia.

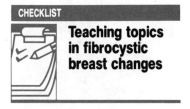

CHECKLIST

Teaching topics in fibrocystic breast changes

☐ Signs and symptoms of fibrocystic breast changes and their relation to the menstrual cycle
☐ Differences between benign and malignant breast lumps
☐ Preparation for diagnostic tests, such as mammography, ultrasonography, and breast biopsy
☐ Dietary modifications, including salt reduction and possible avoidance of methylxanthines
☐ Medications to relieve breast discomfort, such as analgesics, diuretics, danazol or bromocriptine, and hormones
☐ Importance of monthly breast self-examination
☐ Sources of information and support

Understanding cyclical changes in breast tissue

Reassure your patient that some lumpiness of the breasts is normal. To help dispel her fears about fibrocystic lumps or swelling, describe the different breast tissues and their sensitivity to cyclical ovarian hormones.

Inside the breast
Tell the patient that the inside of the breast is made up primarily of fat and milk-producing mammary tissue. Explain that the mammary glands produce the milk, and the mammary ducts transport it to the nipple. Point out how the mammary glands and ducts are sandwiched between layers of fat. These breast structures are held together by fibrous connective tissue.

Fibrocystic breast changes
Teach the patient that cyclical increases in estrogen underlie most benign breast symptoms, although exactly how this happens isn't clear. Just before menstruation, the breasts may retain water, causing painful swelling. During the same time, two other changes may make the breasts lumpier: One or more cysts may form, and the amount of fibrous breast tissue may increase.

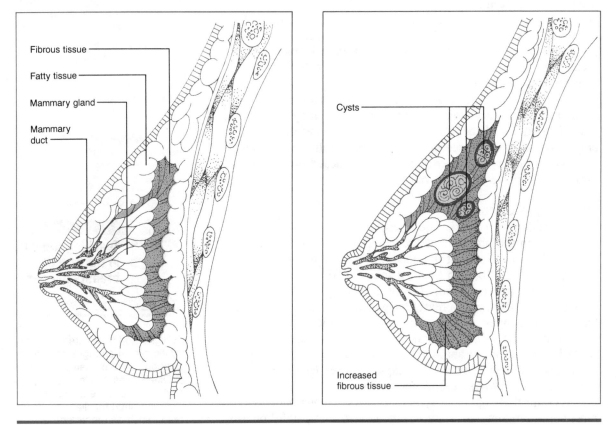

scribed as a full, aching feeling. Breast discomfort may also result from nerve irritation and inflammation associated with edema and fibrocystic breast changes. Typically, the upper, outer quadrants of both breasts become painful in the week before menstruation. Reassure the patient that this discomfort usually subsides with the start of her menstrual period.

Explain that fibrocystic breast changes may be associated with the formation of one or more lumps called cysts—fluid-filled sacs that form in one or both breasts. Cysts tend to enlarge and become tender just before menstruation, then shrink or disappear afterward. Reassure the patient that fibrocystic breast tissue is rarely cancerous. (See *Benign and malignant breast lumps: How they differ*.)

Inform the patient that an increase in fibrous tissue also may cause breast lumpiness, but again, this change does not indicate breast cancer. In some patients, fibrocystic breast changes are associated with nipple discharge. If so, advise the patient to see her doctor, particularly if the discharge is spontaneous, persistent, or unilateral.

Review how symptoms typically change with age:
• Among women in their late teens to early 30s, common signs and symptoms are breast tenderness and fullness with minimal lumpiness in the week before menstruation.
• In women in their late 30s to mid-40s, breast pain typically increases and lasts longer during the menstrual cycle. Increasing breast nodularity prompts many women to seek medical evaluation.
• Women in their late 40s and 50s may experience increasing discomfort and the sudden onset of painful, solitary, or multiple lumps.

Inform the patient that the cause of fibrocystic breast changes is unknown. However, most researchers agree that ovarian hormones are involved. Fibrocystic breast changes may result from abnormal hormone production or from hypersensitive breast tissues that overrespond to normal hormone levels. Mention that fibrocystic breast changes are more common in women with early menarche, late menopause, and irregular or anovulatory cycles. Women with fibrocystic breast changes also are more likely to have symptoms of premenstrual syndrome.

Complications
Tell the patient that fibrocystic breast changes seldom cause complications, although the signs and symptoms may progress. Rarely, a patient who undergoes biopsy for a benign breast lump is found to have atypical hyperplasia. This clinical finding, combined with a family history of breast cancer, does increase the risk of breast cancer. If the patient has atypical hyperplasia, advise her to seek close follow-up care.

Describe the diagnostic workup
Teach the patient that the diagnostic workup begins with a medical history and physical examination. Explain that the doctor will examine her breasts for lumps, tenderness, and other signs and symptoms. If necessary, prepare her for tests, such as mammography, ultrasonography, needle aspiration, and breast biopsy.

Mammography
If the patient has a cyst that can't be easily palpated, the doctor may order mammography. This test also may be performed before a cyst is aspirated. Teach her that mammography uses X-rays to provide an image of breast tissues, which helps the doctor to detect and evaluate lesions. Inform her that the test takes only a few minutes. Give her a copy of the patient-teaching aid *Learning about mammography,* pages 582 and 583.

Benign and malignant breast lumps: How they differ

Although your patient should see her doctor about any suspicious breast lump, remind her that most breast lumps are benign. Point out some of the following characteristic differences between benign and malignant breast lumps.

Benign breast lumps
Inform your patient that benign breast lumps typically occur before menopause. Such lumps may be multiple and found in both breasts. They're characterized as soft, cystic, or nodular. In thin patients, they may be palpable. The patient may complain of a tender, "heavy" feeling. Benign breast lumps usually appear premenstrually and disappear after menstruation.

Malignant breast lumps
In contrast to benign breast lumps, malignant breast lumps usually occur after menopause or after age 40. The lumps are solitary and usually develop on one side only. Rarely tender, they have irregular borders. They're firm, fixed, and may be greater than 2 cm in diameter. Their occurrence is unrelated to the menstrual cycle.

Ultrasonography

Inform the patient that ultrasonography uses high-frequency sound waves to evaluate breast tissue. Explain that this test can help determine if a lump is fluid-filled or solid tissue. If the patient is young (in her teens or early 20s), ultrasonography is preferred over mammography because it uses no radiation and may provide better images. Before the test, provide her with a copy of the teaching aid *Preparing for breast ultrasonography,* page 581.

Needle aspiration

If the doctor suspects the patient has a breast cyst, he may perform needle aspiration. Explain that this procedure determines if a lump contains fluid and is, therefore, a cyst. Tell the patient that needle aspiration often makes a cyst disappear completely. Before this procedure, give her a copy of the patient-teaching aid *Preparing for needle aspiration,* page 584.

Breast biopsy

Tell the patient that the doctor may order a breast biopsy to determine if a breast lump is malignant. Clarify the difference between needle and surgical biopsy. In needle biopsy, the doctor uses a needle to remove a tissue sample from a breast lump. In surgical biopsy, an incision is made in the breast, and the doctor removes the entire lump or a slice of it.

Needle biopsy. Before needle biopsy, prepare the patient for routine blood studies, urinalysis, and chest X-ray, as ordered. Tell her that she need not restrict food or fluids and that she will probably receive a local anesthetic. Instruct her to undress to the waist and remain in a sitting position during the test. Explain that the doctor will insert the biopsy needle into the breast lump to obtain a tissue sample. Warn her that she may feel some pressure when he inserts the needle. Then he'll withdraw the needle and send the sample to the laboratory. Mention that after the test a nurse will assess her vital signs and give her pain medication, if necessary. Instruct the patient to watch for bleeding, redness, or tenderness at the biopsy site.

Surgical biopsy. If the patient's scheduled for surgical biopsy, prepare her for general or local anesthesia, as ordered. Explain that after the procedure her vital signs will be checked frequently, and she'll receive an analgesic to relieve postsurgical pain. Instruct her to watch for and report bleeding, tenderness, and pain at the biopsy site.

Teach about treatments

Reassure the patient that much can be done to relieve her signs and symptoms. Discuss dietary changes and the use of mild analgesics to minimize breast discomfort. If stronger medications are prescribed, review their proper administration and possible adverse effects. Emphasize the importance of performing monthly breast self-examinations to detect suspicious breast changes.

Diet

Advise the patient to cut down on salt in the week before her menstrual period. Explain that reducing salt intake can help prevent the fluid retention that causes breast discomfort. Instruct her not to add salt to foods during cooking or at the table. Also caution her to avoid the many processed foods with hidden salt. Such foods include canned soups, pickles, bacon, baked goods, and commercially prepared foods.

Mention that some patients notice that their signs and symptoms subside when they avoid foods and medications containing caffeine and other methylxanthines. If the patient wants to try this treatment, recommend dietary changes to eliminate methylxanthines. However, point out that this treatment is medically unproven. (See *Should your patient avoid methylxanthines?*)

Medication

Explain that the use of medication varies for each patient, depending on her signs and symptoms. Drug therapy may include analgesics, mild diuretics, danazol, bromocriptine, and hormonal therapy. Vitamin E also has been prescribed by some doctors for fibrocystic breast changes.

Analgesics and diuretics. If the patient suffers breast discomfort, suggest that she take aspirin or acetaminophen during the week before her menstrual period. The doctor also may prescribe a mild diuretic, such as chlorothiazide (Diuril) or hydrochlorothiazide (HydroDIURIL), during this time. Explain that the diuretic will relieve breast fullness by reducing the amount of fluid in her body. Caution the patient about the potential effects of fluid and electrolyte imbalance.

Danazol. If the patient has severe breast pain that can't be relieved by conservative measures, the doctor may prescribe the synthetic androgen danazol (Danocrine). Danazol reduces hormonal stimulation of the breast, thereby helping to reduce breast pain and nodularity. However, warn the patient that danazol can cause harsh adverse reactions, including acne, clitorimegaly, decreased breast size, edema, hot flashes, increased facial hair, menstrual irregularities, voice changes, and weight gain. Also point out that her signs and symptoms may return, requiring another course of therapy.

Bromocriptine. A prolactin blocker, bromocriptine mesylate (Parlodel) helps some women—but it also causes adverse reactions. Caution the patient that possible adverse reactions include dizziness, headache, and nausea. Like danazol, bromocriptine usually is reserved for patients with severe pain.

Hormonal therapy. Oral contraceptives (estrogen-progestin combinations) or progesterone therapy helps to relieve breast tenderness in some patients. For example, medroxyprogesterone acetate (Provera) blocks estrogen's effects on the breast. Instruct the patient to take Provera on days 15 through 25 of her menstrual cycle or as her doctor prescribes. Inform her of potential adverse effects.

Should your patient avoid methylxanthines?

A popular treatment for fibrocystic breast changes involves removing caffeine and other sources of methylxanthines from the patient's diet. But does this treatment really work? Some medical experts think not. They point to the lack of studies supporting the notion that caffeine or any other methylxanthine-containing products worsen fibrocystic breast symptoms. They also criticize early studies, which reported a correlation between benign breast symptoms and caffeine, as being subjective and uncontrolled.

Nevertheless, some women do find that giving up coffee and related products relieves their symptoms.

What advice should you give?
First, make sure your patient's aware of the lack of scientific evidence supporting this treatment. However, if she believes it's worth a try, suggest she avoid common sources of methylxanthines, listed below.

Food and beverages
- Chocolate and cocoa
- Coffee and tea
- Colas

Nonprescription medications
- Anacin (Maximum Strength)
- Aqua-Ban
- Cope
- Excedrin
- Midol
- No Doz
- Vanquish
- Vivarin

Prescription medications
- All medications containing theophylline, aminophylline, or oxtriphylline
- Cafergot
- Darvon Compound
- Fiorinal or Fioricet
- Repan

Surgery

As a last resort, the patient may need to have a cyst surgically removed. Usually, this operation is necessary only if a cyst can't be aspirated or if a solid mass remains after aspiration. Tell the patient that the procedure usually is done under local anesthesia in an outpatient unit.

Other care measures

Recommend that the patient wear a support bra—even while sleeping—when she experiences breast discomfort. Tell her that a firm bra is especially important during exercise.

Encourage the patient to perform monthly breast self-examinations. Advise her to examine her breasts at the same time in each menstrual cycle, so she doesn't become confused by her normal cyclical fibrocystic changes. Ideally, she should examine them 2 or 3 days after her menstrual period. Instruct her to contact her doctor if she notices any new or unusual lumps or increased tenderness.

Sources of information and support

American Cancer Society
1599 Clifton Road, NE, Atlanta, Ga. 30329
(404) 320-3333

National Cancer Institute
9000 Rockville Pike, Bethesda, Md. 20314
(800) 4-CANCER

Further readings

"Benign Breast Disease," *Patient Care* 24(12):85, July 15, 1990.
"Breast Masses in Adolescence: Fibroadenoma Is the Most Common Tumor," *Hospital Medicine* 23(10):121-22, October 1987.
Bullough, B., et al. "Methylxanthines and Fibrocystic Breast Disease: A Study of Correlations," *Nurse Practitioner* 15(3):36, 38, 43-44, March 1990.
"Easing the Discomfort of Fibrocystic Condition," *Patient Care* 21(6):137, March 30, 1987.
Ellerhorst-Ryan, J.M., et al. "Evaluating Benign Breast Disease," *Nurse Practitioner* 13(9):13, 16, 18+, September 1988.
Ettinger, D.S., and Wilcox, P.M. "Benign Breast Disorders: A Symptomatic Approach," *Hospital Practice* 22(9):75-77, 80-82, September 30, 1987.
Love, S.M. "Fibrocystic Disease: What's in a Name?" *Patient Care* 24(12):65-70, 75, 78-79+, July 15, 1990.
Norwood, S.L. "Fibrocystic Disease: An Update and Review," *Journal of Obstetric, Gynecological, and Neonatal Nursing* 19(2):116-21, March-April 1990.
Reifsnider, E. "Educating Women About Benign Breast Disease," *AAOHN* 38(3):121-26, March 1990.
Russell, L.C. "Caffeine Restriction as Initial Treatment for Breast Pain," *Nurse Practitioner* 14(2):36-37, 40, February 1989.

PATIENT-TEACHING AID

Preparing for breast ultrasonography

Dear Patient:

Your doctor wants you to undergo breast ultrasonography. This test provides an image of the inside of your breasts and is helpful for detecting and evaluating breast lumps.

Usually, the test can determine if a lump is fluid-filled or solid. However, the test can't distinguish whether or not a lump is cancerous.

How the test works

This test uses a small instrument called a transducer that will send a beam of high-frequency sound waves toward your breast. When the sound waves bounce back from breast tissue, they are picked up again by the transducer. Then this information is processed by a computer and displayed as an image of the inner breast on a TV screen.

Ultrasound is painless and poses no known health risk. It's also safe if you're pregnant because it uses no radiation.

Before the test

You'll be asked to remove your clothes from the waist up and to put on a hospital gown. Generally, you need not restrict your diet, medications, or activities. If you have questions, ask them now. During the test, it's important to rest quietly so the operator can concentrate on the images.

During the test

The procedure varies at different hospitals and clinics, so check with your doc-tor about how the test will be performed at the facility where you'll be examined. A doctor or an ultrasonographer may perform the test.

In most places, you'll be asked to lie on your back, with a pillow placed under the shoulder on the same side as the breast to be examined. Then a water-soluble gel will be applied to your breast. The test operator will glide the hand-held transducer back and forth over your breast. Unless your breasts are very tender, the test should feel painless, like a light massage.

In some hospitals and clinics, you'll be asked to lie on your back while a water-filled chamber is lowered over your breasts. Or you may be asked to lie on your stomach with your breasts submerged in a warm-water bath. In these methods, the sound waves are sent through water. You should feel no discomfort, although if you're asked to immerse your breasts in a water bath, the water may feel a bit cool.

During the test, don't expect to hear the high-frequency sound waves, which are inaudible to the human ear.

You'll probably be able to see images of your breast on the TV screen, but they'll look obscure, something like a satellite weather map.

After the test

You may resume your normal activities immediately. To find out your test results, you'll typically wait a day or two until a report is sent to the doctor who referred you for the test.

PATIENT-TEACHING AID

Learning about mammography

Dear Patient:

Your doctor wants you to undergo mammography. This test is simply an X-ray of your breast. It can be used to screen for breast cancer or to diagnose the cause of a breast complaint.

Although the test uses radiation, the amount is negligible. The health risk is no greater than that of riding in a car.

Who should have mammography?

Recommendations from the American Cancer Society include the following:
• Every woman between the ages of 35 and 40 should have a *baseline mammogram* to screen for breast cancer.
• Women ages 40 to 49 should be screened every 2 years.
• Women age 50 and older should have an annual mammogram.

The National Cancer Institute also recommends *annual screening* for women in high-risk groups. These women include:
• all women over age 50
• all women over age 40 with a family history of premenopausal breast cancer (a mother, sister, or grandmother)
• women over age 35 with cancer in one breast.

In addition, your doctor may order mammography to help determine the cause of a breast change, such as a lump or nipple discharge.

Before the test

Because the breast must be compressed during the X-ray, you may want to ask your doctor if you can schedule mammography during the time of month when your breasts are less tender.

Tell your doctor if you might be pregnant or are breast-feeding. Ask if you should avoid using deodorant on the test day. Some deodorants contain substances that may interfere with test results. Also avoid lotions, which may make the breasts slippery.

You'll be asked to take off your clothing above your waist, put on a gown, and remove jewelry from your neck.

During the test

Depending on the type of X-ray machine used, you'll be asked to sit, stand, or lie still for the test.

A technician will help you position your breast on an X-ray plate.

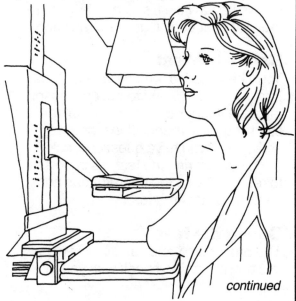

continued

PATIENT-TEACHING AID

Learning about mammography — *continued*

Then another plate will be pressed firmly down toward the first one to help flatten the breast tissue. You'll probably feel a cold sensation where your breast touches the plate, and the compression may cause some discomfort. Generally, the flatter your breast is squeezed, the more accurate the picture.

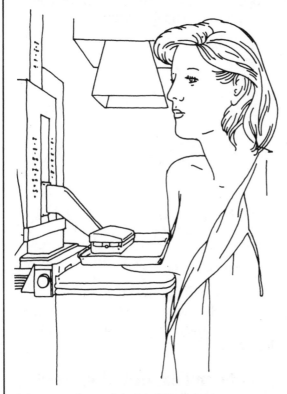

You may be asked to lift your arm or to use your hand to hold your other breast out of the way.

While the X-ray is being taken, you'll be told to hold your breath for a few seconds. Usually, two pictures are taken, one from the top and the other from the side.

Then the procedure will be repeated for the other breast.

After the test
The technician may ask you to wait a few minutes before leaving the test area, in case an X-ray needs to be repeated. In some centers, the radiologist will show you the X-ray pictures immediately and discuss the results. In others, a report will be sent to the doctor who referred you. He will then discuss the results with you.

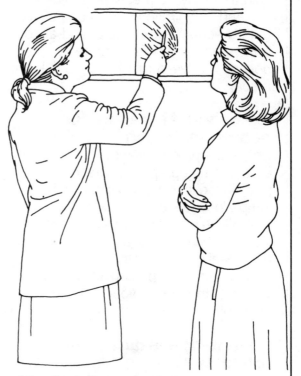

After the test, you may resume your normal diet and activities.

A reminder
Keep in mind that mammography is not a substitute for regular breast self-examinations. Occasionally, mammography fails to detect a suspicious lump. That's why you should continue examining your breasts for unusual changes once a month.

Preparing for needle aspiration

Dear Patient:

Your doctor wants to perform needle aspiration on your breast lump or cyst. This procedure involves inserting a needle into the lump to remove any fluid that may be present.

Needle aspiration may sound scary, but it's actually quick, safe, and almost always painless. What's more, it doesn't involve surgery and won't leave a scar.

How should I prepare for needle aspiration?

Before the procedure, your doctor may order mammography or ultrasonography. These tests help to pinpoint the lump's location and characteristics.

You'll be asked to remove your clothing from the waist up, and you'll be given a hospital gown to wear.

Just before the procedure, the doctor will clean the skin on your breast with an antiseptic solution.

What happens during the procedure?

Usually, your doctor can do the procedure in his office. It takes 5 to 10 minutes. You'll be asked to lie on an examination table.

You may receive a local anesthetic to numb the area. Except for a brief sting when the anesthetic is injected, you should feel little or no discomfort during the procedure.

The doctor will use one hand to steady the lump between his fingers.

With his other hand, he'll quickly insert a small, hollow needle into the lump. If the lump is a cyst, he'll be able to remove fluid—anywhere from a few drops to several ounces. After the cyst is aspirated, it usually disappears.

FLUID ASPIRATION

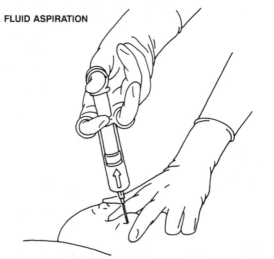

Usually, the withdrawn fluid is discarded. However, if the fluid is bloody, the doctor may send a sample to the lab for analysis.

What can I expect afterward?

The doctor will remove the needle and apply a bandage.

Be sure to keep all appointments for follow-up visits. Typically, your doctor will want to examine your breasts again 1 month and 6 months after the aspiration. Sometimes, a cyst recurs or a new one forms. If this happens, you may need to undergo another aspiration.

If the doctor was unable to remove fluid during the aspiration, he may order more tests to evaluate the lump.

Endometriosis

If you've taught patients about endometriosis, you know that apprehension and misunderstanding are common responses to this disease. A patient, for instance, may justifiably fear that endometriosis will cause infertility, yet she may wrongly believe that it can cause cancer or be life-threatening. By clearly explaining the disease, its possible complications, various diagnostic tests, and the impact of treatment options on childbearing, you can correct your patient's misunderstandings and help her make informed decisions about her care.

Discuss the disorder

Begin by reassuring the patient that endometriosis *isn't* life-threatening or cancerous (although, rarely, an endometrial mass becomes malignant). Explain that it's a benign growth of endometrial tissue outside the uterus.

Using an anatomic drawing of the female reproductive system, show her that tissue growths, also known as endometrial implants, are usually confined to the pelvic area but can appear anywhere in the body. Explain that hormones secreted during the menstrual cycle influence this misplaced tissue, causing profuse menstrual bleeding and, sometimes, pain in the lower abdomen, vagina, posterior pelvis, and back. Typically, the patient feels suprapubic pain that begins several days before menses and lasts possibly throughout menstruation. Associated symptoms include dyspareunia and painful bowel movements. As the tissue grows and spreads, it irritates and scars surrounding structures, leading to fibrosis, with adhesions and blood-filled cysts.

What causes endometriosis? The definitive cause remains unknown, although several theories exist. If appropriate, discuss them with the patient. Tell her that retrograde menstruation is the most widely held explanation. According to this theory, some blood "backs up" during every menstrual cycle, flowing up through the fallopian tubes and spilling into the pelvic cavity instead of flowing out through the cervix. Endometrial cells from this menstrual flow attach to structures in the pelvic cavity (for example, the ovaries), where they grow and respond to monthly hormonal changes, causing bleeding into the pelvic cavity.

Another theory claims that endometrial cells spread through the lymph and circulatory systems and become implanted throughout the body. A third theory purports that some endometrial cells are misplaced outside the uterus during embryonic development;

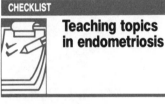

CHECKLIST

Teaching topics in endometriosis

☐ The pathophysiology of endometriosis and possible causes
☐ Importance of treatment to prevent or postpone such complications as infertility or endometrioma rupture
☐ Description of internal pelvic examination and abdominal palpation
☐ Preparation for diagnostic laparoscopy
☐ Medications to relieve pain
☐ Rationale for using oral contraceptives and other hormonal therapies
☐ Surgery, including therapeutic laparoscopy, total hysterectomy and bilateral salpingo-oophorectomy, and presacral neurectomy
☐ Other care measures, including the effects of pregnancy on endometriosis, dyspareunia relief, and dietary prevention of anemia
☐ Sources of information and support

Janet Akin, RN, MSN, and **Miriam Horwitz, RN, MS,** wrote this chapter. Ms. Akin is an instructor at the Research College of Nursing, Kansas City, Mo. Ms. Horwitz is president of Executive Search Consultants, a nursing administration career service in Westwood, Mass.

after puberty, they respond to cyclic hormonal activity. A fourth theory, now under scrutiny, asserts that endometriosis is an auto-immune disease.

Tell the patient that while the causes of endometriosis are controversial, the risk factors are indisputable. Women with short menstrual cycles (fewer than 27 days) and long menstrual periods (more than 7 days) are prone to endometriosis. So are women who have a family history of the disease, have children late in life (endometriosis is sometimes called the "career woman's disease"), and have a retroflexed (tilted) uterus.

Complications

Inform the patient that complying with prescribed treatment may help prevent or postpone complications of endometriosis, such as infertility, ruptured endometrioma, and anemia. Explain that endometrial implants cause inflammation. Consequently, fibrosis (scar tissue and adhesions) usually involves the fallopian tubes, ovaries, uterus, bladder, and intestines, binding these organs and contributing to infertility.

Warn the patient that sudden, excruciating abdominal pain may signal a life-threatening complication: ruptured endometrioma (typically an ovarian cyst composed of endometrial cells) and possible peritonitis. Instruct her to go to the hospital emergency department immediately. To prevent a misdiagnosis of acute appendicitis, advise her to alert the emergency department doctor that she has endometriosis.

Inform the patient that excessive bleeding during menstruation may lead to anemia.

Describe the diagnostic workup

Teach about diagnostic procedures to detect and confirm endometriosis, including a pelvic examination, abdominal palpation, and laparoscopy.

Pelvic examination and abdominal palpation

Inform the patient that the doctor will take her history and then perform an internal pelvic examination. He'll look for endometrial implants—small bluish areas on the cervix and in the vagina. To do this, he'll palpate the abdominal areas most often affected by endometriosis. For example, he'll check the uterosacral ligaments and cul-de-sac for nodules and tenderness, the ovaries for enlargement and tenderness, and the adnexa for fullness and nodules. He'll also palpate over the uterus to check its position, and if necessary for accuracy, he'll palpate through the rectum. Mention that this bimanual examination may feel uncomfortable but that her discomfort will subside when the examination ends.

Laparoscopy

If the patient's health history and examination findings suggest endometriosis, teach her about laparoscopy. Explain that this procedure allows the doctor to view the pelvic organs and to determine

Staging endometriosis

Inform your patient that during laparoscopy, the doctor will judge the degree of her endometriosis. Called "staging," this system scores the disease in four stages from minimal to severe. This establishes a baseline for determining treatment.

Staging by points
Developed by the American Fertility Society, the staging system assigns numerical values to endometrial implants or adhesions by their size (less than 1 cm to more than 3 cm); degree of implantation (superficial or deep); characteristic (filmy or dense); and degree of obstructiveness (partial or complete).

Interpreting the score
Compare your patient's total number of assigned points to the staging scale below:
● Stage I (minimal), 1 to 5 points
● Stage II (mild), 6 to 15 points
● Stage III (moderate), 16 to 40 points
● Stage IV (severe), more than 40 points.

the extent of endometrial tissue growth. It also permits him to classify the disease's severity. (See *Staging endometriosis.*) Add that the doctor may remove endometrial implants during laparoscopy.

Tell the patient who will perform the procedure, where it will be done, and how she should prepare for it. Then give her the patient-teaching aid *Learning about laparoscopy,* pages 591 and 592, to reinforce your explanation.

Other tests
Inform the patient that the doctor may occasionally order other tests, such as a barium enema, cystoscopy, or cul-de-sac aspiration, to pinpoint sites of endometrial tissue growth.

Teach about treatments
Advise the patient that treatment usually depends on her age, her desire for childbearing, and the disease's stage or the severity of symptoms. (Some patients with Stage I endometriosis have severe symptoms, while others with Stage IV have only mild symptoms.) Explain that treatment usually begins conservatively, then progresses to more aggressive measures as needed.

Common treatments include medications to relieve pain, reduce inflammation, and suppress ovulation or surgery to remove endometrial implants and adhesions. Or the doctor may recommend combined therapy: medication to shrink the implants, allowing easier surgical removal. This treatment may also prevent adhesions.

Medication
Tell the patient that the doctor may prescribe analgesics and anti-inflammatory drugs to relieve symptoms and reduce inflammation. Examples include ibuprofen (Advil, Motrin), mefenamic acid (Ponstel, Ponstan), and naproxen (Anaprox). Inform her that hormonal agents may be the primary treatment.

Oral contraceptives. Inform the patient that oral contraceptives treat endometriosis, not just its symptoms. Explain that sup-

Comparing procedures for implant removal

Tell your patient that during laparoscopy, the surgeon may remove endometrial implants and adhesions without using a knife. This spares healthy tissues, causes little or no bleeding, decreases the risks of infections and swelling, and reduces pain by sealing nerve endings.

Laser surgery

Laser energy can destroy deep-seated, widespread implants and adhesions. The surgeon may use an *argon laser* beam directed through a fiber-optic wave guide. This beam penetrates 1 to 2 mm but causes minimal scarring.

For shallow implants or adhesions, the surgeon may use a *carbon dioxide laser*. Focused through the laparoscope, this beam travels only 0.1 to 1.2 mm into the target tissue as it raises the tissue's intracellular water temperature to the flash point. In turn, the tissue vaporizes, and the intense heat coagulates blood vessels. Suctioning through the laparoscope removes the vapor.

Cryosurgery

To destroy tissue by freezing, the surgeon uses the laparoscope to introduce a probe into the target area. Then he instills a refrigerant (such as liquid nitrogen or Freon) through an insulated tube to the probe's uninsulated tip. This causes intracapillary thrombosis and tissue necrosis as a frozen tissue ball forms around the tip.

Electrocautery

The surgeon uses laparoscopy to apply a small, wire loop heated by a steady, direct electrical current to implants. This destroys a small amount of tissue on contact. The intense heat coagulates vesicular blood.

pressing ovulation with oral contraceptives has the same effect as pregnancy, which helps resolve endometriosis or cause remission.

Tell her that the doctor usually prescribes low-dose oral contraceptives for 6 to 9 months, depending on the patient's response. These drugs reduce menstrual flow and endometrial implants. However, they may also cause breast tenderness, dizziness, headache, and nausea. So advise her to observe safety precautions. For example, if she feels dizzy, she shouldn't drive a car. Mention that this therapy may improve her condition only temporarily.

Androgens. Explain that danazol (Danocrine), a synthetic androgen, stops ovulation and menstruation, which induces pseudomenopause. As a result, endometrial cells atrophy, improving endometriosis. The patient can start therapy immediately after her last menstrual period. Tell her that she'll probably take danazol twice a day for 6 to 9 months.

Make sure that the patient understands danazol's possible adverse effects, including acne, decreased breast size, edema, flushing, mild hirsutism, sweating, voice deepening, and weight gain. Explain that these effects result from the drug's androgenic (male hormone) effects and that some effects may be irreversible. She may also experience depression, dizziness, fatigue, and light-headedness.

Gonadotropin-releasing hormone analgesics. If the doctor prescribes nafarelin or another similar drug, tell the patient that reduction of circulating estrogen levels induces pseudomenopause. Nafarelin is thought to be as effective as danazol in halting the progression of endometrial implants. Be sure the patient understands how this drug works and that its use in treating endometriosis is still experimental. Also warn her about adverse effects related to low estrogen levels, including bone loss, decreased libido, hot flashes, and vaginal dryness.

Surgery

Explain that surgery's goal is to remove as many endometrial implants, adhesions, or endometriomas as possible and still preserve healthy, functioning tissue. Answer questions about anesthesia, and tell the patient how to follow preoperative and postoperative procedures to prevent complications and ensure recovery.

Therapeutic laparoscopy. Inform the patient that the doctor may remove endometrial implants if he finds them during diagnostic laparoscopy. Then explain how the surgeon may combine laparoscopy with such procedures as electrocautery, cryosurgery, or laser surgery to remove the implants. For more information, see *Comparing procedures for implant removal.*

Laparotomy. If the doctor finds an ovarian cyst that contains endometrial implants, he may remove it. First he'll make an abdominal incision to open the pelvic cavity. Then he'll aspirate the cyst, palpate the ovary to determine the cyst's depth, and cut the cyst from the ovarian cortex. Explain that cyst removal typically relieves dysmenorrhea, abnormal bleeding, and dyspareunia and preserves normal tissue. This helps to maintain reproductive function, with minimal scarring and adhesions.

INQUIRY

Questions patients ask about endometriosis and pregnancy

Will endometriosis prevent me from becoming pregnant?

That depends on how severe it is and where the implants and adhesions are located. If severe endometriosis affects your ovaries or fallopian tubes, it might make conception difficult or impossible. For instance, extensive blood-filled cysts around an ovary may prevent the egg from leaving. Or adhesions in the fallopian tubes, pelvic peritoneum, or cul-de-sac may obstruct the ovum's path from the ovary to the uterus.

How can treatment help me get pregnant?

Medication can shrink the endometrial implants or suppress their growth. And laparoscopy can remove implants that interfere with conception. If you want to become pregnant, the doctor can prescribe drugs that don't affect your ability to ovulate. And if you need surgery, he'll leave your uterus intact and preserve at least part of one ovary and fallopian tube.

Will I be able to get pregnant after laparascopy?

With mild endometriosis, the pregnancy rate after surgery is about 70%; with moderate endometriosis, it's about 50%; and with severe endometriosis, it's about 30%. You can usually resume sexual intercourse a few days after a laparoscopy, when the bleeding stops. You can try to become pregnant as soon as the doctor gives his okay, usually when healing's complete and you have a better chance for a viable pregnancy. Until then, use a reliable means of contraception.

Hysterectomy and bilateral salpingo-oophorectomy. For widespread endometriosis in a patient who doesn't want to become pregnant, the doctor may advise total hysterectomy and bilateral salpingo-oophorectomy. Explain that this surgery prevents recurrent endometriosis by removing the uterus, cervix, fallopian tubes, and ovaries. Discuss the aftereffects of surgery, including decreased estrogen levels leading to bone loss, decreased libido, hot flashes, and vaginal dryness. Then, if appropriate, discuss possible treatments, such as estrogen replacement therapy, which reduces the severity of these aftereffects.

Presacral neurectomy. For severe pain with endometriosis, the doctor may perform a presacral neurectomy. Make sure the patient understands that this procedure relieves pain by removing a nerve, but that it doesn't cure endometriosis. Also explain that after this operation she may have decreased bowel and bladder control and heavier menstrual periods because of vasodilation. If appropriate, teach bowel and bladder retraining techniques.

Other care measures

If you're teaching a young woman with mild endometriosis who wants to have children, tell her that pregnancy may not always cure endometriosis, but it does delay its progression. Explain that the hormones of pregnancy cause the implants to soften and atrophy. More than 50% of patients with mild-to-moderate endometriosis are able to become pregnant (see *Questions patients ask about endometriosis and pregnancy*).

Caution patients who want to have children not to postpone pregnancy because infertility is a common complication of endometriosis.

If your patient has dyspareunia, suggest that she take an analgesic or apply a vaginal lubricant before sexual intercourse. Also suggest that she use a superior or side-lying position for greater control over pressure exerted during intercourse to help prevent dyspareunia.

If your patient feels exceptionally weak and tired or has other symptoms suggesting anemia, urge her to discuss this with her doctor. Then suggest that she include iron-rich foods in her diet—for example, mozzarella or American cheese, whole or enriched grains, milk, salmon, broccoli, liver, and clams. Also remind her to get adequate rest.

Finally, help the patient cope with endometriosis by acquainting her with a support group, such as the Endometriosis Association. If she asks for help dealing with endometriosis-related infertility, refer her to a support group, such as Resolve, for infertile couples.

Sources of information and support

Endometriosis Association
c/o Bread and Roses Women's Health Center
238 W. Wisconsin Avenue, Milwaukee, Wis. 53202
(414) 278-0260

Resolve, Inc.
P.O. Box 474, Belmont, Mass. 02178
(617) 484-2424

Further readings

Breitkopf, L.J., and Bakoulis, M.G. "Can't Get Pregnant? Endometriosis Can Lead to Infertility in Several Ways," *Health* 20(8):56-59, August 1988.

"Endometriosis: Clinical Features," *Hospital Medicine* 23(8):93-94, August 1987.

Few, B.J. "Treating Endometriosis with Nafarelin," *MCN* 13(5):323, September-October 1988.

Kettel, L.M., and Murphy, A.A. "Combination Medical and Surgical Therapy for Infertile Patients with Endometriosis," *Obstetric and Gynecology Clinics of North America* 16(1):167-75, March 1989.

Petersen, N.F., and Rhoe, J. "Endometriosis: Obtaining Relief via 'Near Contact' Laparoscopy," *AORN Journal* 48(4):700-01, 703, 705-07, October 1988.

Treybig, M. "Primary Dysmenorrhea or Endometriosis?" *Nurse Practitioner* 14(5):8, 10, 15-16, May 1989.

Learning about laparoscopy

Dear Patient:

Your doctor has scheduled you for a laparoscopy. This procedure lets him see your reproductive and upper abdominal organs through a slender, telescope-like instrument. Laparoscopy allows the doctor to diagnose and, sometimes, to treat your disorder during the same procedure.

Laparoscopy takes about 1 hour. It's performed in the operating room, and you'll probably receive a general anesthetic. Usually, you can go home the same day.

Getting ready
Beforehand, the doctor will order a few routine laboratory tests to assess your general health. These tests include a complete blood count, blood chemistry studies, and a urinalysis.

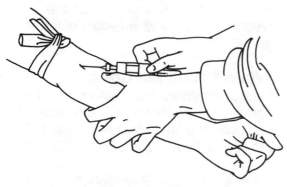

Because you'll be receiving an anesthetic, don't eat or drink anything after midnight on the night before the procedure. If you happen to be a smoker, don't smoke for about 12 hours before surgery. Also, remove any eye makeup or nail polish beforehand.

During the procedure
When the anesthetic takes effect, the doctor will make a small incision in the lower part of your navel. Then he'll insert a needle through the incision and inject carbon dioxide or nitrous oxide into your pelvic area. This inflates the area. It creates a viewing space by lifting the abdominal wall away from the organs below.

Next, the doctor will insert a thin, flexible, optical instrument—called a laparoscope—through the incision. This instrument magnifies the doctor's view of your organs.

Removing implants during laparoscopy
If the laparoscopic findings confirm endometriosis, the doctor may decide to remove the implants and adhesions then and there.

If so, the doctor will make a second, smaller incision just above your pubic hairline. Then he'll insert a special instrument for moving your internal organs aside. He may also insert a blunt instrument called a cannula through your vagina and into your uterus, allowing him to move your uterus. He'll remove as many implants and adhesions as possible by inserting instruments through the laparoscope.

continued

Learning about laparoscopy — *continued*

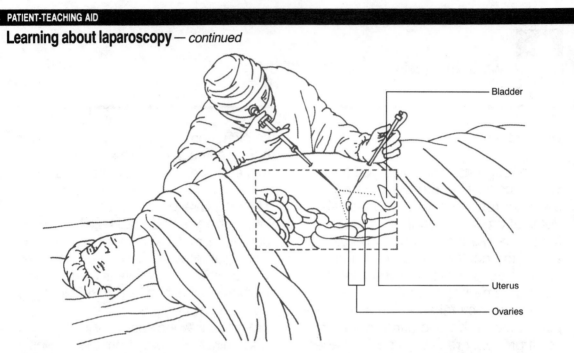

Bladder

Uterus

Ovaries

Next, the doctor will release the gas through the incision and remove the laparoscope. Then he'll close the incision and apply a large adhesive bandage.

After the procedure

After laparoscopy, you'll go to the recovery room, where nurses will monitor you until you're fully alert. If necessary, the doctor will prescribe an analgesic for any minor discomfort in the incisional area when the anesthetic wears off. Expect vaginal bleeding similar to a menstrual period for a few days.

Tips for recovery

When you get home, keep these points in mind:
• Wait until the day after surgery to remove your bandage and to bathe or shower.
• Eat lightly because some gas will remain in your abdomen; you'll probably belch or feel bloated for 1 or 2 days.
• Take aspirin or acetaminophen

(Tylenol) to relieve any shoulder pain. Called "referred pain," this results from the remaining gas in your abdomen, which can irritate your diaphragm and cause a pain in your shoulders.
• Expect to resume your normal activities after 1 or 2 days, but avoid strenuous work or sports for about 1 week.
• Resume sexual activity when the bleeding stops or when your doctor gives approval.

When to call the doctor

In rare instances, laparoscopy may be complicated by infection, hemorrhage, or a burn or a small cut on an organ. Call the doctor if you experience any of the following:
• A fever of 100.4° F. or higher
• Persistent or excessive vaginal bleeding
• Severe abdominal pain
• Redness, puffiness, or drainage from your incision
• Nausea, vomiting, or diarrhea.

Infertility

Teaching a couple about infertility and its treatment requires many skills. For instance, you'll need to guide them sensitively through rigorous tests and treatments—some of which may be painful and embarrassing. At the same time, you'll need to help them deal with their own emotions. After all, a diagnosis of infertility may stir up many feelings and conflicts, such as anger, guilt, and blame, which may disrupt relationships and shake self-esteem. What's more, although treatment heightens the hope of conception, it can also lead to deep disappointment if measures fail.

You'll need to foster open communication with the couple and help build their trust and confidence in the health care team. Understandably, many couples feel uncomfortable discussing their sex life, let alone having intercourse on a rigid schedule designed to take advantage of peak fertile days.

Discuss the disorder

Defined as 1 year of unprotected intercourse without conception, infertility affects between 10% and 15% of American couples (see *What's behind rising infertility rates?* page 594). Tell your patients that more than half of these infertile couples eventually become biological parents. Then inform them of the necessary conditions for conception:
• sufficient and motile sperm
• mucus secretions that promote sperm movement in the reproductive tract
• an unobstructed uterus and open fallopian tubes that allow the sperm free passage
• regular ovulation and healthy ova
• hormonal sufficiency and balance that support implantation of the embryo in the uterus
• sexual intercourse timed so that sperm fertilize the ovum (egg) within 24 hours of the egg's release.

Next, let the couple know about the wide-ranging causes of male and female infertility (see *Sex-specific causes of infertility,* page 594).

Complications

Inform the couple that without treatment, conditions that cause infertility will continue—and may worsen. For example, infections in the vagina, pelvis, scrotum, or prostate gland pose general health risks; and endometriosis or varicocele may progress, causing increasing discomfort and possible dysfunction.

Ruby Diane Fischer, RN,C, MPH, and **Janet Akin, RN, MSN,** contributed to this chapter. Ms. Fischer is program coordinator of the In Vitro Fertilization and GIFT Program, St. David's Hospital, Austin, Tex. Ms. Akin is an instructor at the Research College of Nursing, Kansas City, Mo.

CHECKLIST

Teaching topics in infertility

☐ Definition of infertility
☐ Possible causes, such as ovulatory dysfunction and structural abnormalities
☐ Diagnostic tests, such as semen analysis, hysterosalpingography, hysteroscopy, laparoscopy, cervical mucus analysis, and postcoital test.
☐ Fertility drugs, including menotropins and clomiphene citrate
☐ Explanation of in vitro fertilization-embryo transfer and gamete intrafallopian transfer, if appropriate
☐ Artificial insemination, if appropriate
☐ Surgery to promote fertility, including varicolectomy, hysteroscopy, laparoscopy, and laparotomy
☐ Psychological counseling
☐ Sources of information and support

What's behind rising infertility rates?

Childless couples need to feel that they're not alone. Let them know that the number of such couples has doubled in recent years. Among the factors that may contribute to rising infertility rates:
• the aging process—more and more couples postpone childbearing until age 30 or over, allowing age and concomitant disease processes to affect fertility
• sexually transmitted diseases (STDs), which may be responsible for up to 20% of infertility
• intrauterine devices (IUDs), which can cause pelvic inflammatory disease and consequent infertility
• environmental factors, such as toxins
• complications of abortion or childbirth.

Sex-specific causes of infertility

Many conditions can cause infertility in men or women. When explaining possible causes to a couple, choose your words carefully. For example, be sure to use the word "cause" rather than "personal problem" or "fault."

What causes male infertility?
While some causes of male infertility remain unknown, others are:
• structural abnormalities, such as varicoceles (enlarged, varicose veins in the scrotum), which can affect sperm number and motility
• infection, possibly from a sexually transmitted disease (STD)
• hormonal imbalances that reduce sperm produced or disrupt its ability to travel effectively in the female reproductive tract
• heat produced by wearing tight underwear or jeans; sitting in a hot tub or hot bath water; driving long distances; and fever-producing illnesses—causing adverse effects on sperm number and motility
• penile or testicular injury or congenital anomalies that diminish sperm
• some prescription drugs known to affect sperm quality and, possibly, such substances as alcohol, marijuana, cocaine, and tobacco suspected of affecting sperm quality
• coital frequency—either too often or too seldom, which may decrease sperm number and motility
• environmental agents, such as exposure to radiation and to other industrial and environmental toxins
• psychological and emotional stress.

What causes female infertility?
Female infertility usually stems from ovulatory dysfunction, fallopian tube obstruction, uterine conditions, or pelvic abnormalities caused by one or more of the following:
• hormonal imbalances, preventing the ovary from releasing an egg regularly or at all, or from producing enough hormone (progesterone) to support growth and to maintain the uterine lining needed for implantation of the embryo (the fertilized egg)
• infection or inflammation (past, chronic, or current) that damages the ovaries and fallopian tubes, such as from pelvic inflammatory disease, STDs, appendicitis, childhood disease, or surgical trauma
• structural abnormalities—for example, a uterus scarred by infection or one that's abnormally shaped or positioned since birth, deformed by fibroid tumors, exposed to diethylstilbestrol, or injured by conization
• mucosal abnormalities caused by infection, inadequate hormone levels, or antibodies to sperm, which may create a hostile environment that prevents sperm from entering the uterus and continuing to the fallopian tubes
• endometriosis (in some women) in which the endometrial tissue—normally confined to the inner lining of the uterine cavity—is deposited outside the uterus on such structures as the ovaries or fallopian tubes, causing inflammation and scarring
• endocrine abnormalities, such as elevated prolactin levels or pituitary, thyroid, or adrenal dysfunction.

Describe the diagnostic workup
Explain that the workup begins with a thorough history and physical examination of the woman and, ideally, the man, too. Mention that the doctor may defer examining the man if a semen analysis uncovers no abnormalities.

Urge both patients to be present during these initial consultations. This will help them establish a relationship with the health care team and improve their understanding of infertility and its treatments. Forewarn them that the questions their doctor will ask about their sexual histories will be deeply personal.

Male fertility tests

Tell the male patient that he may be referred to a urologist for a physical examination. Explain that the urologist will delve deeply into the patient's sexual and health history. He'll ask questions about the patient's use of lubricants during intercourse and use of prescription drugs, alcohol, tobacco, marijuana, and cocaine. Outline several tests that the patient may undergo to evaluate infertility, including a semen analysis, hormone testing, sperm penetration assay, and sperm antibody tests.

Semen analysis. A microscopic examination, this test measures seminal volume and the number and percentage of motile and normally formed sperm. The test also detects signs of infection, including white blood cells; bacteria; and abnormal color, odor, and liquefaction time.

Inform the patient that he'll provide a semen sample after abstaining from sexual intercourse for 3 to 6 days. Then instruct him to clean his genital area. Depending on his doctor's instructions, he may be allowed to apply a nonspermicidal lubricant to his penis. Next, he should masturbate, depositing semen into a sterile container. Advise him to report whether any semen is not deposited in the container, which may postpone the test until he can supply a complete sample on another day. Also instruct him to report the collection time for the record.

Keep in mind that semen collection can be emotionally and physically difficult. If the patient seems anxious about masturbating at a specific time and place required by the laboratory, suggest that he ask the doctor if he can collect the semen in a nonspermicidal condom during intercourse. For more information, see *Questions men ask about semen analysis.*

Hormone tests. If semen analysis confirms a low sperm count, explain that the doctor may order blood tests to measure follicle-stimulating hormone (FSH), luteinizing hormone (LH), and testosterone levels. Then describe the venipuncture procedure.

Sperm penetration assay and sperm antibody tests. If the semen analysis shows impaired sperm function or if infertility persists for unknown reasons, tell the patient that he may need to provide a semen sample for a sperm penetration assay or a sperm antibody test. Not commonly available, these costly tests require expert explanation and interpretation.

Female fertility tests

Tell the female patient about tests to assess her ovarian function, fallopian tube patency, and uterine condition. Also explain what to expect in a cervical mucus analysis and a postcoital test.

Ovarian function studies. Advise the patient that monitoring her morning temperature for 3 months when she wakes up—called the *basal body temperature*—may help her to determine that she ovulated. Explain that a few women ovulate without a temperature change. But in most women, ovulation raises proges-

INQUIRY

Questions men ask about semen analysis

What's a normal sperm count?
Typically, it's at least 60 million, or about 20 million sperm per milliliter of semen. Your sperm has a normal fertility potential if at least 60% have normal shape and motility.

Why must I take my semen to the lab within an hour?
If your semen stays in a container for more than 1 hour, some of the sperm may no longer be suitable for testing. Only live, motile, healthy sperm count. Sperm should be as close to body temperature as possible, so you can't store them in a refrigerator. Refrigeration will interfere with accurate results and possibly kill normal sperm.

What if my sperm count's low, or the sperm aren't active?
Your doctor will probably ask you to have another test to check if the first test results were reliable. Because your sperm count and motility vary naturally, you'll have the second test in about 90 days—the sperm's complete life cycle. The doctor may also order blood tests to evaluate your hormone levels.

Keep in mind that a low sperm count may indicate possible impairment or dysfunction but not sterility. Many men with low sperm counts still impregnate their mates.

What happens in hysterosalpingography

Inform your patient that the doctor may perform hysterosalpingography to evaluate her uterus or fallopian tubes for abnormalities that prevent conception. Advise her that this test may detect adhesions, occlusions, or other malformations.

Preparation
Begin by describing how the patient will lie in the lithotomy position on a table in the radiology department. Tell her that some patients experience moderate cramping from the procedure. To ensure her comfort, the doctor may give her an analgesic or an anesthetic.

Procedure
Explain that first the doctor will X-ray the pelvic area. Then he'll use a speculum and cannula to inject contrast medium through the cervix into the uterus. As the contrast medium outlines the uterine shape and spills through the fallopian tubes (if they're open), the doctor will take more X-rays.

Instruct the patient to report any cramping or reactions to the contrast medium, such as itching, hives, or light-headedness.

Then offer encouragement, especially if the X-rays show possible obstruction in a tube, explaining that sometimes the contrast medium takes the path of least resistance, spilling out of only one tube even if the other is open. Or, muscle spasms may cause a tube to close temporarily.

terone levels, which resets the the brain's thermoregulatory mechanism and raises waking temperature about 0.3° F. or more.

Instruct the patient to take her temperature at the same time each morning, and offer her a copy of the patient-teaching aid *How to take your basal body temperature*, page 602.

Inform the patient about over-the-counter *ovulation prediction* kits. Explain that unlike other tests that look for evidence of ovulation, these tests predict ovulation by measuring a surge of LH excreted in the patient's urine just before ovulation. (When this happens, advise the patient to have intercourse on the day that LH levels peak and on the day after.) Suggest that she bring the test kit to you for help in reviewing the instructions.

Tell the patient that *serum progesterone levels* also suggest whether ovulation occurred. Explain that these levels should peak when progesterone prepares the uterine lining for an embryo—about midway between ovulation and menses. Inform her that the test requires analysis of a venous blood sample taken during the third quarter of her menstrual cycle.

If test results prove inconclusive, the doctor may perform an *endometrial biopsy* to determine whether the ovary produced enough progesterone after ovulation to prepare the uterine lining for implantation of an embryo. Explain that with normal results (called "in phase"), the doctor presumes that ovulation occurred. On the other hand, with abnormal results (called "out of phase"), showing inadequate or incorrect development of the uterine lining, he suspects a luteal phase dysfunction.

Inform the patient that the biopsy can be performed in the doctor's office. Then explain how the doctor passes an instrument through the cervix into the uterus and removes a tiny tissue sample for microscopic examination. Because the procedure can hurt, suggest that she ask her doctor about pain medication.

Tests of fallopian tube patency and uterine condition. Inform the patient that the doctor may perform *hysterosalpingography* (HSG) to examine uterine shape and detect fallopian tube blockage. Tell her that the test takes 15 to 45 minutes and is usually done early in the monthly cycle—before ovulation. For more information, see *What happens in hysterosalpingography*.

Tell the patient scheduled for *hysteroscopy* that the doctor may use this procedure to identify uterine cavity abnormalities or to treat abnormalities detected by HSG. She'll have the procedure in the operating room and be anesthetized before the doctor passes a fiber-optic hysteroscope through the vagina and cervix into the uterus.

If appropriate, explain that *laparoscopy* may follow hysteroscopy. In this abdominal procedure, the doctor makes a small incision and inserts a fiber-optic laparoscope in the pelvic cavity. Then he manipulates organs to look for scar tissue (adhesions), cysts, uterine fibroid tumors, endometrial implants, and damaged fallopian tubes. Sometimes he injects a dye into the uterine cavity to see whether it flows out of the fallopian tubes. If it does, he assumes the fallopian tubes are patent.

Cervical mucus analysis. If the doctor orders this test, tell the patient that he'll inspect a mucus sample obtained during her peak fertile days just before ovulation. Test timing is crucial; diagnostic errors can occur if the examination takes place too early or late in the fertile period. The doctor will inspect the mucus, which is normally abundant, clear, slippery, and stretchy during fertile days. Then he'll examine it microscopically. Abnormalities may indicate an estrogen deficiency, chronic inflammation or infection, or other disorders that interfere with sperm passage.

Explain that in a *postcoital test* the doctor obtains a cervical mucus sample usually between 2 and 8 hours after intercourse on the days of peak preovulatory mucus production. He counts how many active sperm are moving progressively. A commonly accepted normal result is more than 20 sperm per high power field (HPF). Lower counts call for a repeated test.

Teach about treatments
Tell the patients that the doctor can treat infertility in several ways. He may prescribe drugs for conditions that inhibit fertility—for example, antibiotics for infections and danazol for endometriosis (see *How danazol affects fertility*). And he may prescribe drugs designed to initiate ovulation, improve cervical mucus, or stimulate sperm production. He may recommend surgery, for instance, to repair or remove a varicocele or to treat fallopian tube disease, endometriosis, uterine polyps, pelvic adhesions, or cysts. Or he may suggest procedures—for example, in vitro fertilization–embryo transfer (IVF–ET), gamete intrafallopian transfer (GIFT), or artificial insemination.

Medication
Fertility drugs for men with abnormal endocrine levels and compromised sperm include such hormones as clomiphene citrate (Clomid), thyroid, human chorionic gonadotropin (HCG), and menotropins (Pergonal). These drugs may increase testosterone levels and sperm counts. Tailor your teaching to the drugs the doctor orders.

Fertility drugs for women include clomiphene citrate, estrogen, progesterone, and menotropins or urofollitropin (Metrodin) with HCG.

Clomiphene citrate. Explain that this drug, taken on cycle days 5 through 10, may produce ovulation 6 to 11 days after the last dose. Advise the patient to have sexual intercourse every other day for 1 week beginning 5 days after she takes her last dose. Explain that the initial dose may not cause ovulation and that the doctor may adjust the dosage later. Advise her to document the ovulatory process by keeping a basal body temperature chart or by using an ovulation prediction kit (or both). Explain, too, that the drug may trigger multiple egg development and release, but that the incidence of multiple births (mostly twins) stays near 5%. Mention, too, that she may feel moody from fluctuating hormone levels. If she fails to have a normal menstrual period, she should contact the doctor, who will probably withhold the drug and order a pregnancy test.

Then tell her that she may also expect slight bloating and hot flashes (caused by a release of LH, which indicates the drug is working). And mention that she may experience dysmenorrhea because the drug may trigger her first ovulatory cycle in a while.

How danazol affects fertility

If the doctor finds that endometriosis interferes with your patient's ability to conceive, he may recommend treatment with danazol (Danocrine).

Effects of hormonal suppression
Inform the patient that danazol suppresses her hormonal cycle, so she won't menstruate while she's taking it. This gives the uterine endometrial tissue, which usually swells and bleeds during her monthly period, a rest. And the endometrial implants deposited on her ovaries or fallopian tubes should also recede and not bleed, helping inflammation subside as well.

Then the patient can stop taking the drug and try to become pregnant. Or, the doctor may suggest surgery to remove the implants while they're small.

Adverse reactions
Warn the patient to report voice changes or other signs of virilization promptly. Some androgenic effects, such as deepening of the voice, may not be reversible after stopping the drug.

Caution the patient to report these rare drug reactions to her doctor at once: blurred vision and other visual changes, such as spots or flashing lights, and severe headaches unrelieved by acetaminophen (Tylenol). Warn her to contact the doctor if abdominal distention, bloating, pain, or weight gain occur. These effects may signal ovarian enlargement or ovarian cysts, which usually require cessation of treatment.

Estrogen. Inform the patient that the doctor may order this drug for cycle days 10 through 16—alone or with clomiphene citrate—to improve cervical mucus. At typical low dosages, she should experience no adverse reactions.

Progesterone. Explain that this drug, taken after ovulation to supplement the luteal phase, may improve the uterine environment and balance a short luteal phase.

Advise the patient that she may notice heightened premenstrual symptoms, such as tender breasts, increased appetite, and increased whitish yellow cervical mucus. Tell her that the drug may postpone menstruation, so she doesn't assume that a delayed period necessarily signals pregnancy.

Menotropins or urofollitropin with HCG. Tell the patient that these drugs promote ovarian follicular growth (ovarian follicles propel the eggs into the fallopian tube). Prepare her for intensive and expensive therapy with one or the other drug. Explain that the drug must be injected into the buttock muscle daily for about 8 to 10 days followed by one dose of HCG after the last dose of either drug. If appropriate, teach her partner to give the injections.

Inform the patient that she'll need nearly daily monitoring (ultrasonography and blood tests) to regulate the dosage and to time ovulation stimulation. Advise her to have sexual intercourse on the night of drug adminstration and on the next 2 nights.

Explain that this drug should stimulate one or more ovarian follicles for ovulation. In fact, it may work too well—producing multiple eggs. Inform her that too many released eggs may cause multiple gestation, which carries the risk of prematurity and infant mortality. Also discuss possible hyperstimulation syndrome, which occurs only after ovulation. Marked by enlarged, fragile ovaries, this syndrome causes potentially life-threatening fluid and electrolyte imbalances. Explain that daily monitoring may detect this syndrome. If the doctor suspects it, he'll stop therapy until her ovaries return to normal size.

Caution the patient to report immediately any severe headaches unrelieved by acetaminophen, extreme abdominal distention, excessive postovulatory weight gain (5 to 10 lb), and shortness of breath. Forewarn her also that she may feel moody.

Procedures
Discuss advances in fertilization options, such as in vitro fertilization–embryo transfer (IVF–ET), gamete intrafallopian transfer (GIFT), embryo donation, and artificial insemination.

In vitro fertilization–embryo transfer. Tell patients that IVF–ET circumvents the need for a fallopian tube to pick up an egg or to propel a fertilized egg to the uterus. (See *How in vitro fertilization works.*)

How in vitro fertilization works

For suitable patients, in vitro fertilization-embryo transfer (IVF-ET) bypasses the barriers to in vivo fertilization.

In IVF-ET, after the ovaries receive hormonal stimulation, the doctor may use laparoscopy to visualize and aspirate fluid (containing eggs) from the ovarian follicles. (Or to eliminate using laparoscopy and a general anesthetic, he may use an ultrasound technique, first to visualize the ovarian follicles and then to guide a needle through the back of the vagina to retrieve fluid and eggs from the ovarian follicles.) He then deposits the eggs in a test tube or a laboratory dish containing a culture medium.

Next, the doctor or a technician adds the sperm from the patient's husband (or a donor) to the dish. One to two days after insemination, the doctor transfers the now-fertilized egg or embryo into the patient's uterus, where it may implant and establish a pregnancy.

**IN VITRO FERTILIZATION
AND EMBRYO TRANSFER**

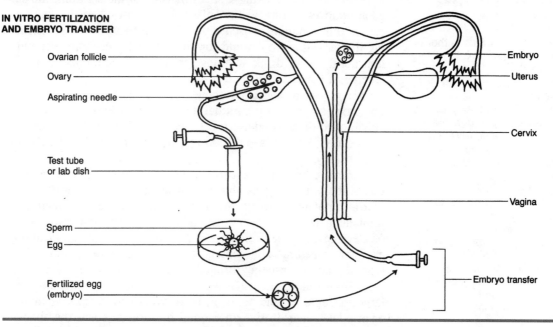

Gamete intrafallopian transfer. If the patient has one functioning fallopian tube, tell her about GIFT. In this procedure, the ovaries are stimulated with fertility drugs and the results are monitored. Next, the doctor collects eggs from the ovaries either by laparoscopy or by vaginal needle aspiration. Then he places them in a catheter with sperm and transfers this gamete mix into the fallopian tube, allowing fertilization and implantation to occur naturally from that point.

Embryo donation. Discuss the possibility of receiving a donated egg or an embryo fertilized in vitro, especially if the woman has ovarian failure but a functioning uterus. Also discuss whether the husband's sperm can be used to fertilize a donated egg so that the embryo will contain half of the couples' gene pool. Some couples see this alternative as an advantage over adoption because they'll experience a pregnancy and possibly have a shorter wait for a child.

Artificial insemination. Encourage patients to express their feelings about artificial insemination, especially if cervical mucus prevents sperm from moving progressively through the reproduc-

Dispelling common myths about infertility

As infertile couples search for answers as to why pregnancy eludes them, tell them that they're likely to hear some popular but misleading explanations for their situation. Set the record straight for them by distinguishing myth from reality; for example:

• *Myth 1:* "You need to relax. Go on vacation; then you'll get pregnant."

Reality: Tension *follows* the recognition of infertility. It doesn't cause it.

• *Myth 2:* "Adopt—you'll get pregnant."

Reality: Although a few previously infertile couples *do* achieve pregnancy spontaneously after they adopt a child, so do an equally few infertile couples who choose not to adopt. Adoption in no way increases fertility.

• *Myth 3:* "Ask your doctor to give you a thyroid hormone. That should work."

Reality: Studies have repeatedly shown that thyroid hormone has no value for treating infertility in men or women with normal thyroid hormone levels.

• *Myth 4:* "Have a D&C—maybe that will help."

Reality: Invasive and expensive, dilatation and curettage neither increases fertility nor diagnoses disorders that can't be detected in a routine evaluation.

• *Myth 5:* "Maybe you have a tilted uterus. If you do, you'll never get pregnant."

Reality: A "tilted," or retroverted, uterus does not cause infertility—although it may be found with other conditions that do. Women who have a retroverted uterus *can* and *do* get pregnant.

tive tract, if sperm counts remain low, or if sperm have poor motility. Describe how the doctor will pass washed sperm from the male partner or donor through a catheter into the uterus.

Surgery

If either patient requires surgery to enhance fertility, you'll need to explain the procedure. Typical surgeries include varicolectomy, laparoscopy, and laparotomy.

Varicolectomy. Advise the male patient that he may need surgery to repair or remove a varicocele. The varicocele allows blood to pool in the scrotum and raises the temperature around the sperm. This, in turn, may reduce sperm production and motility. Explain that after making a small incision in the scrotum, the surgeon removes or ties off the enlarged, varicose-like vein that causes this condition. Discuss possible risks and benefits, instructing the patient as you would for any surgical procedure. Remind him not to eat or drink anything for at least 8 hours before he receives a general anesthetic.

Laparoscopy and laparotomy. Tell the female patient that she may need surgery to treat tubal disease, endometriosis, or such pelvic conditions as adhesions. If she'll receive a general anesthetic, advise her to avoid food and fluids for at least 8 hours before surgery.

Prepare her for *laparoscopy,* which visualizes the pelvic and upper abdominal organs and peritoneal surfaces to identify endometrial implants. Explain that the surgeon removes endometrial implants using the laparoscope and a laser beam or a cryosurgical or electrocautery device. Discuss possible complications including excessive bleeding, abdominal cramps, and shoulder pain resulting from the abdomen being inflated with carbon dioxide.

Advise the patient that if the surgeon finds the implants too large for laparoscopic removal, he may perform a *laparotomy* then or at a later date. In this operation, the surgeon opens the abdomen to remove the larger implants. While operating, he may remove pelvic adhesions or perform microsurgery or laser surgery on damaged fallopian tubes. Advise her that a laparotomy is major surgery and that a lengthy recovery period may follow.

Inform the patient that complications, including an increased risk for infection, are the same as those for other abdominal surgeries. Show her the postoperative care measures she'll need to perform.

Inform the patient that the surgeon may perform a *hysteroscopy* to remove uterine polyps and small fibroid tumors. Explain that after he anesthetizes the patient, he will pass a fiber-optic hysteroscope through the vagina and cervix and into the uterus, where he'll remove the lesions.

Other care measures

Counseling infertile patients may be your greatest teaching challenge. Let them know that surprise and shock are common first reactions. Typically, denial and "why me?" questions follow. Warn couples that they may receive unhelpful, insensitive, and even inaccurate advice from well-meaning family members and friends (see *Dispelling common myths about infertility*). Encourage them to discuss their feelings, and help them address feelings of exclusion and isolation. Suggest appropriate support groups or associations with other infertile couples.

If all efforts at conception fail, help the couple recognize and deal with grief. Reassure them that their loss is real—even for a child they will never have. Realize that your task will be complicated—especially if the health care team can't detect the reasons for infertility and, therefore, can't predict the chances for conception. In such situations, the couple may be caught between giving up prematurely and postponing grief and acceptance indefinitely.

As appropriate, help them accept and resolve their situation. Confirm that acceptance doesn't mean they won't grieve at times or feel angry. It may simply help them to get on with their lives.

Mention adoption. If the patients express interest, direct them to appropriate resources. Caution them against waiting until they exhaust their medical options because advancing age or reduced finances may make adoption difficult.

Recognize also that patients who achieve conception may still need help. After all they've been through, they may distrust their bodies and fear miscarriage.

Sources of information and support

American Fertility Society
2140 11th Avenue, South, Suite 200, Birmingham, Ala. 35205
(205) 933-8494

Fertility Research Foundation
1430 Second Avenue, Suite 103, New York, N.Y. 10021
(212) 744-5500

Resolve
5 Water Street, Arlington, Mass. 02174
(617) 643-2424

Further readings

Breitkopf, L.J., and Bakoulis, M.G. "Can't Get Pregnant?... Endometriosis Can Lead to Infertility in Several Ways," *Health* 20(8):56-59, August 1988.
"Female Infertility: Differential Diagnosis," *Hospital Medicine* 24(9):109-12, 114-15, September 1988.
Fincham, E. "Gift of Life...Gamete Intrafallopian Transfer (GIFT)," *Nursing Times* 83(48):51-53, December 2-8, 1987.
Frank, D.I. "Treatment Preferences of Infertile Couples," *Applied Nursing Research* 2(2):94-95, May 1989.
Pace-Owens, S. "Gamete Intrafallopian Transfer (GIFT)," *Journal of Obstetric, Gynecologic, and Neonatal Nursing* 18(2):93-97, March-April 1989.
Swatfield, L. "The Baby Boom...Infertility," *Nursing Times* 84(33):16-17, August 17-23, 1989.
Woods, S. "Myths and Realities of the Biological Time Clock: The Childbearing Years," *Health Values* 11(15):21-25, September-October 1987.
Zion, A.B. "The Process of Developing Patient Education Materials for Infertile Couples," *Journal of Obstetric, Gynecologic, and Neonatal Nursing* 17(4):259-63, July-August 1988.

PATIENT-TEACHING AID

How to take your basal body temperature

Dear Patient:

Here are some tips to help you record your basal body temperature. This temperature may dip just before you ovulate, then rise about three-tenths of a degree, and dip again before your next period. The rise indicates that progesterone's in your system, which, in turn, means that you've ovulated. Here's how to start:

1 Chart the days of your menstrual flow by darkening the squares above the 98-degree mark. Start with the first day of your period (day 1). Take your temperature each day after your period ends.

2 Use a thermometer that measures tenths of a degree. If you're using a glass oral thermometer, shake it down to 94 degrees before using it.

3 When you wake up and before you get out of bed or do anything else, place the thermometer under your tongue for 5 minutes. *Try to do this at the same time each morning.*

4 Now, place a dot on the graph's line that matches your temperature reading. (Don't be surprised if your waking temperature before ovulation is 96 or 97 degrees.) If you forget to take your temperature on one day, leave that day blank on the graph, and don't connect the dots.

5 Make notes on the graph if you miss taking your temperature, feel sick, can't sleep, or wake up at a different time. Note, too, if you're taking any medicine—even aspirin, which may affect your temperature. Remember to mark the dates when you had sexual relations.

SAMPLE TEMPERATURE CHART

Look over this sample temperature chart, recorded by Susan Jones. Mrs. Jones used an *S* to record sexual relations and made notes showing she had insomnia on September 27. She forgot to take her temperature on September 19. Notice that she didn't connect the dots during these times. Her temperature dipped on September 24 (day 15 of her cycle). Then it began rising.

Of course your own chart will be larger, including temperatures over 99.3° and under 97°.

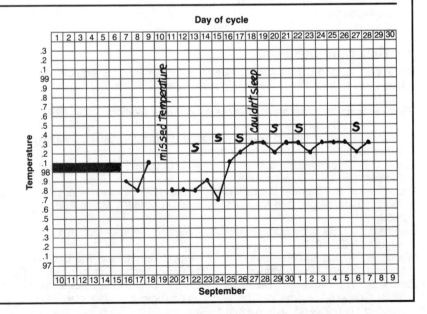

CHAPTER

10

Musculoskeletal Conditions

Contents

Osteoporosis

Sometimes called the "silent disease," osteoporosis often goes undetected until the patient sustains a fracture and seeks medical attention. This makes your first opportunity for patient teaching more complicated than usual. You'll have to ensure that the fracture heals properly and, at the same time, teach the patient how to avoid new fractures. Meanwhile, because osteoporosis has long been viewed as an inevitable part of aging, you may have to overcome the belief that little can be done to slow or prevent the disorder. Accordingly, you'll emphasize the roles played by proper diet, vitamin and mineral supplements, and regular exercise in controlling osteoporosis. You'll also need to emphasize proper body mechanics and new ways to perform daily activities safely. (See *Teaching the patient with advanced osteoporosis,* page 606.)

Discuss the disorder

Tell your patient that osteoporosis—which means "porous bone"—causes a gradual loss of bone mass, leaving bones brittle and prone to fractures. Explain that over a lifetime, the body continuously forms and resorbs bone. For the patient's first 30 to 35 years, this process remains in balance (for more information, see *Reviewing calcium regulation,* page 607). Then, when bones reach maturity between ages 30 and 35, the rate of bone resorption starts exceeding that of bone formation. The result: gradual bone loss.

Inform the patient that osteoporosis occurs in two forms: *postmenopausal (Type I)* and *senile (Type II) osteoporosis.* Related to the loss of estrogen's protective effect on bone, *Type I* affects postmenopausal women between ages 55 and 75. Trabecular bone loss is greater than cortical bone loss, with fractures of the vertebrae and wrist most common.

Explain that several factors appear to affect the rate of bone loss. Naturally, as the rate increases, so does the patient's risk of developing osteoporosis (for more information, see *Identifying osteoporosis risk factors,* page 608). In menopausal women, for instance, estrogen loss poses a significant risk factor. That's because estrogen plays a crucial role in maintaining the balance between bone formation and bone resorption. (For more information, see *How menopause intensifies osteoporosis,* page 609.)

Affecting men and women equally, *Type II* osteoporosis occurs most commonly between ages 70 and 85. This type of osteoporosis is characterized by both trabecular and cortical bone loss,

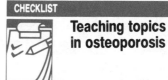

CHECKLIST

Teaching topics in osteoporosis

☐ How an imbalance between bone formation and resorption leads to osteoporosis
☐ Explanation of osteoporosis types: Type I or Type II
☐ Risk factors
☐ Diagnostic studies, such as X-rays, single- or dual-photon absorptiometry, transiliac bone biopsy, and blood and urine tests
☐ Exercise program based on weight-bearing activities
☐ Ensuring adequate dietary calcium and vitamin D intake
☐ Drug therapy, including vitamin and mineral supplements, estrogen, and calcitonin
☐ Observing safety practices and proper body mechanics to prevent fractures
☐ Source of information and support

Madeline Albanese, RN, MSN, ONC, Marianne K. Ostrow, RN, BSN, and **Karin K. Roberts, RN, MN,** contributed to this chapter. Ms. Albanese, manager of patient education, and Ms. Ostrow, clinical nurse, work at Thomas Jefferson University Hospital, Philadelphia. Ms. Roberts is an assistant professor at the Research College of Nursing in Kansas City, Mo.

Teaching the patient with advanced osteoporosis

Most osteoporosis patients don't realize how brittle their bones are until they're hospitalized with a fracture and their bone mass is considerably diminished. Even at this late stage, though, you can teach the patient measures to halt the disease's progression and to prevent additional fractures. Just take a standard teaching plan and mold it to the patient's needs. To learn how to do this, read over the account of 68-year-old Hazel Greenwood, a retired school guidance counselor.

Assess first
Mrs. Greenwood was admitted to the orthopedic unit soon after back pain and muscle spasms forced her to abandon her basement-cleaning project. Spinal X-rays showed compression fractures of three thoracic vertebrae. Dual-photon absorptiometry of the spine confirmed advanced Type I osteoporosis.

As you collect health history data, Mrs. Greenwood tells you, "I went through 'the change' early. I was only 45. They didn't prescribe estrogen then." You also learn that she's lactose intolerant, she rarely goes outdoors, and she gets little exercise. "Between church work, my book group, and three grandchildren, I hardly have time to walk the dog around the yard," she confides.

She says that the doctor has prescribed 3 days of bed rest, heat therapy, pain relievers, calcium and vitamin D supplements, and exercise instruction. And she's anxious about her future: "My mother spent her last years hunched over and practically crippled. Is that what's happening to me?" she asks.

What are Mrs. Greenwood's learning needs?
To decide what to teach Mrs. Greenwood, compare her knowledge of osteoporosis with standard teaching plan topics, which include:
• pathophysiology of Type I osteoporosis
• osteoporosis risk factors
• tests (X-rays and photon absorptiometry)
• exercise program featuring weight-bearing activities, such as walking
• diet planning to boost calcium intake
• safety and proper body mechanics.

Clearly Mrs. Greenwood doesn't recognize the factors contributing to her condition. She's also uninformed about treatments, such as how to increase calcium intake without consuming dairy products she's allergic to. You decide that your teaching plan for Mrs. Greenwood should include a review of risk factors, a discussion of how osteoporosis develops, and full instructions on exercise, diet, and safety. Be-

cause Mrs. Greenwood should avoid milk, you decide to ask a dietitian to teach her about calcium-rich foods and help her plan appropriate menus.

Set learning outcomes
Using the standard teaching plan as a guide, you and Mrs. Greenwood choose suitable learning outcomes. Both of you agree that she should be able to:

```
-discuss how osteoporosis develops
-identify her risk factors for osteoporosis and specify
those that can be altered
-describe her exercise program
-identify nondairy calcium sources
-develop a meal plan that meets her calcium needs
-list safety measures and demonstrate proper body mechanics.
```

Select teaching tools and techniques
Because Mrs. Greenwood will be hospitalized at least 3 more days, you'll have time for several teaching sessions. To avoid overwhelming her with information, you choose to portion each day's teaching into a morning and an afternoon session.

You'll use *explanation and discussion* to portray what happens in osteoporosis and to show how Mrs. Greenwood's personal risk factors contribute to her condition. You'll include *demonstrations* of safety measures and body mechanics, and you'll arrange *consultations* with a dietitian (for menu planning) and a physical therapist (for exercise planning).

Because Mrs. Greenwood worked with students, she should be receptive to *printed teaching aids* like *pamphlets, illustrated handouts,* and *books*. She may also benefit from *diagrams* that illustrate the disease process. Remind her to ask the dietitian for *sample menus* and a list of calcium-rich foods.

Evaluate your teaching
Has Mrs. Greenwood learned enough about osteoporosis to ensure that she'll make healthful life-style changes? Can she avoid new fractures? *Questions and answers* can help you decide just how much she comprehends. For example, ask her to list the osteoporosis risk factors. Or initiate a *discussion* about exercise to determine the extent of her commitment to therapeutic activity.

Return demonstration and *simulation* can help you evaluate what she's learned about menu planning and proper body mechanics. For example, review the hospital menu she's selected, or have her describe how she'll put on her shoes when she's allowed out of bed. Her responses will help you to judge her progress and modify your teaching plan as needed.

Reviewing calcium regulation

Tell your patient that strong bones depend on a delicate mechanism that keeps the body's calcium levels in balance. Explain that parathyroid hormone (PTH), vitamin D, and to a lesser extent, calcitonin and adrenal steroids regulate blood levels of calcium by influencing its absorption and excretion. They also regulate the mobilization of calcium from bones and teeth (which together store more than 98% of the body's calcium).

The body absorbs calcium from the GI tract (provided sufficient vitamin D is present) and excretes calcium in the urine and feces. When calcium levels fall, PTH and vitamin D work to enhance intestinal absorption of calcium, promote renal retention of calcium, and advance mobilization of calcium from the bones and teeth. When calcium levels rise, calcitonin— secreted by the thyroid gland—inhibits the release of calcium from the bones and teeth but enhances renal excretion of calcium.

Here's a graphic description of what happens:

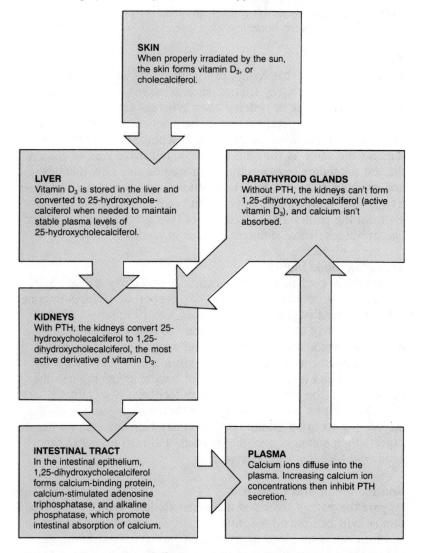

SKIN
When properly irradiated by the sun, the skin forms vitamin D_3, or cholecalciferol.

LIVER
Vitamin D_3 is stored in the liver and converted to 25-hydroxychole-calciferol when needed to maintain stable plasma levels of 25-hydroxycholecalciferol.

PARATHYROID GLANDS
Without PTH, the kidneys can't form 1,25-dihydroxycholecalciferol (active vitamin D_3), and calcium isn't absorbed.

KIDNEYS
With PTH, the kidneys convert 25-hydroxycholecalciferol to 1,25-dihydroxycholecalciferol, the most active derivative of vitamin D_3.

INTESTINAL TRACT
In the intestinal epithelium, 1,25-dihydroxycholecalciferol forms calcium-binding protein, calcium-stimulated adenosine triphosphatase, and alkaline phosphatase, which promote intestinal absorption of calcium.

PLASMA
Calcium ions diffuse into the plasma. Increasing calcium ion concentrations then inhibit PTH secretion.

Identifying osteoporosis risk factors

Everyone loses some bone tissue with age. However, some people are more likely to have extensive bone loss. The following factors affect a person's risk for osteoporosis:
• sex — osteoporosis affects four times as many women as men
• age — after age 50 the osteoporosis risk increases
• race — Whites and Asians are at greater risk than Blacks
• body frame — osteoporosis affects more petite, small-framed persons than average-sized, large-framed persons
• onset of menopause in women — the earlier the onset (whether natural or surgically induced), the higher the risk
• a calcium-deficient diet
• a sedentary life-style
• a family history of osteoporosis
• regular alcohol and tobacco use or excessive caffeine consumption
• long-term corticosteroid, heparin, or certain antibiotic and anticonvulsant drug use
• multiparity, breast-feeding more than one nontwin offspring, or both
• medical conditions, such as chronic renal failure; Cushing's syndrome; eating disorders, such as anorexia; hyperparathyroidism; hyperthyroidism; intestinal absorption disorders requiring special therapy, such as intestinal bypass or gastrectomy; liver disease; or rheumatoid arthritis.

with resultant vertebral, hip, and long-bone fractures. Mention that a calcium-poor diet may be a cause of Type II osteoporosis.

Complications
Stress that failure to observe safety measures, proper body mechanics, and other treatment measures increases the risk of fractures. Explain that a fracture can result from minor traumatic injury—a fall, for example—or from a simple activity, such as rising from a chair, bending over, or raising a window. That's why you'll urge the patient to report even minor injuries to the doctor, especially if pain, swelling, or stiffness persists.

Describe the diagnostic workup
Teach the patient about tests that she may have to confirm osteoporosis and to differentiate Type I from Type II. Besides routine blood tests, urinalyses, and X-rays, she may undergo special X-ray studies, transiliac bone biopsy, or quantitative computed tomography (CT) to measure bone loss precisely.

X-ray studies
Inform the patient that X-rays can identify fractures and advanced bone loss. Special X-ray studies, such as *single-* or *dual-photon absorptiometry* may be ordered also. Whereas single-photon studies measure the mineral content of long bones, dual-photon studies measure bone mass (or density). Teaching for these studies remains the same as for routine X-rays, but make sure to discuss the test procedure. Explain that both studies take only minutes and produce no discomfort. Both studies use an external radioactive photon source and a camera. The camera records energy levels from the photon beam as it passes through the bone. Different energy values denote different degrees of disease.

Transiliac bone biopsy
If the patient's scheduled for transiliac bone biopsy, explain that this test allows direct examination of osteoporotic changes in bone cells. Tell her that the actual test takes 5 to 10 minutes. Tell her that a nurse will cleanse the skin over the iliac crest (the bony protrusion just above the buttock) and apply a topical anesthetic. Then the doctor will make a small skin incision, introduce a hollow needle, and remove a tiny core of bone marrow through the needle. Warn the patient that she may feel brief discomfort.

Tell her that after the needle's withdrawn, pressure applied to the site for 10 to 15 minutes will stop any bleeding. Advise her to expect slight soreness over the incision, and instruct her to report additional bleeding or severe pain.

Routine blood and urine tests
Prepare the patient for blood and urine studies. Typically, a blood sample will be drawn for serum protein electrophoresis studies and for evaluating blood urea nitrogen and serum calcium, phosphorus, triiodothyronine, and thyroxine levels. If the doctor orders serum alkaline phosphatase and creatinine tests, instruct the patient to fast before the blood sample's drawn. If the doctor orders

a 24-hour urine collection to assess calcium, creatinine, and hydroxyproline levels, tell the patient how to collect the sample.

Quantitative CT scan
Unlike conventional CT, which uses serial images to produce three-dimensional results, quantitative CT provides images of only a "slice" of bone. However, you'll prepare the patient as you would for a conventional CT scan. Tell her that the scan causes no pain and may take about 30 minutes.

Explain that during the test the patient will lie on an X-ray table. Instruct her to lie still and remain quiet because movement will blur the image. Describe how the scanner will take pictures of her bone. Reassure her that she can resume her usual activities after the test.

Teach about treatments
Treatment for osteoporosis aims to control bone loss and prevent fractures. As appropriate, you'll teach the patient about a calcium-rich diet, weight-bearing exercise, and medications. To help her avoid falls and other injuries, you'll discuss daily safety practices and proper body mechanics.

Activity
Urge the patient to plan a weight-bearing exercise program to prevent bone loss. Emphasize that exercise increases the bone formation rate; improves muscle strength, which increases bone density; and promotes circulation, which enhances intestinal absorption of such nutrients as calcium.

Recommend such weight-bearing activities as walking, jogging, bicycling, or aerobic exercises. Mention that swimming—a popular but non-weight-bearing activity—isn't effective at controlling osteoporosis. If the patient's unaccustomed to regular exercise, suggest that she begin with walking. At first, for example, she can take short walks, increasing her activity until she can cover 1 or 1½ miles at least three times a week. To avoid falls and support regular exercise, encourage her to walk inside rather than outside in poor weather. For instance, if she has access to a shopping mall or a gymnasium, she could walk there. If not, she can map out a course in her home. Point out that 1 hour of walking indoors is equivalent to about 1 mile.

Warn the patient to be especially cautious while exercising. Advise her to avoid such activities as tennis and bowling, which involve twisting, jumping, or straining the back. Explain that these activities may cause fractures.

Diet
Although daily dietary calcium can't replace lost bone, it may retard or prevent bone loss. Point out that daily calcium requirements vary, especially among women. For example, children and young adults require about 800 mg of calcium each day. Pregnant women need about 1,200 mg/day and breast-feeding women about 2,000 mg/day. Men and nonmenopausal women need about 1,000 mg/day; but with menopause, a woman's calcium need jumps to

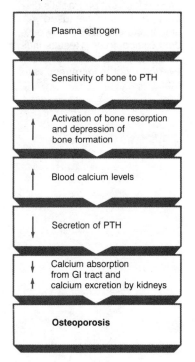

How menopause intensifies osteoporosis

As a woman goes through menopause, circulating estrogen levels fall. As estrogen decreases, the bone's sensitivity to parathyroid hormone (PTH) increases. PTH stimulates resorption of calcium from the bone by activating the bone-resorbing cells and depressing the bone-forming cells.

The subsequent increase in circulating calcium then depresses PTH secretion. In turn, the intestines absorb less dietary calcium, and the kidneys excrete more circulating calcium.

Eventually, the bones become so weak that they can't withstand force, and fractures result from minimal traumatic injury.

The flow chart below summarizes the physiological sequence that accelerates osteoporosis.

↓ Plasma estrogen

↑ Sensitivity of bone to PTH

↑ Activation of bone resorption and depression of bone formation

↑ Blood calcium levels

↓ Secretion of PTH

↓ Calcium absorption from GI tract and
↑ calcium excretion by kidneys

Osteoporosis

Possible new drugs for osteoporosis patients

Two drugs offer potentially dramatic results for patients with osteoporosis.

Calcitonin
Already recommended to slow the progression of osteoporosis, calcitonin must be given by injection. This makes the drug, which prevents bone loss after menopause, too inconvenient and expensive for most patients. Now, calcitonin in a trial nasal spray form — already approved for use in Europe — promises to overcome these drawbacks. Additionally, calcitonin in this form may offer an alternative to a woman who can't or won't take estrogen.

Etidronate
Another drug, etidronate (Didronel), is the first agent proven to restore lost bone. Already approved for treating Paget's disease, etidronate was used safely and effectively in two recent clinical trials. Results indicate that just 2 weeks of use every 4 months increases bone mass.

about 1,500 mg/day. To help guide the patient's menu selections, provide a copy of the teaching aid *Planning a calcium-rich diet,* page 612. Review these guidelines with the patient, and schedule time to answer any questions.

Medication
Inform the patient that calcium and vitamin D supplements, calcitonin, or estrogen (for menopausal women) may be prescribed to prevent or slow bone loss. Review how to take these medications, and discuss possible adverse effects. If appropriate, mention that certain new drugs may improve the long-term prospects for successful osteoporosis treatment (see *Possible new drugs for osteoporosis patients*).

Vitamin and mineral supplements. Inform the patient who's not getting enough calcium in her diet that the doctor may recommend an over-the-counter calcium supplement. Refer to *Choosing a calcium supplement* to help the patient select an appropriate supplement.

Instruct the patient to take the calcium supplement 1 hour before meals to ensure maximum absorption. Should this decrease digestive acid production, however, advise her to take the supplement with meals. Recommend that she avoid laxatives and multivitamins containing zinc. These preparations decrease calcium absorption.

Point out that the doctor may recommend taking a vitamin D supplement along with the calcium to maximize intestinal absorption.

Estrogen. For the postmenopausal patient, or for the menopausal patient at high risk for osteoporosis, the doctor may recommend estrogen replacement therapy. Explain that estrogen can prevent further bone loss but that it can't replace bone that's already lost. Add that estrogen replacement therapy is usually begun within 6 years of menopause for maximum effectiveness.

Tell the patient that a short-acting oral estrogen—for example, a conjugated estrogen—is commonly prescribed. Explain that she'll take the drug daily for 3 weeks and then wait a week before beginning the medicine again.

Inform her that long-term estrogen replacement therapy may increase her risk for endometrial cancer. And while she's taking estrogen, stress that she'll need regular checkups to detect early cellular changes, such as endometrial hyperplasia. Add that the doctor may prescribe a progestin to accompany estrogen replacement therapy. Explain that taking both hormones may minimize her risk for uterine cancer. Also point out that estrogen replacement therapy may increase the patient's risk for breast cancer, especially if she's already at high risk or if she's taken estrogen for more than 15 years. Urge the patient to have a mammogram before starting estrogen replacement therapy and yearly thereafter. Review also how to perform a monthly breast self-examination.

Calcitonin. Explain to the patient that the hormone calcitonin (Calcimar) prevents bone loss by inhibiting resorption. Advise the patient to ask the doctor if calcitonin—usually administered by injection—must be taken this way or whether another form is available. Instruct the patient to report nausea, rash, and swelling or tenderness of the hands to the doctor.

Other care measures

In osteoporosis, safety practices and proper body mechanics go hand in hand in preventing fractures. Advise the patient to wear comfortable, well-fitting shoes with rubber heels to help cushion and protect the spine during walking. Discourage high heels.

To prevent falls, suggest removing throw rugs, placing a non-skid mat in the bathtub, and installing handrails on stairs. Caution the patient to avoid walking about in dimly lit rooms. Also caution against lifting heavy objects, twisting suddenly, or bending from the waist. Describe devices that may make daily activities easier—for example, a shoe horn, long-handled sponge, or a reacher-grabber. If appropriate, suggest a cane or walker to help the patient maintain balance and decrease lower back pain.

Source of information and support

National Osteoporosis Foundation
2100 M Street, NW, Suite 602, Washington, D.C. 20037
(202) 223-2226

Further readings

Carter, L.W. "Calcium Intake in Young Adult Women: Implications for Osteoporosis Risk Assessment," *Journal of Obstetric, Gynecologic, and Neonatal Nursing* 16(5):301-08, September-October 1987.

Chesnut, C.H., et al. "New Options in Osteoporosis," *Patient Care* 22(1):160-64, 167, 171-73, 187, January 1988.

Dalsky, G.P. "The Role of Exercise in the Prevention of Osteoporosis," *Comprehensive Therapy* 15(9):30-37, September 1989.

Ettinger, B. "Estrogen and Postmenopausal Osteoporosis," *American Association of Occupational Health Nursing* 35(12):543-46, 559-61, December 1987.

Glowacki, G.A. "A New Look at Osteoporosis and Estrogen Replacement Therapy," *Comprehensive Therapy* 14(2):49-53, February 1988.

Goodman, C.E. "Osteoporosis and Physical Activity," *American Association of Occupational Health Nursing* 35(12):539-42, 559-61, December 1987.

Guinan, M.E., et al. "Osteoporosis and ERT—The Jury Is Still Out," *Journal of the American Medical Women's Association* 42(3):92-93, May-June 1987.

Lufkin, E.G., and Ory, S.J. "Estrogen Replacement Therapy for the Prevention of Osteoporosis," *American Family Physician* 40(3):205-12, September 1989.

Marcus, R. "Understanding and Preventing Osteoporosis," *Hospital Practice* 24(4):189, 192, 194-96, 201-03+, April 1989.

McDonnell, J.M., et al. "Osteoporosis: Definition, Risk Factors, Etiology, and Diagnosis," *American Association of Occupational Health Nursing* 35(12):527-30, 559-61, December 1987.

National Institute of Arthritis and Musculoskeletal and Skin Diseases, National Institutes of Health. "Osteoporosis: Cause, Treatment, Prevention," *Orthopedic Nursing* 5(6):29-38, November-December 1986.

Thorneycroft, I.H. "The Role of Estrogen Replacement Therapy in the Prevention of Osteoporosis," *American Journal of Obstetrics and Gynecology* 160(5):1306-10, May 1989.

Vogler, J.B., and Martinez, S. "Non-Invasive Procedures: Pros and Cons," *American Association of Occupational Health Nursing* 35(12):547-61, December 1987.

Choosing a calcium supplement

When the doctor recommends an over-the-counter calcium supplement, your patient may ask which preparation is best. Offer some guidelines for choosing a suitable supplement.

• Advise him to read the product label to learn how much elemental calcium the product contains. Explain that different supplements contain different amounts of *elemental calcium* (the amount of calcium that the body actually uses). For example, calcium carbonate products, such as Cal Sup, Caltrate 600, Os-Cal, Biocal, oyster shell calcium, and antacids (such as Tums) contain the most elemental calcium—about 40%. Another form of calcium—calcium lactate—contains about 13% elemental calcium. Still another form, calcium gluconate, contains only 9%.

• Instruct the patient to avoid dolomite and bone meal products. These preparations may contain lead.

• Inform the patient that calcium carbonate supplements may cause gas and constipation. To reduce these effects, suggest that he drink more fluids and increase his fiber intake—between meals. (Extra fiber with meals interferes with calcium absorption.)

PATIENT-TEACHING AID

Planning a calcium-rich diet

Dear Patient:

Your body needs calcium for strong bones and teeth. Eating calcium-rich foods is one way to make sure your body gets enough of this vital mineral. Here are some things to consider.

What's enough?

How much calcium you need changes throughout your lifetime. For example, teenagers need extra calcium to meet the needs of their rapidly growing bones. Women need more calcium after menopause, as well as during pregnancy and while breast-feeding.

Ask your nurse or doctor to help you determine exactly how much calcium you need each day.

Where to get calcium

Dairy products (milk, cheese, yogurt, and ice cream) are potent calcium sources. If you're avoiding cholesterol or watching your weight, you can still have skimmed or powdered milk and low-fat yogurt.

If you have trouble digesting milk, you may still be able to eat yogurt, hard cheeses, acidophilus milk, or lactose-reduced milk. (Ask your grocery store manager to order a product, such as Lactaid, if your store doesn't carry it.) Or ask your pharmacist about adding *lactobacillus acidophilus* to regular milk. Also called by such trade names as Bacid and Lactinex, this substance makes milk easier to digest.

Certain vegetables, such as collards, turnip greens, and broccoli contain lots of calcium. Oysters, salmon, sardines, and tofu are other foods with a high calcium content.

Other tips

Some foods, especially very fibrous foods, can interfere with your body's uptake of calcium. So, to get the most calcium from the foods you eat, avoid eating calcium- and fiber-rich foods at the same meal.

Also, eat less red meat, chocolate, peanut butter, rhubarb, sweet potatoes, and fatty foods. And cut down on caffeine-containing drinks, such as coffee, tea, and colas.

Calcium's most effective when your body has enough vitamin D. Spending just 15 minutes in sunshine every day will fill your daily requirement. Besides, most manufacturers add vitamin D to milk and cereals. And egg yolks, saltwater fish, and liver also have this vitamin.

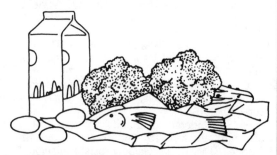

Avoid taking a vitamin D supplement, though, unless your doctor specifically tells you to do so. Too much vitamin D may do more harm than good.

Osteoarthritis

Because the chronic joint pain of osteoarthritis has no cure, your teaching will feature compliance with a program designed to manage pain, restore or maintain joint mobility, and preserve independence. For pain relief, you'll help the patient to combine medication, heat or cold therapy, and massage. For joint mobility, muscle strength, and independence, you'll emphasize ways to balance exercise and rest in daily life. This may be difficult, especially if the therapy disrupts the patient's routine. But with your encouragement, he can learn to discipline himself and pace his daily activities. By learning how not to "overdo it," he'll help himself to maintain independence.

Occasionally, the effects of osteoarthritis require surgery to correct deformity or to improve function. Then, you'll need to teach the patient about such procedures as joint fusion or replacement. As appropriate after surgery, you'll show the patient how to care for his brace or cast and how to resume safe exercise.

Discuss the disorder

Inform your patient that osteoarthritis is a common degenerative disorder in which the smooth elastic cartilage of his joints gradually wears down or erodes. The bones underneath this worn cartilage stiffen, and bony spurs develop around the joint, narrowing the joint space. For example, osteoarthritis of the interphalangeal joints produces bone spurs in the distal joints (known as Heberden's nodes) and in the proximal joints (where they're known as Bouchard's nodes). During movement, the bones rub together. Inflammation, pain, and loss of joint function may result. For more information, see *What happens in osteoarthritis*, page 614.

Tell the patient that of the primary and secondary forms of osteoarthritis, *primary osteoarthritis* appears to be related to aging, although researchers don't understand why. This form of the disorder isn't attributable to predisposing factors. In some cases, however, it may be hereditary. Point out that more than 50% of persons over age 30 have some features of primary osteoarthritis. And nearly 100% of persons over age 60 have X-ray evidence of the disorder, although only about 40% actually experience symptoms.

Tell the patient that *secondary osteoarthritis* results from a predisposing factor—most commonly, traumatic injury or a congenital abnormality such as hip dysplasia. Endocrine disorders

Madeline Albanese, RN, MSN, ONC, Marianne K. Ostrow, RN, BSN, and **Patricia Mosko, RN, BSN, MSN, CRNP,** contributed to this chapter. Ms. Albanese, manager of patient education, and Ms. Ostrow, clinical nurse, work at Thomas Jefferson University Hospital, Philadelphia. Ms. Mosko is a certified registered nurse practitioner in rheumatology at Temple University School of Medicine, Philadelphia.

CHECKLIST

Teaching topics in osteoarthritis

☐ The osteoarthritis disease process
☐ Types of osteoarthritis: primary or secondary
☐ How exercise preserves joint function
☐ Preparing for tests, such as blood and urine studies, X-rays, joint aspiration, magnetic resonance imaging, and radionuclide bone scan
☐ Range-of-motion, extension, flexion, and isometric exercises
☐ Medications and their administration
☐ Epidural block to relieve pain from osteoarthritis in the lumbar spine
☐ Surgery, such as debridement, osteotomy, arthrodesis, or joint replacement
☐ Appropriate postoperative exercises and activity restrictions
☐ Other pain-relief measures, including heat or cold therapy and massage
☐ Using protective and assistive devices to avoid joint fatigue
☐ Source of information and support

What happens in osteoarthritis

Tell your patient that osteoarthritis doesn't happen suddenly. The characteristic breakdown of articular cartilage is a gradual response to aging or predisposing factors, such as joint abnormalities or traumatic injury. Use the illustrations below to help you describe the disease process to your patient.

Normal anatomy
Begin with normal joint anatomy. Show the patient how the bones fit together and how cartilage—a smooth, fibrous tissue—cushions the end of each bone. Also point out that synovial fluid fills each joint space. Explain that this fluid lubricates the joint to ease movement, much like brake fluid functions in a car.

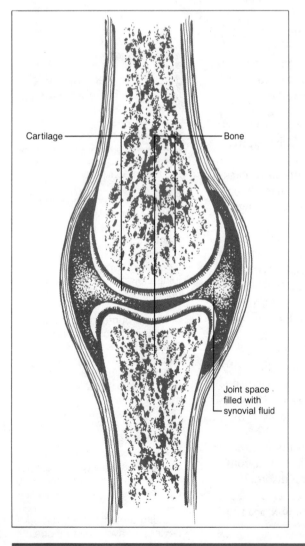

Early stage
Usually cartilage begins to break down long before symptoms surface. Typically, in early osteoarthritis the patient either has no symptoms or has a mild, dull ache when he uses the affected joints, but rest relieves the discomfort. Or he may feel stiffness in the affected joint, especially in the morning. The stiffness usually lasts 15 minutes or less.

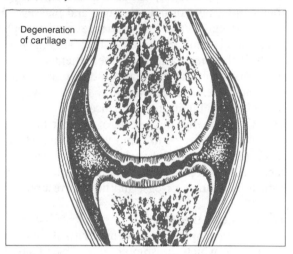

Later stage
As the disease progresses, though, whole sections of cartilage may disintegrate, osteophytes (bony spurs) form, and fragments of cartilage and bone float free in the joint. More common now, pain may arise even during rest, typically worsening throughout the day. Movement becomes increasingly limited and stiffness may persist even after limbering exercises.

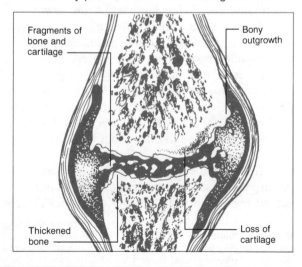

(such as diabetes mellitus), metabolic disorders (such as chondrocalcinosis), and other types of arthritis also can lead to secondary osteoarthritis.

Emphasize that the nature and severity of osteoarthritis vary from one person to another. Because of this, advise the patient not to compare his condition with the conditions of others who have osteoarthritis. For more information, see *Questions patients ask about osteoarthritis.*

Complications
Repeat, if necessary, that a prescribed treatment plan aims to alleviate pain and promote mobility. Without such treatment the patient risks both permanent loss of function and deformity in the affected joint.

Describe the diagnostic workup
Prepare the patient to undergo tests to confirm the osteoarthritis diagnosis, to evaluate the disease's underlying cause, or to monitor its progress. Explain that the doctor may order routine laboratory tests (for example, a complete blood count, a blood chemistry profile, and a urinalysis) to rule out other forms of arthritis or to detect metabolic disorders associated with secondary osteoarthritis. Accordingly, describe what happens in venipuncture and instruct the patient in how to provide a urine sample. Other scheduled tests may include X-rays, joint aspiration, magnetic resonance imaging (MRI), and a radionuclide bone scan.

X-rays
Explain to the patient that X-rays of the affected joint can detect or monitor bone erosion and deformity. Tell him who will take the X-rays and when and where they'll be taken. Add that the procedure takes only minutes although the patient may have to wait while the technician or a doctor checks the quality of the X-ray films.

Tell the patient that before having the test, he may need to remove clothing that covers the affected joint. If appropriate, instruct him to remove all jewelry from his neck, chest, and arms.

Explain that if the studies will take place in the radiology department, the patient will stand or sit in front of an X-ray machine. If they'll be taken at bedside, a nurse will help the patient to a sitting position. Then she'll place a cold, hard film plate behind the affected joint. Emphasize that he'll need to remain still for a few seconds while the X-rays are taken because movement will blur the X-ray images. Reassure him that radiation exposure remains minimal. Explain, however, that hospital personnel will leave the area while the X-rays are taken because they're potentially exposed to radiation many times a day.

Joint aspiration
In this test, a fluid sample is removed from the joint space for laboratory analysis. Tell the patient that the test takes about 10 minutes.

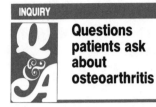

I've been a typist for 30 years. Is that why I have osteoarthritis in my hands?
It's possible. Years of excessive use may trigger secondary osteoarthritis in a joint or group of joints. That's why osteoarthritis typically affects individuals in such fields as typing, construction, and athletics. Other predisposing factors include obesity, a family history of arthritis (especially with hand and finger involvement), a history of joint injury or congenital abnormality, and certain diseases.

Will the arthritis in my knee spread to my hip?
Probably not. Osteoarthritis typically affects only one joint, usually a weight-bearing joint, such as the knee. In some cases, the disease affects several joints, but it doesn't spread in the usual sense of the word.

Will I eventually be crippled by my osteoarthritis?
Unlike rheumatoid arthritis, osteoarthritis isn't a systemic, crippling disease. Many patients with osteoarthritis have only mild symptoms that don't interfere significantly with their daily activities. By avoiding activities that increase the risk of joint injury and by following your doctor's guidelines on rest and exercise, you can help retard further deterioration of the affected joint.

At first he'll be asked to assume a position and then to remain still. After cleansing the skin over the joint, the doctor will insert a needle to withdraw fluid from the joint space. When he's done, he'll apply a small bandage to the puncture site.

If the doctor removed a lot of fluid, tell the patient that he may need to wear an elastic bandage. To prevent damaging the joint after the test, advise him to avoid using it excessively. Instruct him to contact his doctor if he has any fever or any increased pain, tenderness, swelling, warmth, or redness in his joint. Add that these signs may indicate infection if they persist after 2 days.

Magnetic resonance imaging

Inform the patient that this painless, noninvasive test relies on a powerful magnet, radio waves, and a computer to produce clear, cross-sectional images of the affected joint and the adjacent bones. Mention that the test will be done in a special laboratory that shields the MRI scanner's powerful magnetic field.

Instruct the patient to remove all jewelry and to take everything out of his pockets before the test. Emphasize that there must be no metal in the test room. The scanner's magnetic field is powerful enough to erase the magnetic strip off a credit card or to stop a watch. Instruct the patient to make sure he's notified his doctor if he has any metal inside his body—for example, a pacemaker or orthopedic pins or disks.

Advise the patient that he'll lie on a table that slides into a tunnel-like opening inside the magnet. To avoid distorted results, instruct him to breathe normally but not to talk or move during the test. Warn him that the machinery will be noisy, with sounds ranging from an incessant ping to a loud bang. He may feel claustrophobic or bored. Encourage him to relax. Suggest that he try concentrating on a favorite subject or image, or even on his breathing.

Radionuclide bone scan

Tell the patient that this painless test helps the doctor to rule out inflammatory arthritis or to monitor the progression of osteoarthritis. Name who will perform the test and when and where it will take place. For comfort's sake, advise the patient to avoid eating a full meal or drinking a lot of fluid right before the test because the test takes several hours. Instruct the patient to void before the test begins.

Explain that the doctor will wrap a tourniquet around the patient's arm before injecting a small dose of a radioactive isotope into the patient's vein. Add that the isotope emits less radiation than a standard X-ray machine. Mention that the patient will wait for 2 or 3 hours after the isotope's injected. During this time while the isotope circulates, he'll need to drink 4 to 6 glasses of fluid. Then he'll be asked to lie on a table within the radionuclide scanner. The scanner will move slowly back and forth, recording images for about 1 hour. Instruct the patient to lie as still as possible during the test. Remind him that he may be repositioned several times.

Teach about treatments

Adequate rest, an appropriate exercise program, and medication to relieve pain and reduce inflammation are the mainstays of osteoarthritis treatment. If these measures fail to control the disease's progression or to relieve pain, you may need to teach the patient about epidural block or surgery if the doctor recommends these therapies.

Activity

Perhaps more than any other treatment measure, an exercise program that balances activity and rest remains the key for restoring, maintaining, and improving joint function and for sustaining as much independence as possible. Assure the patient that together you'll plan a program to meet his needs. Add that the amount and type of recommended exercise will depend on the disease's severity, the specific joints affected, and his life-style.

Explain that exercise maintains joint mobility and muscle strength whereas rest prevents undue joint fatigue. Demonstrate how to perform full, active range-of-motion (ROM) exercises daily (as prescribed), and give the patient a copy of the teaching aid *Performing active range-of-motion exercises,* pages 622 to 624. Emphasize that his usual daily activities won't put his joints through full ROM.

Because many osteoarthritis patients—especially elderly patients—tend to hold themselves in a flexed position, encourage your patient to promote flexibility by exercising. Urge him to do extension and flexion exercises at least three times a day. These exercises can easily be performed almost anywhere—for example, if the patient's sitting in a chair, he can periodically stretch his arms.

To maintain muscle strength, show the patient how to do isometric exercises, and give him a copy of the patient-teaching aid *Doing isometric exercises,* pages 625 and 626. These exercises place little stress on the joints and require few repetitions for maximum effect. Tell the patient to count out loud during each exercise to prevent holding his breath and to get the most benefit from the exercise.

Caution the patient to avoid excessive exercise, which can increase joint inflammation. For instance, advise him to adjust his exercise program if he notices increased joint pain or swelling or decreased ROM or muscle strength. For increased joint pain or swelling, instruct him to reduce the repetitions of his exercises. For decreased ROM, however, instruct him to increase the repetitions. If these changes don't help, or if new joints become involved, advise the patient to consult the doctor. Also urge the patient to have regular checkups to monitor ROM and muscle strength.

Make sure your patient understands that rest doesn't mean

bed rest. In fact, he should avoid prolonged immobility, which will only increase joint pain and stiffness. Explain how recommended assistive or protective devices—such as reachers, splints and braces, or a crutch, cane, or walker—can rest joints and prevent stressing them during daily activity. Show the patient how to use recommended devices, as necessary. Teach him how to use relaxation techniques to reduce pain and relieve stress.

Diet
Because excess weight adds stress to already painful joints, advise the patient to follow a weight-reduction diet, if appropriate.

Medication
Drugs of choice for osteoarthritis include aspirin and other salicylates and nonsteroidal anti-inflammatory drugs (for more information, see *Teaching about drugs for osteoarthritis*). Discuss how taking these drugs before exercise can help the patient adhere to his prescribed activity program.

Procedures
Tell the patient with osteoarthritis of the lumbar spine that if drug therapy fails to relieve his pain, the doctor may perform an *epidural block*. Explain that in this procedure, the doctor injects a corticosteroid (usually methylprednisolone acetate) into the fluid sac or dura that surrounds the spinal column. Before the patient has the block, be sure to ask him if he's ever had an adverse reaction to any local anesthetic.

Inform the patient that he'll remain awake and alert during the injection. If he's nervous, however, he may be given a sedative to help him relax. Explain that the doctor will ask him to lie on his side. Then he'll insert a needle into the dura, possibly using fluoroscopy to verify proper placement. Once the needle's in place, the patient will receive a test dose of the medication. If no adverse reactions occur, he'll receive the rest of the corticosteroid, usually in small increments. Urge the patient to stay still to confine the corticosteroid and to avoid injury. Instruct him to report any pain to the doctor.

When he finishes giving the injection, the doctor will remove the needle and apply pressure over the puncture site. Tell the patient he'll need to remain lying on his side for at least 30 minutes, or longer if the doctor orders. Explain that this prevents the drug from diffusing out of the treatment area.

Before the patient goes home, help him assess the procedure's effectiveness by rating his pain. Ask him to compare his current pain level with his pain level before the epidural block. Instruct him to tell his doctor immediately if he experiences any bleeding, fainting, breathing difficulties, or decreased motor function.

Teaching about drugs for osteoarthritis

DRUG	ADVERSE REACTIONS	TEACHING POINTS
Aspirin and salicylates		
aspirin (Bayer Aspirin, Ecotrin, St. Joseph's Aspirin for Children) **aspirin and caffeine** (Anacin) **buffered aspirin** (Ascriptin, Bufferin) **choline and magnesium salicylates** (Trilisate) **magnesium salicylate** (Doan's Pills) **salsalate** (Disalcid) **sodium salicylate** (Pabalate)	• Watch for abdominal pain, breathing problems (for example, unusually rapid or deep breathing), bloody stools, bloody urine, chest tightness, confusion, hallucinations, hearing loss, seizures, severe diarrhea, severe drowsiness, severe nausea, tinnitus, uncontrollable flapping of the hands, unusual sweating, unusual thirst, visual disturbances, vomiting (especially bloody or resembling coffee grounds), and wheezing. • Other reactions include heartburn and indigestion.	• Tell the patient that this drug helps to relieve pain and joint inflammation associated with osteoarthritis. • Inform him that he may have to take this drug for 2 to 3 weeks until he experiences initial relief. • Advise him to call the doctor if the drug doesn't relieve his symptoms. Caution him not to adjust the dosage himself. • If he's on a sodium-restricted diet, inform him that buffered aspirin, effervescent tablets, and sodium salicylate may contain large amounts of sodium. • Tell him that he can chew, crush and dissolve, or swallow whole *chewable* aspirin tablets. To take *effervescent* tablets, advise him to dissolve them in water, immediately drink all of the water, then add more water to the glass and drink that also. He shouldn't crush *regular* tablets, although his pharmacist may allow the aspirin to be gently broken. To take an aspirin *suppository,* he should moisten the suppository with water or lubricant, then insert it well into the rectum. • Instruct him to take this drug with food or a full glass of water if he experiences gastric upset. • Tell him to take a missed dose as soon as he remembers. But if it's almost time for the next dose, tell him to skip the missed dose. Caution him not to double-dose. • Advise the patient to discontinue aspirin and other salicylates for 5 days before any surgery or dental work to avoid increased bleeding. • Inform him that the doctor may order biweekly serum tests until tests show that his blood contains optimal levels of the drug. • Tell him to inform the doctor if he's taking acetaminophen, other aspirin or salicylate products, such as bismuth subsalicylate (Pepto-Bismol), or cellulose-containing laxatives. • Advise against taking this drug with alcohol.
Nonsteroidal anti-inflammatory agents		
diclofenac (Voltaren) **flurbiprofen** (Ansaid) **ibuprofen** (Advil, Motrin, Nuprin) **indomethacin** (Indocin, Indocin SR) **meclofenamate** (Meclomen) **naproxen** (Anaprox, Naprosyn) **piroxicam** (Feldene) **sulindac** (Clinoril) **tolmetin** (Tolectin)	• Watch for unusual bleeding, bloody or tarry stools, bloody urine, bruises, decreased urine output, fever, rash, sore throat, wheezing, and yellowing of skin and eyes. • Other reactions include diarrhea, dizziness, drowsiness, heartburn, indigestion, nausea, and vomiting.	• Explain that this drug should help to relieve the patient's osteoarthritis symptoms and joint inflammation. • Tell the patient to take a missed dose as soon as he remembers. However, if it's almost time for the next dose, tell him to skip the missed dose. Caution him not to double-dose. • Inform him that he may have to take the drug for 2 to 3 weeks before he experiences the drug's benefits. • Suggest that he take the drug with an antacid if he experiences gastric upset. • If this drug makes him feel drowsy, recommend that he avoid driving, operating machinery, or undertaking other activities that require alertness. • Advise him not to take this drug with aspirin, acetaminophen, or alcohol. • Tell him that if he's at high risk for gastric ulcer complications, he may receive concomitant therapy with misoprostol (Cytotec).

Surgery

Although not a cornerstone of treatment, surgery may be recommended to correct deformity or to restore mobility. Typical surgical procedures include debridement, osteotomy, arthrodesis, and partial or total joint replacement.

Debridement. Tell the patient that this surgery's usually done to smooth irregular joint surfaces and to remove loose bone or cartilage particles and inflamed synovium. After surgery, the affected joint will be immobilized for a few days. Then the patient will do ROM exercises to restore joint mobility. Show the patient how to bear partial or full weight on the joint, as the doctor instructs.

Osteotomy. To correct joint misalignment, explain that the doctor may recommend an osteotomy. Usually performed on the knee, this procedure involves cutting the bone to remold the weight-bearing surfaces. Reassure the patient that osteotomy usually relieves joint pain and improves joint mobility and stability. Describe the bulky dressing and knee immobilizer that he'll wear for 2 to 3 days after surgery until swelling subsides. Also discuss the long leg cylinder cast that the doctor will apply.

Arthrodesis. Also called fusion, arthrodesis involves fusing a joint to relieve pain or to provide support. Although typically performed on the cervical or lumbar spine, this surgery also can treat other joints. After surgery, the affected joint must be immobilized until X-rays confirm healing (which usually takes from 3 to 6 months). Accordingly, prepare the patient to wear a halo vest or cervical collar (for cervical vertebrae); a brace, body cast, or clam shell cast (for other spinal vertebrae); a hip spica cast; an external fixation device; a long leg cast; or a knee immobilizer. Instruct him how to apply and care for his device.

Joint replacement. Inform the patient with severe joint pain and disability that the doctor may recommend partial or total joint replacement. Explain that this surgery involves replacing some or all of the joint with a prosthesis made of plastic or metal or both. Tell the patient that this operation can be done on all joints except those in the spine. Add that hip and knee replacements are performed most often. Results usually include pain relief and improved joint function. Urge the patient to begin his exercise program immediately to maintain joint mobility.

After a *total knee replacement,* the doctor will usually recommend continuous passive motion (CPM). Explain that this may involve using stationary, electrically controlled exercise apparatus or a series of suspended pulleys and ropes. Advise the patient also that CPM promotes healing. Explain that the degree of flexion will increase gradually until he achieves full flexion. Inform him that he probably won't be allowed out of CPM for more than 4 hours a day for meals, bathroom visits, and other activities of daily living. Add that he probably won't leave bed until 2 or 3 days after surgery. Then once he's up, introduce him to the knee immobilizer that he'll need to wear, and show him how to apply it.

After a *total hip replacement,* advise the patient to keep his hips abducted and not to cross his legs. By observing these measures, he will avoid dislocating the prosthesis. Also show him how to get in and out of bed or a chair so that he flexes his hips no more than 90 degrees. Reinforce your instruction with a copy of the patient-teaching aid *Adjusting to a total hip replacement,* pages 627 and 628. Review these guidelines with the patient. Make sure to schedule time to answer any questions.

Other care measures

Teach the patient other measures to relieve discomfort, including massage and heat or cold therapy. Heat and cold can temporarily relieve pain and increase joint ROM, making prescribed exercises easier to do. Heat also can help relieve morning stiffness.

Emphasize safety measures and use of assistive devices to compensate for restricted mobility. Mention that he can obtain aids for personal care, eating, driving, and walking, to name a few. Suggest that he consider adapting his home, if necessary. And refer him to the Arthritis Foundation for additional information and support.

Source of information and support

Arthritis Foundation
1314 Spring Street, NW, Atlanta, Ga. 30309
(404) 872-7100

Further readings

Blechman, W.J., et al. "Are You Up-to-Date on Osteoarthritis?" *Patient Care* 22(6):57-62, 69, 73-74, March 30, 1988.

Brick, G., and Poss, P. "Long-Term Follow-up of Cemented Total Hip Replacement for Osteoarthritis," *Rheumatic Disease Clinics of North America* 14(3):565-77, December 1988.

Olivo, J.L. "Developing an Exercise Program for the Elderly with Osteoarthritis," *Orthopaedic Nursing* 6(3):23-26, May-June 1987.

Rippey, R.M., et al. "Computer-Based Patient Education for Older Persons with Osteoarthritis," *Arthritis and Rheumatism* 30(8):932-35, August 1987.

Schank, J.A., et al. "Physical Therapy in the Multidisciplinary Assessment and Management of Osteoarthritis," *Clinical Therapy* 9(Suppl. B):14-23, September 1986.

Performing active range-of-motion exercises

Dear Patient:

Review the following guidelines before you begin doing active range-of-motion exercises.

Some guidelines
- Do your exercises daily to get the most benefit from them.
- Repeat each exercise three to five times or as often as your doctor recommends. (As you get stronger, he may tell you to increase your activity.)
- Impose order on your routine. If you're exercising all your major joints, begin at your neck; then work toward your toes.
- Move slowly and gently, so you don't injure yourself. If an exercise hurts, *stop doing it.* Then ask your doctor if you should keep doing that particular exercise.
- Take a break and rest after an exercise that's especially tiring.
- Consider spacing your exercises over the day if you prefer not doing them in a single session.

Neck exercise
Slowly tilt your head as far back as possible. Next, move it to the right, toward your shoulder.

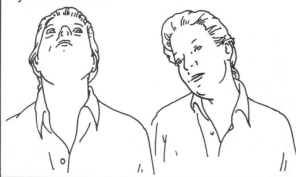

Still with your head to the right, lower your chin as far as it will go toward your chest. Then move your head toward your left shoulder. Complete a full circle by moving your head back to its usual upright position.

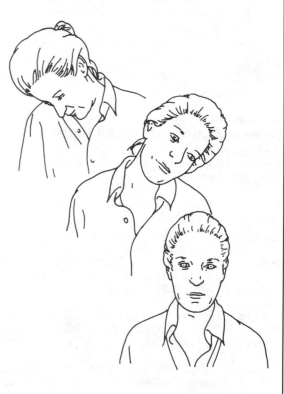

After you do the recommended number of counterclockwise circles, reverse the exercise, doing an equal number of clockwise circles.

Shoulder exercise
Raise your shoulders as if you were going to shrug. Next, move them forward, down, then up, in a single circular motion.

continued

PATIENT-TEACHING AID

Performing active range-of-motion exercises — *continued*

Now move them backward, down, then up again in a single circular motion.

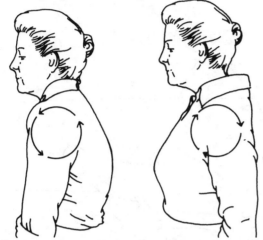

Continue to alternate forward and backward shoulder circles throughout the exercise.

Elbow exercise

Extend your arm straight out to your side. Open your hand, palm up, as if to catch a raindrop. Now, slowly reach back with your forearm so that you touch your shoulder with your fingers. Then slowly return your arm to its straight position. Now repeat with your other arm.

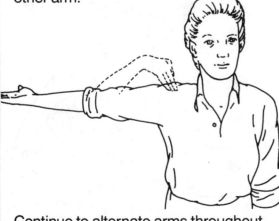

Continue to alternate arms throughout the exercise.

Wrist and hand exercise

Extend your arms, palms down and fingers straight. Keeping your palms flat, slowly raise your fingers and "point" them back toward you. Then slowly lower your fingers and "point" them as far downward as you comfortably can.

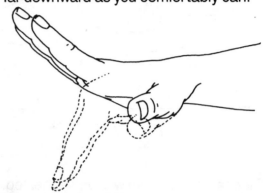

Finger exercise

Spread the fingers and thumb on each hand as wide apart as possible without causing discomfort. Then bring the fingers back together into a fist.

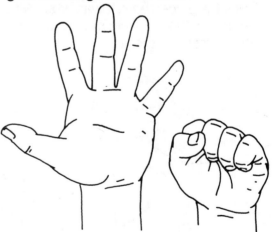

Leg and knee exercise

Lie on your bed or on the floor. Bend one leg so the knee is straight up and the foot is flat on the bed or floor.

Now, bend the other leg, raise your foot, and slowly bring your knee as far

continued

Performing active range-of-motion exercises — *continued*

toward your chest as you can without discomfort.

Then straighten this leg slowly while you lower it.

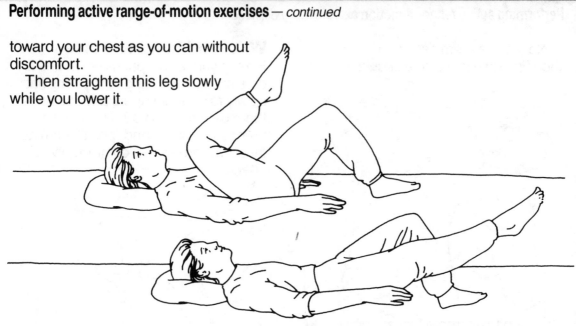

Repeat this exercise with your other leg.

Ankle and foot exercise

Raise one foot and point your toes away from you. Move this foot in a circular motion — first to the right, then to the left.

Point your toes back toward you. With your foot in this position, make a circle with it, first right, then left.

Toe exercise

Sit in a chair or lie on your bed. Stretch your legs out in front of you, with your heels resting on the floor or the bed. Slowly bend your toes down and away from you. Next, bend your toes up and back toward you. Finally, spread out your toes so that they're totally separated. Then squeeze your toes together.

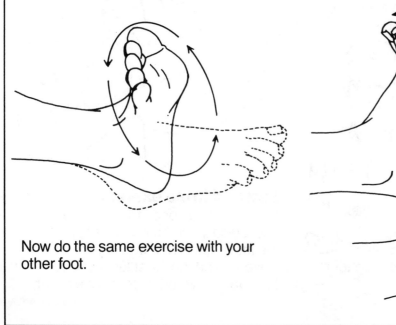

Now do the same exercise with your other foot.

Doing isometric exercises

Dear Patient:

To perform isometric exercises properly, you'll exercise against resistive force to increase the muscle-strengthening effect of the exercises. Remember to repeat each exercise as many times (typically three) as your doctor directs. Then review the following tips.

Some guidelines

In isometric exercise, you don't move your joints; instead, you contract your muscles against the resistance of a stationary object, such as a bed, a wall, or another body part. If you press your palms together (pushing with one, resisting with the other) until you feel a tightness in your chest and upper-arm muscles, you're doing a basic isometric exercise.

You don't have to be in any special position for most isometric exercises, so you can do them anytime and anywhere. Hold each contraction from 3 to 5 seconds. Repeat the entire series at least five times a day.

For the first week, don't contract your muscles fully; this will give them a chance to get used to the exercises. After that, contract them fully.

Neck exercises

● Place the heel of your right hand above your right ear. Without moving your head, neck, or arm, push your head toward your hand. Then duplicate this exercise with your left hand above your left ear.

● Clasp your fingers behind your head. Without moving your neck or hands, push your head back against your hands.

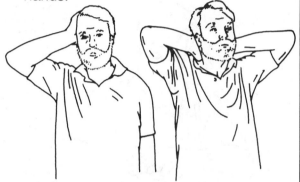

Shoulder and chest exercise

First, hold your right arm straight down at your side. Grasp your right wrist with your left hand. Then try to shrug your right shoulder, but prevent this by keeping a firm grip on your right wrist.

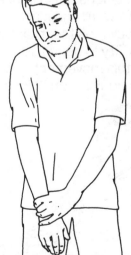

Next, do a reverse version of this exercise with your left arm and shoulder.

continued

Doing isometric exercises — *continued*

Arm exercise

With your right arm straight down at your side, bend your elbow at a 90-degree angle. Turn your right palm up and place your left fist in it. Then try to bend your right arm upward while you resist this force with your left fist.

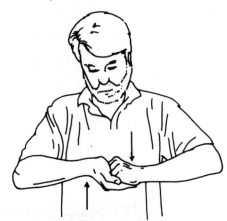

Do a reverse version of this exercise with your left arm and right fist.

Abdominal exercise

Begin by sitting on the floor or on a bed with your legs out in front of you. Then bend forward and place your hands palm down on the midfront of your thighs. Try to bend further forward, but resist this movement by pressing your palms against your thighs.

Buttocks exercise

While standing, squeeze your inner thighs and buttocks together as tightly as possible. If you're doing this exercise in bed, place a pillow between your knees to make this exercise more effective.

Thigh exercise

For leg support, sit on the floor or on a bed. With your legs completely straight, vigorously tighten the muscles above your knees so that your kneecaps move upward.

Calf exercise

Sitting up in bed, bend down and grasp your toes. Then pull gently backward, and hold this position briefly. Still touching your toes, push them forward and down as far as possible, and hold this position briefly.

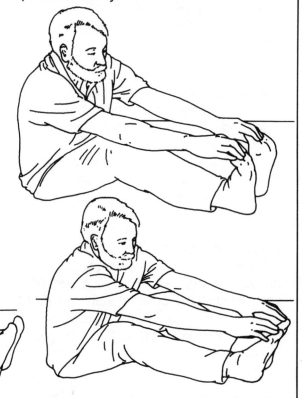

Adjusting to a total hip replacement

Dear Patient:

Your new artificial hip should eliminate hip pain and help you get around better. But go easy at first.

To give your hip time to heal and to avoid too much stress on it, follow these "do's and don'ts" for the next 3 months, or for as long as your doctor orders.

Do's
• Sit only in chairs with arms that can support you when you get up.

When you want to stand up, first ease to the edge of your chair. Place your affected leg in front of the unaffected one, which should be well under your chair. Now, grip the chair's arms firmly, and push up with your arms — not with your legs. You should be supporting most of your weight with your arms and your unaffected leg.

• Wear your support stockings (except when you're in bed at night).
• Keep your affected leg facing forward, whether you're sitting, lying down, or walking.
• Exercise regularly, as ordered. Stop exercising immediately, though, if you feel severe hip pain.
• Lie down and elevate your feet and legs if they swell after walking.
• Rent or purchase a raised toilet seat for use at home, and use public toilets designated for the disabled.
• Turn in bed only as directed by your doctor.

continued

628

Adjusting to a total hip replacement — *continued*

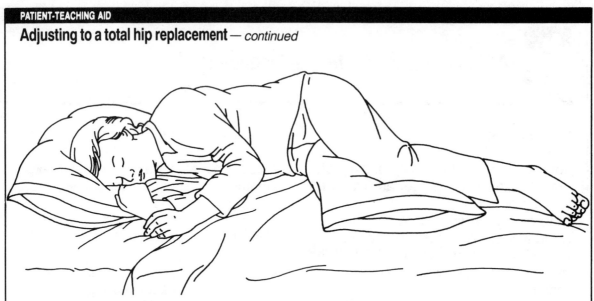

- Place a pillow between your legs when you lie on your side and when you go to bed at night. (This keeps your leg from twisting and dislodging your new hip.)
- Sit on a firm pillow when riding in a car, and keep your affected leg extended (should your knee suddenly hit the dashboard, your hip prosthesis could be dislodged).

Don'ts
Make sure not to:
- Lean far forward to stand up.
- Sit on low chairs or couches.
- Bend way over when picking up objects or tying your shoes. (To pick up dropped objects, position yourself as your therapist taught you.)
- Cross your legs or turn your hip or knee inward or outward. This could dislodge your hip. Avoid this by placing a pillow between your knees.
- Scrub your hip incision.
- Take a tub bath.
- Lift heavy items.
- Have sexual intercourse until your doctor says you can.

- Play tennis, run, jog, or do other strenuous activities.
- Drive a car.
- Reach to the end of the bed to pull the blankets up.

When to call your doctor
Call your doctor if you have:
- redness, swelling, or warmth around your incision
- drainage from your incision
- fever or chills
- severe hip pain uncontrolled by prescribed pain medicine
- sudden sharp pain and a clicking or popping sound in your joint
- leg shortening, with your foot turning outward
- loss of control over leg motion or complete loss of leg motion.

An important precaution
You'll need to take antibiotics just before and 2 days after any tooth extractions, dental procedures other than routine fillings, any other surgery, and some diagnostic procedures.

Chronic low back pain

Experts estimate that 70% to 80% of the world's population will suffer from disabling low back pain at some time in their life. What's more, once a person sustains one low back injury, the risk of reinjury rises. Because chronic back pain can have a far-reaching impact on a person's life-style and productivity, you'll need to provide comprehensive teaching about the condition.

First, you'll help the patient identify what triggers his low back pain. Then, together you'll develop strategies to help him avoid or live productively with recurrent pain. (See *Teaching about life-style changes in chronic low back pain,* page 630.) Careful instruction is crucial because the patient's progress and comfort hinge on how well he learns to care for himself and comply with treatment.

Discuss the disorder

Explain that chronic low back pain is characterized as pain that lasts for more than 6 months or that recurs every 3 months to 3 years. Inform the patient that low back pain can result from disease or injury caused by occupational hazards, stress, poor body mechanics, or other factors. Explain back anatomy to help identify possible pain sources.

Inform the patient that the *spinal column,* composed of 33 vertebrae, extends from his neckbone to his tailbone. The vertebrae are stacked one atop the other—curving S-like—providing a superstructure that supports his upright position. Identify the cervical, lumbar, and thoracic vertebrae, explaining the areas most often injured.

Tell the patient that all but the first two vertebrae have a disk between them. The disks absorb the shock generated by walking and allow for movement of the spinal column—forward, backward, and sideways. (For more information, see *Understanding the spine,* page 631.)

Explain that the spinal cord, a thick, cablelike structure about 18″ (46 cm) long, runs the length of the spine. Like a dispatcher, the spinal cord relays messages from the muscles to the brain and back again, controlling all body movement from the neck down. Spinal nerves exit from the spinal cord and enervate the arm, leg, and trunk muscles. The spinal column houses and protects the spinal cord and nerves.

Next, tell the patient about the facet joints, which also help the back move forward, backward, and sideways. Located up and

Marilyn A. Folcik, RN, BA, MPH, ONC, who wrote this chapter, is a staff development instructor in orthopedics, neurosurgery, and rehabilitation nursing, Hartford Hospital, Hartford, Conn.

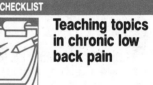

CHECKLIST

Teaching topics in chronic low back pain

☐ Explanation of back anatomy
☐ Risk factors and causes of low back pain
☐ Preparation for diagnostic tests, including laboratory tests, computed tomography and magnetic resonance imaging scans, and myelography
☐ Proper body mechanics for activities of daily living, such as standing, lifting, sitting, and driving
☐ Exercises to strengthen the back
☐ Drug therapy, including non-steroidal anti-inflammatory agents, muscle relaxants, and other medications
☐ Relaxation, physical therapy, and other pain management techniques, including massage and transcutaneous electrical nerve stimulation
☐ When to call the doctor
☐ Sources of information and support

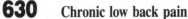

Teaching about life-style changes in chronic low back pain

How do you help the patient with chronic low back pain change his life-style to avoid further pain? One way is to follow a three-step process: First, assess the patient; second, review a standard teaching plan for chronic low back pain; and third, adapt the plan to meet the patient's needs. Here's one example.

Gather assessment data

Ivan Jacoby, a 41-year-old vice president of a large sporting goods firm, enters the outpatient clinic barely able to walk. Holding himself stiffly and grimacing as he lowers himself into a chair, he describes his low back pain brought on by raking leaves.

An avid golfer, he says he considers himself physically fit. Today, though, he moves hesitantly, and he walks with stooped shoulders. He appears to carry about 250 lb on his 6-foot frame. He recounts earlier bouts of back pain but none severe enough to keep him home from work. His first episode occurred years ago when he built an outdoor deck on his home. Mustering some enthusiasm, he relates how he lugged the lumber unassisted until his "back went out," and he had to find a helper.

But it isn't just lifting and pulling that aggravate Mr. Jacoby's condition. He says that he feels twinges of pain when he works at his desk for long periods. So far, his back hasn't bothered him on the golf course.

He states emphatically that he knows his excess weight aggravates his pain, and he intends to lose some weight to lessen the strain on his back. Clearly, Mr Jacoby's current episode of severe pain has motivated him to avoid future pain episodes.

What are Mr. Jacoby's learning needs?

What does Mr. Jacoby already know about chronic low back pain? Compare this with the contents of a standard teaching plan. Such a plan for the patient with chronic low back pain includes the following:
• basic anatomy of the lower back
• diagnostic tests, such as computed tomography and magnetic resonance imaging scans and myelography, to detect possible causes of low back pain
• a body mechanics program, focusing on proper standing, sitting, lying down, and lifting
• an exercise program to strengthen the back
• drug therapy during acute episodes of back pain
• other treatments for back pain, including a weight-loss program and relaxation techniques.

After reviewing the standard teaching plan, you decide that first you'll give Mr. Jacoby information about diagnostic tests and medication. Once he obtains pain relief, he could profit from a lesson in basic back anatomy, so that he'll understand why he's having pain and how his actions aggravate his condition.

You're sure that he'll benefit from learning how to sit, stand, and even sleep defensively. So you'll teach him proper body mechanics and special exercises, too, to help make his back less vulnerable to injury.

Because he has already committed to losing weight, you'll include information about a weight-loss diet. Now's a good time to get a baseline weight.

Mr. Jacoby did not volunteer any information regarding stress at work other than increased pain when sitting at his desk for long periods. Explore whether instructions in mental or physical relaxation techniques may be helpful.

What learning outcomes will you set?

After discussing your assessment findings with Mr. Jacoby, you and he identify specific learning outcomes. You agree that he'll be able to:

```
-describe the basic structure of his back and how
each component can contribute to low back pain
-discuss the tests he'll have and their purposes
-list medication side effects
-demonstrate proper body mechanics, for instance,
when sitting, standing, lifting, and pulling
-participate in an exercise program that
strengthens his back against injury
-plan a diet to lose weight.
```

Which teaching methods and tools will you use?

Discuss his tests and medication schedule, using illustrations and patient-teaching aids to reinforce your explanations. Then with an illustration or a model, explain back anatomy to help Mr. Jacoby picture his back and its structures. Assisted by a videotape or using yourself as an example, rehearse proper ways to sit, walk, lie down, lift, pull a rake, and push a lawn mower. Also show Mr. Jacoby the proper way to perform prescribed back exercises. Give him a printed low-calorie diet, and discuss menu planning.

How will you evaluate your teaching?

At the follow-up appointment, question Mr. Jacoby about possible adverse effects of medications he's taking. Are his body mechanics improving? Return demonstration will help you evaluate whether he's learned the correct way to sit at a desk, walk, stand tall, lie down, lift a package, or pull a rake. Can he demonstrate the proper technique for his back exercises? Have Mr. Jacoby show you lists he's developed to monitor his diet. Then, together review his food-intake record and pinpoint possible trouble spots. Weighing the patient at this time will help to document his progress. It also may be an added incentive to stick to the diet if he knows that he will be weighed at each visit.

Understanding the spine

Using an illustration or a skeletal model, identify for the patient the *lumbar* (or low back) vertebrae, explaining that this area and the *cervical* vertebrae are the most often injured. That's because these areas have few or no supportive structures. Because the lumbar vertebrae are most often used—or mis-used—during lifting, pushing, and other labors, they are at increased risk for injury. By contrast, the *thoracic* verte-brae attach to the ribs, which provide support. Thus braced, the thoracic area sustains injury less fre-quently.

Show the patient the posi-tion of the disks between the vertebrae. Explain that the disk is composed of a fluid-filled center surrounded by a tough fibrous ring.

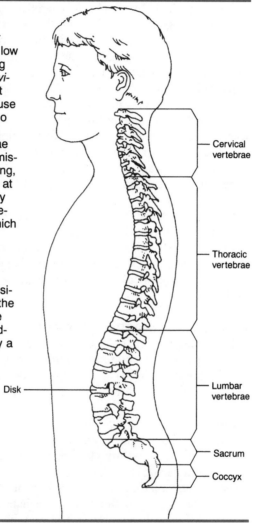

Cervical vertebrae

Thoracic vertebrae

Lumbar vertebrae

Disk

Sacrum

Coccyx

down the spine, these joints are covered with cartilage to help blood and its nutrients reach the disks.

Explain how the back ligaments, flexible bands of fibrous tis-sue, extend the length of the spinal column from vertebra to ver-tebra, creating extra stability. Finally, discuss the three layers of back muscle. The first layer, long and thin, supports the verte-brae. The second layer, broader and thicker, is used in lifting. The third layer, broad and flat, provides the strength to lift, push, carry, and pull.

Finding the pain source

As the patient begins to understand back structure, he may recog-nize the difficulties involved in identifying the primary cause of low back pain.

Injuries and inflammation. Inform the patient that injury or inflammation in any one of the spinal structures may cause pain—

What's a pinched nerve?

Tell the patient that normally spinal nerves pass through a small notch between the vertebrae. This notch can be a treacherous point on the nerves' pathway to the spinal cord. Why? Because many conditions can close off part of the notch, thereby trapping, or pinching, the nerve.

Explain that poor posture—for example, swayback—can pinch a spinal nerve by putting the vertebrae closer together. Add that tumors, broken vertebrae, or a disk problem can cause swelling in the area or shift the vertebrae's alignment and pinch the nerve, too.

Inform the patient that a pinched nerve in the lumbar spine typically causes low back pain.

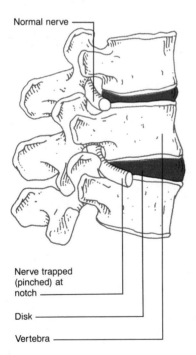

Normal nerve

Nerve trapped (pinched) at notch

Disk

Vertebra

for example, pain may result from a herniated disk, a slipped facet joint, a sprained or strained ligament, a torn muscle, or a pinched nerve (see *What's a pinched nerve?*). Other common causes include arthritis and degenerative disorders.

Psychological stress. Explain that stress results from the body's response to external events. If the patient feels pressure from his job or personal life, he may internalize it, hoping it will disappear or at least be deferred. Caution him that if he does this consistently, his body may respond by displaying physical symptoms, such as ulcers, hives, and back pain.

Tell the patient that his back muscles may tighten in response to stress, causing pain. Then a cycle begins: Stress causes tension, which causes pain, which causes more stress, and so on. Unbroken, this cycle can immobilize the patient, causing physical, personal, and job-related problems. (See *When low back pain persists.*)

Physical stress. Tell the patient that certain physical factors put him at risk for low back pain. These include poor posture and poor body mechanics, a low level of physical fitness, and certain jobs, such as a truck driver, materials handler, or nurse, that require intense physical labor or awkward positioning for prolonged periods.

Describe the diagnostic workup

Tell the patient that the doctor may order laboratory tests and imaging tests, such as computed tomography (CT) and magnetic resonance imaging (MRI) scans or, possibly, myelography to help determine the cause of chronic low back pain.

Laboratory tests

Inform the patient that laboratory tests may include a complete blood count and erythrocyte sedimentation rate, HLA-B27, and rheumatoid factor tests. Explain that these tests will help determine if a rheumatoid disease, such as arthritis, is causing the patient's back pain or if the pain is mechanical or structural in origin. A Bence Jones protein test may be ordered to rule out multiple myeloma.

Imaging tests

Tell the patient that routine X-rays can identify any structural defects that may be contributing to his back pain. Sometimes CT and MRI scans are performed to detect soft-tissue defects. Inform him that because of the complexity of the spine, these imaging studies may not reveal the exact cause of his back pain.

If the patient is having a radiologic test, tell him to remove all metallic objects, such as jewelry, from the test site. Also instruct him to report any adverse reactions, such as hives and difficulty breathing, especially for tests using a contrast medium.

CT scan. Inform the patient that a CT scan uses X-ray images to detect structural abnormalities. Mention that the test takes 30 to 60 minutes and causes little discomfort, although he may feel chilled because the equipment requires a cool environment.

When low back pain persists

Counsel your patient that chronic low back pain can lead to problems that may affect him physically, emotionally, and economically. This illustration shows some devastating effects of chronic low back pain.

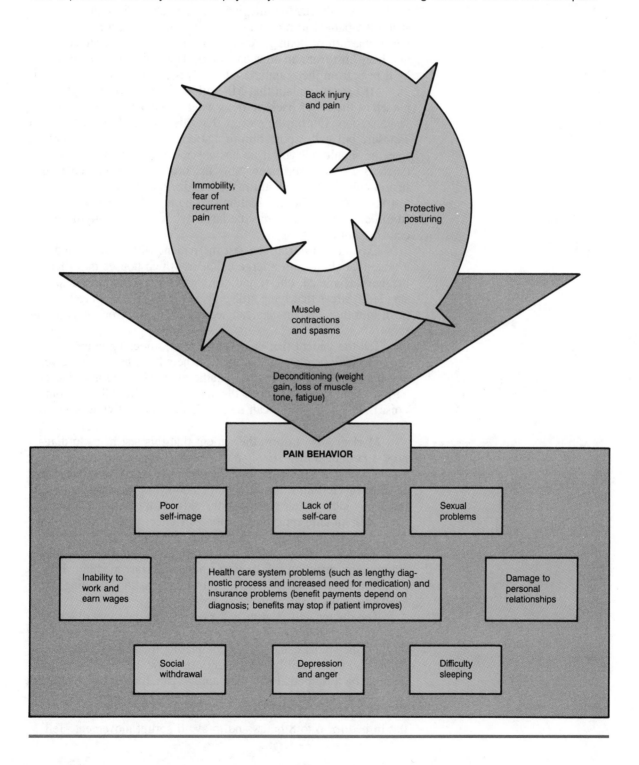

He won't be allowed food or fluids for 4 hours before the scan if the test requires using a contrast medium.

Explain that during the test he'll be positioned on an X-ray table and a strap will be placed across the body part to be scanned. This restricts his movement to ensure a clear image. The table then slides into the scanner's tubelike opening. If a contrast medium is ordered, the infusion will take about 5 minutes. Instruct the patient to report immediately any discomfort or a feeling of warmth or itching. Assure him that the technician can see and hear him from an adjacent room. Then describe the noises he'll hear from the scanner as it revolves around him.

MRI scan. Explain that MRI allows imaging of multiple planes of the lower back in areas where bone normally obscures visualization. Inform the patient that this test involves no radiation exposure but will expose him to a strong magnetic field. Therefore, he should tell you if he has any metal objects in his body (such as a pacemaker, aneurysm clip, prosthesis, or implanted infusion pump), which could make him ineligible for the test. The test takes about 1 hour. Mention that he may feel some discomfort from being enclosed within the large cylinder, especially if he's claustrophobic.

Explain that during the test the patient will be positioned on a table that slides into a large cylinder, which houses the MRI magnets. His head, chest, and arms will be restrained to help him stay still. Stress that lying still prevents blurring the images. Inform him that a technician can see and hear him from an adjacent room.

Tell the patient that he'll hear a loud, knocking noise while the machine operates. If the noise bothers him, he may be given earplugs or pads for his ears. A radio encased in the machine or earphones may help to block the sound (but he'll still hear some noise). Tell him that he can resume his normal activities after the test.

Myelography. Inform the patient that this test helps to diagnose a herniated disk. Explain that it takes about 1 hour. If he's taking a phenothiazine, he must temporarily discontinue the drug, as ordered. Tell him that he'll be positioned on his back on a tilting X-ray table. After cleansing the skin on the patient's lower back with an antiseptic, the doctor will inject an anesthetic. Warn the patient that he may feel a stinging sensation. The doctor will then insert a needle between two vertebrae of the patient's spinal column and inject an oil- or water-based contrast medium. Prepare him for a possible transient burning sensation, flushing, headache, salty taste, nausea, or vomiting.

The doctor will then take X-ray films as the table tilts vertically and then horizontally to allow the contrast medium to flow through the spinal canal. After completing the test, the doctor will withdraw the oil-based medium or allow the water-based medium to be absorbed. He'll then apply a small dressing or bandage to the puncture site.

Instruct the patient who's had an oil-based medium to remain flat in bed for 6 to 8 hours and to avoid abrupt movement. Tell him that he can resume his normal diet but that he must drink plenty of fluids. Advise him to notify the doctor if he has a headache for more than 24 hours after the test or if weakness, numbness, or tingling develops in his legs.

Teach about treatments

Inform the patient that medication is the primary treatment for acute low back pain. Otherwise, treatment mainly consists of measures to prevent recurring pain episodes. Such measures include modified ways to use the back in moving and lifting and an exercise program to strengthen and stretch the muscles that support the back. Other treatments involve weight loss, mental and physical relaxation techniques, and physical therapy.

Activity

Teach the patient proper body positions for most routine activities, such as standing, walking, sitting, driving, lying down, lifting, pulling, and pushing. Tell him that his old habits may be straining his back structure. Give him a copy of the patient-teaching aid *Using good posture to protect your back,* pages 640 and 641.

Explain that a regular exercise program will increase blood flow to the tissues and strengthen his back. Stress that appropriate exercise will help the patient stay physically and emotionally fit.

Tell the patient that most back exercises strengthen abdominal muscles, strengthen and stretch back muscles, and stretch the ligaments that attach the muscles to bone. They also keep the joints moving smoothly and help maintain the normal curvature of the spine (excessive curvature can cause back problems).

Inform the patient that the doctor may prescribe Williams flexion and McKenzie extension exercises. Warn him to perform only the ones ordered by his doctor or physical therapist, or he could risk further pain and injury. (See *Exercises for a stronger back,* pages 642 to 644.)

Advise the patient that he can participate in sports if the activity doesn't hurt his back. For example, in cycling or swimming the back doesn't absorb a lot of shock or take a pounding as it may in running or playing basketball. Suggest that he consult the physical therapist or the doctor for recommendations.

Medication

Tell the patient that the doctor may prescribe drug therapy for acute pain. Therapy commonly begins with a nonsteroidal anti-inflammatory medication and a muscle relaxant. Inform him that he may also receive acetaminophen or aspirin or other salicylates. If these drugs fail to relieve his pain, the doctor may order narcotics and tranquilizers (see *Teaching about drugs for chronic low back pain,* pages 636 to 638).

Other care measures

Recommend a weight-loss program for the overweight patient. Explain that excess weight increases stress on spinal structures. If

continued on page 638

Teaching about drugs for chronic low back pain

DRUG	ADVERSE REACTIONS	TEACHING POINTS
Aspirin and salicylates		

DRUG	ADVERSE REACTIONS	TEACHING POINTS
aspirin (Bayer Aspirin, Ecotrin, St. Joseph Aspirin for Children) **aspirin and caffeine** (Anacin) **buffered aspirin** (Ascriptin, Bufferin) **choline and magnesium salicylates** (Trilisate) **magnesium salicylate** (Doan's Pills) **salsalate** (Disalcid) **sodium salicylate** (Pabalate)	• Watch for abdominal pain, bloody stools, bloody urine, chest tightness, confusion, diaphoresis, hallucinations, hearing loss, severe diarrhea, severe drowsiness, severe nausea, seizures, thirst, tinnitus, uncontrollable flapping of the hands, unusually fast or deep breathing, visual disturbances, vomiting (containing blood or resembling coffee grounds), and wheezing. • Other reactions include heartburn and indigestion.	• Tell the patient that aspirin and other salicylates relieve mild to moderate pain. • Advise parents against giving aspirin to children without the doctor's approval. • If the drug doesn't relieve the patient's symptoms, tell him to call the doctor and not to adjust the dosage himself. • If he's on a sodium-restricted diet, inform him that buffered aspirin, effervescent tablets, and sodium salicylate may contain excessive sodium. • Tell the patient that he can chew, crush and dissolve, or swallow whole chewable aspirin tablets. To take effervescent tablets, he should dissolve them in water, immediately drink all of the water, then add more water to the glass and drink that, also. He shouldn't crush aspirin, although his pharmacist may allow the aspirin to be broken gently. To take an aspirin suppository, he should moisten the suppository with water or lubricant, then insert it well up into the rectum. • If he experiences GI upset, instruct him to take the drug with food or a full glass of water. • If he misses a dose, but remembers within an hour, advise him to take the missed dose. If he doesn't remember until later, he should skip the missed dose. Warn him not to double-dose. • Advise him to avoid aspirin and other salicylates for 5 days before any surgery or dental work to avoid increased bleeding. • Inform him that the doctor may order biweekly serum tests until optimal blood levels of the drug are achieved.
Nonnarcotic analgesic		
acetaminophen (Acephen, Anacin-3, Bromo-Seltzer, Datril, Datril-500, Tempra, Tylenol, Valadol, Valorin)	• Watch for agitation, bleeding or bruising, confusion, fatigue, stupor, weakness, and yellow skin and mucous membranes. • Other reactions include abdominal cramps and pain, bloody or cloudy urine, diarrhea, difficult or painful urination, erythema, hives, itching, loss of appetite, nausea, rash, sudden decrease in urine volume, unexplained sore throat or fever, and vomiting.	• Tell the patient that this drug relieves mild pain. Teach him how to take the prescribed form (capsules, tablets, liquids, suppositories, or effervescent granules). • Warn the patient with a history of rectal bleeding to avoid using rectal acetaminophen suppositories. If they are used, they must be retained in the rectum for at least 1 hour. • Caution him that high doses or unsupervised chronic use of acetaminophen can cause liver damage. Use of alcoholic beverages increases the risk of liver toxicity. • Tell him to avoid using the drug for a fever above 103.1° F. (39.5° C.), a fever persisting longer than 3 days, or a recurrent fever, unless directed by a doctor. • Advise patients on sodium-restricted diets to check with the doctor before taking buffered acetaminophen effervescent granules because of their high sodium content. • Tell the patient not to take nonsteroidal anti-inflammatory drugs together with acetaminophen on a regular basis. • Warn the patient to avoid taking tetracycline antibiotics within 1 hour of taking buffered acetaminophen effervescent granules. • Instruct him not to use this medication for arthritic or rheumatic conditions without notifying his doctor. This medication may relieve pain but not other symptoms. • Advise the adult patient not to take this medication more than 10 days without consulting his doctor. • Tell him to notify his doctor if symptoms don't improve or if fever lasts more than 3 days. • Advise the patient on high-dose or long-term therapy that regular visits to his doctor are essential.

continued

Teaching about drugs for chronic low back pain—*continued*

DRUG	ADVERSE REACTIONS	TEACHING POINTS
Nonsteroidal anti-inflammatory agents		
diflunisal (Dolobid) **ibuprofen** (Advil, Motrin, Nuprin) **indomethacin** (Indocin, Indocin SR) **meclofenamate** (Meclomen) **naproxen** (Anaprox, Naprosyn) **piroxicam** (Feldene) **sulindac** (Clinoril) **tolmetin** (Tolectin)	• Watch for bleeding, bloody or tarry stools, bloody urine, bruises, decreased urine output, fever, rash, sore throat, wheezing, and yellow skin and eyes. • Other reactions include diarrhea, dizziness, drowsiness, heartburn, indigestion, nausea, and vomiting.	• If the patient misses a dose, tell him to take the dose as soon as he remembers. However, if it's almost time for the next dose, tell him to skip the missed dose; warn him not to double-dose. • If he experiences GI upset, tell him to take the drug with meals or with an antacid. • If the drug makes him drowsy, advise him not to perform activities that require alertness.
Skeletal muscle relaxants		
carisoprodol (Rela, Soma)	• Watch for blurred or double vision; fever; fast, slow, or pounding heartbeat; hives; itching; rash; shortness of breath; swollen lips, tongue, and face; and wheezing. • Other reactions include dizziness, drowsiness, hiccups, nausea, stomach cramps, and vomiting.	• Explain to the patient that this drug relaxes certain muscles in his body. • If the patient misses a dose but remembers within an hour, advise him to take the missed dose. If he doesn't remember until later, he should skip the missed dose. Warn him not to double-dose. • Because this drug may cause dizziness or drowsiness, caution the patient to get out of bed and change positions slowly. Have him lie down whenever he feels dizzy. • Caution the patient not to perform tasks requiring mental or physical alertness (driving a car, for example) if he feels dizzy or drowsy.
chlorzoxazone (Paraflex, Parafon Forte DSC, Strifon Forte DSC)	• Watch for hives, itching, rash, and yellow skin and mucous membranes. • Other reactions include agitation, constipation, depression, diarrhea, dizziness, drowsiness, epigastric distress, irritability, headache, insomnia, nausea, tremor, and vomiting.	• Explain to the patient that this drug relaxes certain muscles in his body. • Caution him to avoid hazardous activities that require alertness or physical coordination until central nervous system (CNS) depression is determined. • Warn him to avoid alcoholic beverages and to use caution when taking cough and cold preparations, because they may contain alcohol or other CNS stimulants. • Advise him to take a missed dose only if remembered within 1 hour of the scheduled time. If beyond 1 hour, the patient should skip the dose and go back to his regular schedule. Warn him not to double-dose. • Instruct him not to stop taking this medication without first consulting with the doctor. • Tell him to be sure to store the drug away from direct heat or light (not in the bathroom medicine chest or in a kitchen cabinet). • Inform him that his urine may turn orange or reddish purple, but this is a harmless effect.

continued

Teaching about drugs for chronic low back pain — *continued*

DRUG	ADVERSE REACTIONS	TEACHING POINTS
Skeletal muscle relaxants — *continued*		
cyclobenzaprine (Flexeril)	• Watch for breathing difficulty, buzzing in ears, confusion, severe drowsiness, fainting, fever or decreased temperature, hallucinations, unusually fast or irregular heartbeat, hives, muscle stiffness, and severe vomiting. • Other reactions include dizziness, slight drowsiness, and dry mouth.	• Explain to the patient that this drug relaxes certain muscles in his body. • If the patient misses a dose but remembers within an hour, advise him to take the missed dose. If he doesn't remember until later, he should skip the missed dose. Warn him not to double-dose. • Because this drug may cause dizziness or drowsiness, caution him to get out of bed and change positions slowly. Have him lie down whenever he feels dizzy. Warn against driving or operating machinery when he feels this way. • If he experiences dry mouth, tell him that sucking on ice chips or sugarless candy or chewing gum may provide relief.
diazepam (Valium)	• Watch for confusion, severe drowsiness, hallucinations, hostility, insomnia, restlessness, severe weakness, slurred speech, and staggering. • Other reactions include constipation, transient drowsiness, dry mouth, nausea, vomiting, and weakness.	• Explain to the patient that this drug relaxes certain muscles in his body and should relieve muscle spasms. • Advise the patient to take the drug with food or a full glass of water. He should swallow capsules whole and not crush or chew them. • If he misses a dose but remembers within an hour, advise him to take the missed dose. If he doesn't remember until later, he should skip the missed dose. Warn him not to double-dose. • Instruct him not to drive or operate machinery when he's taking this drug. • Inform him that diazepam may be habit-forming.
methocarbamol (Robaxin)	• Watch for fever, hives, itching, and rash. • Other reactions include blurred vision, dizziness, drowsiness, headache, light-headedness, nausea, nervousness, unsteadiness, and vomiting.	• Explain to the patient that this drug relaxes certain muscles in his body. • Tell the patient that this drug can be taken by mouth or injection. For easy swallowing, instruct him to crush the tablets and mix them with food or liquid. • If he misses a dose, advise him to take it as soon as he remembers. But if it's almost time for the next dose, tell him to skip the missed dose. • If the drug makes him drowsy, instruct him not to drive or operate machinery.

the patient's excess weight contributes to a poor body image, discuss how psychological stress can increase his back pain.

Suggest the use of mental or physical relaxation techniques to alleviate psychological stress that may contribute to his pain. Explain that one common method of mental relaxation is meditation, which helps to bring the mind under conscious control. By doing this, the patient may decrease his pain by "willing it away." Caution the patient that this method doesn't work for everyone and that he may get better results by participating in some type of physical activity.

Explain several methods of physical relaxation, including exercise and physical therapy, such as massage therapy or application of a transcutaneous electrical nerve stimulation (TENS) unit.

Teach the patient other pain relief methods, including rest and the application of heat or ice.

If the female patient is planning to have a family, explain that pregnancy can add strain to the back. Pregnancy may heighten a tendency to swayback as the body's center of gravity changes, which can cause back pain. Advise the patient to avoid gaining more weight than the doctor recommends. Suggest that she learn the pelvic tilt to keep the body in its most healthful position. Mention that back pain may occur if the baby's position in the uterus compresses the sciatic nerve, but that this should disappear once the baby is born.

Advise the patient to contact the doctor if pain grows more severe, is unrelenting, or if it isn't relieved by medication, heat, ice, or rest. Instruct him to contact the doctor immediately if he experiences numbness, tingling, or weakness in an extremity, severe pain radiating down both legs simultaneously, or loss of bowel or bladder control.

Sources of information and support

International Association for the Study of Pain
909 NE 43rd Street, Suite 306, Seattle, Wash. 98105-6020
(206) 547-6409

National Committee on the Treatment of Intractable Pain
P.O. Box 9553, Friendship Station, Washington, D.C. 20016-6717
(202) 965-6717

Further readings

Fredrickson, B.E., et al. "Rehabilitation of the Patient with Chronic Back Pain: A Search for Outcome Predictors," *Spine* 13(3):351-53, March 1988.

Gottleib, H., et al. "Self-Management for Medication Reduction in Chronic Low Back Pain," *Archives of Physical Medicine and Rehabilitation* 69(6):442-48, June 1988.

Kleinke, C.L., and Spangler, A.S. "Predicting Treatment Outcome of Chronic Back Pain Patients in a Multidisciplinary Pain Clinic: Methodological Issues and Treatment Implications," *Pain* 33(1):41-48, April 1988.

Linton, S.J., et al. "The Secondary Prevention of Low Back Pain: A Controlled Study with Follow-up," *Pain* 36(2):197-207, February 1989.

Mayer, T.G., et al. "Progressive Isoinertial Lifting Evaluation: A Comparison with Isokinetic Lifting in a Disabled Chronic Low-Back Pain Industrial Population, Part 2," *Spine* 13(9):998-1002, September 1988.

McQuade, K.J., et al. "Physical Fitness and Chronic Low Back Pain: An Analysis of the Relationships Among Fitness, Functional Limitations, and Depression," *Clinical Orthopaedics and Related Research* 23(3):198-204, August 1988.

Using good posture to protect your back

Dear Patient:

Good posture is a must—whether you're standing, sitting, or lying down. It strengthens the abdominal and buttock muscles that support your hard-working back.

While practicing good posture, remember to maintain the natural curve of the spine by using muscle power, a pillow support, or a towel roll.

Standing and walking

When you're standing correctly, you should be able to draw an imaginary line from your ear through the tip of your shoulder, middle of your hip, back of your knee, and front of your ankle. You won't be able to do this if you stand with your lower back arched, your upper back stooped, or your abdomen sagging forward.

To correct your posture, stand 1 foot away from a wall. Then lean back against the wall with your knees slightly bent. Tighten your stomach and buttock muscles to tilt your pelvis back and flatten your lower back.

Holding this position, inch up the wall until you're standing. Your lower back should still be pressed against the wall. This is the posture to assume when walking.

When walking, wear rubber-soled shoes with moderate heels, if possible. Avoid changing between low and high heels. When standing longer than a few minutes, put one foot on a stool or step, switching legs as necessary for comfort.

Sitting

If possible, choose a hard, straight-backed chair to sit on. Place a towel roll or small pillow behind your lower back. Carry this back support with you when you travel.

To keep your back from tiring when you're sitting for a long time, raise one leg higher than the other by propping it on a footrest.

While you're sitting to read or knit, place a plump pillow on your lap to raise the work up to you. If you're working at a desk, slant a clipboard toward you, supporting it with books. Or sit at an artist's or a draftsman's table, if available.

continued

Using good posture to protect your back — *continued*

When driving a car, support your neck with a towel roll or a neck rest. Build it up if it feels too far back to support your neck comfortably. Position your seat low and close to the wheel so your knees are level with your hips. You should be able to reach the pedals without fully extending your legs.

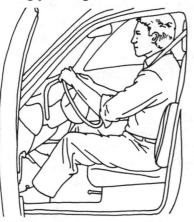

Lying down

Sleep on a firm mattress. If you must sleep on a soft mattress, support it with a bedboard or a piece of plywood placed underneath it.

The best position for sleeping is lying on your side with your knees bent and a pillow between them. This position prevents your spine from twisting when you drop your upper leg. Don't curl up excessively. This can put too much pressure on your back bones.

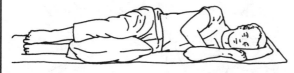

Sleeping on your back is okay if you keep a pillow under your knees or place a small pillow or rolled towel under the small of your back or both. Avoid sleeping on your stomach or on high pillows. These posi-

tions can strain your back, neck, and shoulders. Also avoid foam pillows because they don't allow complete resting support. If you read in bed, support your back and arms with pillows.

Lifting and carrying

Maintain the natural low back curve with your pelvis tucked in while lifting and carrying. Turn and face the object you want to lift. Keeping your feet flat and shoulder-width apart, bend your knees, lower yourself to the object, and place your hands around it. Keeping your knees bent and your back straight, use your arm and leg muscles (instead of your back muscles) to lift the object. Avoid lifting heavy objects above your waist.

Carry the object by holding it close to your body. Avoid carrying unbalanced loads or anything heavier than you can easily manage. Get help for large or bulky items.

Pushing and pulling

Maintain the natural low back curve with your pelvis tucked in while pushing and pulling. When raking or vacuuming, bend your knees rather than bending or twisting your back. Avoid straining to open windows or doors, and don't attempt to move heavy furniture.

Exercises for a stronger back

Dear Patient:

The doctor has prescribed special exercises to strengthen your back and help relieve your lower back pain. (They're called Williams flexion and McKenzie extension exercises.) Perform only the exercises your doctor has recommended. If you do the others, you could aggravate your back condition, causing more pain.

If your doctor approves, do each exercise 10 times every day. After 2 weeks increase each by 10 times until you are doing each exercise 30 times every day, then cut back to 30 times every other day.

Head and shoulder lift

Lying on your back with your knees bent, your feet flat on the floor, and your arms folded across your chest, lift your head and shoulders off the floor. Do not elevate your head and chest more than 45 degrees. Hold for a count of 5 and relax back to the floor.

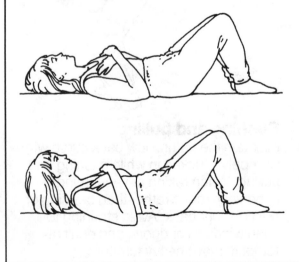

Pelvic tilt, while lying on your back

The pelvic tilt is the basic starting point for most back exercises. Lie on your back with your knees bent and your feet flat on the floor. Pull in your stomach, and pinch your buttocks together to flatten your lower back to the floor. Hold for a count of 5 and relax.

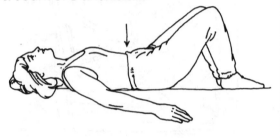

Foot flex and leg lift

Lie on your back with your knees bent and your feet flat on the floor. Straighten one knee without moving your thighs. Then bend (flex) the foot of the straight leg toward your head.

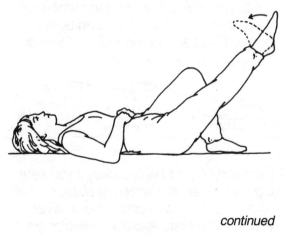

continued

Exercises for a stronger back — *continued*

Next, lift your straight leg as far as you can, keeping the knee straight and the foot flexed toward your head.

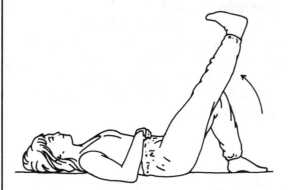

Hold for a count of 5, lower the straight leg, relax your foot, and bend your knee until the foot is flat on the floor. Perform the exercise with the other leg, too.

Foot flex and bent leg lift
Lie on your back with one knee bent so that the foot is flat on the floor. Hold the other leg firmly to your chest with your hands under the knee. First, bend (flex) your elevated foot toward your head.

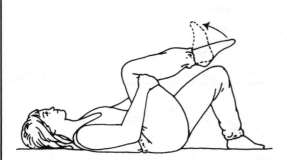

Then straighten that leg, keeping your thigh close to your chest.

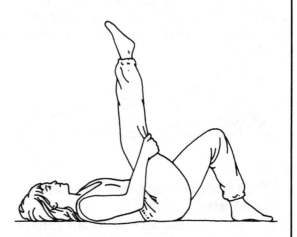

Hold for a count of 5 and relax to the starting position. Do the same exercise with the other leg.

Leg stretches
Hold the ends of a towel in each hand, place your foot against the middle of the towel, and extend your leg to stretch out your hamstring muscles. Then do the same stretching exercise with your other leg.

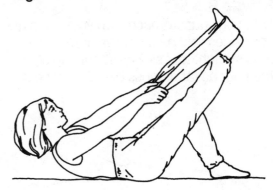

continued

PATIENT-TEACHING AID

Exercises for a stronger back — *continued*

The pelvic tilt, while lying on your stomach

Lying on your stomach with your hands at your sides, tighten your buttocks as much as you can. Hold for a count of 5 and relax.

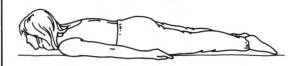

Shoulder blade squeeze with head and chest lift

Lying on your stomach with your arms at your sides and palms down, squeeze your shoulder blades together, and raise your head and chest as far as you can. Hold for a count of 5 and relax.

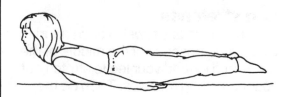

Single leg lift

Lying on your stomach with your arms at your sides and palms down, keep your legs straight and slowly lift one leg off the floor as far as possible. Do not hold

the position. Return your leg slowly to the floor, and perform the exercise with the other leg.

Double leg lift

Lying on your stomach with your arms at your sides and palms down, keep your legs straight and raise both of them off the floor together as far as possible. Do not hold the position. Return your legs *slowly* to the floor.

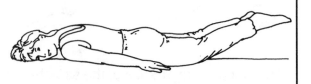

Alternate arm and leg lift

Lying on your stomach with your arms extended past your head and palms down, raise one arm and the opposite leg from the floor as high as possible without bending either. Do not hold the position. Return your arm and leg *slowly* to the floor. Perform the exercise with the other arm and leg.

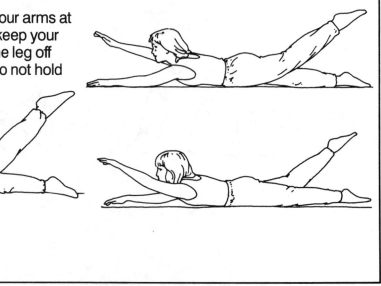

Scoliosis

Affecting nearly 4% of school-aged children, scoliosis is identified most often during the adolescent growth spurt between ages 10 and 13. The disorder appears equally in boys and girls; however, spinal curve progression is more common in girls.

Because early detection and follow-up are critical in treating scoliosis, your teaching should focus on two areas. The first consists of alerting parents to scoliosis signs to prevent progression. The second involves helping children and their parents manage the disorder—with observation if scoliosis is mild or with a brace and sometimes surgery if the curve progresses. If necessary, you'll discuss potential health problems and physical deformity to encourage scrupulous compliance with treatment.

In families with a history of scoliosis, parents may already be screening their children carefully. Even so, they probably have many questions and will need careful teaching to clear up any misconceptions about the disorder and its treatment. Parents unfamiliar with scoliosis may need more extensive teaching.

In any case, be prepared to encourage and support patients and parents—possibly through years of treatment. Parents may need reassurance, especially if they blame themselves for their child's disorder. Adolescent patients may need extra reassurance, especially if scoliosis makes them feel different from their peers.

Discuss the disorder
Teach the patient and his parents that scoliosis refers to a lateral curvature of the spine in which vertebrae rotate into the convexity of the curve. This rotation causes rib prominence in the thoracic spine and waist asymmetry in the lumbar spine. (For more information, see *Spinal curvature: Normal and abnormal,* page 646.) Explain that scoliosis can affect the spine at any level but that right thoracic curves occur most commonly.

Inform the patient that scoliosis can be classified as nonstructural or structural or by age of onset (see *Classifying scoliosis by age,* page 647).

Nonstructural or structural scoliosis
In *nonstructural scoliosis,* the spinal curve appears flexible, straightening temporarily when the patient leans sideways. It's commonly related to leg-length discrepancies, posture, paraspinal inflammation, or acute disk disease. In contrast, *structural scoliosis* is a fixed deformity that doesn't correct itself when the pa-

---

Hannah Brosnan, RN, MS, a clinical nurse specialist in orthopedics, wrote this chapter. Ms. Brosnan is an instructor at the College of Nursing, Rush University, Rush Presbyterian–St. Luke's Medical Center, Chicago.

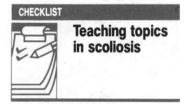

CHECKLIST

Teaching topics in scoliosis

☐ Comparison of a normal spine and a scoliotic spine
☐ Scoliosis classifications, including infantile, juvenile, and adolescent; nonstructural and structural (idiopathic, congenital, and neuromuscular)
☐ Potential complications of untreated scoliosis and importance of follow-up care
☐ Diagnostic tests, such as school screening, X-ray and bone growth studies, and integrated shape imaging system tests
☐ Braces used for scoliosis and tips for adjusting to them
☐ Surgery—spinal fusion and instrumentation
☐ Observation for mild scoliosis
☐ Sources of information and support

Spinal curvature: Normal and abnormal

When describing scoliosis to your patient, use pictures to compare the normal spine with the scoliotic spine.

The normal spine

Point out normal spinal curvatures. For example, in the sagittal plane (lateral view), the cervical spine has a slight anterior or forward curve (called lordosis), and the thoracic spine has a slight posterior or backward curve (called kyphosis). The lumbar spine curves slightly forward also. Explain that this alignment provides symmetry, an upright position, and flexibility.

The scoliotic spine

In contrast, identify how scoliosis disturbs normal alignment and symmetry. For instance, as the spine curves and the thoracic vertebrae rotate, the ribs nearest the curve's convexity become more prominent than the ribs on the opposite side. Likewise, lumbar vertebral rotation accounts for unilateral waist fullness.

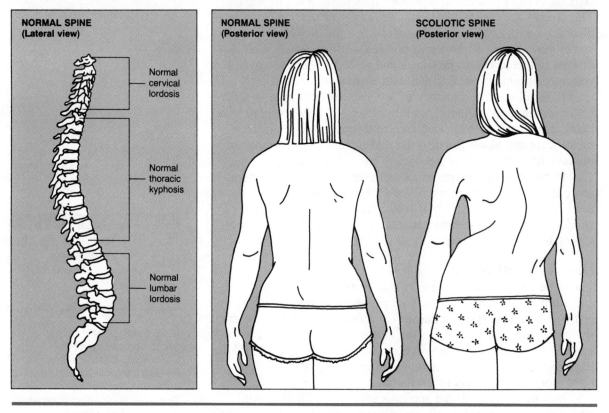

NORMAL SPINE (Lateral view)
- Normal cervical lordosis
- Normal thoracic kyphosis
- Normal lumbar lordosis

NORMAL SPINE (Posterior view)

SCOLIOTIC SPINE (Posterior view)

tient leans sideways. Spinal X-rays may show vertebral body rotation and wedging. This type of scoliosis may have no known cause (called idiopathic scoliosis). It may be congenital or be related to a neuromuscular problem.

Idiopathic scoliosis. Tell the patient and his parents that this most common type of scoliosis affects otherwise healthy children for no known reason. Mention that some researchers believe that parents with idiopathic scoliosis have a 25% chance of passing the problem on to their children.

Congenital scoliosis. Explain that in congenital structural scoliosis, the vertebrae or the rib cage develop abnormally before birth, leaving the spine with a potential for curving. Common abnormalities include wedge-shaped and block (unseparated) vertebrae. Spinal abnormalities can occur separately or together to cause abnormal curvature, and sometimes multiple spinal abnormalities balance each other, making treatment unnecessary.

Neuromuscular scoliosis. Inform the patient that weakened muscles surrounding the spine may cause neuromuscular scoliosis. For instance, a patient with Duchenne type muscular dystrophy (marked by a long, C-shaped spinal curve), polio, cerebral palsy, or spinal muscular atrophy may also have neuromuscular scoliosis.

Other causes
Explain that some types of scoliosis fit no specific category, such as scoliosis resulting from neurofibromatosis (Recklinghausen's disease). Typically, the patient has a short, sharp-angled, rigid spinal curve that eventually requires surgical stabilization. Rarely, scoliosis may be radiation-induced or caused by trauma, degeneration, or benign osteoid osteoma. Radiation-induced scoliosis may occur in growing children who've been treated with radiation for a tumor condition. Traumatic scoliosis may stem from vertebral fractures or disk disease. Degenerative scoliosis may develop in older patients with osteoporosis and degenerative joint disease of the spine. And benign osteoid osteoma may develop in a child. Because of paraspinal inflammation, this patient may experience painful scoliosis.

Complications
Advise the patient and his parents that untreated or inadequately treated extreme spinal curvature can eventually result in debilitating back pain, severe deformity, and other complications. For example, thoracic curves exceeding 60 degrees result in decreased pulmonary function. Worse yet, thoracic curves exceeding 80 degrees heighten the risk for cor pulmonale in middle age. Besides affecting physical health, advanced scoliosis can affect the patient's socioeconomic well-being—many employers, fearing potential liability, prefer not to hire a person with back problems.

Describe the diagnostic workup
Discuss the tests that detect and monitor scoliosis. Include school screening, X-ray films, and the integrated shape imaging system (ISIS) test. Because most patients are children, take special care to explain exactly what happens during tests. Be brief, and use terms that children understand.

School screening
In most states, specially trained examiners screen school children between ages 11 and 14 (grades 5 through 9) for scoliosis signs (see *A simple test for scoliosis,* page 648). If the examiner suspects the disorder, she refers the child for follow-up medical care.

School screening may or may not include testing with a scoliometer, a hand-held, oblong, gauged instrument that measures degrees of spinal curvature. Explain that the examiner moves the scoliometer over the spine as the patient bends forward. She

---

Classifying scoliosis by age

Inform parents that children risk developing scoliosis for as long as the spine continues growing. Explain that scoliosis is classified by age of onset as infantile, juvenile, or adolescent.

Infantile scoliosis occurs most often in boys ages 1 to 3. The disorder may resolve spontaneously, or it may progress and require treatment.

Juvenile scoliosis equally affects boys and girls ages 3 to 10. The disorder usually requires long-term follow-up and treatment during these peak growing years.

Adolescent scoliosis occurs after age 10 and during adolescence. Typically, curves progress more markedly in girls than in boys. In girls, they more commonly require treatment.

A simple test for scoliosis

Explain to the patient that a brief examination can detect signs of scoliosis. In this examination, the patient removes her shirt and stands as straight as she can with her back to the examiner, putting her weight evenly on each foot. While she does this, the examiner observes both sides of the patient's back from neck to buttocks, checking for these signs:
• uneven shoulder height and shoulder blade prominence
• unequal distance between the arms and the body
• asymmetrical waistline
• uneven hip height
• a sideways lean.

Next, with the patient's back still facing the examiner, the patient does the "forward-bend" test. The examiner instructs the patient to place her palms together and slowly bend forward, reminding her to keep her head down. As she complies, the examiner checks for these signs:
• asymmetrical thoracic spine or prominent rib cage (rib hump) on either side
• asymmetrical waistline.

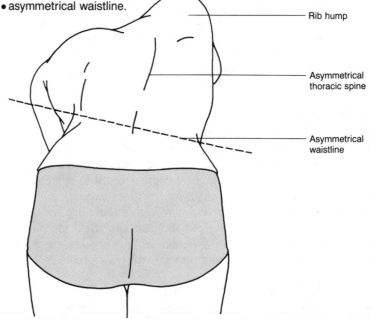

Rib hump

Asymmetrical thoracic spine

Asymmetrical waistline

watches the gauge carefully at the thoracic and lumbar areas. As the device passes along a curve, a metal ball in the gauge swings right or left to register the degree of curvature. If the curve measures more than 5 degrees, the examiner recommends further evaluation.

Spinal X-rays

Inform the patient and the family that X-ray films of the spine remain the standard method for detecting and confirming scoliosis. They also help the doctor determine the bone's maturity and predict remaining bone growth. Emphasize the importance of bone maturity. (For more information, see *Seeking signs of bone*

Seeking signs of bone maturity

Explain to the patient that the less mature his bones, the greater the likelihood that scoliosis will progress. So before deciding on treatment, the doctor takes X-ray films to determine the maturity of the patient's spine.

Tell the patient that the doctor looks for radiographic evidence of excursion of the iliac apophyses (called the Rissor sign). As the bones mature, the osseous centers of the iliac crest move posteromedially toward the sacrum. When the excursion covers the iliac crest and fuses, the bones are mature.

Posteromedial movement of iliac crest   **Excursion complete**   **Maturation complete**

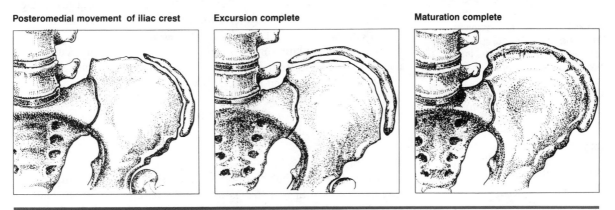

maturity.) Explain that the thoracic and lumbar vertebral end plates can also yield information about maturity. When the end plates unite with the vertebral body, maturity is complete.

If the patient's never had X-ray films taken, explain that the technician will take X-ray films of the spine while the patient stands and again while he bends laterally. The technician will also take X-ray films of the thoracolumbar spine from the front and from the back (anteroposterior view). From this view, the doctor can compute the degree of spinal curvature—the Cobb angle (see *Computing the Cobb angle,* page 650). In follow-up studies, he'll chart the curve's progression or stability. X-ray studies can also identify curve flexibility and can show whether the patient has nonstructural or structural scoliosis.

Bone growth studies

Tell the patient and his parents that the doctor may order X-ray films of the hand for more information about bone maturity. A growing child's hand has multiple growth plates, which serve as good indicators of overall bone growth. By comparing the patient's bone growth with established standards, the doctor can estimate whether chronological and skeletal age match.

ISIS test

If the patient's having an ISIS test, reassure him that this test uses no radiation, causes no pain, and requires little time. Explain that he'll remove his clothing from the waist up and stand within a stabilizing, H-shaped metal frame. Then the nurse or technician will place small, disposable markers on his spine over the spinous processes. He'll remain standing during the test. Next, a scanner

Computing the Cobb angle

Inform the patient with scoliosis that the doctor identifies the curvature angle from a spinal X-ray.

First he locates the curve's top vertebra (T6 in the illustration). This is the uppermost vertebra whose upper face tilts toward the curve's concave side. Then he finds the curve's bottom vertebra (T12). This is the lowest vertebra whose lower face tilts toward the curve's concave side.

The angle at which perpendicular lines (drawn from the top vertebra's upper face and bottom vertebra's lower face) intersect reflects the curvature angle — or the Cobb angle.

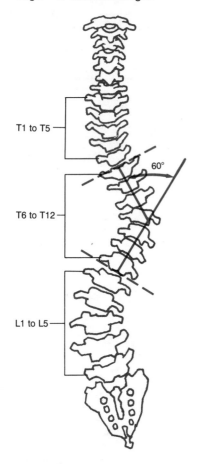

T1 to T5

60°

T6 to T12

L1 to L5

will direct a light beam along the markers on his spine. Finally, transformed by a computer into a printout, the scanned information will depict a surface image of the patient's spine and back shape (see *Explaining ISIS*).

Teach about treatments

Advise the patient and his family that the usual scoliosis treatments include observation, a brace, and surgery. The doctor chooses and combines these treatments based on the curve's angle, the patient's bone maturity, and the risk of curve progression.

Because scoliosis typically affects adolescents, you'll need to devise teaching plans that motivate teenagers to comply with treatment—even if the treatment consists of watching the curve until it stabilizes or requires more aggressive measures. Keep in mind that adolescents may delay or resist treatment, not wanting to be "different" from their peers and not fully appreciating possible scoliosis complications.

Procedures

Inform the patient that bracing is the most common nonsurgical treatment procedure. If the patient or his parents ask about lateral electrical surface stimulation (LESS), explain that this treatment is less common (and is also controversial) because bracing provides more predictable and more consistent results.

Bracing. Rarely used for adults (except after surgery), bracing is typically recommended for patients who have a 20-degree curve or more and who have a substantial growth period remaining. State clearly that bracing can't straighten the spine. It may, however, prevent the curve's progression during the growing years—making surgery unnecessary in later years. Emphasize the long-term patient commitment required for effective bracing.

Discuss braces used to control scoliosis, explaining that the doctor will determine the type of brace and the number of hours a day the patient will need to wear it (see *Braces for scoliosis*, page 652). Once the patient has the brace, describe how it works.

Also discuss activity restrictions. Tell the patient that once he's used to the brace, he should be able to ride a bike, run, jump, and participate in most school or team sports—depending on his doctor's recommendations. However, he may have to come out of his brace while doing some strenuous activities, such as gymnastics or skiing.

Explain to the patient that he'll learn to do special exercises while wearing the brace. These include stretches to maintain flexibility and pelvic tilts to strengthen the stomach muscles. He'll also learn how to "work with the brace" by pulling his body away from the curve (or away from the brace pads).

Inform the patient that adjusting to a brace also requires making changes in diet and skin care. Shaped to fit his body exactly, the brace may feel snug at first, especially during meals. Advise him to loosen it for 30 minutes after a meal. Or suggest that eating smaller meals and snacking more often may help. Also show him how to prevent skin irritation at pressure points under

Explaining ISIS

If your patient's having an integrated shape imaging system (ISIS) examination, show him the end result—a printout. Explain that this three-part document records curves in the surface image of the back. What's more, it helps the doctor estimate the degree of spinal curve without using X-ray radiation. The illustration below represents a typical printout of ISIS test results.

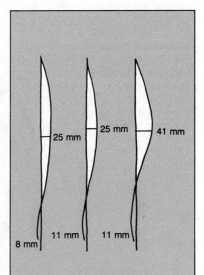

This computer image depicts the degree of spinal asymmetry in a forward-bending patient. The back's asymmetry is depicted in degrees on the scale at right.

This posterior spinal view clearly shows waist and shoulder asymmetry. The curved line in the center is the spine; the slanted lines show the tilt angles. Measurements for the curve form part of the printout.

These computer images show three different lateral views of the back's shape—right, middle, and left. They represent the asymmetry of the back's sagittal contour in millimeters.

the brace. Make sure to offer him the patient-teaching aid *Adjusting to your brace,* page 656.

Last, encourage the patient to voice his feelings about wearing a brace and about being "different." Acknowledge his feelings, yet affirm the benefits of complying with treatment. If the patient and his parents express interest, arrange a meeting with another family or a support group that has experienced bracing for scoliosis.

Lateral electrical surface stimulation
If the patient undergoes LESS, explain that this treatment works while the patient sleeps. Each night the patient will have electrodes placed on his paraspinal muscles. The electrodes lead to a battery pack that the patient wears to bed. As the patient sleeps, the device stimulates the paraspinal muscles with a mild electrical charge. This current "pulls" the muscles away from the curve—theoretically preventing curve progression.

Surgery
If bracing or other measures don't prevent progression or if the

Braces for scoliosis

Explain that the doctor may order a brace during the patient's growing years to prevent the spinal curve from progressing and possibly to avoid surgery.

Point out that these braces apply dynamic physical forces to control a deformity. Commonly used braces include the Milwaukee brace, the Lyon brace, and the Boston brace.

If the doctor has ordered a brace, such as the thoracolumbar sacral orthosis (TLSO), to be worn after surgery, explain that this brace supplies added stability while the spine heals.

Milwaukee brace
This brace helps control high thoracic scoliotic curves and kyphosis. The Milwaukee brace extends from the hip area to the chin and imposes a stretched, upright posture.

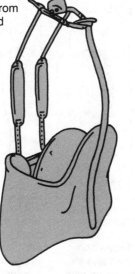

Lyon brace
To control thoracic and lumbar curves (or thoracolumbar curves), the doctor may order a Lyon brace, the most commonly used device. Similar to the Milwaukee brace in the hip and waist areas, the Lyon brace extends to the underarms but not to the neck. Pads placed on the brace over the curve's convexity supply external force to prevent curve progression.

Boston brace
Used for lower thoracolumbar curves and lumbar curves, this device fits over the hips, waist, and some of the trunk. It also pads the curve's convexity to prevent progression.

Thoracolumbar sacral orthosis
Used to immobilize the spine after surgery, the TLSO is molded to a cast of the patient's body. This bivalved brace has two closures on each side and an abdominal opening to allow for normal expansion.

spine curves 50 degrees or more, the doctor may recommend surgery. Typically, this involves spinal fusion with instrumentation. These procedures prevent progression by stabilizing or partially correcting the curve—without damaging the spinal cord and nerves. Reassure the patient and his family that improved anesthesia techniques, advanced technology, and preoperative planning add to surgical safety.

What happens before surgery. Inform the patient that he'll do preoperative mobilization exercises to promote flexibility. Explain that the doctor tailors the exercise plan to the patient, but most exercises involve stretching, bending, and doing pelvic tilts. Also make sure to give the usual preoperative instructions. For instance, tell him he'll receive a general anesthetic, so he won't be allowed any food or beverages after midnight before the operation. Inform him also that the surgical site may be shaved. Also inform him that he will need blood for surgery. Mention that the best blood for this elective surgery is his own blood. In general, the patient may donate between 6 and 10 units, depending on how much blood his doctor estimates he will need. Explain that he may bank about 1 unit of blood bimonthly. Add that he may need iron supplements during this time. Then describe the operation.

What happens during surgery. Explain that the surgeon will fuse the curved portion of the patient's spine in a partially corrected position and insert a metal, rodlike instrument to maintain correction until the fusion heals (see *Reviewing spinal surgery and instrumentation,* page 654).

What happens after surgery. Alert the patient that he'll return from surgery with various tubes and drains in place, including an indwelling catheter and an I.V. line. Assure him that he'll receive adequate medication for pain relief.

For the first day after surgery, he's likely to have complete bed rest. Then he'll gradually increase his activity. As his condition improves, the nurse will remove any tubes and drains. About 5 or 6 days after surgery, an immobilizing brace may be molded for him to wear for added stability while the spine heals. Called a thoracolumbar sacral orthosis (TLSO), this molded brace may be worn for up to 7 months. If the patient's an adolescent, the doctor may not order a brace if he thinks the surgical instrumentation provides sufficient stability. The patient may also begin physical therapy with mild upper- and lower-extremity exercise and stair walking.

Tell the patient that he'll be discharged about 10 to 12 days after surgery. (Some patients—children, usually—can go home sooner.) If the patient had a two-stage surgery (involving anterior and posterior incisions), he'll stay in the hospital longer. The surgeon usually schedules two-stage operations from 7 to 10 days apart.

Before discharge, teach the patient to recognize signs of infection—fever and redness, swelling, and tenderness at the incision site. Instruct him to call the doctor if he suspects an infection.

Activity restrictions. Most children recovering from surgery will stay home from school for 4 to 6 weeks. Most adults will stay home from work for 2 to 3 months, depending on their occupation. Caution the patient to avoid extreme bending, twisting, or stooping during the first 2 months and not to lift more than 10 lb (after 2 months, he can generally lift up to 25 lb).

During the patient's first 2 weeks at home, advise him to rest frequently, pacing himself. Suggest a general increase in activities as tolerated. By his first follow-up doctor's visit, he should be walking 1 to 2 blocks a day. He should also continue doing the mild strengthening exercises he learned in the hospital. Instruct a sexually active patient to support his back during sexual intercourse, either by lying supine or by lying on his side. Add that most patients don't feel well enough for sex until 4 to 6 weeks after surgery.

Diet modification. Advise the patient to consume foods containing iron, such as spinach, broccoli, and red meat, to build up his blood counts. And suggest he have dairy products three or four times daily. Explain that he needs adequate calcium to promote bone healing. Explain further that fresh fruits, vegetables, bran, and other fibrous foods will help prevent constipation. Add

Reviewing spinal surgery and instrumentation

If the patient's scheduled for spinal surgery, give him a careful explanation of his operation—spinal fusion combined with instrumentation. As appropriate, review the selected instrumentation systems described below.

Spinal fusion
To prevent spinal curves from progressing, the surgeon performs a spinal fusion (arthrodesis) by stripping the paraspinal muscles from the spinal area to be fused and by decorticating the bone. Then he obtains a bone graft—usually from the iliac crest—to place along the fusion area. After healing is complete, the fusion mass prevents the spine from curving further.

For a curve caused by a congenital defect, spinal fusion may be all that's needed. Usually, however, the surgeon combines fusion with instrumentation. The type of instrumentation depends on the patient, the curve's degree and location, and the surgeon's preference.

If appropriate, review instrumentation with your patient. Explain that surgeons may use instrumentation for young patients with curves ranging over 45 degrees and for adult patients with curve progression.

Harrington rod
To hold the spine in the corrected position, the surgeon combines spinal fusion with insertion of a Harrington rod. This device relies on distraction to correct the curve. Explain that the surgeon aligns the instrument—two hooks and a rod—along the spine through an incision on the patient's back.

If the fusion doesn't heal well, the rod may crack or a hook may come loose, requiring further surgery. Attaching the rod to only two points on the spine slows the rate at which most patients can return to activity. And patients must wear a brace—a thoracolumbar sacral orthosis—for about 7 months after surgery.

Luque rod
Explain that the surgeon may use Luque rod (also called L-rod) instrumentation for patients with paralytic or neuromuscular curves. He fixes this metal rod and wiring to multiple points on the patient's spine to increase stability. However, the risk of neurologic damage increases because he must thread the wires under the vertebral laminae near the neural elements.

Cotrel Dubousset technique
This technique involves placing a series of rods and hooks to distract, compress, and derotate the spine. Cross-linking devices provide further stability. Tell the patient that this apparatus can be adapted to normal sagittal spinal alignment and lumbar lordosis. Because the surgeon attaches it to many points, the patient may not need to wear a brace after the operation.

Zielke instrumentation
Zielke instrumentation is attached to the spine with screws and cables. Through an anterolateral incision, the surgeon removes the involved intervertebral disks. Then he excises a rib and chops it into small blocks, which he places in the intervertebral spaces. Then he tightens the cable to obtain correction. This instrumentation may be used alone or combined with the second stage of the operation to treat a double spinal curve. Advise the patient that he may have to wear a brace for about 7 months after this surgery.

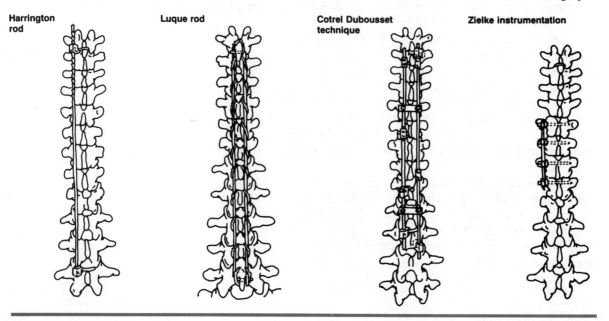

Harrington rod   **Luque rod**   **Cotrel Dubousset technique**   **Zielke instrumentation**

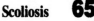

that irregularity may result from decreased physical activity, iron supplements, and some pain medications.

Emotional changes. Last, prepare the patient to deal with possible mood changes or depression after surgery. Adult patients, especially, may worry about their jobs or their households. What's more, they may fear becoming overly dependent on friends and family members. Younger patients may feel bored or depressed from inactivity. Encourage patients and families to express their fears and concerns, and offer them information and support.

Other care measures

Most patients with mild scoliosis require no treatment other than observation and reevaluation. In most cases, the patient with a spinal curve measuring 20 degrees or less simply has an examination every 4 to 6 months for several years to be sure the curve doesn't progress. If the curve progresses between 5 and 10 degrees and if the patient's still growing, the doctor may recommend bracing.

Reassure the patient under observation that he may participate in any school or recreational activities. The doctor may prescribe an exercise program that includes pelvic tilts, spine hyperextension, push-ups, and breathing exercises to strengthen torso muscles. Then dispel any myths he or his parents may have about exercise. Confirm that exercise alone won't eliminate the curve or stop scoliosis from progressing.

Sources of information and support

National Scoliosis Foundation
93 Concord Avenue, P.O. Box 547, Belmont, Mass. 02178
(617) 489-0880

Scoliosis Association
P.O. Box 51353, Raleigh, N.C. 27609
(919) 846-2639

Further readings

Block, C.E. "Scoliosis: School Screening Specifics," *School Nurse* 4(2):7-10, March-April 1988.

Bridwell, K.H. "Cotrel Dubousset Instrumentation," *Orthopaedic Nursing* 7(1):11-16, January-February 1988.

Francis, R.S. "Scoliosis Screening of 3,000 College-aged Women: The Utah Study—Phase 2," *Physical Therapy* 68(10):1513-16, October 1988.

Lonstein, J.E., and Winter, R.B. "Adolescent Idiopathic Scoliosis: Nonoperative Treatment," *Orthopedic Clinics of North America* 19(2):239-46, April 1988.

Poussa, M., et al. "Spinal Mobility in Adolescent Girls with Idiopathic Scoliosis and in Structurally Normal Controls," *Spine* 14(2):217-19, February 1989.

Rodts, M.F. "Surgical Interventions for Adult Scoliosis," *Orthopaedic Nursing* 6(6):11-17, November-December 1987.

Voznak, L. "My Life with Scoliosis," *Orthopaedic Nursing* 7(1):22-26, January-February 1988.

Weisz, I., et al. "Back Shape in Brace Treatment of Idiopathic Scoliosis," *Clinical Orthopaedics and Related Research* (240):157-63, March 1989.

Adjusting to your brace

Dear Patient:

Now that you have a brace to help control scoliosis, here are some tips to help you wear it more comfortably and effectively.

Getting used to your brace
Adjusting to your brace may take about 2 weeks. Don't be discouraged if it feels awkward at first. As you gradually build up to wearing the brace full time (the time your doctor recommends), it will feel more natural.

Caring for your skin
Wear your brace just the way your nurse and doctor say. If you wear it incorrectly, you can irritate your skin. Always wear a soft, snug undershirt between your brace and your skin. A loose one can wrinkle under the brace and irritate your skin.

LYON BRACE

Change your undershirt at least once a day and more often if you perspire. This will help you avoid skin irritation or acne.

Watch your skin for red marks or other irritation whenever you remove your brace. Especially check the skin under the brace pads and over your hip bones. Apply rubbing alcohol to these areas regularly to toughen your skin and help prevent blistering and skin breakdown. Don't apply lotions or powders to the skin under your brace.

Wash your brace with mild soap and water every few days. And make sure it's dry before you put it back on.

Dressing to cover the brace
If your usual clothing doesn't fit over the brace, look for looser-fitting clothing.

If your brace's metal hardware tears your clothing, cover the metal parts with moleskin (available at drugstores).

Resuming activities
Once your brace feels more comfortable, you can resume most of your former activities. If you're a student, the doctor may let you remove your brace for gym class or special occasions. And he won't recommend wearing the brace for vigorous activities that require a lot of flexibility—like gymnastics.

Doing special exercises
Do the special exercises your physical therapist taught you. These exercises will promote muscle tone and flexibility.

Be sure to do them as often as recommended. And always practice standing tall.

Index